AF520519

Trends in Small Ruminant Production : Perspectives and Prospects

Trends in Small Ruminant Production : Perspectives and Prospects

Editors

Dr A. Sahoo

Dr. S.K. Sankhyan

Dr. C.P. Swarnkar

Dr A.K. Shinde

Dr. S.A. Karim

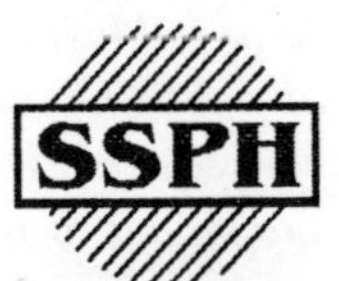

SATISH SERIAL PUBLISHING HOUSE

403, Express Tower, Commercial Complex, Azadpur, Delhi-110033 (India)

Phone : 011-27672852, Fax : 91-11-27672046

E-mail :info@satishserial.com, hkjain1975@yahoo.com

Website : www.satishserial.com

Published by :

SATISH SERIAL PUBLISHING HOUSE
403, Express Tower, Commercial Complex, Azadpur, Delhi-110033 (INDIA)
Phone : 011-27672852 Fax : 91-11-27672046
E-mail : info@satishserial.com, hkjain1975@yahoo.com

ISBN 978-93-81226-10-0

Typeset at: Harminder Singh Kharb *for* Laxmi Art Creation
Printed at: Salasar Imaging Systems, Delhi-110035

Preface

Livestock is emerging as a driving force of agricultural sector in India by contributing towards the income and employment of rural households well as by imparting sustainability to the production system. Among livestock sectors sheep, goat and rabbits bear an important role in providing livelihood to the rural mass, especially to the socio-economically weaker section of the society. The rapidly changing patterns of demand for livestock and livestock products point to livestock production being an increasing component of the agricultural economies of India. The extent to which the rural poor will benefit from these changes depends on how livestock can be integrated into developing markets and whether cheaper livestock products benefit the rural poor as consumers as well producers. Nonetheless, the research and development needs to be integrated and/ or modified to suit the field applicability and easy adoption by the farmers. The past growth in many of the livestock sector has been driven more by population growth than by technological change. Given the constraints in increasing the population of livestock, technological change is imperative for increasing the output growth in these livestock sectors. There is scope for small ruminants to play as important role for smallholder farmers in accessing these new markets. To meet the growing demand for meat, meat products and wool, the production level of these commodities has to be increased many fold. The increasing domestic and export demand for the meat and meat products from India open a great opportunity for commercial rearing. However, this is not easy considering the supply side constraints like the present low productivity, feed and fodder scarcity, deterioration of common property resources, inappropriate disease management, poor infrastructure, socio-cultural and legal rigidities and unfavorable external market conditions.

The Central Sheep and Wool Research Insitute (CSWRI), Avikanagar and Central Institute for Research on Goats (CIRG), Makhdoom in pursuit towards excellence has produced technology matrix aimed at increasing the production and productivity at comparatively low resource utilization for adoption by the farmers. However, the extent and rate of adoption of many of the technologies are low, mainly due to the inertia in shifting towards the new technology and the unsuitability of the technologies in the present resource use regime. But, the commercial rearing farms raised on lines of the scientific management principles can adopt many technologies to increase the production level. The contributors tried to provide in-depth knowledge on various production issues in line with breeding, reproduction, nutrition, health, meat and wool products and utilization including value addition and marketing for more return from the livestock produce. Some of the major technologies developed in these institute, which can be adopted by commercial farms are also detailed in this book.

We are grateful to ISSGPU, CWDB and research endeavors of two noble Institutes, CSWRI, Avikanagar and CIRG, Makhdoom for contributing to its publication in the form of a book for the ultimate guidance of end-users. The authors gratefully thank Indian Council of Agricultural Research, being at the helm of affairs that has supported all research and development activities carried out in various platforms.

We would like to admit that the present manuscript may not be free from errors as committing mistakes is human. Therefore, we would be grateful, if, such mistakes are pointed out by the readers for further improvement.

Editors

Contents

Preface .... *v*

Chapter-1 : Small Ruminant Production in India: Issues and Approaches 1
S.A. Karim

Chapter-2 : Genomics and Selection in Small Ruminants 13
Neelam Gupta and S.C. Gupta

Chapter-3 : Issues and Strategies for Sheep Breeding Program in India 23
Anil Kumar Mishra

Chapter-4 : Prolific Sheep: A Promise to Make and Deliver for the Socio-economic Upliftment of Sheep Farmer 49
A.L. Arora, Ashiṣh Chopra and L. Leslie Leo Prince

Chapter-5 : Genomic Selection in Small Ruminants: Global Status, Challenges and Opportunities 71
S.P. Dixit and Dinesh Kumar

Chapter-6 : Techniques for Enhancing Reproductive Efficiency in Small Ruminants 83
A.K. Goel

Chapter-7 : The State of the Art in the Artificial Insemination of Sheep 115
S.M.K. Naqvi and Davendra Kumar

Chapter-8 : Climate Change and Sheep Production: Concept of Multiple Stresses, Adaptation and Mitigation Strategies to Sustain Production 137
V. Sejian and S.M.K. Naqvi

Chapter-9 : Male Reproductive Biotechnology of Goats-Advances and Constraints 169
S.K. Jindal and Priyadharshini Raju

Chapter-10 : Understanding Stress Pathways Involved in Modulation of GnRH/LH Release in the EWE........ 183
J.B. Phogat and S.P.S. Ghuman

Chapter-11 : Stem Cell: Advances and Prospects in Farm Animals 195
Satish Kumar

Chapter-12 : Relevance and Importance of Pasture-based Production System of Small Ruminants in India...... 209
K. Sharma, A.K. Pattanaik and K.Y. Deshpande

Chapter-13 : Effect of Probiotics (Direct fed microbials) on Small Ruminant Production 229
D.N. Kamra and Neeta Agarwal

Chapter-14 : Expanding Feed Resource Base for Nutritional Security of Ruminants 241
R.C. Jakhmola

Chapter-15 : Nutritional Augmentation of Consumer Preferred Trait-specific Quality Enhancement in Meat, Wool and Milk Production 253
A. Sahoo and R.S. Bhatt

Chapter-16 : In vitro Gas Production Technique for Feed Evaluation – An Overview 273
B. Singh

Chapter-17 : Nutritional Management of Sheep Under Thermal, Migratory and Transportation Stress 301
S.K. Sankhyan and O.H. Chaturvedi

Chapter-18 : Stall Feeding System in Small Ruminants: Future Perspectives 325
U.B. Chaudhary, T.K. Dutta, M.K. Tripathi and P. Tripathi

Chapter-19 : Epidemiology and Management of Gastrointestinal Helminths in Small Ruminants – An Update 347
D. Singh and C.P. Swarnkar

Chapter-20 : Genetics of Disease Resistance in Small Ruminants: Scope and Future Application 397
P.K. Rout

Chapter-21 : Neonatal Mortality in Small Ruminants: Issues and Management 409
V.K. Gupta and Ashok Kumar

Chapter-22 : Meat Production and Value Addition - Where we Stand? 421
S. Sureshkumar, D. Santhi and A. Kalaikannan

Chapter-23 : Small Ruminant Meat in India: Production and Export Prospects 443
Suresh A.

Chapter-24 : Pelt Production: Counts and Discounts 465
A.K. Shinde

Chapter-25 : Recent Advances in Wool and Woollen Processing 477
V.S. Goud and J.S. Udakhe

Chapter-26 : Advances in Wool Based Non Woven Technical Textiles 493
G.Thilagavathi, V.R. Giridev, T. Senthilram and A.S.M.Raja

Chapter-27 : Non-conventional Utilisation of Wool and Other Animal Hairs 507
D.B. Shakyawar and A.S.M. Raja

Chapter-28 : Developments in Processing and Product Development of Speciality hair Fibres (Pashmina) 515
Sarfaraz A Wani, D.B. Shakyawar and Asif H Sofi

Chapter-29 : Advances in Eco-friendly Processing of Woollen Textiles 533
A.S.M. Raja and Ajay Kumar

Chapter-30 : Development of Woollen Khadi Spinning System .. 547
R. Chattopadhyay, D.B. Shakyawar and Nishant Kumar

Chapter-31 : Scope, Performance and Current Status of Broiler Rabbit Production in India 561
Rajeev Gulyani

Chapter-32 : Existing Technology Transfer System- Where we Stand? 577
Hema Tripathi and Shabeer Ahmad Hamdani

Chapter-33 : Linking Goat Farmers and Markets for Improving Productivity and Livelihoods 595
Shalander Kumar, Khem Chand and M.M. Roy

Chapter-34 : Current Status and Role of Extension in Promotion and Development of Sheep in India 609
Rajeev Gulyani and L.R. Meena

Chapter 1

Small Ruminant Production in India: Issues and Approaches

S.A. Karim and R.S. Bhatt
Central Sheep and Wool Research Institute
Avikanagar 304501 Rajasthan

There are 1044 million sheep and 746 million goats and represents second and fourth most numerous livestock species in the world (FAOSTAT, 2003). Out of total population, about 65% of the sheep and 76% of the goats are reared in developing countries. Small ruminant in the country contributes 4.8 and 3.4 % of the total world meat and milk production and the contribution is smaller in developed (3.0% and 1.6%) than developing countries (6.2% and 6.1) (FAOSTAT, 2003). The milk products and lean meat produced from small ruminants have special characteristics (flavor, taste and aroma) and composition (proteins, fatty acids, amino acids etc.) which designate as products of extra quality and are in great demand (Boyazoglu and Morand-Fehr, 2001).

In Asia, the rapidly increasing demand of livestock products is contributing toward vital role of livestock in agricultural economies. Their significance among farming community is now exploited in several Asian countries, as they can thrive on low inputs and local resources. A detailed analysis of the distribution of sheep and goats shows that sheep can be adapted to wide varieties of agro-climatic conditions under pasture grazing system. Goats, by contrast, are more concentrated in dry tropical and subtropical areas of poor agricultural potential and even on marginal lands (Morand-Fehr and Boyazoglu, 1999). The relatively small investment is required and increasing size of flock makes sheep production a good choice for the farmers.

In India, livestock sector is emerging as a driving force in agriculture by contributing towards the income and employment of rural households as well as imparting sustainability to the production system. The share of livestock to the agricultural gross domestic product has increased from 14% in 1980-81 to 23% in 1997-98 and further increased to 32% in 2001-02. Sheep and goats constituted 29.47 % of the total livestock population and increased to 38.32% in 2003 (Table 1). Latest census reported by FAO (2009) depicts an increase of 6.91 percent in sheep population and 1.31 percent in goat population and a decrease of 7.19 percent in cattle population.

Table 1 : Livestock population growth rate in India

Species	Population (million) 1951	Population (million) 2003	Population (million) 2009	Annual 1972-82	Compound 1982-92	Growth rate % 1992-2003	Growth rate % 1951-2009	Growth rate % 2003-2009
Cattle	155.3 (53.04)	185.18 (38.18)	172.45	0.76	0.61	-0.99	0.19	-1.37
Buffalo	43.40 (14.82)	96.62 (19.92)	106.63	1.96	1.89	1.38	2.51	2.07
Sheep	39.10 (13.35)	61.47 (12.67)	65.72	2.01	0.40	1.93	1.17	1.38
Goat	47.20 (16.12)	124.36 (25.66)	126.00	3.50	1.93	0.78	2.88	0.26
Livestock	292.80	485.00	472.18	1.73	1.44	0.31	1.05	-0.52

Values in parenthesis depicts the percent contribution of the values

Livestock being an integral component of our social, economic and environmental system, its importance goes beyond the food production function. It is an important source of income and employment generation for millions of landless and small landholders particularly in the resource poor section. As per the 18th livestock census (2007) there are about 71.5 million sheep in our country and about 1.2 million people are involved in sheep rearing. Further 1.3 million people including artisans are employed in activities related to woollen processing and value addition (GOI, 2006).

The country has third highest population of sheep (65.72 million) and the second highest population of goats (126.00 million) and the current trend of sheep and goat population (2003-2009) depicts an annual increase of 1.38 per cent in sheep and 0.26 percent in goat and decrease of 0.52 percent in cattle population. As per the 2003 livestock census, India possesses 61 million sheep and produce 229 million kg of mutton and 51 million kg of wool. However, the productivity of Indian sheep is low as compared to the world production standards and there is tremendous scope for increasing looking to impending demand for mutton in the country. In rain-fed areas dependency on agriculture is always at stake and investment in livestock seems the only alternatives for livelihood of the farmers. In rain fed area, where other livestock are difficult to raise due to feed scarcity, small ruminants can sustain and contribute towards livelihood and economic sustenance of poor farmers in dry zones of the country.

Among livestock sector, sheep bears as important role in providing livelihood to the rural mass, especially to the socio-economically weaker section of the society. The ability of sheep to thrive in the adverse climatic condition of arid and semi-arid regions on the sparse vegetation and minimal external inputs makes the sheep rearing an important component of livestock farming. During the frequent drought conditions, affecting many parts of India, the sheep act as a liquid asset, which can be cashed easily to meet urgent financial requirement. The role of sheep and goat in reducing the interpersonal and interregional inequalities existing in the rural areas is also well appreciated. Sheep is mainly reared on extensive system on availability pasture land and common property resources with minimal or no supplementation of concentrate mixture. To meet the growing demands of meat and wool, the production level of existing sheep breeds need to be increased many fold. The increasing domestic and export demand for the meat from India open the great opportunity for commercial sheep rearing. However, this is not an easy with present status of low productivity, feed and fodder scarcity, deterioration of common property resources, inappropriate disease management, poor infrastructure, socio-cultural and legal rigidities and unfavorable external market conditions (Birthal *et al.*, 2002).

Goat has distinct social, economical, management and biological advantages over other livestock species. They significantly contribute to the agrarian economy and play a very vital role in the livelihood security of the small and marginal farmers and landless labors especially in arid, semi-arid and mountainous regions of the country. Goats have several advantages over other animals. They are widely adapted, thrive and reproduce well in tropical, cold, humid as well as dry regions. The small size compared to cattle and buffaloes permit them to be maintained on a limited area. Goats consume a wide variety of grasses, weeds, forbs, bushes, shrubs, tree leaves and crop residues that would otherwise go waste. Goat milk is prescribed for children, old and sick as it is easily digestible and has medicinal value. Goat meat (chevon) is preferred over other meats because it is lean and there are no religious taboos against its consumption.

Mutton Production from Cull Animals

Under Indian condition, about 40 % of sheep put to slaughter belonges to spent category with low body score, dressing yield and carcass fat (Jacob *et al.,* 2005). Meat from such aged sheep is usually tough and fibrous in texture and is not preferred by the consumers (Mendiratta *et al.,* 2008). Aged and spent ewes constitute nearly 40 % of the animals put to slaughter and have usually low body score and general appearance due to the burden of repeated pregnancies, lambing and poor nutrition resulting in their poor market weights and values. At present spent sheep irrespective of sex, age, breeds, body weights, body conditions and production stages are sold off without fattening which in turn results in low meat yield and low income (Galmessa *et al.* 2004). Thiruvenkadan *et al.* (2004) has reported that aged animals are sold at about 50 % of the price fetched by the young animals due to poor carcass attributes. Due to growing demand of meat in the country, more thrust should be given for improving meat yield and quality of growing lambs by better feeding to bridge the gap of demand and supply. The meat yield and quality of cull sheep can be improved by supplementary feeding, however not much has been done on these aspects in the country.

Issues

Small ruminant makes an important contribution to the sustenance of small and marginal landholders and landless rural people in India. They also contribute substantially (Rs 24,000 million per annum) to the rural economy. The contribution of agriculture sector to national GDP was 25% during 1990s and the share of livestock in agricultural GDP was 23%, of which small ruminants contribution was 10% to the total value of livestock sector. At the national level, small ruminant accounts for 14% of the meat output, 4% of the milk output and 15% of hides and skin production in the country. But small ruminates have received only 2.5% of allocation in livestock sector, which is much less than the share of small ruminants in livestock sector. Small ruminant production is providing sustenance to the poorest people.

1. *Selling the Lamb at early age*: Most of the sheep breeders, sell their lambs at weaning age (2.5 to 3 month of age) due to poor availability of grazing resources, fear of mortality losses, financial requirement for household and lack of financial credit and support from government agencies. The research conducted at institute clearly indicated that the active growth phase of lambs falls between 3-6 months of age. Disposal of lambs at an early age reduced the mutton production potential of animals by half. Further, the lambs sold at 3 months of age do not contribute to wool production thus, losses to nation in terms of mutton as well as wool production. This is one of the setbacks for growth of meat industry in the country, which is growing at an annual rate of 10 % (Annual report, Department of Animal Husbandry, Dairy and Fisheries, Govt. of India, 2009). Further, in the WTO regime, the opening of markets has created both opportunities for growth based on demand from foreign markets as well as threat from external competition.

2. *Poor awareness regarding the importance of small ruminants in the livelihood security*: Small ruminant rearing provides significant self-employment opportunities and is a source of supplementary income for the landless, tribal and poor section of people. During migration, animals are often kept on moving with little or no attention to supplementary feed inputs, or to disease control, housing and security of animals as well as farmers. In spite of its important contribution in poverty reduction, the small ruminant sector has received little attention in the country.

3. *Absence /lack of active farmer organizations*: Small ruminant farmers are unorganized and unable to raise their voice. The ignorance of social organization is barring their development. Absence of active organizations for the mobilization of the farmers is another reason contributing to poor development of the small ruminant sector. NGOs and semi-organized institutions representing the cause of pastoralists are mostly unable to trace them during migration to lobby them for their rights.

4. *Pressure on fodder resource base*: A vast majority of small ruminant farmers belong to small and marginal farmers, pastoralists and landless labourers largely depend on common property resources to feed their animals. Common property resources mainly consist of village pastures belonging to the Panchayats, revenue land and forest land. Over the period land under grazing is declining on the other hand livestock population is increasing resulting in deterioration of grazing resources and vanishing of important plant species.

5. *Inadequate veterinary health services*: The small ruminant sector in India receives low funds allocation and attention for veterinary services. The services available are, not reaching most of the farmers as majority of them are either in the remote resource poor areas or are on migration. Even though the number of veterinary hospitals, polyclinics and dispensaries increased almost doubled during the last 15 years, still health care for small ruminant receives low priority, possibly due to lack of infrastructure facilities, shortage of trained personnel, non-availability of medicines / vaccine, overall lack of information on small ruminants etc.

6. *Lack of adequate focus on genetic improvement*: Development of small ruminant breeds in the Indian context is relatively difficult and slow because the animals are either under constant migration or under free grazing situation and remain under low plane of nutrition, flock size is small and males are sold at relatively younger age making selection difficult. In a free grazing situation where there is no possibility of performance recording, improvement of feeding and management, controlled mating, genetic improvement of the animals is comparatively difficult. Instead of AI, selected males of the indigenous breeds can be used by the communities under such conditions but the genetic progress will be much slower. Productivity enhancement among sheep and goat through crossbreeding with exotic breed is fraught with the danger of the sheep / goat populations loosing their inherent sturdiness, vitality and the ability to withstand stress.

7. *Poor access to credit and insurance*: Access of small ruminant farmers to institutional credit and its flexibility to match the requirement are limited and in majority of cases, they are under the clutches of money lenders. Poorer households have little or

no capital resources to invest in their livestock enterprise. Investments for upgrading breeds, improving health care, feeding and management practices are too luxurious on their existing resources. Similarly insurance support to livestock, especially small ruminants is also very weak. As goats and sheep are important productive assets and a source of livelihood for millions of poor farmers, any loss of animal is a direct threat to their livelihood. It has not received much attention from the insurance agencies or banks. Even though, there are many practical difficulties, horizons of livestock insurance may be extended to poor farmers rearing small ruminants.

8. *Lack of efficient marketing mechanisms*: Rapid urbanization combined with continued economic growth is creating an increase in market demand for livestock products in India. It is well known fact that as income rises people diversify their diet from cereals to meat and other livestock products. The massive growth in demand for livestock products, especially meat is a great opportunity for the Indian livestock keepers, especially the small ruminant farmers. Marketing of live animal is unorganized while wool marketing is partly organized with a chain of intermediaries and commission agents linking the primary producers to industrial houses/ end users. Leaving aside the metropolitan, in rural areas the slaughter of sheep and goat by butcher is taken as a back yard enterprise as meat is sold to the consumers on per kg basis irrespective of the cost/ cut concept prevalent in developed countries. Traditionally, the middle man involved in live animal trade loan out required to the farmers for meeting their social obligation and family emergencies. While giving loans the trader generally accept verbal commitment of the farmer that he will sell off his animals to the trader, at a later date, in the price fixed on that date. In such transaction benefits accrued by occasional upwards trend in market is pocketed by middleman while the slump in price is directly passed on to the farmers by lowering purchase price. Butchers involved in the trade are largely benefited as the market price of the meat does not follow the downward trends in consonance with the fall in live animal cost (Karim, 1996). Small farmers find it difficult to penetrate these markets because of the nexus. Absence of strong farmer organizations and their network to address the marketing needs

of the farmers and consumers is one of the bottlenecks in capturing the markets.

9. *Poor inter-departmental coordination*: Non-convergence of policies and programs of different departments is a matter of serious concern in small ruminant development. For instance, the Department of Rural Development promotes goat rearing whereas the Forest Department bans on goat rearing. When grazing policy is made by the Forest Department, it is normally done with no consultation with other relevant stakeholders like AH Department, Panchayats, Revenue Department, Agricultural Department etc. The local community is also not often involved in the policy making.
10. *Lack of inter-state coordination*: This is also a matter of serious consideration in respect of migratory farmers and their movement to neighboring states in search of grazing resources.

Approaches

1. *Involvement of Self Help Group*: There is a need for private entrepreneur/ unemployed innovative youth among farmers who could play a key role in purchasing the lambs from farmers at weaning stage. Rearing them on scientific lines up to six month of age which is the most productive age. The best one should be selected for breeding purposes. The interaction with agencies involved in export of mutton should be developed and quality lambs should be sold for slaughter at remunerative prices.
2. *Establishment of Small Ruminant Farmer Organizations*: Establishment of strong sheep and goat farmer organization at the district and state level is an essential need for exploiting the market potential. A vertically integrated two-tier structure, owned, controlled and managed by rearers' Self Help Groups or Associations or Co-operatives at the grass root level federated into a state level Unit /Federation will be the ideal structure for rearer organizations. It should be a democratic structure with well defined roles and responsibilities for each tier and adequate infrastructure owned and controlled by the rearers through professional Managers. An integrated approach to production, procurement, processing/marketing and productivity enhancement under which all the infrastructure are owned and controlled by the rearers themselves would be the ideal way of

stimulating production and growth. Such an organization should be able to provide extension and inputs for production, assured market round the year and assure a reasonable price band to the rearers and build brand equity in the long term.

3. *Inter-departmental committee*: An inter-departmental committee consisting of key stakeholders should be formed to give them opportunity to understand programs of related departments and to explore possible areas of synergy.

4. *Inter-state coordination*: The Animal Husbandry Department (in the states where large scale migratory animals are present) with the help of pastoral communities, NGOs and rearer associations should take initiative to coordinate with concerned department in the recipient states for fixing migratory routes, norms of migration, code of conduct, services during migration and other related issues faced by the rearers during the course of migration.

5. *Linking individual farmer and farmer groups with institutional credit and insurance*: The AH Department may facilitate linkages between small ruminant rearing groups (SHGs) and sources of institutional credit. Access to market and feed resources, as well as borrowers' experience on related production activity shall be considered as prerequisite for lending. Credit should also be linked with insurance for covering the risk of loss of production and life. Short-term credit facility available for livestock sector should be extended to small ruminant sector as well. Sheep farmers may be given bank loans to establish pastures and growing fodder trees on their own lands. The Kisan Credit Card Scheme presently does not allow withdrawal of credit for livestock rearing. The facility of credit for livestock production may be extended on these cards also. For insurance protection innovative ideas like "Community insurance" through interest groups (SHGs) can be implemented where compensation is paid to the claimant from funds generated out of the premium paid by the members.

6. *Selective Breeding*: As the primary objective of small ruminant farming is meat production, the recommended breeding policy is selective breeding for faster growth and higher body weights for which enormous selection differential exists among indigenous breeds. Superior breeding males in the identified breeding tracts should be selected from elite flocks. The selection intensity can be enhanced with the involvement of farmer flocks. The farmer

flocks can be regulated to form a goat / sheep breeder cooperative to function as an elite open nucleus herd. The high producing animals of the cooperative herd should be pooled to form the nucleus herd, which will produce proven bucks / rams, which can be sold to farmers.

7. *Disease prevention*: Prevention of diseases to avert risk shall be central to the provision of livestock services to sheep / goat farmers and herders. Prevention strategies against important diseases such as Blue Tongue, PPR etc. should be developed. Greater coverage should be provided for vaccination against diseases like Enterotoxaemia, Sheep Pox etc. There is a need for speedy, effective and accessible diagnostic services.

8. *Services to animals on migration*: In case of migratory small ruminant flocks the approach for providing veterinary services may be through border / migratory route posts where basic preventive veterinary medicine such as vaccination shall be provided. The veterinary care to migratory flocks may include advice on deworming and anthelmintic use, protection against endemic diseases prevalent in the area where the animals are migrating to and prevention of spread of disease through these animals.

9. *Training community based para-vet workers*: Training of 'para-vets' from within the rearer/pastoral communities who can treat minor ailments, recognize epizootic conditions and major traumas.

10. *Institutional development*: If rearer organizations already exist, strengthen them. Otherwise support and mobilize the rearers to get them organized in the form of Associations / Cooperatives / Federations / Networks. Initially there is a need to have an outside agency (NGOs or other agencies) to initiate and extend support to rearers, village leaders and groups in bringing them together. These NGOs should play a role in creating awareness, capacity building, advocacy, building networks, bringing synergies / convergence and empowering the rearers through rearer SHGs, networks etc. All NGOs working in the same area for the same cause should network to form a consortium and synergies their efforts rather than working in isolation.

11. *Small Ruminant Cell*: may be formed within the Department of Animal Husbandry (Central level as also in the States, where small ruminant population is high). Within this cell special

responsibility may be entrusted to handle issues of pastoralists such as conflicts related to operational issues with Forest Department, migration to adjacent states, health services during migration, training on breeding, health care and management practices etc.

References

Birthal, P.S., Joshi, P.K., and Kumar, A. 2002. Assessment of research priorities for livestock sector in India. Policy paper 15. New Delhi, India: National Centre for Agricultural Economics and Policy Research. p. 75.

Boyazoglu, J. and Morand-Fehr, P., 2001. Mediterranean dairy sheep and goat products and their quality. A critical review. Small Ruminant Research 4: 1-11.

FAO, 2009. Food and Agriculture Organization. FAO Production Year Book . Rome Italy

FAOSTAT, 2003. http://www.apps.fao.org/page/collections?subset= agriculture.

Galmessa, Ulfine; Dhuguma, Gammada; Abegaz, Solomon; Aboma, Girma; Gizaw, Solomon, Prasad, Shiv and Terefe, Fiqiru. 2004. Pre-market supplementary feeding in aged Horro sheep in relation to weight gain, carcass yield and economic response in Western Oromia. Indian Journal of Anim. Science 74 (3): 327-329.

Government of India 2006. Compendium of Textile Statistics, Ministry of Textiles, New Delhi.

Govt. of India, 2009. Annual report, Department of Animal Husbandry, Dairy and Fisheries, New Delhi.

Jacob. R. H., , P. J. Walker J. W. Skerritt, R. H. Davidson, D. L. Hopkins, J. M. Thompson and D. W. Pethick. 2005. The effect of lairage time on consumer sensory scores of the *M. longissimus thoracis et lumborum* from lambs and lactating ewes. Australian Journal of Experimental Agriculture (45) 535-542.

Karim, S.A. (1996). Market trends in live animal transaction. Proceeding, Advances in sheep production, CSWRI, Avikanagar, pp.186-195.

Mendiratta, S.K., N. Kondaiah, A.S.R. Anjaneyulu and B.D. Sharma. 2008. Comparisons of handling practices of culled sheep meat for Production of Mutton Curry. Asian Australation Journal of Animal Science (21):738-744.

Morand-Fehr, P., Boyazoglu, J., 1999. Present state and future outlook of the small ruminant sector. Small Ruminant Research 34: 175–188.

Thiruvenkadan, A.K., Karunanithi, K. and Purushothaman, M.R. 2004. Socio-economic status of the Mecheri sheep farmers and economics of rearing under farmer's management. Indian Journal of Small Ruminant 10 (2) : 117-122.

□□□

Chapter 2

Genomics and Selection in Small Ruminants

Neelam Gupta[1] and S.C. Gupta[2]
[1]Principal Scientist (AG & B), [2]Assistant Director General (AG & B), Animal Science Division, Indian Council of Agricultural Research, New Delhi – 110 114

Genome science and genomic tools have led to revolutionary biological breakthroughs that dramatically affect and continue to advance animal agriculture. In a short period of time, costs have fallen while technology has improved to make possible the reality that assembled genome sequences can be produced for any species of interest, particularly agricultural species. Research focused on small ruminant genomes will be able to make rapid progress by leveraging resources, tools, and knowledge gained from bovine and other species' genome projects. The cattle and sheep genome research consortia have recently completed high density gene maps, genome assemblies, haplotype maps and related analyses. Research in goat genomics can take advantage of comparative genome similarity, as well as lessons learned from bovine and ovine studies, to make progress toward development of caprine-specific genome tools. Currently, several efforts are underway for construction of radiation-hybrid gene maps, SNP discovery, and genome sequence assembly. All of these projects present challenges for production of high quality data, storage and management of data, and bioinformatics analyses, but goat genome research can potentially move quickly as a result of previous findings. The future availability of genomic resources for goat provides great opportunity for application in the goat industry.

Genomics is the study of DNA. DNA encodes the instructions on how an animal grows, reproduces and responds to its changing environment. This includes how it digests and stores nutrients and counters disease challenges. In farmed animals these instructions are encoded in chromosomes or segments of DNA. Each letter or nucleotide of DNA potentially stores an instruction and there are about 2.7 billion of them in every cell of a cow. In fact there is double that number, because each animal gets a copy of the instructions from its mother and another from its father. The instructions are not exactly the same. On average, if two segments of DNA are compared about one nucleotide in every 500 to 1000 differs. That is about 2.7 to 5.4 million differences. In fact, these differences are constantly generated and each offspring also has 20-50 new variants. These differences underlie the observed genetic variation. How these differences affect the performance of an animal is the key area of study in genomics. Most of the variants, perhaps as many as 93 percent, have little or no effect, another 6 percent have only minor effects, with only perhaps less than 1 percent contributing the majority of the observed genetic variation for all traits. However, that is still 50 to 100 thousand variants plus perhaps a new one naturally created each generation. For a given trait it has been estimated that typically 5-50 variants control more than 50% of the observed genetic variation.

There are several different kinds of DNA variants, but only two kinds are commonly measured. The first are Single Nucleotide Polymorphisms (SNPs), where individual nucleotides are altered. The second are microsatellites where short repetitive segments of repeating bases, typically in units of 2 to 5 nucleotides long, vary in length. The latter typically have little effect on performance, but are highly variable and have historically been used for that reason. More recently SNPs are becoming more widely used for reasons detailed later. The ability to predict the total genetic merit of livestock using molecular or biochemical markers would allow the opportunity to completely redesign animal breeding and management programs.

Genomics technologies

Candidate gene approach: The candidate gene approach studies the relationship between the traits and known genes that may be associated with the physiological pathways underlying the trait (Liu *et al.*, 2008). In other words, this approach assumes that a gene involved in the physiology of the trait could harbour a mutation causing variation in the trait. The gene or part of gene, are sequenced in a number of different animals, and any variation found in the DNA sequences, is tested for association with variation in the phenotypic trait. This approach has had some success. For example a mutation was discovered in the estrogen receptor locus (ESR) which results increased litter size in pig. There are 2 problems with the candidate gene approach.

Firstly, there are usually a large number of candidate genes affecting the trait, so many genes must be sequenced in several animals and many association studies carried out in a large sample of animals. Secondly, the causative mutation may lie in a gene that would not have been regarded prior as an obvious candidate for this particular trait. Candidate gene approach is performed in 5 steps:

- Collection of resource population.
- Phenotyping of the traits.
- Selection of gene or functional polymorphism that potentially could affect the traits.
- Genotyping of the resource population for genes or functional polymorphism.
- Lastly, one is statistical analysis of phenotypic and genotypic data (Da, 2003).

This is an effective way to find the genes associated with the trait. So far a number of genes have been investigated. Candidate gene approach has been ubiquitously applied for gene disease research, genetic association studies, biomarker and drug target selection in many organisms from animals (Tabor *et al.*, 2002).

The traditional candidate gene approach is largely limited by its reliance on existing knowledge about the known or presumed biology of the phenotype under investigation, unfortunately the detailed molecular anatomy of most biological traits remain unknown (Zhu and Zhao, 2007). Recently, a new developing method on candidate gene approach [digital candidate gene - DigiCGA) has emerged and is primarily applied to identify potential candidate gene in some studies. DigiCGA, which also named in Koopaei and Koshkoiyeh 127 silico candidate gene approach or computer facilitated candidate gene approach, is a novel web resource based candidate gene identification approach. DigiCGA approach is included to ontology-based identification approach, computation-based identification approach and integrated identification approach (including literature based meta-analysis). The ontology-based identification approach is mainly involved in the bioinformatics analyses for in silico identification of candidate gene for specific interest in case of the semi structured, structured and controlled vocabularies for systematic annotation of gene function information from biological ontology source available through internet. A typical example of this approach is the prioritization of positional candidate gene by using gene ontology (Harhay and Keele, 2003).

The computation-based identification includes those computational candidate gene identification methods that describe computational framework to prioritize the most likely candidate gene through a variety of web resource based data sets. There are many statistical algorithms or computational methods, and of which some included data mining analysis, hidden Markov analysis, cluster analysis and kernel-based data fusion analysis. There have been reported many candidate gene prioritized by the integrated identification approach such as pathway and gene ontology combined analysis.

Genome scan approach: The genome scan approach studies the relationship between a trait and markers selected across the genome to identify chromosomal locations associated with the trait. The genome scan will find out the map location of a trait locus with major effect. It involves the following steps:

- Design and construction of resource population.
- Phenotyping traits of resource population.
- Selection of genetic markers.
- Genotyping of the population for selected markers.
- Construction of linkage maps, and
- Statistical analysis of the phenotypic and genotypic data derived from the resource population (Da, 2003).

Using the genome scan, a large amount of quantitative trait loci (QTL) can be obtained in farm animals that can provide a useful bridge to link genome information with phenotype. There is an animal QTL data base, which contains all publicly available QTL data on farm animal species for the past decade.

Scottish Blackface sheep: The population studied was a double backcross between lines of sheep divergently selected for carcass lean content (LEAN and FAT lines), comprising nine half-sib families. Carcass composition (600 lambs) was assessed non-destructively using computerized tomography (CT) scanning, while meat quality measurements (initial and final pH of semi-membranous, colour, shear force value, carcass weight, lamb flavour, juiciness, tenderness and overall liking) were taken on 300 male lambs. Lambs and their sires were genotyped across candidate regions on chromosomes 1, 2, 3, 5, 14, 18, 20 and 21. QTL analyses were performed using regression interval mapping techniques. In total, nine genome-wise was significant and 11 chromosome-wise and suggestive QTL were detected in seven out of eight chromosomes. Genome wise significant QTL were mapped for lamb flavour on sheep chromosome 1 (OAR1); for muscle densities (OAR 2 and OAR3); for colour (redness) (OAR3); for bone density (OAR 1); for slaughter live weight (OAR 1 and OAR 2) and for the weights of cold and hot carcass (OAR5). The QTL with the strongest statistical evidence affected the lamb flavour of meat and was on OAR 1, in a region homologous with a porcine chromosome 13 (SSC13) QTL identified for pork flavour. This QTL was segregated in four of the nine families. This study provides new information on QTL affecting meat quality and carcass composition traits in sheep, which may lead to novel opportunities for genetically improving these traits. Although, a genome scan can give full genome coverage for a trait, it will fail to detect trait loci with smaller effects if they do not reach the stringent significance of the threshold.

Fine mapping: It involves the identification of markers that are very tightly linked to a targeted gene. A genetic fine map of a specific locus will usually give us its goal by the identification and location of marker that flank the targeted gene within one or fewer cent Morgan (cM) with a fine map, and assisted selection precise. Several problems are associated with the generation of fine map around any animal gene. First, mapping marker to a resolution of one cM requires the investigation of a few hundred sexual progeny. Second, marker polymorphism can be low in mapping population and third, recombination rate per chromosome arm in sexual generation. The ultimate goal of genome scan approach is to identify the genes that underlie polygenic trait and gain better understanding of their physiological and biochemical functions. In fact a region of QTL often spans 5 to 30 cM and it is too large to find the target genes, so fine mapping needs to be done. It is a step towards restricting the region of interest and the number of potential candidate genes. The goal of fine mapping is mapping QTL to a narrow chromosome region so that the physical QTL affecting the phenotype can be identified and cloned. Finally fine mapping a gene is usually an essential step in map-based gene isolation.

Characterization of expression QTL : The central paradigm of molecular biology states that DNA is transcribed into RNA and RNA is translated into the proteins that affect cellular function and ultimately determine phenotype. This simplistic model allows extension to numerous layers of complexity including variation in coding and regulatory DNA sequence, alternate splicing of RNA to mRNA, the regulation by small RNA of translation through transcript degradation and the posttranslational modification of proteins *en route* to the determination of phenotype. The extent to which these layers of genomic complexity underlie a phenotype might be measured by the narrow sense heritability. Traits with high heritability's, such as growth, may have relatively few major pathways through the complex network of regulatory processes that connect genotype to phenotype, whereas traits with low heritability such as fertility may have many environmentally sensitive pathways, all of small effect. We already know from QTL mapping studies that genes of large effect underlie variation in most phenotypes, even for traits with low heritability. The key question therefore is to what extent are QTL explained by cis-acting mutations that regulate the expression level of nearby genes vs. mutations, which act by alternative means such as charged amino acid substitutions, which may affect protein structure. All of the methods used to examine the expression levels of genes possess an inherent measurement error.

Furthermore, the level of expression of individual genes is dependent on both the environmental circumstances of the individual (tissue or cell line) and the character state of other genes within the genome. Therefore, measures of gene expression can be considered to be quantitative traits, much as we think about production traits in livestock and agriculture.

Understanding the roles of epigenetic effects

"Epigenetic modifications at the DNA, nucleosomal and chromosomal level affect gene expression and ultimately phenotypes, by providing differential access to the underlying genetic information" (Richards, 2006).Epigenetic modi?cations are potentially reversible and do not alter the underlying DNA sequence, but rather exert an in?uence on phenotypes by permitting differential access of the transcriptional machinery to the DNA by altering chromatin structure. Epigenetic mechanisms (such as DNA and histone modi?cations) in?uences numerous processes including parental imprinting, gene silencing, X-inactivation and embryonic reprogramming. To make genetic progress in livestock, we must consider how epigenetic mechanisms influence economically important phenotypes. Breeding strategies that make use of imprinting information, diet adjustments, that in?uence methylation patterns in offspring, and the elucidation of DNA and histone modification patterns to improve cloning rates could all impact livestock improvement and management.

The DNA can be methylated at the 5-position of cytosine residues in CpGdi nucleotides to convert cytosine to 5-methylcytosine via the action of enzymes known as DNA methyl transferases (Dnmt). This epigenetic event occurs globally in the normal genome and affects70 to 80% of all CpGdi nucleotides in human cells. These dinucleotides are not uniformly distributed in the genome, but occur in clusters such as large repetitive sequences or in short CG-rich DNA stretches known as CpG islands (CGI). The majority of affected CpGdi nucleotides are found in intragenic regions that harbour repetitive sequences such as satellite sequences and centromeric repeats while CGI, which are preferentially found in the promoter regions of genes, appear to be protected from this modification in somatic cells.

Exceptions to this rule include CGI located on the inactive X chromosome in females and those associated with imprinted genes (where only the paternally or maternally inherited allele is expressed) that are methylated in the normal state. It is common for methylation status to vary among regions of the promoter CGI, and gene silencing has been attributed to both the density of CpG methylation (proportion of methylated CpGdi nucleotides within a CGI) and with site-speci?c CpG methylation (methylation of specific CpGdi nucleotides). Histones create a compact conformation with the methylated region that renders the DNA inaccessible to the transcriptional machinery. However, when these regions are unmethylated, the chromatin structure is relaxed and the gene can be expressed.

RNA interference

Messenger RNA, which until recently has been the best-characterized RNA, serves as a transporter of information from DNA to a functional protein. However, there is also an extremely diverse repertoire of small RNA molecules that play an important role in the control of gene expression and cellular function. The RNA silencing pathway is initiated by 2 types of small RNA, small interfering RNA (siRNA) and miRNA. These siRNA and miRNA have been studied using may different methods in many different model systems, including livestock. The first characterized miRNA was a non-protein coding transcript of the lin-4 gene identified in *Caenorhabditis elegans* (Lee *et al.*, 1993).

The RNAi is at the forefront of genomics research. The technique promises to generate useful data in the ?elds of genetic and viral disease, immunology, tumour behaviour, and drug target identi?cation. Exploring the opportunities and limitations of RNAi in model systems, including livestock species, will become increasingly important not only for basic research but also for identifying potential therapeutics for human and livestock applications. The greatest impediment to RNAi is that the knock-down effect is only transient. Attempts are now underway to persistently express siRNA in mammalian systems by using vector delivery systems and constitutively active promoters to persistently knock-down target mRNA.

Genetic and genomic selection

One of the most economically important aspects of genome data is the possibility to use it for improving selective breeding. In comparison to traditional methods of selection - which are based on selecting for quantitative traits using breeding value estimates calculated from measured traits, genetic co-variances among traits, and the pedigree relationships in populations - selection using genome information supplements phenotypic data with knowledge of the genotype of individuals in the population for known relevant gene variants(alleles). Gene-assisted selection is potentially more rapid. It also can be more easily applied to traits where the heritability is low and genetic change is slow, and traits that are difficult to measure. This presupposes, however, that the data on the trait and the QTL or the genes it links to are known. In turn, this means we need more data on genetic markers, particularly on SNPs.

Conclusion

Next generation sequencing technologies appear to be poised to revolutionize livestock genomics. We can soon expect the de novo sequencing of the genomes of most, if not all, agriculturally important species, which will provide the fundamental reagents for important comparative analyses and for the development of technology platforms for whole genome SNP genotyping, mRNA and mi-RNA expression, and DNA methylation analysis within each species. We can expect dramatic reductions in per sample reagent costs and even more dramatic increases in the per sample data volumes that will be generated by these platforms. The livestock genomics research community is certainly ready for the former, but is ill prepared for the latter situation, and the limiting factor in research discovery will move from technology availability to the ability to appropriately integrate, analyse and interpret huge volumes of disparate forms of data. Fortunately, human and model animal species researchers face identical problems and have greater access to resources to arrive at solutions. Coming decade will be characterized by greater changes and challenges to livestock improvement systems than have occurred since the introduction of arti?cial insemination.

References

Da, Y. 2003. Statistical analysis and experimental design for mapping genes of complex traits in domestic animals. Bioinformatics 30: 1183-1192.

Harhay, G.P. and Keele, J.W. 2003. Positional candidate gene selection from livestock EST databases using gene ontology. Bioinformatics 19: 249-255.

Lee, R.C., Feinbaum, R.L. and Ambros, V. 1993. The *C. elegans* heterochronic gene *lin-4* encodes small RNAs with antisense complementarity to *lin-14*. Cell 75: 843-854.

Liu, X., Zhang, H., Li, H., Li, N., Zhang, Y., Zhang, Q., Wang, S., Wang, Q. and Wang, H. 2008. Fine mapping quantitative trait loci for body weight and abdominal fat traits: Effects of marker density and sample size. Poultry Science 87: 1314-1319.

Richards, E.J. 2006. Inherited epigenetic variation [mdash] revisiting soft inheritance. Nature Reviews Genetics 7: 395-401.

Tabor, H.K., Risch, N.J. and Myers, R.M. 2002. Candidate-gene approaches for studying complex genetic traits: Practical considerations. Nature Reviews Genetics 3: 391-397.

Zhu, M. and Zhao, S. 2007. Candidate gene identification approach: Progress and challenges. International Journal of Biological Sciences 3: 420-427.

□□□

Chapter 3

Issues and Strategies for Sheep Breeding Program in India

Anil Kumar Mishra
Central Avian Research Institute, Izatnagar- 243 122 (UP)

The focus of sheep breeding in past was on the improvement of quality and quantity of wool by using different types of exotic fine wool breeds. A number of strains were developed through crossbreeding of native breeds with exotics. The developed genetic groups demonstrated their production potential in terms of body weight, wool quantity and quality under experimental farm management conditions but these could not outdo the natives in field conditions barring few crosses due to non-availability of required plane of nutrition and other managemental and climatic conditions. In addition to the All India Coordinated Research Project/ NetWork programme on Sheep Improvement, the genetic improvement of indigenous breeds of sheep in their home tracts at present is being mostly done through state Government which are maintaining small populations and thus neither can bring any genetic improvement in the farm populations nor can meet the requirement of breeding rams for the improvement in the farmers flocks. State wise sheep breeding policy were first proposed in 1970 by the Ad-hoc committee on sheep breeding policy set up by the Government of India. Improvement of sheep through breeding strategy should involve decision on objectives and approaches in bringing genetic improvement. This will also depend upon socio-economic and ecological considerations, existing genetic resources, their productivity, possibility of their improvement through selection within a breed, grading with indigenous improver breeds, or replacing an indigenous breed with an existing breed if it is arising from similar ecological region and thus will be adaptable, or cross-breeding for evolving new breed combining the adaptation and hardiness of local breed and higher productivity of the exotic breed. Major objectives for improving sheep production should qualitative and quantitative improvement in carpet wool, apparel wool and meat production.

In mutton breeds body weight gain, efficiency of feed conversion, carcass yield and quality, reproductive performance and lamb survival are major characters of importance. However, kg of lamb weaned/ ewe/year can be used as an index combining most of these characteristics. The index can also be used in selecting rams and ewes in farmers' flocks. In carpet wool although greasy fleece weight, scoured fleece yield, average fibre diameter and percentage of heterotypic and completely medullated fibres, are characters of interest, but to make the selections under field conditions, simple and feasible, first 6-monthly greasy fleece weight and medullation percentage may be considered in selecting breeding rams. In apparel wool major characteristics of importance are greasy fleece weight, scoured fleece yield, average fibre diameter and staple length, the later where wools are combed for use in worsted system but to make the selection under field conditions simple and feasible, first 6-monthly greasy fleece weight and average fibre diameter with some emphasis on staple length if the wools are used in worsted sector may be used in selecting rams.

Diversities in Indian sheep breeds

According to the FAO World Watch List (1995), there are 57 breeds of sheep in India. This list includes both well-recognized and lesser-known breeds along with some wild species. Although there are about 42 breeds of sheep, majority of sheep population do not belong to any of the defined breeds. India's share to total number of breeds of World is 6.41%. India is endowed with large and biologically diverse sheep population comprising of sheep producing fleeces having fibre diameter below 30 μ to totally hairy sheep. Some of the breeds from the adjoining areas have been identified as separate breeds although they may be similar to each other genetically. The phenotypic differences may be due to selection for adaptation to specific agro-climatic conditions. The Madras Red in Tamil Nadu, Red Nellore in Andhra Pradesh and Ganjam sheep in Orissa although identified as separate breeds appear to be similar but their actual genetic differences are not known. Similarly in Rajasthan Marwari, Jaisalmeri and Kheri are black face sheep. The so-called Bikaneri sheep include brown face breeds, viz. Chokla, Magra and Nali and the phenotypic differences might have been due to assortative mating. Real genetic differences, if any, among similar groups need to be established.

Breeds exhibiting more than one strain

There are more than one strains in some of the breeds viz. Deccani, Patanwadi, Nellore etc. The sheep of Deccani breed are not uniform and their coat colour varies from black to white and the mixture of the two. It has been estimated that about 57% of Deccani are black, 28% white and 15% have a mixed coat colour. The varieties of Deccani are Lonad, Sangamneri, Solhapuri (Sangola) and Kolhapuri. Sangamneri type sheep has a stronger body constitution and higher wool yield. The wool is coarser and of longer staple. Sangola type sheep have higher proportion of black colour sheep and produce finer fleece. Madgyal strain of Deccani is also available in native area. Patanwadi sheep has three types (a) non-migratory- small bodied and fine fleeced Patanwadi, (b) migratory- leggy with long tubular ears and relatively coarse fleeced-Kathiawadi and (c) low stuttered, meat type, very coarse fleeced-Charotari also called Sonadi in Rajasthan However, looking to the phenotypic appearance of Sonadi and Patanwadi their genetic similarity needs to be verified. Nellore sheep in Andhra Pradesh has three varieties distinguished primarily on the basis of colour viz., Jodipi, Palla and Dora (a) Jodpi (also called Jodimpu) with black spots particularly around the lips, eyes and lower jaw and also on belly and legs (b) Pala completely white or white with light brown spots on head, neck, back and legs and (c) Dora, completely brown. The differences between the strains at genetic level need to be looked into to name them as separate breeds.

Breeds with unique characteristics

All the indigenous sheep breeds are known for adaptability under varied climate conditions, which is obvious from their long struggle against the natural forces (Table 1). Garole sheep are reputed for multiple births and are found in the Sunderban area of West Bengal. These sheep are reported to have contributed prolificacy to the Booroola Merino sheep. Litter size at first lambing is two and at subsequent lambing is 2 to 3. Prolificacy reported is singles 25-30%, twin's 55-60%, triplet's 15-20% and quadruplet's 1-2%. Kendrapada sheep is identified as another prolific sheep of India after Garole of West Bengal. It is 2nd sheep breed of India and 6th in world which carry *FecB* mutation. Kendrapada is distributed in Bhadrak, Konark and Puri district of coastal area of Orissa. The survey reveals that Kendrapada is a prolific and excellent medium stature meat type sheep. In the flocks surveyed more than 75% ewes produces multiple births and the adult body weight of sheep was about 23 kg. The coat color varies from white to dark brown. Some black animals and black/ white spot on body are also found during survey (Report, 2007). Munjal sheep is the least discussed among Indian sheep breeds. Information on population and production performance of this breed is scanty. Munjal is one of the important mutton type sheep. Animals of this breed are quite big and tall. Average adult body weight is around 45 kg.

Table 1 : Breeds with unique characteristics

Breed	Unique characteristics
Magra	Lustrous wool, excellent for carpet manufacture
Changthangi	Alpine sheep of high altitude for fine wool
Chokla	Fine carpet quality fleece
Garole	High fecundity- twins and triplets common. Survival under saline conditions
Mecheri, Madras Red	High quality skin and mutton
Mandya	Excellent meaty conformation, high quality and meat palatability
Patanwadi	Carpet wool and good milk producer
Nellore	Tallest sheep breed of India
Muzaffarnagari	Best mutton producing breeds
Marwari, Deccani Jaisalmeri	Hardy and capable of walking long distances during migration
Kendrapada	High fecundity- twins and triplets common

Special characteristics of indigenous breeds

Indigenous animals during its evolution have developed superior heat tolerance as well as disease resistance. Most of the breeds are very well adapted to harsh climate, long migration, tropical diseases and ability to thrive and produce with poor nutrition and shortage of drinking water and its poor quality. These qualities are found lacking in the exotic sheep breeds and crosses developed from them.

Heat stress: Indigenous sheep breeds are hardy and are relatively better adapted to local climatic conditions and can sustain extremely high temperature during summer season. Crossbred sheep can't be sent for migration and start panting during hot summer months. Hence crossbred and exotic sheep have to be grazed during cooler hours i.e. morning, evening and night grazing.

Disease Resistance: Indigenous sheep breeds have been found to have better resistance against endoparasites whereas crossbreds and exotic sheep are relatively more susceptible to diseases. There are substantial evidences for genetic variation between indigenous sheep and exotic crosses in resistance to internal parasites such as *Haemonchus contortus, Ostertagia circumcincta* and *Trichostrongylus colubriformis*. Studies conducted on some of the indigenous sheep and exotic crosses with respect to infection with gastrointestinal nematodes revealed that there is significant differences in FEC (faecal egg count), haematological and biochemical parameters between the breeds. Indigenous sheep excreted fever worm eggs in faeces and had lower morbidity and mortality rates compared to exotic breed and their crosses. Garole sheep are naturally resistance to haemonchosis.

Imrovement programmes

As a result of crossbreeding, improved strains were evolved, e.g. Hissardale by crossing Bikaneri ewes with Merino rams at Hisar, and Kashmir Merino by crossing indigenous breeds like Gaddi, Bhakarwal, Rampurbushair, Poochhi, Kamah and Gurez with Merino. Under the All India Co-ordinate Research Programme (AICRP) on sheep breeding initiated by the ICAR in 1971 and institutional research programmes undertaken by CSWRI, Avikanagar, a number of strains for fine/ carpet wool and mutton production have been evolved. These new strains of sheep were named as Avivastra, Nali-Synthetic, Chokla-Synthetic, Nilgiri-synthetic, Patanwadi-synthetic and Gaddi-synthetic. Merino type sheep were also evolved by *inter-se* mating of 75% grade and stabilizing the exotic inheritance at this level through inter-breeding and selection for wool weight and quality. This strain has been named as Bharat Merino and is a substitute of exotic fine wool breed. Avikalin strain, evolved from Rambouillet x Malpura half-breds has a significant improvement in carpet wool production and quality and rams of this strain have been extensively distributed in Rajasthan, UP and Haryana. Crossbreeding experiments for improving mutton involved exotic mutton breeds viz. Dorset and Sufflok with indigenous breeds, viz. Malpura, Sonadi, Muzzafarnagari, Nellore, Mandya, Deccani and Madras Red and crossbreds shown improvement in meat production as reflected by improvement in body weight gains, efficiency of feed conversion and dressing percentage. Avimaans (Mutton Synthetic) lambs at CSWRI could attain 25 kg body weight at 130 days but have tendency to deposit fat during terminal part of feedlot. Poor reproduction was the serious limitation with this strain. Similarly, crossbreds of different exotic breeds like Rambouillet, Dorset, Suffolk, and Corriedale were generated in number of states. Crossbreds evolved along with their genetic composition are presented in table 2.

From the available reports it is revealed that percent improvement in body weight up to 6 months of age is conspicuous in different crossbreds over contemporary natives but only marginal improvement is observed at 12 months of age. This is indicative of the fact that crossbreds/new synthetics required high plane of nutrition and if they are managed on the same feeding regimen as for natives, the differences that are conspicuous up to 6 months age, narrow down gradually and become marginal at the age of one year. An improvement in fleece quality has been reflected by a decrease in the percentage of medullated fibres and average fibre diameter, but in some cases a decline in fleece weight and reproductive performance was reported.

Cross-breeding among indigenous breeds has been extensive in Andhra Pradesh, Karnataka, Tamil Nadu and UP for improving wool production and quality and, to some extent, for improving mutton production. Most of the wool breeds involved were from Rajasthan (Bikaneri, Magra and Nali). This programme was not fully successful in the Southern States, since the Bikaneri rams did not survive long, presumably because, except in Uttar Pradesh, they adapted poorly to the hot humid climate. There was however an improvement in wool production and quality, reflected in an increase in staple length and a decrease in medullation percentage and average fibre diameter. Cross-breeding work carried out in the country in general indicated the superiority in body weight, greasy fleece weight and fleece quality of half-breds over the indigenous pure-breds involved in crosses, except for Polwarth crosses with Rampur Bushair in UP. The survival of half-breds was similar to that of indigenous breeds involved in the crosses, but crosses containing higher exotic inheritance did show problems of survival. Rambouillet appeared to be superior to other exotic breeds in cross-breeding experiments. When more than one indigenous breed was used with the same exotic breed, carpet-wool breeds - particularly Magra (Bikaner) - showed superiority.

Table 2 : Sheep strains developed in India

Genotype with utility / location	Parent breeds		Level of exotic inheritance (%)
	Indigenous	Exotic	
Bharat Merino, for fine wool CSWRI, Avikanagar	Chokla, Nali, Malpura, Jaiselmeri	Rambouillet, Russian Merino	75
Avivastra, for fine wool CSWRI, Avikanagar	Chokla, Nali	Rambouillet, Russian Merino	50
Nilgiri Synthetic, for apparel wool, TNVASU Sandynallah	Nilgiri	Rambouillet, Soviet Merino	62.5/75
Patanwadi Synthetic, for carpet wool, GAU, Dantiwada	Patanwadi	Rambouillet, Soviet Merino	50
Avikalin, for carpet wool, CSWRI, Avikanagar	Malpura	Rambouillet	50
Avimaans, for mutton, CSWRI, Avikanagar	Malpura, Sonadi	Dorset, Suffolk	50
Indian Karakul, for pelt, CSWRI, ARC Bikaner	Marwari, Malpura, Sonadi	Karakul	75
Kashmir Merino, for fine wool, J &K	Gaddi, Bhakarwal, Poonchi	Delaine Merino Rambouillet, Soviet Merino	50-75
Hisardale, for apparel wool, Haryana	Bikaneri	Australian Merino	75

Sheep-breeding work under AICRP for fine wool, involving exotic fine-wool breeds (Soviet Merino and Rambouillet) and indigenous breeds (Gaddi, Nali, Chokla, Patanwadi, Nilgiri and Bonpala), yielded improvement in greasy wool production and fleece quality in the half-breds over the native breeds involved in crosses, but the improvement in greasy wool production was minimal where the native breed was already producing relatively high quantities of fleece (e.g. Nali and Chokla). Similarly, the improvement in fleece quality was minimal in breeds with already reasonably fine fleece, such as Nilgiri. At CSWRI, Avikanagar in a breeding experiment involving Rambouillet and three different indigenous breeds, Chokla, Jaisalmeri and Malpura, the half-breds were substantially superior in body weight, greasy fleece yield and fleece quality, but beyond 50% exotic fine-wool inheritance, there was little improvement in body weight and greasy fleece weight though there was some further improvement in wool quality. The performance of progeny produced from inter-breeding half-breds was not much inferior to that of the first generation half-breds.

Research has been undertaken at CSWRI for breeding sheep for pelt and Karakul is being crossed with indigenous extremely coarse carpet-wool breeds. The results achieved have been very encouraging. The Network Project on Sheep Improvement (NWPSI) was initiated on 1.4.1990 for survey, evaluation and improvement of indigenous sheep breeds under native environment. All the centres of All India Coordinated Research Project on Sheep Breeding (AICRP-SB) were converted into NWPSI Centres. Different breeds of sheep are being improved through selection and inter-se mating for wool and mutton production. Presently, there are eight ongoing centres of NWPSI including farm based units at CSWRI, Avikanagar (Chokla, carpet Wool), ARC (CSWRI), Bikaner (Marwari, carpet wool), CIRG, Makhdoom (Muzaffamagri, Dual type), MPKV, Rahuri (Deccani, Dual type) and ANGRAU, Palamner (Nei lore, Mutton) and field-based units at RAU, Bikaner (Magra, Carpet wool) and TNVASU, Kattupakkam (Madras Red, Mutton) and OUAT Bhubaneswar (Garjam, mutton). Recently during 11th Five year plan under Mega seed project the rams of Chotanagpuri (BAU Ranchi), Sonadi (Vallabhnagar), Mecheri (TANUVAS Chennai) and Mandya have been distributed to sheep farmers for genetic improvement.

Recent advances in sheep breeding

Genetic improvement of sheep: Considering the importance of heavy body weight and milk yield in economic mutton production, a pilot project on crossbreeding of Awassi rams with Malpura ewes was started in 1994. A need was felt to enhance milk and mutton production in Malpura sheep by crossing it with Awassi rams (well known for heavy body weights and milk production). Awassi x Malpura (AM) half-bred lambs exhibited 18.75, 27.05, 19.56 and 14.92 % improvement over Malpura lambs at birth, 3, 6 and 12-month weights. These crossbreds produced 37% more 1st six monthly wool yield compared to Malpura lambs. Crossbred wool was found to have better wool quality with 36 μ diameter and 45% medullation compared to 45 μ diameter and 60% medullation in Malpura wool. Crossbred wool is also lustrous and can be used as carpet wool. Awassi x Malpura ewes produced 29% more milk than that of Malpura ewes. Awassi rams were used to cross Malpura ewes in farmer's flocks and local farmers are interested in crossbreeding of their animals with Awassi rams. The information generated at CSWRI indicated that six-month weight is the simplest criterion for improving mutton production.

Improving Prolificacy: Considering the importance of multiple births in sheep breeding in special reference to mutton production, Garole a prolific breed of sheep has been introduced at CSWRI, Avikanagar in 1997. Recently in the year 2010 the Kendrapada sheep of coastal Orissa was also introduced at CSWRI, Aviaknagar for improving the prolificacy of Malpura sheep. The results indicated that twining percent in Garole X Malpura (GM) half-breeds ewes were 52.24% and lamb born, as triplets were 7.46%. The average number lambs born per ewe lambed was 1.64 in GM sheep (Kumar *et al*.., 2004, 2006; Mishra *et al*., 2007a). The overall percent gain in prolificacy in GM was 52.38 which increased to 75.73 in third parity (Mishra *et al*., 2007a, 2008). The GM compared to Malpura ewes also weaned more lambs per ewe lambed (1 vs. 1.41). It was observed that the body weights at different ages of GM half-bred were on little lower side compared to contemporary Malpura lambs. The survivability of GM sheep is almost at par with native Malpura sheep (Mishra *et al*., 2007a). Similar study was also carried out at Nimbkar Agricultural Research Institute (NARI), Phaltan (Maharashtra) using Deccani and Bellary breed (Nimbkar, 1995; Nimbkar *et al*., 2000). Nimbkar *et al*. (2003) reported that crossing with Garole reduces liveweight and growth rate significantly compared with Deccani. The *FecB* genotyping was carried out by Forced-Restriction Fragment Length Polymorphism PCR technique in Garole, GM and Malpura. The results showed that a majority of animals (~98.0%) carrying mutated *FecB* allele in Garole sheep. The results indicated that the single copy mutation in *FecB* gene increased extra litter size by about 0.93 in GM ewes. The introduction of *FecB* gene from Garole to non-prolific Malpura improved the multiple births and enhanced the prolificacy in GM crosses (Kumar *et al*., 2006). Mishra *et al*. (2009) reported that *FecB* genotypes were significantly associated with the cumulative litter size and cumulative number of weaned lambs. There is a tremendous potential to exploit the *FecB* gene possessing GM germplasm for backcrossing with Malpura sheep to further propagate the fecundity gene and enhance the body weight gains in progeny having 25% Garole and 75% Malpura inheritance. The *FecB* gene carrier GM sheep were used in backcrossing breeding programme (i) as sires with Malpura ewes as dams to produce the GM x Malpura (GMM) and reciprocal (ii) as dams with Malpura rams to produce M x GM (MGM) progeny. The growth performance of backcross progenies and contemporary Malpura and GM lambs were compared. There were 53.76, 49.13 and 33.52% increase in body weight of GMM lambs over GM half-breds at birth, weaning and 6-month of age, respectively. The results indicate that there is pronounced higher gain in the body weight and growth rate of lambs produced after backcrossing of GM rams with Malpura ewes compared to the reciprocal backcrossing (Mishra and Arora, 2003; Arora *et al.*, 2009; Singh *et al.*, 2006; Annual Report, 2007, 2008). In GMM X Patwandi lambs the average body weight at birth, 3, 6 and 12 months were 3.34, 20.34, 30.15 and 41.00 kg, respectively (Annual Report, 2010).

Improving milk yield: To improve the growth rate as well as milk yields the Awassi rams were crossed with Malpura ewes at CSWRI, Avikanagar and with Deccani at NARI, Phaltan. A need was felt to enhance milk and mutton production in Malpura sheep by crossing it with Awassi rams (well known for heavy body weights and milk production). Hence, a pilot project on crossbreeding of Awassi rams with Malpura ewes was started in 1994, at CSWRI, Avikanagar. Awassi x Malpura (AM) half-bred lambs exhibited improvement over Malpura lambs at birth, 3, 6 and 12-month weights. These crossbreds produced more 1st six monthly wool yield compared to Malpura lambs. Crossbred wool was found to have better wool quality compared to Malpura wool. Awassi x Malpura ewes produced 29% more milk than that of Malpura ewes. Awassi rams were used to cross Malpura ewes in farmer's flocks and local farmers are interested in crossbreeding of their animals with Awassi rams (Arora *et al.*, 1998, 2004; Maurya *et al.*,1997). The results reveal that Awassi blood can be introduced in native sheep like Malpura to enhance wool and mutton production. Some farmers were fascinated by fat tail of Awassi and they showed interest in crossbreeding of native Malpura ewes with Awassi rams. The significant improvement in crossbreds was observed over native with respect to growth and milk yield (Nimbkar, 1995; Report, 1998;

Narula *et al.,* 1999). Recently the crossing of Paranwadi with Garole X Malpura was started at CSWRI, Avikanagar to increase milk yield in prolific sheep.

Fat lamb production: Malpura weaner lambs (2 months age) are capable of achieving 25 kg body weight at about 5 months of age under intensive feeding on composite ration of the ratio of 60 concentrates and 40 roughage. The major advantage is that sheep owners need to rear the animals only for about 5 months with earning of about Rs. 370/- per lamb on slaughter basis and Rs. 100/- on live animal sale basis.

Animal biotechnology: Genome analysis of sheep breeds reveals that Avikalin and Chokla are closer whereas Malpura and Garole were more distant to each other. DNA isolation protocol has been standardized from sheep wool follicles and can be used for identification of *FecB* mutation eliminating need of blood. The identification of *FeB* mutation was carried out in Garole, Kendrapada and Garole x Malpura crosses. The introduction of *FecB* gene from Garole to non-prolific Malpura improved the multiple births and enhanced the prolificacy in GM crosses. The results showed that a majority of animals (~98.0%) carrying mutated *FecB* allele in Garole sheep.

Implementation of breeding programs

Selection in institutional flocks: Hitherto most of the sheep farms under the Central and State Animal Husbandry Departments in the country have been supplying rams to the private flock owners. The best males are first used in the institutional flock and after that these rams along with other rams are made available to farmers for use in their flocks. In majority of the cases, however, the flock size in the government farms is small allowing little selection within the flock. Males produced on such farms may not be superior to those in the farmers' flocks because of small size not allowing effective selection and maintained essentially under limited hours of grazing supplemented with cultivated fodder/hay/dried tree leaves/ concentrates and are thus not acceptable to farmers whose flocks have to walk long distances in search of feed whether such flocks are stationary or migratory. Moreover, if the flocks are closed (as is generally the case), they will have larger risk of inbreeding and random genetic drift causing loss of genetic variability because of small size and a few rams being used for breeding. The State/Central sheep breeding farms will not be in a position to supply breeding rams in desired numbers. In that conditions, farmers generally use their own breeding rams for couple of years altogether without paying due attention towards adverse effect of inbreeding in their flocks or manage other rams that may be inferior in terms of reproduction and other characteristics like true to the breed etc. In certain areas sheep farmers use the rams of enroute migratory flocks and consequently there is dilution in the purity of breed. As a result of all these, sizeable non-descript type of sheep population has been generated in the field.

Selection in farmers' flocks: Sheep farmers in India are having small to medium sized flocks. Farmers need to be motivated to cooperate and allow/adapt recording of their flocks for objective assessment to identify flocks which are better than average. Performance recording in the farmer's flocks may be difficult and laborious but it is essential. At least first 6-monthly greasy fleece weight and kg of lamb weaned/ewe/year are the two characters which must find a place for recording in farmers' flocks and for this purpose farmers will also have to be persuaded to adopt some method for identification. Farmers' flocks thus identified will be used for producing genetically superior males which could subsequently be distributed to the flocks which are inferior to the average of the population. This will require identification of superior males and females based on the characters of importance and mating them to produce male progeny. Following either of the two approaches given below can rear the male progeny thus produced:

(a) *Rearing of ram lambs in farmers' flocks:* The farmers from whose flock, selected ram lambs have been produced will rear them up to breeding age of 18 months. These farmers will be given incentives in the form of subsidized feeds, free health cover and when the ram lambs have reached the breedable age, these will be purchased at three times the prevailing market price per kg live weight and distributed among the farmers' flocks having below average performance at subsidized rates. This scheme will be cheaper compared to purchasing and rearing them at the ram lamb rearing centers or at some state farms. Such rams will also be more acceptable and will have little problem of adaptation in the farmers' management condition.

(b) *Ram lamb rearing centres:* This could be an alternative to scheme mentioned above. The selected ram lambs are purchased from the farmers' flocks after weaning and reared up to breedable age in the ram-lambs rearing centres. These centres will have to be established in large numbers to cover the maximum number of farmers' flocks. These centres should also be used as performance testing units wherein 6-monthly body weight, first 6-monthly greasy fleece weight and fibre diameter could be recorded and used for selection of rams. The rams will then be distributed to flocks which are inferior.

Selection in open nucleus breeding system (ONBS): This breeding programme essentially consists of organizing farmers into cooperative breeding groups so that the combined strength of many small to medium flocks in a single village or a group of contiguous villages will form a sufficiently large population, say, 1,000 breedable females. Majority of sheep farmers in India are small holders and so within flock selection will not be possible, particularly when flock owners are lacking in formal skills for performance recording and flock being too small. After an initial screening of the associated flocks, better performing animals (males and females) are selected on the basis of objective assessment from the farmers' flocks. The animals thus selected are placed in a central breeding nucleus farm where these are utilized for producing males. The flock is also subjected to intra-population selection. The best males from the nucleus are used in the nucleus flock itself and rest of better-than-average rams/male lambs are distributed to the cooperating farmers. Keeping the flock 'open' through regular cycles of bringing in better performing animals from the associated farms would help in making greater improvement and will also reduce chances of inbreeding. After distributing the males in the co-operating flocks the rest would be distributed to other flocks to be improved. Subsequently, flocks of co-operating farmers could also be utilized in breeding males (multiplier flocks) using the selected males from the nucleus flock.

Central and State breeding farms support the present breeding policy by producing acclimatized exotic and superior crossbred rams under specialized management conditions to avoid recurrent import. Exotic rams from the Central, ICAR and selected State farms are provided to different States for production of half-bred rams in the farms maintained by them. The half-bred rams produced in the sheep breeding farms of the States are supplied to the fanners in the concerned breeding tracts to produce quarter-breds initially and to make further improvement to 50% level of exotic inheritance. However, such policy is not being followed strictly and some of the large scale sheep breeding farms meant for rearing of exotic animals are also producing half bred rams. The production and supply of superior breeding males from the Central farm at Hisar and the seven Centre aided large farms in the states and 70 other state farms are a part of this support system. However, this entire farm capacity can be significantly multiplied by converting as many of the 70 state farms as possible to open nucleus breeding farms and ram rearing units. Thus the large Central Breeding Farm, Hisar will have to maintain exotic nucleus germ plasm and supply exotic males to the centrally aided farms situated in different states and other states farms for production and distribution of cross bred stock using the local females of the respective localities. The seventy state farms will be primarily used as open nucleus breeding farms to improve local breeds of the respective tracts through pure breeding and selection. They may be strengthened wherever necessary to meet the objectives of their respective breeding policy.

Region wise sheep breeding recommendations

Sheep breeding approach (which involves decision on criterion for selection and mating plans) for each of the four agro-climatic regions of the country is based on the problems related to sheep improvement and production type found in each of these regions.

Northern temperate region: The region comprises states of Jammu and Kashmir, Himachal Pradesh, Uttarakhand and Arunachal Pradesh. This region has a large potential for apparel wool production, 75-80% of the flocks are already crossbreds involving a number of exotic fine wool breeds. Crossbreeding with exotic fine wool breeds has been successfully carried out in almost all the local breeds, viz., Gaddi, Bhakarwal, Poonchi, Karnah, Rampur Bushair and Gurez breeds. Crossbreeding programmes may be further intensified to cover all the farmers' flocks in the region. The exotic inheritance may be stabilised at 75% and further improvement in greasy fleece weight may be brought through selection on first annual greasy fleece weight. Wherever crossing of indigenous sheep is required it may involve Rambouillet, Kashmir Merino and Bharat Merino for improving staple length by taking it into selection of rams in addition to greasy fleece weight and average fibre diameter. The farmers should also be encouraged to adopt annual shearing in this region. Changthangi breed of Ladakh which is hardy and yields good carpet/medium apparel wool has relatively longer staple length than other breeds of this region. The breed may be improved through selection for annual greasy wool production. In Sikkim and Arunachal Pradesh, Tibetan sheep are available which have good carpet quality fleece and could be crossed with Rambouillet for improvement in wool production and quality for apparel wool. Level of exotic inheritance may be stabilized at 75%.

North-western arid and semi-arid region: This region comprises states of Punjab, Haryana, Rajasthan, Gujarat and plains of UP and MP. Chokla, Magra, Nali, Jaisalmeri, Pugal, Pattanwadi and Marwari breeds should be brought under large-scale selection by involving majority of farmers' flocks for improvement in body weight and carpet wool production and quality. Malpura, Sonadi, Muzaffanagri and Jalauni breeds should be similarly brought under selection involving the farmers' flocks mainly for improvement of 6-month body weight with little emphasis in selected rams for greasy wool production and against medullation percentage.

Southern penninsular and eastern region: The Southern region comprises states of Maharashtra, Andhra Pradesh, Kamataka, Tamil Nadu, Kerala and other nearby Union Territories. The Eastern region comprises of the states of Bihar, West Bengal, Orissa, Assam, Meghalaya, Arunachal Pradesh, Mizoram, Manipur, Tripura, Nagaland and Sikkim. Most of the sheep breeds in this region are used for meat and the wool is extremely coarse and hairy; the wool production is very low and has low market price. Improvement in their meat production may be brought through inter-breeding and selection involving farmers' flocks preferably through open nucleus breeding schemes. Deccani, Bellary, Nellore and Mandya breeds may be selected in the farmers' flocks on the basis of 6-monthly body weight. Since there is a large incidence of cryptorchadism in Mandya rams, no ram should be selected from flocks showing incidence of cryptorchadism. Rams of these breeds should also be used for improving mutton production through upgrading non-descript population. Madras Red and Macheri breeds could also be used for this purpose in grading non-descript population in contiguous areas in an organised manner, besides being improved through selection for 6-month body weight. Selected rams of Shahabadi breed are relatively heavier in body weight and may be used for upgrading Chhotanagpuri sheep. Other non-descript sheep may be improved through selection of rams for 6-monthly body weight in farmers' flocks preferably following ONBS involving farmers' flocks and Government Sheep Breeding Farms in the Eastern region. Ganjam and Bolangir breeds should be improved through selection of rams in farmers' flocks for 6-monthly body weight.

Nellore and Mandya may also be used for grading non-descript population. Rams of these breeds could be purchased from the breeding tracts of these breeds on 6-month body weight basis and raised on institutional farms or preferably got raised in farmers' flocks and purchased at breeding age and distributed to flocks to be improved.

Major issues related to sheep improvement

Keeping in view the above facts, in sheep development programmes there are certain issues, which need to be addressed. The following issues have been identified and addressed in strategies and recommendations part of this chapter:

- Indiscriminate breeding
- Inadequate availability of improver breeding rams
- Breed registration society
- Reproduction problem
- Conservation programmes
- Large proportion of non-descript sheep
- Poor exploitation of genetic potential of native stock
- Shortage of feed resources and nutritional deficiency
- Poor health coverage and disease monitoring and reporting system
- Lack of training and education facility to sheep farmers
- Inadequate marketing and credit support
- Socio- economic conditions of sheep farmers
- Migration
- Problems faced by sheep farmers during migration
- Lack of grazing policy in most of the states
- Lack of subsidy on wool

Strategies/ recommendations

Sheep breeding

- Sheep breeding policy needs to be reviewed keeping in view the global liberalization, farmers needs and perception, demand and supply of animal products like wool and meat, availability of feeds and fodder, existing species/breeds and their performance, infrastructure and support system in different agro climatic zones. Development of fine wool production in arid and semi arid region has negligible scope. In view of current trends in globalization of trade, import of apparel quality wool will continue to fill the gap in the requirement for value addition.

- Past experience shows that it has not been possible to get fine wool with desirable staple length from the higher crosses in the arid and semi arid region, apparel wool production may be intensified only in the temperate areas such as northern temperate hilly region and Nilgiri and Kodai hills of southern region. In these areas 3/4th crosses of Rambouillet or Merino including Bharat Merino may be propagated and annual clips may be obtained to meet the requirements for apparel manufacture.
- The carpet wool type breeds such as Nali, Chokla, Patanwadi, Marwari, Magra, Pugal, Gaddi and Jaisalmeri etc. may be further improved through selective breeding by distribution of good quality rams of the respective breeds. Wool quality traits of these breeds meet closer to the requirements of industry for carpet wool.
- Efforts should be made to introduce lusture in indigenous carpet wool breeds to harvest maximum return through sale of quality carpet wool.
- Selection index incorporating six-month body weight and first six monthly greasy fleece weight has yielded encouraging results towards enhancing body weight besides fleece production.
- There is a tremendous potential and demand of meat both in local market and for export especially to Middle-eastern countries. Therefore, strategy to fulfill this potential is to breed for more efficient, sturdy, prolific type of animals for both extensive (low input) and intensive (feedlot) systems. The intensive systems will be developed for feeding lambs for fattening from selected areas where organized breeding will be possible. Areas having extensive system of management could serve as resource areas for availability of lambs to be reared under intensive feeding conditions in feed surplus areas. Elite male germ plasm centres should be developed for providing good breeding rams.
- Within breed selection may be taken up systematically in the recognized breeds in the country. Selection of anyone of the

following schemes may be adopted in descending order of preference: (i) Selection and rearing of ram lambs in the farmers' flocks and their use in their flocks and for distribution to other flocks which are to be improved. (ii) Selection of ram lambs in the farmers' flocks and rearing them in the ram lamb rearing centers for distribution to the farmers' flocks. (iii) Establishment of an open nucleus breeding flocks through animals selected objectively on the basis of trait(s) of interest and selection within the nucleus to produce genetically superior rams for use in the nucleus flocks and for distribution to farmers' flocks be improved. The existing state sheep breeding farms may also be considered for conversion into ONBS. The productivity of each breed may be improved by bringing as large a number of farmers' flocks as possible under the improvement programme which may not only take up improvement through different breeding approaches but may involve provision of a totality of inputs and services related to genetic improvement, health cover, feed resources development, conservation and their strategic utilization, management and marketing of the produce.

- Grading up of non-descript sheep through their continuous breeding with selected rams of the desired descript breed(s), depending on characters to be improved should be under taken. As far as possible the rams of a breed from tracts close in agro-ecology of the flock to be improved should be selected.

- The country is short of good and elite rams and to cover whole sheep population of breedable ewes (around 25 million) about 60,000 elite rams are required in order to improve their productivity. Efforts need to be required in this direction. This can be accomplished by establishing ram production units and also young rams can be selected based on their own and parent's performance and record up to the age of maturity for distribution in the farmers flocks. Hence, there is a need to strengthen the ram raring centers and open nucleus system involving local sheep farmers should be followed.

- For profitable meat production, we need to evolve a breed, which must have fast and efficient growing lambs/kinds. The ewes/does should be prolific and must have good mothering ability. Fast growth and early maturity are the most important characteristics for meat production. Selection programs were undertaken in indigenous stock to increase their productivity. Malpura Muzaffarnagri, Madras Red and Mandya sheep exhibited considerable improvement through selective breeding which indicated that these are promising sheep breeds for increasing mutton production and they can also be used as improver breed for upgradation of native stock.

- Potential mutton type breed such as Malpura, Sonadi, Muzzaffarnagari, Madras Red, Mandya, Nellore, Deccani, Mecheri, Ganjam etc., may be restricted to selective breeding by using superior rams of the respective breeds for enhancing mutton production.
- Crossbreds may be tried in the area where feed and fodder are available adequately and they are not required to travel long distances in search of food.
- Data base, pertaining to breed-wise (descript and non descript) population, animal productivity, production of forage crops, industrial by-products and non-conventional feeds, grasses available in forest areas and grazing lands, is grossly inadequate. This needs to be updated through periodic surveys and livestock censuses. Important indigenous breeds of sheep should be properly characterised both phenotypically and genetically. Experiments should be undertaken to assess their population, production performance and to exploit their production potential under ideal feeding and health management conditions. Elite flock of different native breeds should be developed for producing genetically superior rams.
- Development and transfer of appropriate viable technologies of livestock production systems and farming systems deserve urgent attention by researchers involving farmers.
- Garole and Kendrapada indigenous prolific sheep breeds should be used for crossbreeding of sheep belonging to different locations of country subject to sufficient milk availability for multiple lambs. At CSWRI, Avikanagar, Garole x Malpura half-breds have been successfully developed and further research is in progress to strengthen this programme for increasing lambing rate but not at the cost of body weights.

Sheep conservation

- Livestock census gives information on sex ratio, population of different age groups and production status. However, it should be conducted on breed basis so that the population of sheep breeds showing declining trend can be monitored and conservation programs are undertaken.
- Breed societies be created and should get patronage, funding and scientific support for the conservation and sustainable utilization of sheep genetic resources. An expert panel should also be appointed at National level to determine the basic norms for a breed registration.
- A National Watch List of endangered breeds of livestock should be established like that of wild life and plants supported by strict legislation.
- The facilities available in the Government farms should be improved to keep the recognized indigenous breeds of livestock for in-situ conservation.
- Genetic improvement programs with high intensity of selection should be adopted for each breed. These selected elite animals would thus be economically viable and would be preserved/ conserved by the farmers due to their utility.
- Wherever feasible, live animal reserves for keeping to limited number of animals of a rare breed should be encouraged.
- A large infrastructure is available in the country for the semen/ embryo collection, storage and deep freezing. It should be mandatory for them to keep sample of semen doses/embryos in addition to their development needs.

Sheep health

- Inadequate information on various aspects of sheep diseases is available such as epidemiology, economics of disease and its control, diagnosis and prevention including those of exotic origin. There is a need for a standard disease reporting system which provides database for planning of disease control programmes and for immediate intervention at various levels, viz. village, tehsils, district and state. Surveillance system should be established for reporting diseases in small ruminants. The Central and State

Governments should initiate measures that provide the required information for effective control of sheep diseases at priority.

- Diagnostic facilities for small ruminant diseases need improvement. States those have significant populations of sheep, should develop special cells in existing diagnostic laboratories, equipped fully to diagnose the diseases. Animal Health Divisions of the CSWRI, Avikanagar and CIRG, Makdoom should be strengthened to provide referral services for disease diagnosis at the National level.
- The importance of veterinary extension to educate farmers on the prevention and control of disease is stressed to run of major disease control programs successfully in the country.
- Research in the development of appropriate health care delivery systems for varying production systems in the country is required. These delivery systems should be implemented along with all development programs envisaged for sheep.

Feed and nutrition

- Country has about 121 million hectares of grazing land, which includes pastures, forests, miscellaneous tree crops and crops cultivable wastelands, and fallow land. These areas have to be developed exclusively under pastures and forest. A national policy has to be framed to develop these lands and manage them suitably for grazing purposes. Individual farmers owning such land should be given incentive and material inputs for bringing such lands in their control under such silvi-pastoral development.
- Top feed resources constitute important feed resources for sheep, which require greater attention for their propagation, collection, conservation and utilization. The tree fodders should be incorporated in the complete feeds for intensive feeding. Complete feeds containing Ardu, Khejari and Pala leaves have been given satisfactory results for meat lamb production.
- Feeding strategies should be developed to utilize various resources of straws and crop residues, grasses and by product feeds in complete feeds. Methods need to be developed for alleviating deleterious factors of anti-nutritional factors present in top feeds, by product feeds etc. Simultaneously, intensive and semi intensive

systems of feeding management for small ruminant production may be developed.

- Tree and their provenances suitable to that locality be encouraged and preference should be given to indigenous fast growing species.
- Crop combination in agri-silvi-pastoral systems should be selected with minimum negative interaction. Multi-tier system of crop combination could be practiced for effective utilization of land as well as non-food crop production could be balanced.
- Imparting training to farmers in crop and animal Husbandry for better management of farming.
- The shrub and tree fodder tree have extensive value in arid and semi-arid zones because of feed shortage. In the humid regions, leguminous fodder shrubs and trees are especially valuable protein supplements and in reducing cost of production; hence these need to be developed.
- The two-tier concept, providing forage to the small ruminants and increasing the carrying capacity of the grazing lands must be promoted with different silvi-pastoral system.
- Conservation methods of seasonal surplus to feed and forage from the silvi-pastoral systems to be developed.

Reproductive physiology

- Research efforts are needed for developing the non-invasive transcervical technique to determine the factors controlling the servical penetration and lambing percentage after deposition of thawed semen for making this technology more relevant and wide acceptance.
- Studies of the augmentation of fertility in sheep breeds should be undertaken. Cryopreservation of semen of superior breeding rams and utilization of frozen semen with improved conception rate should be emphasized.
- The reproductive efficiency of farm/field flocks should be assessed and suitable methods be developed to enhance lambing rate in these flocks.

Sheep migration

- For regulating sheep migration in an organized way there should be coordination at the administrative heads level of different department of the states related to sheep migration for providing proper security and other facilities to the sheep farmers like health cover, watering and marketing of wool, meat, animals etc.
- The matters and disputes relating to sheep migration may be brought under the preview of Inter state council and grazing tariff charged should be nominal.
- Sheep farmers may be given subsidy and bank loans for establishing pastures and growing fodder trees on their own lands.
- Sheep should be included in the list of the animals entitled for fodder subsidy and other concessions during famine as applicable to cattle.
- Presently no national grazing policy exists in the country. Madhya Pradesh has grazing policy, which imposes several restrictions and grazing fees but that does not discuss pasture development. In the absence of a grazing policy, only forest regulations cover grazing restriction and these often contradicts the fodder policy. All these factors lead to an imbalance between grazing pressure and carrying capacity of grazing lands.

Wool marketing

- Wool should be declared as an agricultural commodity to introduce a price support system on the lines of cotton, jute and other commodities. Inclusion of wool in the National Cooperative Development Council list to help refinancing at lower rates of interest to marketing organization and soft loan to growers by NABARD.
- Activate and revitalize the state wool marketing Federations Boards/Corporations and provide adequate funds to these organizations to expand their activities with an aim to procure 20 to 25% of the total wool produced in the country.
- Import of wool should be allowed to the actual users only and this facility should be linked with export performance of the user.

- In the manufacturing of carpet 34µ and above quality wool is required, therefore the import of carpet grade wool of 34µ and above should be allowed at concessional rates instead of 32µ and above as at present. The wool development Board should be the sole canalizing agency for import of wool and should use revenue generated from this operation for development of the wool.
- Simple need based grading system should be developed to ensure remunerative prices to wool-growers and encourage quality wool production. Primary processing facilities for scouring, carbonizing, etc. should be made available in the country in rural areas as well as major wool trading centres in the country.

Mutton marketing

- Animal market yards with facilities of regulated marketing of animals may be established. In these market yards the federation/ corporation may provide market support system based on prevailing mutton prices and provide support price of live animals.
- Disease free zone of sheep may be created in states.
- Minimum export price should be reviewed periodically for matching with actual purchase price of animals in India.
- To provide hygienic meat to the consumers, modern slaughterhouses should be established. Specific refrigerated vans and cold storage may be established.
- Modern tanneries and other by-product processing units should be established near large slaughterhouses.
- In export of chilled/frozen meat to Gulf and other countries, federations/corporations may be given priority in getting space from Airlines.
- A market study may be undertaken for the processed meat products in the international market because it is a highly sensitive product oriented market.

References

Report Annual 2007. Annual progress Report, CSWRI, Avikanagar, Rajasthan.

Report Annual. 2008. Annual progress Report, CSWRI, Avikanagar, Rajasthan.

Report Annual. 2010. Annual progress Report, CSWRI, Avikanagar, Rajasthan.

Arora, A.L., Narula, H.K. and Sharma, R.C. 1998. Production performance of Malpura sheep *vis-a-vis* Awassi x Malpura halfbreds in semi-arid region of India, In: Proc. 4th Global Conference on Conservation of Domestic Animals Genetics Resources, Kathmandu (Nepal), 17-21 August, pp 151-152.

Arora, A.L., Sharma, R.C. and Narula, H.K. 2004. Evaluation of Awassi X Malpura half-brd sheep in semi-arid region of Rajasthan. Indian Journal of Animal Sciences 74: 1219-1222.

Arora, A.L., Mishra, A.K., Prince, L.L.L., Kumar Sushil and Gowane, G.R. 2009. Productivity efficiency of Prolofic garole X Malpura half-breeds. Indian Veterinary Journal 86: 217-218.

Kumar, A., Arora, A.L. and M.K. Srivastava. 2004. Annual Report, 2003-2004, CSWRI, Avikanagar, India.

Kumar, S., Kolte, A.P., Mishra, A.K., Arora, A.L and Singh, V.K. 2006. Identification of *Fec B* mutation in Garole x Malpura sheep and its effect on litter size. Small Ruminant Research 64: 305-310.

Maurya, V.P., Naqvi, S.M.K. and Mittal, J.P.1997. Performance of Awassi crossbred lambs in farmers' flocks of semi-arid region. Indian Journal of Animal Sciences 67: 438-440.

Mishra, A.K. and Arora, A.L. 2003. Evaluation of Garole X Malpura half-breds. *Indian* Journal of Animal Genetics and Breeding 24: 8

Mishra, A.K., Arora, A.L., Kumar, S., Kumar, S. and Singh, V.K. 2007a. Improving productivity of Malpura breed by crossbreeding with prolific Garole sheep in India. Small Ruminant Research 70: 159-164.

Mishra, A.K., Kumar, S., Arora, A.L. and Karim, S.A. 2007b. Kendrapada sheep of coastal Orissa: needs to be conserved, ISSGPU NEWS Letter, July, pp. 1-2.

Mishra, A.K., Arora, A.L., Kumar, S., Prince, L.L.L. and Singh, V.K. 2008. Productive and reproductive efficiency of Malpura and prolific Garole ewes and their crosses in semi-arid region, India Journal of Animal Sciences 78: 70-74.

Mishra, A.K., Arora, A.L., Kumar, S. and Prince, L.L.L. 2009. Studies on effect of Booroola (FecB) genotype on lifetime ewes productivity efficiency, litter size and number of weaned lambs in Garole X Malpura sheep, Animal Reproduction Science 113: 293-298.

Narula, H.K., Arora, A.L. and Sharma, R.C. 1999. Assessment of milk yield in Malpura sheep. Indian Journal of Small Ruminants 5: 62-64.

Nimbkar, B.V. 1995. The role of voluntary organizations. In: Proc. III National Seminar on Sheep and Goat Production and Utilization, Avikinagar, 8-10 April, pp 203-209.

Nimbkar, C., Ghalsasi, P.M., Walkden-Brown, S.W., Kahn, L.P. and Gray, G.D. 2000. A comparison of the growth performance and worm resistance of lambs produced by diallel crossing of three Indian sheep breeds. Asian-Australasian Journal of Animal Sciences 13: 72-75.

Nimbkar, C., Ghalsasi P.M., Maddox, J.F., Pardeshi, V.C., Sainani, M.N., Gupta, V. and Walkden-Brown, S.W. 2003. Expression of *FecB* gene in Garole and Crossbred ewes in Maharastra, India. In: Proc. Fifteenth Conference of AAABG, Melbourne, Australia, p.111-114.

Report, 1998. 35-Years of Research. CSWRI, Avikanagar, India.

Singh, V.K., Arora, A.L., Mehta, B.S., Mishra, A.K., Kumar Sushil and Prince, L.L.L. 2006. New strains of sheep evolved, CSWRI, Avikanagar.

□□□

Chapter 4

Prolific Sheep : A Promise to Make and Deliver for the Socio-Economic Upliftment of Sheep Farmer

A.L. Arora, Ashish Chopra and L. Leslie Leo Prince
Division of Animal Genetics and Breeding, Central Sheep and Wool Research Institute, Avikanagar- 304 501 (Rajasthan)

Improved animal genetic resources with versatile characteristics are the need of the day to meet the growing human demand. India is endowed with wide diversity of sheep genetic resources, which forms the backbone of its rural livelihood security systems. Sheep rearing now faces a dilemma to produce more mutton and wool for the growing human population against the reality of shrinking grazing resources, creating a major constraint to the further growth of sheep population. In the present scenario the demand for meat in India has increased rapidly and the emphasis has shifted from wool towards mutton as the main produce from sheep rearing (Mishra, 2008). There is acute shortage of meat for domestic needs besides huge demand in the international market. The gap between the demand and production of mutton could be bridged by augmenting the reproductive rate of low producing Indian sheep breeds. Improving prolificacy in sheep flock can increase the profitability of sheep production. Lamb production has become a most important source of income for sheep rearer. In order to improve the fecundity of sheep, incorporation of genetic material of prolific sheep is an ideal approach to evolve a large size breed capable of multiple births for economic and remunerative mutton production.

Most of the domestic sheep breeds of the world are reported to deliver only one or two lambs at each lambing. The increase in production associated with litter size is controlled by both genetic and environmental factors. Since the heritability of litter size is low in sheep, attempts were made to discover the gene(s) controlling ovulation rate and thus litter size (LS). Turner (1969) concluded that litter size seemed to be the most useful selection criterion for genetic improvement of reproduction. Ewe productivity is dependent upon the component traits of fertility, litter size, lamb survival and growth (Fogarty *et al.*, 1984) and is a major concern for the sheep industry. Improving female reproductive performance is an important objective for increasing the prolificacy of sheep (Abdulkhaliq *et al.*, 1989). There is greater potential for increasing both biological and economic efficiency of lamb production through genetic improvement in reproductive rate than through improvement in growth rate or body composition (Dickerson, 1978). The ovulation rate analysis of the first recorded highly prolific breed, 'Booroola Merino' (BM) of Australia, provided strong evidence for the presence of a single gene governing it (Davis *et al.*, 1982). In 1982, Dr Helen Newton Turner suggested that the Garole sheep from Sunderbans, West Bengal, India, could be the source of the *FecB* mutation in highly prolific BMs. Later, in 1996, Piper and Bindon reported the inclusion of the prolific Bengal sheep in an early Australian BM flock. Davis *et al.* (2002) detected the *FecB* mutation in Garole and Indonesian Javanese sheep, thereby confirming the hypothesis that the *FecB* gene in the Garole is the same as that reported in Australian BMs.

Realizing the importance of *FecB* mutation, extensive work has been done all over the world including India improving prolificacy and its effects and economics in sheep production traits. The *FecB* gene has spread from the Booroola Merino to some 40 breeds of sheep worldwide. It is now also spreading from the Garole, Hu and Han breeds in India and China, from one of which it probably originated. Many country of world imported or utilized prolific sheep in cross breeding program to introgress the prolificacy gene in non-prolific breeds of their native tract and faces diverse type of experiences.

World wide experiences of prolificacy improvement through introgression of *FecB* (Booroola) gene

The *FecB* mutation has probably been present in Australia since 1792 or 1793 when the first shipments of the diminutive but highly fecund 'Bengal sheep' arrived from Calcutta (Turner, 1982). These sheep were likely the same as or related to the diminutive but highly fecund Garole sheep from West Bengal, in which the *FecB* mutation occurs at a very high frequency. BM rams carrying the *FecB* gene were made widely available to industry by CSIRO, Australia in late 1980s. In 1987 only 20 flocks were actively incorporating the gene into their sheep. Today the prolificacy gene has been present in Australia for more than 200 years and has been deliberately introgressed into various Merino sheep. The heterozygous carrier produces sufficient additional lambs weaned (26%) to be economically viable (albeit with excessive lamb mortality), but that the homozygote is commercially disastrous, exhibiting significantly lower conception rates and lamb survival rates despite similar litter size (LS) as the heterozygote (Brown *et al.*, 2008). The experience of *FecB* introgression into Awassi and Assaf sheep in Israel, commenced in 1986 (Gootwine, 2008). Apart from central institutional flocks, rams of both breeds carrying *FecB* (Afec in the author's terminology) have been quite widely disseminated to industry. The improved genotypes have been most successful to date in fully intensive dairy and non-dairy production systems with artificial rearing of lambs. As in the Australian experience, the heterozygote is more productive than the homozygote carrier due to higher lamb survival despite similar LS. Typical LSs of the Awassi are 1.31, 1.90 and 1.92 for 0, 1 and 2 copies of *FecB* respectively. *FecB* is generally associated with reduced birth weight, growth and milk production but remains economically viable for intensive system of rearing.

In USA, Introgressions of $FecB^B$ into a Rambouillet genetic background occurred in the mid-1980s at the University of Wisconsin (after transfer of the Illinois BM flock to that location) and at San Angelo, and resulting 'Booroola Rambouillet' populations are being maintained at both locations. Results from the first two backcrosses of BM × Rambouillet ewes to Rambouillet rams were reported by Southey *et al.* (2002), and provided estimates of effects of a single copy of $FecB^B$ in a 75% or 87.5% Rambouillet genetic background. The effect of a single copy of $FecB^B$ on ovulation rate (OR) did not change in a systematic way during upgrading, averaging 1.61 ova. The effect on $FecB^B$ on LS was relatively consistent in 50% and 75% Rambouillet ewes, averaging 0.90 lambs, but was reduced to only 0.26 lambs in a small group (34 heterozygous and 17 wild-type) of young 87.5% Rambouillet ewes. Ewes with one copy of the *FecB*^{B} allele had lambs with significantly lower survival rates and weaning weights, and produced a similar weight of lamb per ewe exposed when compared to ewes of similar breed composition without the *FecB*^{B} allele. Production of commercial Rambouillet ewes carrying a single copy of *FecB*^{B} is achieved in the Wisconsin flock by continual backcrossing of Rambouillet–BM ewes to Rambouillet rams and differentiation of heterozygous ewes from wild-type ewes. Comparisons of effects of *FecB*^{B} in a predominantly Rambouillet genetic background (Crooks *et al.*, 1999, 2000) confirm no effect of *FecB*^{B} on fertility or average lamb weaning weight, but a 5 kg (9.2%) reduction in realised lamb weight (i.e. without adjustment for birth type) at 120 days. Effects of *FecB*^{B} were observed for OR (1.54 ova), LS (0.59 lambs), lamb survival (-8.5%) and ewe productivity at weaning (9.7%) at a lamb age of 180 days (8.9%) and at a lamb weight of 54.4 kg (20.8%). Moreover, Notter *et al.* (2008) reviewed many studies conducted in USA showed little opportunity for future use of *FecB*^{B} in commercial sheep production in the USA. This outcome mainly reflects the relatively high prolificacy levels already present in several US sheep breeds and the desire by most US producers to avoid high frequencies of triplet births. However, if the mean LS of local breeds is below 1.3 lambs/litter, use of *FecB*^{B} has the potential to rapidly increase the frequency of twinning with only modest increases in numbers of triplet births.

The Indonesian production system is semi-intensive, more like that in India. Under Indonesian conditions when nutrition is good, ewes carrying one copy of *FecB* exhibit the highest gross margin, followed by homozygotes then non-carriers. Under conditions of poor nutrition there was no economic benefit of *FecB* at all. Typical LSs of the Indonesian Thin Tailed sheep are 1.22, 2.02 and 2.5 for 0, 1 and 2 copies of *FecB*, respectively, with respective lamb survival to 90 days being 84.3, 71.9 and 59.2% (Inounu and Priyanti, 2008). *FecB* Introgression into French Mérinos d'Arles sheep in France was commenced in 1983. Teyssier *et al.* (2008) reported on datasets collected from both an institutional farm and a commercial producer. There was a clear economic advantage for *FecB* heterozygote ewes based on consistent production of 50-65% additional lambs for sale or replacement. However, under the French system the homozygote carrier is undesirable, and comparatively complex breeding systems are required to use only the heterozygote.

Experiences in India to evolve a prolific strain through *FecB* (Booroola) introgression of Garole inheritance

At NARI, Phaltan: Nimbkar Agricultural Research Institute introduced the *FecB* mutation from the Garole sheep into the Deccani breed to increase lamb production and incomes of smallholder shepherds. Artificial insemination was used because the small size of Garole rams precluded natural mating. Two fecund strains were developed - the NARI Suwarna, with contributions from only Garole and Deccani breeds, and the NARI Composite, with additional contributions from Awassi and/or Bannur breeds. At NARI during 2002-2007, there were 808 non-carrier (++) ewes including 306 Deccani, 111 Bannur and 391 crossbred ewes (104 with only Deccani and Garole breed proportions and 287 Composite). There were 532 heterozygous (B+) ewes (200 fecund Deccani (NARI Suwarna) and 332 NARI Composite) and 47 homozygous (BB) ewes (9 NARI Suwarna and 38 NARI Composite). In smallholder flocks 2,465 and 325 lambing records were available from ++ and B+ ewes respectively. These records were of 959 ++ and 115 B+ ewes born in those flocks and 51 ++ ewes and 52 B+ ewes introduced by NARI from February 2004 to January 2008 (Nimbkar *et al.,* 2008). Study revealed that one copy of *FecB* led to an increase in live LS at birth from 1.0 to 1.6 in the NARI flock and from 1.0 to 1.4 in smallholder flocks. Less than 5% of the litters of B+ ewes were triplets. The increased LS was found to be manageable under the existing production system of smallholders by keeping young lambs behind in the pens when ewes went grazing, and by providing lambs with a small amount of supplementary feed. The LS at 3 months of B+ ewes was 1.3 and 1.2 in NARI and smallholder flocks, respectively, compared to 0.9 of ++ ewes. In a smallholder flock with 8, 41 and 50 B+ ewes in 2005 to 2008, respectively, the gross margin per B+ ewe over the 3-year period was found to be 37–50% higher than the gross margin per ++ ewe. It is likely that the significantly larger LS of B+ ewes in the NARI flock, compared to B+ ewes in smallholder flocks, was due to the 100 g/day supplementary feed given to all ewes at NARI for 2 months at breeding and to the better body condition of ewes owing to longer lambing intervals. It could be termed a *FecB* genotype by environment interaction because the supplementary feeding did not influence the LS of non-carrier ewes. In conclusion, the introduction of the *FecB* mutation in Deccani sheep proved to be successful in increasing both lamb production and incomes. NARI also began to disseminate *FecB*-carrier rams and ewes and surveyed 23 participating sheep owners. In general, the sheep owners' responses to twin lambs were positive. Twin lambs were viewed as more profitable than single lambs, with the main disadvantage cited as the need to undertake supplementary feeding and management to ensure adequate growth rates and survival of twin lambs (Prior *et al.*, 2008).

At CSWRI, Avikanagar: Keeping all the view in consideration, Central Sheep and Wool Research Institute, Avikanagar, also took the opportunity to conduct the research on prolificacy introgression from Garole sheep into native Malpura sheep. A cross breeding scheme was initiated in 1997 to introgress the *FecB* gene from India's most valuable germ plasm "Garole sheep" of a hot and humid environment into the non-prolific and large size mutton sheep breed "Malpura" best adapted of a semi-arid tropical environment to produce the Garole X Malpura (GM) crossbred carrying *FecB* gene. Encouraging results have been obtained in GM half-breds in terms of twinning percent and growth of quarterbreds (GMM; backcross of GM with Malpura; Arora *et al.* 2008). The viable benefits accrued by gene infusion are reflected by 45.7% increase in the prolificacy and 35.05% in weaning rate of GM compared to that of Malpura. A single mutated copy of *FecB* gene produced 0.70 and weaned 0.58 extra lambs in GM sheep (Mishra *et al.*, 2009). The improved *FecB* carriers (BB and B+) are proposed to be sold to the interested sheep farmers for making genetic improvement and increasing prolificacy in their flocks without compromising with the growth rate.

Having developed prolific GM half-bred sheep, there was scope to exploit the prolific GM sheep for relatively better growth by backcrossing with native Malpura. In the backcrossing programme the *FecB* gene carrier GM rams were used as sires and Malpura ewes as dam breed to produce the GM x Malpura (GM (M); 75% Malpura and 25% Garole) and reciprocal crosses were also attempted to produce M (GM). The 3/4th crosses so produced are able to produce twins and also have higher body weight compared to half-breds but problem of low milk yield from the dam persisted in the 3/4th crosses. In year 2009 Patanwadi sheep inheritance was introduced in the GM (M) to increase the milk yield of dams.

Crossbreeding for production of Garole x Malpura (GM)

Garole inheritance was introduced into native Malpura sheep in the year 1997-98, for enhancing prolificacy. From 1997, Malpura ewes were mated with Garole rams and this crossbreeding programme was continued in subsequent years (Sharma *et al.*, 2004; Mishra *et al.*, 2007a). GM ewes started giving birth to young ones since year 2000 onwards. At CSWRI, Avikanagar, Garole sheep was purchased from the native tract i.e. hot humid region of West Bengal in 1997. Malpura, native mutton type sheep breed usually gave single birth and it was used as dam breed whereas Garole was used as sire breed in developing GM half breds that was supposed to segregate *FecB* gene in crosses. The GM sheep included in the study was obtained by either crossing Malpura ewes with Garole rams or from interbreeding among GM half breds. Ewes were bred in two breeding season i.e. autumn (August-September) and spring (March-April). The contemporary Malpura lambs were produced through selective breeding within that breed (mating of selected males and females). Reproduction traits on GM ewes started to become available from the year 2000 onward. Initially all the sheep were raised under semi-intensive management system and provided similar grazing/feeding conditions. An extra allowance of concentrate @ 250g/ewe/day was provided under group feeding for three months every year i.e. from last month of pregnancy to completion of 2nd month of lactation over and above of 8-10 hrs grazing in the field interspersed with seasonal shrubs and forbs. The diet was supplemented with minerals and vitamins. The lambs were allowed to suck their dams from birth until weaning at 3 months of age. All the prophylactic measures against various sheep diseases were carried out as per prescribed health calendar of the Institute in addition to curative treatment of sick animals as and when required. The presence of *FecB* gene in GM sheep ($FecB^{BB}$, $FecB^{B+}$ or $FecB^{++}$) was determined using DNA typing. The DNA was isolated by standard proteinase K digestion followed by phenol–chloroform extraction and ethanol precipitation. The *FecB* mutation assay was carried out by the forced RFLP-PCR technique (Wilson *et al.*, 2001). The traits studied were litter size at birth, percentage of multiple births, body weights of the lambs at birth, 3, 6 and 12 months of age. The "Ewe Productivity Efficiency" (EPE) was calculated as sum of total lambs weight harvested at birth, weaning, 6 or 12 months of age/ number of ewes lambed.

Reproductive Performance: There was a tremendous increase in multiple births and in other reproductive efficiency traits in GM ewes compared to contemporary Malpura ewes. These results provided the first evidence for increased litter size in GM, with the possibility of further exploitation using appropriate breeding and selection strategies. The average litter size at birth was 1.56 with highest litter size of 1.68 was rerecorded in year 2008 and 2010 (Table 1). There was significant improvement in multiple births in GM crosses compared to Malpura. The GM ewes had 49% (1.56 vs 1.05) advantages over Malpura for litter size at birth. Average twinning and triplet in last 6 years was 40.09% and 9.80% respectively in GM. Sharma *et al.* (2004) reported prolificacy of GM as 1.19. Arora *et al.* (2009) reported that GM ewes had 45.7% (1.53 vs 1.05) advantages over Malpura ewes for litter size at birth. Mishra *et al.* (2007a) reported overall percent gain in prolificacy of GM as 52.38. Kumar *et al.* (2006) also reported that crossing of Garole with Malpura improves litter sizes in GM crosses. Above reviews are also the reports from the same flock maintained at CSWRI studied on earlier data set. Other studies (Nimbkar *et al.*, 1998; 2003b) have also shown Garole crosses to have high reproductive efficiency.

Table 1 : Type of birth and litter size at birth in Garole x Malpura (GM)

Year	Type of birth Single	Twin	Triplet/quad	Litter size (at birth)
2004	35.3	55.3	9.4	1.67
2005	57.8	34.9	7.3	1.50
2006	54.6	38.0	7.4	1.52
2007	58.1	37.6	4.3	1.41
2008	46.8	39.7	12.1/1.4	1.68
2009	59.8	35.0	5.1	1.48
2010	41.2	50.0	8.8	1.68

Growth performance: The growth performance of GM was studied in terms of body weights recorded at birth, 3, 6, and 12 months age and their least squares means are presented in table 2. Least-squares means for these body weights were 1.87, 10.13, 15.27 and 20.59 kg respectively. A little higher value for body weights were reported by Kumar *et al.* (2008) in GM crosses. Significant effect of year, sex and type of birth was found. The body weights of single born lambs were relatively higher than twins and triplets as expected. It was obvious that on crossing the small sized Garole rams with large sized Malpura ewes the half-bred progenies would weigh less than the dam parent and higher than the sire parent. The main purpose was to attain multiple births from the *FecB* introgressed GM sheep. Malpura lambs were always heavier than GM lambs at all stages of growth up to 1 year (Arora *et al.,* 1999, Mishra *et al.,* 2005). Two reasons contributed to these differences, (i) the fact that the cross contained genes from a significantly lighter breed and (ii) many of the crossbred lambs were born twins or triplets which are mostly lighter than single-born lambs.

Table 2 : Least squares means for body weight (kg) in Garole x Malpura (1998-2011)

Particulars	Birth weight	3-m weight	6-m weight	12-M WT
Over all mean	1.87±0.02(1578)	10.13±0.14 (1303)	15.27±0.20 (1137)	20.59±0.29 (791)
Year	**	**	**	**
1998	1.86±0.06 (46)	8.40±0.37 (42)	11.72±0.51 (43)	17.47±0.75 (27)
1999	1.86±0.06 (47)	9.50±0.36 (42)	14.71±0.50(41)	18.76±0.71 (28)
2000	1.65±0.07(37)	10.19±0.41(32)	15.27±0.57(32)	20.47±0.79(23)
2001	1.80±0.04(110)	9.00±0.26(99)	13.83±0.37 (96)	19.81±0.60 (48)
2002	1.85±0.04 (114)	9.53±0.26(101)	15.10±0.38 (87)	23.34±0.52 (69)
2003	1.82±0.04 (125)	10.44±0.23 (115)	15.83±0.32(114)	19.36±0.43 (99)
2004	1.85±0.03 (141)	9.41±0.22(121)	14.52±0.33(103)	19.40±0.48 (69)
2005	1.97±0.04 (99)	9.96±0.26 (77)	13.96±0.38 (67)	18.13±0.57 (42)
2006	1.90±0.04(104)	10.36±0.26 (84)	14.96±0.36(81)	20.06±0.48 (66)
2007	1.87±0.04(129)	11.25±0.25(96)	16.65±0.36(88)	20.15±0.52(58)
2008	1.90±0.03(158)	9.85±0.23(119)	13.68±0.32(117)	18.16±0.45 (85)
2009	1.91±0.03 (154)	10.46±0.22 (126)	17.18±0.31 (119)	26.72±0.47 (87)
2010-11	1.94±0.03 (314)	11.30±0.21 (249)	18.57±0.32 (149)	24.48±0.47(90)
Sex	**	**	**	**
Male	1.92±0.02 (796)	10.72±0.15(670)	16.53±0.22(574)	22.42±0.33(368)
Female	1.81±0.02 (782)	9.73±0.16(633)	14.03±0.22(563)	18.91±0.31(423)
Type of birth	**	**	**	**
Single	2.22±0.02 (707)	11.49±0.12 (620)	16.54±0.17 (556)	22.51±0.27 (385)
Twin	1.81±0.02(748)	9.83±0.14(593)	15.22±0.20 (499)	20.37±0.30 (329)
Triplet	1.58±0.05(123)	9.11±0.30 (90)	14.90±0.43 (82)	19.93±0.590 (57)
Reg. Ewe wt.	**	**	**	**

Survivability: Survivability is a very crucial factor in deciding the economic viability of any breed improvement programme. It is the indicator of adaptability of a genetic group under prevailing climatic and management conditions of a particular region. The survivability was lowest up to weaning in GM. The pre-weaning survivability ranged from 87.94 to 93.36%. Mishra *et al.* (2007b) reported pre-weaning survivability ranging from 93.58 to 94.59% in GM animals. Overall survivability of the GM over the years was greater than 89.90% (Table 3). The overall lambs' survivability of GM has almost similar survivability as observed in case of Malpura sheep (Sharma *et al.*, 2004). These results further indicated that the progenies of GM crossbred were inheriting traits of adaptation from Malpura sheep and the prolific genes from Garole.

Table 3 : survivability (%) in different age group in Garole x Malpura sheep

Year	Age Group 0-3 month	3-12 month	Adults	Overall
2003	93.36 (241)	95.90(122)	97.52(242)	95.54(605)
2004	88.00 (200)	89.21(139)	94.65(243)	91.07(582)
2005	92.07 (164)	87.50(88)	94.04(235)	92.20(487)
2006	87.94 (199)	87.61(113)	92.37 (262)	89.90 (574)
2007	88.98 (245)	83.33 (114)	93.54 (294)	90.06 (653)
2008	90.30 (268)	90.67 (150)	91.74 (327)	91.01(745)
2009	93.53 (378)	96.13(155)	93.62(329)	94.09 (762)
2010	92.56(309)	96.92(292)	97.71(350)	95.79 (951)

Wool yield: Basically this strain was developed with the aim to evolve mutton type sheep, wool production traits were also analysed during the study. The 1st 6 monthly greasy fleece weight (GFY) and adult annual fleece weight is presented in Table 4. The 1st 6 monthly GFY ranged from 0.29 to 0.38 kg over the years. Wool produced was generally a coarser type (even hairy type many times) may be suitable for Namda preparation by local artisans.

Ewe productivity efficiency: It was calculated as sum of total lambs weight harvested at birth, weaning, 6, 9 or 12 months of age/ number of ewes lambed. It shows the litter weight produced by the ewe at different stages of growth of its lambs. The twin and triplet bearing ewe has higher EPE leading to more profit per ewe reared. The EPE of GM was significantly affected by year of lambing and type of lamb produced by the ewe (Table 5). GM ewes bearing twins and triplets produced 34.61 and 37.47 kg of lamb weight at 12 month of age. Mishra *et al.* (2007b) reported that at yearling stage on an average GM ewes bearing twin and triplet lambs produces a total of 32.21 and 32.51 kg lambs weight. In accordance with these results, Nimbkar *et al.* (2003a) reported similar findings in Garole x Deccani and Bannur crosses. Other studies have found that Finn cross ewes weaned more total lamb weight (Thomas and Whiteman, 1979; Fogarty *et al.*, 1984; Iman and Slyter, 1996).

Table 4 : Least squares means for greasy fleece yield (kg) in Garole x Malpura sheep

Year	1st 6 monthly GFY	Adult annual GFY
2003	0.32±0.01 (101)	0.60±0.03 (74)
2004	0.31±0.02 (110)	0.46±0.02 (90)
2005	0.29±0.02 (151)	0.50±0.02 (119)
2006	0.33±0.02 (80)	0.46±0.02 (119)
2007	0.38±0.01 (85)	0.46±0.02 (146)
2008	0.29±0.12 (121)	0.41±0.02 (114)
2009	0.36±0.01 (107)	0.43±0.02 (108)
2010	037±0.01 (116)	0.45±0.02 (106)

Table 5 : Least squares means for EPE (kg) in Garole x Malpura sheep

Particulars	Birth	3-M	6-M	12-M
Over all mean	3.25±0.05 (681)	14.71±0.33 (603)	23.53±0.51 (587)	31.52±0.68 (557)
Type of birth	**	**	**	**
Single	2.05±0.04(380)	10.67±0.28 (323)	16.44±0.42 (311)	22.47±0.58 (294)
Twin	3.25±0.04 (272)	15.57±0.31 (251)	24.96±0.47 (248)	34.61±0.64 (236)
Triplet	4.46±0.12 (29)	17.88±0.79 (29)	29.20±1.21 (28)	37.47±1.16 (27)

Performance of backcrosses (GMM / MGM)

Having developed prolific GM half-bred sheep, there was scope to exploit the prolific GM sheep for relatively better growth by backcrossing with native Malpura. Backcrossing of GM with Malpura was employed to make gain in body weights and growth performances and at the same time maintaining the prolificacy level comparable to GM sheep. In the backcrossing programme the *FecB* gene carrier GM rams were used as sires and Malpura ewes as dam breed to produce the GM x Malpura (GM (M); 75% Malpura and 25% Garole) and reciprocal crosses were also attempted to produce M (GM) and their reproductive and productive performances were analyzed.

Reproductive performance: Percentage of multiple births ranged from 6.7 to 40.0 in GMM and from 14.3 to 27.3 in MGM (Table 6). The litter size at birth ranged from 1.07 to 1.42 in GMM and from 1.14 to 1.29 in MGM crosses. The incidence of multiple births is low compared to GM mainly due to lower *FecB* gene frequency in population and retention of more number of non-carrier females in flock. Once a sizeable population of GMM ewes are reached more rigorous selection for *FecB* gene will be carried out to further increase the prolificacy.

Table 6 : Type of birth and litter size at birth in GMM and MGM

Year of birth	Type of birth (%)				Litter size (at birth)	
	Single		Twin/Triplet			
	GMM	MGM	GMM	MGM	GMM	MGM
2007	93.3	85.7	6.7	14.3	1.07	1.14
2008	60.0	72.7	40.0	27.3	1.40	1.27
2009	71.11	73.17	28.89	24.39/2.44	1.29	1.29
2010	61.45	-	38.55	-	1.42	-

Survivability: The survivability of the back crosses (GMM/ MGM) is better than the GM and at par with the native Malpura sheep. The survivability for all age group over the year was greater than 92% in GMM animals. The overall survivability has been greater than 95% in GMM over the years (Table 7). The higher survivability indicates better adaptability of GMM under prevailing climatic and managemental conditions.

Table 7 : Survivability (%) in different age group in GMM and MGM

Year	GMM			
	0-3 month	3-12 month	Adults	Overall
2005	95.45 (88)	94.44 (36)	100.00 (26)	99.6 (150)
2006	98.10 (103)	92.16 (51)	95.89 (73)	96.07 (229)
2007	95.63 (160)	95.38 (65)	97.35 (113)	96.15 (338)
2008	98.62 (145)	96.19 (105)	94.05 (185)	95.86 (435)
2009	96.60 (206)	94.12 (102)	95.74 (235)	95.76 (543)
2010	94.00 (293)	97.54 (284)	95.58 (317)	95.45 (770)

MGM				
2005	90.00 (130)	92.31 (52)	100.00 (33)	92.09 (215)
2006	85.04 (127)	91.94 (62)	95.45 (88)	89.89 (277)
2007	91.72 (157)	93.33 (45)	94.39 (107)	92.88 (309)
2008	97.90 (143)	92.31 (104)	95.71 (163)	95.61 (410)
2009	97.12 (104)	98.11 (53)	94.92 (177)	96.11 (334)

Growth performance: The growth performance was studied in terms of body weights recorded at birth, 3, 6, 12 months age (Table 8 and 9). Least-squares means for these body weights were 2.54, 13.68, 20.00 and 26.15 and 2.13, 12.16, 16.59 and 21.10 kg, respectively in GMM and MGM crosses. Arora *et al.* (2009) reported average body weight at birth, weaning and six months as 2.85, 13.7 and 19.6 and 2.14 11.0 and 17.1 kg, respectively of GMM and MGM crosses with 49.2, 35.3 and 27.9% increases in body weight of GMM lambs over GM half-bred at birth, weaning and 6-month of age, respectively. Significant effect of year, sex and type of birth was found. The results indicate that there is pronounced higher gain in the body weight and growth rate of lambs produced after backcrossing of GM rams with Malpura ewes. This also reflects the major role of large uterine capacity of Malpura ewes in producing heavier GMM lambs compared to lighter MGM lambs borne by GM ewes. At present backcrossing is in progress to produce only GMM and production of MGM is stopped.

Table 8 : Least squares means for body weight (kg) in GMM sheep

Particulars	Birth	3-M	6-M	12-M
Over all mean	2.54±0.60 (657)	13.68±0.26 (584)	20.00±0.39 (438)	26.15±1.34 (367)
Year	**		**	**
2005	2.76±0.09 (33)	13.73±0.43 (33)	19.44±0.59 (31)	24.48±1.38 (24)
2006	2.56 ±0.09 (47)	13.57 ±0.41 (47)	19.91±0.55 (46)	24.45±1 47 (43)
2007	2.39 ±0.08(65)	14.26 ±0.34(65)	21.59±0.46(64)	24.77±1.49(42)
2008	2.47±0.08 (84)	13.31±0.34(84)	19.03±0.47 (73)	24.19±1.41 (71)
2009	2.46±0.07 (90)	13.57±0.32 (90)	21.03±0.44 (81)	32.23±1.42 (73)
2010-11	2.54±0.03(338)	13.65±0.18 (265)	19.60 ±0.21 (143)	26.39 ±0.28(114)
Sex	**	**	**	**
Male	2.59±0.07 (327)	14.05±0.29 (290)	20.81±0.41(217)	27.84±1.38(180)
Female	2.46 ±0.06 (330)	13.31±0.29 (294)	19.19 ±0.40 (221)	24.34±1.34 (187)
Type of birth	**	**	**	**
Single	2.86±0.05 (494)	14.65±0.26 (437)	21.02±0.37 (334)	27.19±1.33 (282)
Twin	2.19±0.08 (163)	12.63±0.35 (147)	18.61±0.50 (104)	24.92±1.44 (85)
Reg. Ewe wt.	**	**	**	**

Table 9 : Least squares means for body weight (kg) in MGM sheep

Particulars	Birth	3-M	6-M	12-M
Over all mean	2.13±0.05 (370)	12.16±0.37 (293)	16.59±0.40 (273)	21.10±1.20 (217)
Year	**	**	**	**
2005	2.37±0.07 (62)	12.65±0.47 (50)	16.04±0.53 (47)	19.86±1.31 (32)
2006	2.25 ±0.07 (76)	12.19 ±0.46 (60)	17.27±0.51(58)	20.34±1.26 (52)
2007	2.03 ±0.07(63)	13.07 ±0.49(44)	17.86±0.56(40)	20.35±1.38(26)
2008	2.08±0.06(115)	11.66±0.44(91)	14.85±0.46 (87)	19.16±1.19 (72)
2009	1.92±0.07 (54)	11.24±0.40 (48)	16.92±0.48 (41)	25.80±1.32 (35)
Sex	**	**	**	**
Male	2.18±0.06 (202)	12.60±0.38(161)	17.76±0.42(147)	22.74±1.22(114)
Female	2.08 ±0.06 (168)	11.73±0.39 (132)	15.43±0.43 (126)	19.46±1.22(103)
Type of birth	**	**	**	**
Single	2.70±0.06 (148)	14.12±0.40 (128)	18.46±0.44 (121)	22.59±1.19 (102)
Twin	2.03±0.06 (174)	12.01±0.39 (131)	16.22±0.42 (121)	20.86±1.22 (93)
Triplet	1.66±0.78 (48)	10.36±0.48 (34)	15.08±0.57 (31)	19.85±1.40 (22)
Reg. Ewe wt.	**	**	**	**

Greasy fleece yield: The GMM animals had comparatively higher yield compared to MGM animals (Table 10). First 6 monthly GFY ranged from 0.43 to 0.59 kg in GMM sheep. The yields were relatively lower than Malpura animals.

Table 10 : Least squares means for first 6 monthly GFY (kg) in GMM and MGM sheep

Year	GMM	MGM
2005	0.50±0.03 (31)	0.37±0.02 (47)
2006	0.51±0.03 (50)	0..47±0.03 (60)
2007	0.59±0.02 (54)	0.48±0.03 (41)
2008	0.44±0.02 (91)	0.33±0.01 (78)
2009	0.59±0.022 (76)	0.50±0.01 (34)
2010	043±0.012 (143)	0.39±0.02 (57)

Wool quality: The wool quality analysis indicated coarser nature of the wool of the GM, GMM and MGM animals (Table 11).

Table 11 : Wool quality attributes of GM, GMM and MGM sheep

Genetic group	Diameter (μ)	Medullation (%)	Staple length (cm)
GM	51.68±4.07 (14)	88.17±2.22 (14)	5.05±0.44 (14)
GM(M)	48.27±2.23 (16)	80.34±4.03 (16)	4.23±0.29 (16)
M(GM)	49.10±2.22 (14)	84.85±3.56 (14)	3.85±0.44 (14)

Ewe's productivity efficiency: The EPE in terms of total litter weight harvested at birth, weaning, 6, 9 and 12 month of age in GMM and MGM ewes bearing single, twin, lambs are given in table 12.The EPE of GMM is comparatively better than MGM at all stages of growth except at weaning.

Table 12 : Least squares means for EPE (kg) in GMM and MGM sheep

Particulars	Birth	3-M	6-M	12-M
		GMM		
Overall mean	2.92±0.10 (100)	15.48±0.80 (93)	23.19±0.80 (92)	32.78±1.14 (85)
Type of birth	**	**	**	**
Single	2.36±0.10 (72)	12.21±0.55 (68)	18.08±0.76 (67)	25.52±1.07 (62)
Twin	3.48±0.17 (28)	18.75±0.96 (25)	28.30±1.31 (25)	40.04±1.84 (23)
		MGM		
Overall mean	3.07±0.10 (89)	17.17±1.19 (77)	22.08±0.79 (73)	30.85±1.22 (68)
Type of birth	**	**	**	**
Single	2.30±0.09 (70)	13.29±1.14 (60)	17.38±0.77 (56)	24.11±1.14 (54)
Twin	3.83±0.17 (19)	23.82±1.92(17)	26.79±1.28 (17)	37.58±2.03 (14)

Comparative performance of different prolific genotype with Malpura

Farmers' in the target area are rearing Malpura sheep in the field. Hence, comparison has been made between the EPE of Malpura and different prolific crosses (GM, GMM and MGM). Malpura ewes usually give single birth and EPE was analysed from contemporary data set taken from project "Genetic Improvement of Malpura Sheep for Mutton Production" at CSWRI, Avikanagar. The first lamb crop from MGM and GMM ewes came in 2007; accordingly data from 2007 onward has been compared (Table 13). The EPE at birth was highest in Malpura. From the weaning onward the EPE of GMM animals are higher than Malpura, mainly due to comparable growth with Malpura and high prolificacy. When comparison was made according to EPE recorded for twin born GMM versus overall Malpura, there was 29.39, 27.59 and 31.0% improvement in GMM over Malpura at weaning, 6 and 12 month weight, respectively. The GMM animals also scored over GM and MGM animals especially at market age of 6 and 12 month in terms of EPE. This is mainly attributed to comparatively higher body weight and better survivability leading to higher litter size at various stages of growth. As of now incidence of multiple births is low in

GMM compared to GM, mainly due to lower *FecB* gene frequency in population, retention of more number of non-carrier females in flock and parity of the females present in the flock.

Table 13 : Comparative EPE for Malpura, GM, MGM and GMM sheep

Particulars	MALPURA	GM	MGM	GMM
		At birth		
Overall	3.13±0.04(741)	2.79±0.04(300)	3.07±0.10 (89)	2.92±0.10 (100)
Type of birth	**	**	**	**
Single	3.09±0.04(713)	2.11±0.05(179)	2.30±0.09 (70)	2.36±0.10 (72)
Twin	4.32±0.22(29)	3.34±0.06 (109)	3.83±0.17 (19)	3.48±0.17 (28)
Triplet		4.67±0.19 (12)	-	-
		At weaning		
Overall	14.49±0.13(643)	13.41±0.27(263)	17.17±1.19 (77)	15.48±0.80 (93)
Type of birth	**	**	**	**
Single	14.26±1.14 (617)	10.56±0.34 (153)	13.29±1.14 (60)	12.21±0.55 (68)
Twin	20.09±1.92(26)	15.86±0.43 (98)	23.82±1.92(17)	18.75±0.96 (25)
Triplet		19.69±1.25(12)		
		At 6 Month		
Overall	22.18±0.19(589)	21.45±0.40(258)	22.08±0.79 (73)	23.19±0.80 (92)
Type of birth	**	**	**	**
Single	21.71±0.17(563)	16.63±0.51(148)	17.38±0.77 (56)	18.08±0.76 (67)
Twin	32.38±0.82 (26)	25.64±0.631 (98)	26.79±1.28 (17)	28.30±1.31 (25)
Triplet		31.77±1.83 (12)		
		At 12 Month		
Overall	30.56±0. 34(384)	29.36±0.55(238)	30.85±1.22 (68)	32.78±1.14 (85)
Type of birth	**	**	**	**
Single	30.12±0.17(364)	22.63±0.70(138)	24.11±1.14 (54)	25.52±1.07 (62)
Twin	39.23±1.42 (20)	35.04±0.88 (89)	37.58±2.03 (14)	40.04±1.84 (23)
Triplet		44.78±1.83 (11)		

Once a sizeable population of GMM ewes are reached more rigorous selection for FecB gene will be carried which will further increase the prolificacy. The combined effect of increased prolificacy and higher body weight of GMM will lead to more EPE in future. The higher ewe productivity will ensures more return from rearing small number of animals. This will also help in overcoming challenges being faced by livestock holders due to frequent drought, reducing feed and fodder resources and shrinking grazing land. The difference in weight between single, twin and triplet lambs support the greater profitability of an ewe bearing and rearing twins and triplets over one bearing and rearing single lamb. The GM, MGM and GMM twins and triplets produced more litter weight from birth to 12 month of age over Malpura which mostly produces single lamb.

Introduction of Patanwadi inheritance for further improving the performance of prolific sheep

Problem of low milk yield from the dam is still persisting in the 3/4th crosses (GMM/MGM), which is one of the major factor for lamb mortality, and if this problem is overcome by any intervention then EPE of prolific sheep can be further improved compared to present level. Hence, Patanwadi inheritance is proposed to be introduced in the GMM to increase the milk yield of dam. In this process, GMM and Patanwadi (P) were crossed to produce 3 breed crosses which will result in higher prolificacy, higher birth weight along with more milk yield of dam to feed larger lamb crop per ewe. The breeding on the above proposed line has been started and initial findings are quite encouraging and results and comparison of different genotypes have been shown in Table 14 and 15. However the data size is very low to reach at any decision but these initial results have given a clear cut indication of scope of improvement in all production and reproduction traits. This intervention will meet the demand of farmers for more body weight and more number of lambs per lambing, resulting in higher economic returns. Screening and retention of carrier lambs and Inter-se mating and selection in different genetic groups will be followed to maintain the prolificacy as well as other desired traits. The new genotypes with traits of high prolificacy, more body weight and more milk per dam will be evaluated at the farm and field level. The improved and proven technology will be delivered at the farmers' door step to enhance his economic returns per unit of sheep for livelihood security.

Table 14 : Comparison of growth performance in different genotypes w.r.t. triple cross

Genetic group	Birth weight	3-M weight	6-M weight	12-M weight
Malpura	3.08±0.02 (520)	15.58±0.17 (369)	25.74±0.24 (237)	31.90±0.31 (181)
GMM	2.54±0.03(338)	13.65±0.18 (265)	19.60 ±0.21 (143)	26.39 ±0.28(114)
GMM x P	3.51±0.08 (57)	20.87±0.55 (44)	31.82±0.93(29)	39.35±1.24(19)
P x GMM	2.68±0.08 (75)	14.83±0.34 (55)	20.42±0.67(23)	29.14±0.89(20)

Table 15 : Comparison of wool traits and survivability in different genotypes w.r.t. triple cross

Genetic group	First 6 monthly GFY (kg)	Pre weaning Survivability (%)	Overall survivability (%)
Malpura	0.619±0.013 (223)	95.01	96.23
GM XM	0.430±0.01 (143)	94.00	95.45
GMM X P	0.737±0.05 (30)	98.25	99.31
P X GMM	0.500±0.03 (20)	94.29	97.33

Conclusion

Almost more than 200 years has been passed with utilization of prolific Booroola gene for increased in ovulation rate thus litter size. Being a major gene and having direct correlation with high fecundity, it became one of the widely studied gene in the World. Most of the developed countries showed initial enthusiasm and expectation of practical application through introgression of *FecB* gene in local breeds. But later on due to low uptake from Industry they showed little opportunity for future use of $FecB^{B}$ in commercial sheep production. This outcome mainly reflects the relatively high prolificacy levels already present in several sheep breeds and the desire of most commercial producers to avoid high frequencies of triplet births. However, if the mean litter size of local breeds is below 1.3 lambs/ litter, use of *FecB* has the potential to rapidly increase the frequency of twinning with only modest increases in numbers of triplet births.

In India and other developing countries where *FecB* appeared a fixed trait in the breed like Garole, Javenese sheep etc and were used in crossbreeding program to improve prolificacy of local sheep flocks in semi intensive conditions, results were very encouraging. Crossbred ewes carrying the *FecB* mutation had increased prolificacy, but increases in ovulation rate and litter size were generally lower than reported elsewhere. The increases appeared manageable under traditional management practices and of economic benefit to smallholder sheep owners. NARI, Phaltan reported successful introgression of *FecB* into non-fecund Deccani sheep in India using genotype-assisted selection. This has not resulted in the unmanageable litter size experienced in other countries and is associated with positive effects on biological and economic efficiency. Similarly CSWRI, Avikanagar reported quite enthusiastic results with the crossing and back crossing of Malpura with Garole. The encouraging trend in production and reproduction performance achieved after backcrossing GM with Malpura sheep indicating scope for further boost in lamb production and to make it more remunerative to the farmers. Initial results with respect to production status and survivability improvement in 3- breed cross (Garole, Malpura and Patanwadi) has paved a new way to further enhance the lamb production and high litter survival up to market age will ultimately lead to socio-economic upliftment of farmers.

References

Abdulkhaliq, A.M., Harwey, W.R. and Parker. C.F. 1989. Genetic parameters for ewe productivity traits in the Columbia, Sufolk and Targhee breeds. Journal Animal Sciences 67: 3250-3257.

Arora, A.L., Sharma, R.C., Narula, H.K. and Kumar Ravindra. 1999. Comparative performance of Avikalin and Malpura sheep. Indian Journal of Small Ruminants 5: 4-8.

Arora, A.L., Mishra, A.K., Prince, L.L.L. and Gowane, G.R. 2008. Back crossing of prolific Garole x Malpura half-breds with Malpura to improve growth and greasy fleece yield production. In: IX Annual Conference of Indian Society of Animal Genetics and Breeding and National Symposium on Livestock Genomics in Productivity Enhancement for Food Security, NASC, New Delhi, 3-4 July, p 55.

Arora, A.L., Mishra, A.K. and Prince, L.L.L. 2009. Consequences of introgression of FecB gene in to Malpura Sheep in Rajasthan. In: Use of the FecB (Boroola) gene in sheep breeding programs (S. Walkden-Brown, J.H.J. vanerWerf, C. Nimbkar and V.S. Gupta, Eds.), ACIAR Proceedings No.133, Australian Centre for International Agricultural Research. Canberra, pp 111-118.

Brown, S.W., Wofenden, D.H. and Piper, L.R. 2008. Biological and economic consequences of introgression of the FecB mutation into Merino sheep in Australia. In: Using the FecB (Booroola) gene in sheep breeding programs: Proceedings of International Booroola Workshop, NARI, Phaltan, 10-12 November, pp 88-98.

Crooks A.E., Thomas D.L., Zelinsky R.D., Gottfredson R.G. and McKusick B.C. 1999. Introgression of the FecB allele of the Booroola Merino into a Rambouillet flock- a progress report. In: 'Proc. 47th Annual Spooner Sheep Day', University of Wisconsin, Madison, pp 61-62.

Crooks A.E., Thomas D.L., Zelinsky R.D., Gottfredson R.G. and McKusick, B.C. 2000. Effect of the FecB allele of the Booroola Merino on weight of lamb marketed per ewe when introgressed into a Rambouillet flock. In: Proc. 48th Annual Spooner Sheep Day, University of Wisconsin, Madison, pp 7–9.

Davis, G.H., Montgomery, G.W., Allison, A.J., Kelly, R.W. and Bray, A.R. 1982. Segregation of a major gene influencing fecundity in progeny of Booroola sheep. New Zealand Journal of Agricultural Research 25: 525–529.

Davis, G.H., Galloway, S.M., Ross, I.K., Gregan, S.M., Ward, J., Nimbkar, B.V., Ghalsasi, P.M., Nimbkar, C., Gray, G.D., Subandriyo Inounu I., Tiesnamurti, B., Martyniuk, E., Eythorsdottir, E., Mulsant, P., Lecerf, F., Hanrahan, J.P., Bradford, G.E. and Wilson, T. 2002. DNA tests in prolific sheep from eight countries provide new evidence on origin of the Booroola (*FecB*) mutation. Biology of Reproduction 66: 1869-1874.

Dickerson, G.E. 1978. Animal size and efficiency: Basic concepts. Animal Production 27: 367-379.

Fogarty, N.M., Dickerson, G.E. and Young, L.B. 1984. Lamb production and its components in purebreds and composite lines II. Breed effects and heterosis. Journal of Animal Science 58: 301-311.

Gootwine, E. 2008. Biological and economic consequences of introgressing the B allele of the FecB (Booroola gene) into Awassi and Assaf sheep. In: Using the FecB (Booroola) gene in sheep breeding programs: Proceedings of International Booroola Workshop, NARI, Phaltan, 10-12 November, pp 107-117.

Iman, N.Y. and Slyter, A.L. 1996. Lifetime and wool production of Targhee or Finn-Dorset-Targhee ewes managed as farm or range flock 1. Average annual ewe performance. Journal of Animal Sciences 74: 1757-1765.

Inounu, I. and Priyanti, A. 2008. Biological and economic consequences of the *FecB* mutation in Indonesian thin tailed sheep. In: Using the FecB (Booroola) gene in sheep breeding programs: Proceedings of International Booroola Workshop, NARI, Phaltan, 10-12 November, pp 126-132.

Kumar, S., Kolte, A.P., Mishra, A.K., Arora, A.L. and Singh, V.K. 2006. Identification of *FecB* mutation in Garole x Malpura sheep and its effect on litter size. Small Ruminant Research 64: 305-310.

Kumar, S., Mishra, A.K., Kolte, A.P., Arora, A.L., Singh, D. and Singh, V.K. 2008. Effect of the Booroola (Fec B) genotypes on growth performance, ewe's productivity efficiency and litter size in Garole x Malpura sheep. Animal Reproduction Science 105: 319:331.

Mishra, A.K. 2008. Significance of prolificacy trait in intensive mutton production., In: Small Ruminant production in India: Strategies for enhancing. (S.A. Karim, M.K. Tripathi, O.H. Chaturvedi and A.K. Shinde, Eds.); Satish Serial Publishing House, New Delhi, pp 267-280.

Mishra, A.K., Arora, A.L., Kumar Sushil, Sharma, R.C. and Singh, V.K. 2005. Malpura: A Mutton type sheep breed. Research Bulletin, CSWRI, Avikanagar.

Mishra, A.K., Arora, A.L., Kumar, S. and Singh, V.K. 2007a. Improving productivity of Malpura breed by crossbreeding with prolific Garole sheep in India. Small Ruminant Research 70: 159-164.

Mishra, A.K., Arora, A.L. Kumar Sushil, Gupta, D.C. and Singh, V.K. 2007b. Ewe productivity efficiency of single and multiple bearing lambs of Garole, Malpura and their crossbred ewes. Indian Journal of Animal Sciences 77: 767-772.

Mishra, A.K., Arora, A.L. and Kumar Satish. 2009. Increasing prolificacy and ewe efficiency in sheep through FecB gene introgression. Current Science 97: 925-930.

Nimbkar, C., Ghalsasi, P.M., Ghatge, R.R. and Gray, G.D. 1998. Establishment of prolific Garole sheep from West Bengal in the semi-arid Deccan plateau of Maharastra. In: Proc. 6th World Congress on Genetics Applied to Livestock Production, Armidale, pp 257-260.

Nimbkar, C., Ghalsasi, P.M., Swan, A., Walkkden-Brown, S.W. and Kahn, L.P. 2003a. Evaluation of growth rates and worm resistance of Deccani and Bannur lambs and their crosses with Garole. Animal Science 76: 503-515.

Nimbkar, C., Ghalsasi P.M., Maddox, J.F., Pardeshi, V.C., Sainani, M.N., Gupta, V. and Walkden-Brown, S.W. 2003b. Expression of FecB gene in Garole and Crossbred ewes in Maharastra, India. In: Proc. Fifteenth conference of AAABG, Melbourne, Australia, pp111-114.

Nimbkar, C., Ghalsasi, P.M, Nimbkar, B.V., Ghalsasi, P.P., Gupta, V.S., Pardeshi, V.C., Maddox, J.F., van der Werf, J.H.J., Gray, G.D. and Brown, S.W. 2008. Biological and economic consequences of introgression of the *FecB* (Booroola) gene into Deccani sheep. In: Using the FecB (Booroola) gene in sheep breeding programs: Proceedings of International Booroola Workshop, NARI, Phaltan, 10-12 November, pp 75-87.

Notter, D.R., Thomas, D.L. and Waldron, D.F. 2008. Biological and economic consequences of the *FecB* mutation in the USA. In: Using the FecB (Booroola) gene in sheep breeding programs: Proceedings of International Booroola Workshop, NARI, Phaltan, 10-12 November, pp 118-125.

Piper, L.R. and Bindon, B.M. 1996. The Booroola Merino. In: Prolific sheep (M.H. Fahmy, Ed) CAB International, Wallingford, U.K.

Prior, J., Ghalsasi, P.M., Brown, S.W., Chavan, K.M., Kulkarni, S.R. and Nimbkar, C. 2008. Shepherd's views on the value and management of Deccani crossbred FecB carrier ewes with a higher twinning percentage: implications for a future introgression extension program. In: Using the FecB (Booroola) gene in sheep breeding programs: Proceedings of International Booroola Workshop, NARI, Phaltan, 10-12 November, pp 175-191.

Sharma, R.C., Arora, A.L., Mishra, A. K., Kumar, S. and Singh, V. K. 2004. Breeding prolific Garole with Malpura sheep for increased reproductive efficiency in semi-arid tropics of India. Asian- Australasian Journal of Animal Science 17: 737-742.

Southey B.R., Thomas D.L., Gottfredson R.G. and Zelinsky R.D. 2002. Ewe productivity of Booroola Merino–Rambouillet crossbred sheep during early stages of the introgression of the FecB allele into a Rambouillet population. Livestock Production Science 75: 33-44.

Teyssier, J., Bodin, L., Maton, C., Bouquet, P.M. and Elsen, J.M. 2008. Biological and economic consequences of the *FecB* gene into the French Merinos d'Arles sheep. In: Using the FecB (Booroola) gene in sheep breeding programs: Proceedings of International Booroola Workshop, NARI, Phaltan, 10-12 November, pp 143-149.

Thomas, D.L. and Whiteman, J.V. 1979. Effects of substituting Finnsheep and Dorset breeding for Rambouillet breeding I. Productivity of young, spring-lambing ewes. Journal of Animal Sciences 48: 256-264.

Turner, H.N. 1969. Genetic improvement of reproduction in sheep. Animal Breeding Abstract 37: 545.

Turner, H.N. 1982. Origins of the CSIRO Booroola. In: The Booroola Merino: Proc. A Workshop (L.R. Piper, B.M. Bindon and R.D. Nethery, Eds.), 24–25 August, Armidale, New South Wales, CSIRO, Melbourne, Australia, pp 1-7.

Wilson, T., Wu, X.Y., Juengel, J.L., Ross, I.K., Lumsden, J.M., Lord, E.A., Dodds, K.G., Walling, G.A., McEvan, J.C., O'Connel, A.R., McNatty, K.P. and Montgomery, G.W., 2001. Highly prolific Booroola sheep have a mutation in the intracellular kinase domain of bone morphogenetic protein IB receptor (ALK-6) that is expressed in both oocytes and granulosa cells. Biology of Reproduction 64: 1225-1235.

□□□

Chapter 5

Genomic Selection in Small Ruminants : Global Status, Challenges and Opportunities

S.P. Dixit* and Dinesh Kumar

• Principal Scientist & I/C, DNA Fingerprinting Unit, National Bureau of Animal Genetic Resources, GT Road By-Pass, Karnal-132001 (Haryana)

Traditional genetic improvement of livestock, using information on phenotypes and pedigrees to predict the breeding values has been very successful. However, breeding values should be predicted more accurately by using information on variation in DNA sequence between animals. Marker assisted selection is mainly important in situations, when the accuracy of classical selection is low especially with low heritability, limited, late-in-life, or after slaughter recording of traits. This can be overcome by approach of genome wide association selection (GWAS). The paper describes the latest status of DNA chip for selection of sheep based on 59,494 SNPs which has been made by allele mining from 71 sheep breeds of the world. The reported 639 QTL of sheep has been presented with figures of trait and trait class wise. In case of goat DNA chip which is based on just seven breeds with limited four country consortium, much information are not available in public domain. The challenges being faced by India is double sworded, the "phenotype gap" owing to limited phenome data generation besides lack of integrated DNA bank for almost all domestic animal species. Indian sheep and goat breeds reflect huge genome diversity having very valuable genotype well selected due to tropical climate and limited veterinary coverage. The genes/genotypes are "genomic gold" very precious and relevant due to climate change and also under new global intellectual property regime. Authors have described the steps needed to reap the benefit of genomics both at planning and implementation level which has been hitherto almost missing in Indian scenario. This approach is badly warranted in long run for the enhancement of sheep and goat productivity of the country and also a rare opportunity to have high dividend of sheep and goat high density chip across the world, at least as goat SNP chip leader.

What is genomic selection?

Genomic selection refers to selection decisions based on genomic breeding values (GEBV). The GEBV are calculated as the sum of the effects of dense genetic markers, or haplotypes of these markers, across the entire genome, thereby potentially capturing all the quantitative trait loci (QTL) that contribute to variation in a trait. The QTL effects, inferred from either haplotypes or individual single nucleotide polymorphism markers, are first estimated in a large reference population with phenotypic information. In subsequent generations, only marker information is required to calculate GEBV.

How genomic selection is different from marker aided selection / gene assisted selection?

Genomic selection (GS) is a form of marker assisted selection in which genetic markers covering the whole genome are used so that all QTL are in linkage disequilibrium with at least one marker. This approach has become feasible due to revolution in SNP discovery method like deep sequencing and throughput SNP genotyping on DNA chip.

Marker assisted selection or marker aided selection (MAS) is a process whereby a marker (morphological, biochemical or one based on DNA/RNA variation) is used for indirect selection of a genetic determinant or determinants of a trait of interest (i.e. productivity, disease resistance, abiotic stress tolerance, and/or quality). This process is used in plant and animal breeding. When the gene sequence itself becomes an identifiable marker it's called GAS (Gene Assisted Selection). Considerable developments in biotechnology have led animal breeders to develop more efficient selection systems to replace traditional phenotypic-pedigree-based selection systems. MAS is indirect selection process where a trait of interest is selected, not based on the trait itself, but on a marker linked to it. For example if MAS is being used to select individuals with a disease, the level of disease is not quantified but rather a marker allele which is linked with disease is used to determine disease presence. The assumption is that linked allele associates with the gene and/or QTL of interest. MAS can be useful for traits that are difficult to measure, exhibit low heritability and/or are expressed late in development.

Problems associated with QTL/MAS?

There are three types of markers used in MAS viz genes, linkage equilibrium (LE), which are located very close to the gene and linkage disequilibrium (LD), which are located farther from the gene. LD markers are easiest to find but hard to use. In selection, LE markers are markedly inferior to genes. There were no markers for low heritability traits as these require a large amount of data for estimation. Finally, benefits from commercial applications were hard to assess (Misztal, 2006).

Advantages of genomic selection

Genomic selection may result in higher rates of genetic gain over traditional selection because genomic EBVs have higher reliabilities than BLUP EBVs, especially for young animals, and secondly because young animals with high genomic EBVs become attractive to be selected as parents, which reduces the generation interval (Meuwissen *et al.*, 2001). The advantages of genomic selection may be highest for dairy cattle breeding programs because the generation interval in traditional progeny testing schemes is large and selection of young bulls for progeny testing is inaccurate (Schaeffer, 2006). Furthermore, thousands of bulls that have been progeny tested in the last decades are available as a reference population with very reliable phenotypes, leading to genomic EBVs with high reliabilities (VanRaden *et al.*, 2009). For these reasons, the uptake of genomic selection in animal breeding in recent years has been very high. Genomic selection may decrease the rate of inbreeding because Mendelian sampling effects can be estimated more accurately, which reduces the co-selection of relatives (Daetwyler *et al.*, 2007). Genomic selection in combination with a reduced generation interval may double the rate of genetic gain while keeping the rate of inbreeding per generation constant. Young bulls will be superior to proven bulls, and the number of progeny test bulls can be greatly reduced drastically reducing the cost of a progeny testing programme.

Status of QTL discovery in sheep

To date, there are 639 sheep QTLs in the database (animalgenome.org, release Sep 2011) from 74 publications representing 184 different sheep traits (Table 1-3).

Table 1 : Trait class of sheep and number of QTL reported

S.No.	Trait Class	Number of QTL reported
1	Exterior	21
2	Health	98
3	Meat	216
4	Milk	143
5	Production	119
6	Reproduction	19
7	Wool	23

Table 2 : Top 20 traits of sheep with number of QTL reported

S.No.	Top 20 traits	No. of QTL
1	*Haemonchus contortus* (FEC2)	18
2	Bone density	14
3	Average daily gain (birth-43 weeks)	9
4	Milk yield	14
5	Milk fat percentage	14
6	Lean meat yield Percentage	13
7	*Haemonchus contortus* (FEC1)	13
8	Ultrasound fat depth	13
9	Muscle depth at 3rd lumbar	11
10	Average daily gain (56-83 weeks)	10
11	Carcass fat percentage	10
12	Hot carcass weight	9
13	Body weight (slaughter)	9
14	Longissimus muscle area	9
15	Milk conjugated linoleic acid content	9
16	Scrapie susceptibility	9
17	Milk lactose yield	8
18	Total lambs born	8
19	Hind leg length	8
20	Muscle depth at 3rd lumbar corrected for live weight	8

Table 3 : Total QTL type and QTL discovered in Sheep

SN	QTL type by sheep traits	No. QTL
1	Blood chemistry	1
2	Carcass	158
3	Coat colour	5
4	Conformation	8
5	Congenital defects	2
6	Disease resistance	22
7	Fat	33
8	Fertility	11
9	Fibre	6
10	Fleece	17
11	Growth	119
12	Horns	3
13	Immune capacity	6
14	Mastitis	6
15	Meat composition	12
16	Meat texture	5
17	Meat color	6
18	Milk composition - other	11
19	Milk fat	92
20	Milk protein	17
21	Milk yield	23
22	Parasite resistance	61
23	Reproductive organ	8
24	Sensory panel	2
25	Udder	5

Status of QTL discovery in goat

There is no specific data base with updates of QTL discovered in goat. Limited information is available as shown in table 4.

Global status of genomic selection in sheep

IGSC is an international group of institutes and companies funded by AgResearch of New Zealand, Australia, UK, and US Department of Agriculture and aimed at developing tools to explore the sheep genome. A 1.5K Illumina SNP array was constructed and used to genotype sheep from 23 domestic breeds and two wild sheep species, as well as the International Mapping Flock (IMF). The first commercially available SNP chip for sheep is for only three breeds. Pfizer Animal Genetics, in collaboration with Ovita, have developed the Sheep 50k (S50K) panel marker test which builds a genetic profile early in an animal's life. It is the first SNP chip panel in the world to be commercialised for sheep. The S50k marker panel was validated in NZ and is suitable only for Romney, Coopworth or Perendale breeds. The test represents a DNA panel marker of more than 50,000 single nucleotide polymorphisms (SNP) which have been identified in the ovine genome. From the 50,000SNP spaced evenly across the entire genome, the test can predict breeding values for economically important traits.

Table 4 : Goat genomic resources database

Database	Name	URL
Goat and sheep database	GoSh dB	http://www.itb.cnr.it/gosh/
Goat map database	GoatMap V 2.0	http://locus.jouy.inra.fr/cgi-bin/lgbc/mapping/common/intro2.pl?BASE=goat
QTLdB	Angora QTL dB	http://www.ajol.info/index.php/sajas/article/viewFile/3967/11914

The four economic traits are expressed as molecular breeding values (MBV). They carry a high level of reliability and precision, explaining the strongest relationship between the MBV and the animal's recorded performance to date. Two traits predicted by the MBV - faecal egg count and number of lambs born - are both difficult and costly to measure. Pfizer says this tool provides producers with the best opportunity to date to make significant gains in traits of economic importance. The other traits, weaning weight and carcase weight, can be used to complement the accuracy of existing breeding value data. In future disease, production and quality traits will be included.

The International Sheep Genomics Consortium's immediate objective has been to skim sequence the ovine genome so as to identify SNPs in order to produce a 50k SNP chip. Roche 454 FLX sequencing technology is a new technology based on pyrosequencing. Simulations based on the limited ovine genomic sequence available, and results from a pilot ovine resequencing project identified the following strategy:

Roche 454 FLX technology to produce a 3x whole ovine genome coverage, consisted of 0.5x shotgun sequence coverage from 6 ewes. Each animal represents a different breed and the resulting sequence was initially assembled using the bovine genome as a framework which has then been reorganized using the virtual sheep genome to create a sheep genome sequence.

The 454 approach has been used to produce more than 9 Gb of ovine sequence and to provide assembled and ordered sequence for approximately 76% of the unique portion of the ovine genome. It also allowed the detection of more than 590,000 probable SNPs with defined genomic locations of which more than 270,000 were classified as "class A" SNPs (both alleles seen in two sheep). This is sufficient to select from for a goal of 50k ovine SNP chip comprising equally spaced SNPs. Based on available information a 50k ovine SNP chip would be a resource where the mean linkage disequilibrium (r2) between adjacent SNPs would be in excess of 0.25, which is suitable for whole genome association studies. The 454 sequencing phase of the project was completed by AgResearch in New Zealand sequencing 3 sheep representing the Romney, Texel and Scottish Blackface breeds and Baylor HGSC in Houston Texas sequencing 3 sheep representing the Merino, Poll Dorset and Awassi breeds.

The project had two additional components added to identify more SNPs as well as to estimate their minor allele frequency more accurately and improve the genome assembly. The first extension was to include ~4 Gbp of reduced representational sequencing (RRS) with an Illumina Genome Analyser (GA) to identify numerous additional SNPs and estimate their minor allele frequency using a technique outlined by Smith *et al.* (2008). The second extension has been to improve assembly by creation of paired end reads of various insert sizes and sequencing lengths using a combination of next generation and Sanger sequencing.

To complement the sheep SNPs discovered from the 454 skim sequencing of the sheep genome deeper, reduced representational sequencing (RRS) was also undertaken using the Illumina Genome Analyzer. Three size ranges of HaeIII digested sheep DNA (pooled from sixty diverse animals) were sequenced to an average depth of ~20 fold. After extensive filtering of the Illumina sequencing reads and mapping to the sheep genome assembly 76,000 high quality SNPs were identified. The 1536 pilot chip SNPs (identified using Sanger resequencing) along with the 454 and RRS-derived SNPs were then remapped to the sheep genome assembly. All SNPs were scored for probability of assay conversion by Illumina and minor allele frequency was calculated for 1536 and Illumina-derived SNPs. SNPs with an assay conversion score of less than 0.8, and/or a minor allele frequency of less than 0.2 were excluded. SNPs for the BeadChip were then selected from adjacent windows of the assembled genome sequence with as close to equal spacing as possible. A hierarchy of selection criteria was applied in each window, choosing Sanger before Illumina before 454, Infinium II (requires one bead on the BeadChip) over Infinium I (requires two beads on the Beadchip), highest assay conversion score and minor allele frequency closest to 0.5. In a final quality control SNPs with identical oligonucleotide sequences and SNPs with oligonucleotides with multiple hits to the sheep genome assembly were removed and replaced with the closest adjacent SNP that met the selection criteria. The final Beadchip carries 59,494 sheep SNPs.

The International Sheep Genomics Consortium is conducting a large experiment into the variable component of the ovine genome. Progress to March 2009 has seen the development of the ovine SNP50 BeadChip and its application to genotype a wide range of breeds, wild sheep and out-group species. A total of 3004 domestic sheep DNA samples from 71 breeds were recruited into the experiment which likely represents the most comprehensive sampling of any livestock species achieved to date. Breeds were collected from Africa, Asia, South America, Europe, the Middle East, Australasia, the USA and Caribbean. Out of these 71 breeds, three Indian sheep breeds viz Garole, Deccani and Changthangi were covered in SNP discovery and hap map panel.

Global status of genomic selection in goat

Presently goat SNP chip has been developed by consortia of four countries and they are not in market or public domain. The consortia partners are

(i) University of Utrecht, Netherlands (H. Heuven and M. Groenen): They made reduced representation libraries of 17 Saanen dairy goats by using 120 million of 32 bp paired-ends sequences i.e. 3 Gb of data.

(ii) Malaysian Agricultural Research and Development Institute, Malaysia and DNA Landmarks, Canada (J.J. Abdullah and T.P. Yu). This group has contributed by more than one million SNP detection on whole genome sequencing in 3 populations of Boer, Savanna and Kacang meat and indigenous goats (20 samples each).

(iii) French National Institute for Agricultural Research (INRA), France (Ph. Mulsant, R. Rupp and C. Moreno-Romieux), they did whole genome sequencing of 13 Alpine, Saanen and Creole goats generating 150 Gb data.

(iv) Bejing Genome Institute / Kumming Institute of Zoology / Inner Mongolia Agricultural University, China (W. Zhang and W. Wang) they did de novo assembly of goat contigs.

Present Goat Illumina SNP chip is based on just 7 breeds (Saanen -dairy goats (Netherland and France), Boer, Savanna, Kacang -meat goat (Malaysia), Alpine, Creole (France) and Chinese goat) single genome sequence, as China has not revealed their number of breeds. Though China is part of goat consortia. September 30th 2011 was the dead line of consortia partners to join with SNP list. India is yet to come out with SNP discovery in indigenous goat breeds to have our indigenous goat hap map. India has not joined any consortia as far as domestic animal genome assembly or hap map is concern. In case of crop sciences like rice, potato and wheat India has been consortium partner.

Status of GWAS in sheep and goat breeding programme in India

Limited attempt has been made by few research groups for molecular characterisation of commercially and economically important genes in small ruminants. Allele mining has been done for limited number of genes in case of sheep and goat and very few reports are available for association studies with limited number of SNP. Genomic selection programme is yet to be initiated in case of sheep and goat. India has diverse breeds of sheep (> 42) and also one of the most diversified goat populations (>20 breeds). The integration of phenotype bank with DNA bank is yet to be initiated. The projects targeting indigenous caprine and ovine hap map are yet to be initiated.

Challenges in implementing GS programme in India

The requirements to implement genomic selection in breeding programmes are relatively simple. Generally there will be a discovery dataset where a large number of SNP have been assayed on a moderate number of animals who have phenotypes for all the relevant traits. A prediction equation that uses markers as input and predicts BV is derived from this data. There should then be a validation sample (which can be smaller than the derivation sample) where a larger number of animals are recorded for the traits and genotyped at least for the markers that are proposed to be used commercially. The prediction equation is tested to assess its accuracy on this independent sample. Then selection candidates are genotyped for the markers and the prediction equation estimated in the discovery data used to calculate GEBV, but their accuracy is assumed to be that found in the validation sample. In practice, the process may be more complex but the distinction between discovery, validation and selection candidates is still useful. For instance, it makes clear that the estimation of QTL effects can be carried out on animals that are completely separate from the selection candidates. In fact the selection candidates do not need to have phenotypes recorded at all. This technology has potential to fetch large changes in the structure of the livestock breeding programmes. The combined discovery and validation datasets are referred as 'reference' population (Goddard and Hayes, 2007).

In India the challenges are double sworded. Firstly, the "phenotype gap" due to limited phenome data generation on sheep and goat, secondly, lack of integrated DNA bank. This holds true for almost all domestic animal species. The genetic infrastructure required in implementing GWAS plan and sheep and goat has to be started from scratch. The data generation and curation with integrated DNA sample is a herculean task. The predictor and predictee reference population of more than 4000 sample size at least, is required in order to establish the GEBV in each major breed. This is going to take very long time thus gestation period for GWAS implementation in sheep and goat is no doubt going to take much longer time.

Opportunities for India in domestic and global context

India has been a melting pot of small ruminant diversity with maximum number of breeds in sheep and significant number of goat breeds. As these domestic animal species are not much in organised sector thus there is not much selection pressure leading to homogeneity in diversity. This is true in case of almost all Southern countries in case of goat at least. The diverse climatic zone of India has selected unique combination of genes/genotype in form of distinct breeds of sheep and goat. The tropical and hot/humid climate with full parasitic load has rendered the germplasm to "resistant" genotype in process of nature's natural selection. Thus, our sheep and goat germplasm are "genomic gold". Global climate change has made the world to look for thermo tolerant germplasm which nature has bestowed our country. India has great opportunity to develop a high density (HD) goat 500KSNP cheap over the existing 50K goat SNP chip likely to be released by end of December 2011. As sheep 50K SNP chip has highest number of breeds covered (71), they are in high demand across the world. India can enjoy a similar situation in case of goat HD-SNP chip fetching IP edge and revenue. The huge investment can have better dividend for the country both in terms of increase in small ruminant productivity as well as IP revenue. Such pragmatic approach with right objectivity and rationality is the need of the hour and critically warranted.

Conclusion

Widespread use of DNA markers will have a major impact on the structure of the breeding programmes and a significant impact on production systems. Breeding animals will be reared cheaply with minimum recording of phenotypes and pedigree. Selection will be based on a prediction equation derived from a reference population that has extensive phenotypic recording and genotype data. To take maximum advantage of the genomic selection, generation intervals will be shortened as much as reproductive technology will allow. The time has come and we have to gear up before it gets further delayed or never!

References

Daetwyler, H., Villanueva, B., Bijma, P. and Woolliams, J. 2007. Inbreeding in genome-wide selection. Journal of Animal Breeding and Genetics 124: 369-376.

Goddard, M. and Hayes, B. 2007. Genomic selection. Journal of Animal Breeding and Genetics 124: 323-330.

Meuwissen, T., Hayes, B. and Goddard, M. 2001. Prediction of total genetic value using genome-wide dense marker maps. Genetics 157:1819-1829.

Misztal, I. 2006. Challenges of application of marker assisted selection – a review. Animal Science Papers and Reports 24: 5-10.

Schaeffer, L. 2006. Strategy for applying genome-wide selection in dairy cattle. Journal of Animal Breeding and Genetics 123: 218-223.

Smith, D.R., Quinlan, A.R., Peckham, H.E., Makowsky, K., Woolf, B., Shen, L., Donahue, W.F., Tusneem, N., Stromberg, M.P., Stewart, D.A., Zhang, L., Ranade, S.S., Warner, J.B., Lee, C.C., Coleman, B.E., Zhang, Z., McLaughlin, S.F., Malek, J.A., Sorenson, J.M., Blanchard, A.P., Chapman, J., Hillman, D., Chen, F., Rokhsar, D.S., McKernan, K.J., Jeffries, T.W., Marth, G.T. and Richardson, P.M. 2008. Rapid whole-genome mutational profiling using next-generation sequencing technologies. Genome Research 18: 1638-1642.

VanRaden, P.M., Van Tassel, C.P., Wiggans, G.R., Sonstegard, T.S., Schnabel, R.D., Taylor, J.F. and Schenkel, F.S. 2009. Reliability of genomic predictions for North American Holstein bulls. Journal of Dairy Science 92: 16-24.

□□□

Chapter 6

Techniques for Enhancing Reproductive Efficiency in Small Ruminants

A.K. Goel
Pr. Scientist, Physiology, Reproduction and Shelter Management Division, Central Institute for Research on Goats, Makhdoom, P.O. Farah-281 122, Mathura (UP)

Marginalized groups including women particularly in dry areas typically rely upon small ruminants for their nutrition and livelihoods. Small ruminants serve as a source to reduce poverty, increase food security and employment generation to a larger section of the society, predominantly of resource poor people of the country. India harbours more than 125 million goats (23 defined breeds) and 65 million sheep (42 defined breeds) adapted to different agro-ecological zones of the country. The growth of world mammalian population since 1980 reflected the largest animal number increase for goats during past 30 years. In the present scenario of changing agro-climatic conditions, it has tremendous potential to be projected as the 'Future Animal' for rural as well as urban prosperity. Traditional goat/ sheep rearing is steadily turning to an enterprise in the country. In inhospitable terrain of cold desert small ruminants, besides meat and milk are important source of fiber and draft power. Goat meat (chevon) is one of the choicest food commodities and fetches high cost in the market. The goat milk is believed to possess numerous scientifically unexplored medicinal and health promoting attributes. Over the years, animal research has generated a vast number of outputs aimed to help the livestock owners to realize higher income through increased production, productivity and animal health care. These outputs in the form of technologies, knowledge and practices (TKP) have been exploited by limited number of users.

Optimum reproductive process is a prerequisite to obtain desirable production from farm animals. Reproductive efficiency of Indian goats and sheep is relatively low compared to exotic breeds. Most of the Indian goat/sheep breeds experience late sexual maturity, longer post-partum oestrus interval, thus increasing inter kidding/lambing interval and low fecundity (sheep). To bridge the gap between the demand and production to provide food and fiber, draught power and financial security, it is imperative to optimize the production of prolific breeds *vis a vis* improving reproduction rate of less prolific breeds besides minimizing post-fertilization wastage (reproductive losses). Enhanced rate of reproduction is generally desirable and economical in farm animal production especially in small ruminants for improving global food and health security. The productivity of food animals largely depend upon their reproductive performance for which there is a necessity to precisely control the timing of sequential reproductive events, maximize kidding/lambing rates and ensure the survival of their neonates through better reproductive management. Rapid advances in the areas of molecular biology and biotechnology and further development in reproductive techniques provide new horizons for enhancing livestock production. Reproduction research in the country has recorded perceivable advancement, which need to be sustained and augmented for optimizing livestock production including small ruminants. The application of knowledge on biotechnology is certainly of immense value in expanding the range of options available in the present century to meet out global food requirements and human medicine. In this backdrop present chapter outlines an overview of advances in the area of reproductive biotechnology and their appropriate integration in small ruminant production system.

Artificial insemination (AI) and frozen semen technique

AI technique has been the key to various breed improvement programmes especially in cattle and buffalo species. On the contrary it has yet to receive universal acceptance in small ruminants due to certain technical and economical reasons. Unlike sheep the symptoms of oestrus in goats are distinct, visible and more pronounced. Among the recognized breeds of goat and sheep, with a population size over 125 million and 65 million, respectively, around 20 to 25% belong to descript category and remaining are non-descript with mixed genotype in the country. Under this situation there is a shortage of breeding males at farmer's flocks. In this context a concrete national breeding policy for small ruminant production is the necessity for launching a breed improvement programme across the country. Keeping in view conserving and propagating our native breeds it is desirable to use quality semen and effective AI services at the door steps of farmers. Considering the paucity of breeding sires there is ample scope to adopt AI in small ruminants. For a small flock of 4-5 goats/sheep, farmers often do not prefer to maintain a breeding male. Farmers normally depend on sharing of available male of unknown genetic merit in the village maintained by a big flock owner of 10-15 animals. These breeding males are seldom of high genetic merit and often sub-fertile. It is therefore a strong need to strengthen the breed improvement/ upgradation of germplasm dissemination programmes by selecting superior breeding males of different breeds of goat and sheep for natural mating and artificial insemination (fresh/frozen). Demand of superior breeding sires is further going to be increased in view of commercialization of small ruminant production in the country.

Technique to enhance reproductive efficiency by male effect

Now days, consumers worldwide are demanding products that are "clean, green and ethical". Consequently, sheep and goat producers are moving into husbandry practices that do not compromise the welfare of animals. In many countries, regulatory authorities have already imposed these conditions on local producers, importers and exporters. In the absence of exogenous hormones, the male effect can be used as oestrus and ovulation synchronizers and inducer. In small ruminants the sudden introduction of buck/ram can induce ovulation in females that are reproductively quiescent. Induced ovulations are sufficiently synchronized among a group of females to allow the use of AI and probably therefore focused feeding for litter size, foetal programming and neonatal survival. The male effect has the added advantage that it allows control over the season of births, so we can take advantage of seasonal changes in kid/lamb marketing. It may be the ideal tool of the tropical countries where the anoestrous condition of the female is most often shallow. Its cost is much less than hormones and can be supported even when the income of the flock is very low (landless to marginal farmers).

Technique of accelerated kidding

Post-partum anoestrus period is an important aspect in the reproduction chain influencing the future reproductive efficiency in small ruminants. This time interval between parturition and the first post-partum oestrus determines how soon after parturition conception can possibly occur. Earlier an animal returns to oestrus after parturition, earlier it can be rebred to enhance life time production. Three times kidding/lambing in 2 years is an ideal target of small ruminant production programme. Tropical goat/sheep are characterized by longer post-partum oestrus interval, requiring more period for re-establishment of ovarian cyclicity. Considerable variations exist with respect to this reproductive trait as influenced by breed, lactation, season of parturition, parity, litter size, level of nutrition after parturition and peri-parturient problems. Interventions are possible for shortening of post-partum oestrus interval by improving manage mental conditions to certain extent and advocating hormonal therapy to a greater extent after completion of uterine involution by day 40-60 after parturition. Research efforts in exotic breeds have been diverted by advocating hormone therapy in order to induce and synchronize oestrus/ ovulation. Research findings suggest that to induce oestrus behaviour in sheep and goats prior conditioning of neural centers with progesterone is necessary. Therefore, a progestagen /prostaglandin combination associated with low doses of equine chorionic gonadotropin (eCG) has been found effective in goats with more than 60% goats kidding after AI with frozen thawed semen at a predetermined time (Baril and Saumande, 2000). Presumably kidding rate may further increase if profile goat breeds are put under hormone therapy. PMSG (now known as eCG) is a hormone of choice considering its affordable cost and easier availability (Ritar *et al.*, 1989; Leboeuf *et al.*, 1994). Recent studies carried out at this institute and other places have shown encouraging results (Goel *et al.*, 2009a; Patil *et al.*, 2009). Efficacy of such treatment was two dimensional i.e. considerable shortening of kidding interval and simultaneous substantial increase in kidding rate in hormonally treated goats as compared to untreated controls.

Immuno-neutralization of reproductive hormones to enhance kid/lamb crop

This approach is based upon neutralization of the biological actions of endogenous hormones by antigen-antibody complex formation *in vivo*. Use of these immunological methods to modify normal physiological state by inducing autoimmunity has been attempted with varying degree of success for a number of reproductive hormones. The number of offspring born per female is a major determinant of sustainability of small ruminant production. Majority of the indigenous sheep breeds are single monotocous, which is major limitation in increasing their productivity. Efforts are on the way to enhance productivity of sheep by introgression of Booroola fecundity gene or by physiological and nutritional manipulations (Naqvi *et al.*, 2007). There has been an increasing interest to increase ovulation rate in sheep by active and passive immuno-neutralization of inhibin hormone (Daroliya *et al.*, 1990). Inhibin is a glycoprotein mainly secreted by granulosa cells of large antral follicles, consisting of two dissimilar disulphide-linked α and β sub-units and acts as a negative feed back regulator of follicle-stimulating hormone (FSH). Various inhibin based preparations/vaccines viz. follicular fluid, synthetic peptides and recombinant inhibin α fusion proteins have been advocated to neutralize endogenous inhibin, leading to increase in circulating FSH levels and consequent increase in ovulation rate and thus litter size in ewe and does (Dietrich *et al.*, 1995). Driancourt *et al.* (1990) and Avdi *et al.* (1991) reported on the effect of active immunization against androgen, androstendione on the reproductive performance of goats. The litter size increased significantly from 1.25 to 1.63. Similarly, inhibin based fecundity vaccines have also shown the potential of increasing ovulation rate in indigenous sheep breeds. Active immunization of Malpura ewes against the synthetic peptide sequence of the α sub-unit of bovine inhibin increased the ovulation rate over 5 fold compared to that of controls (Naqvi *et al.*, 2007).The effect of immunization persisted for about 36 months and expressed in term of increased ovulation rate. Besides, the passive immunization against synthetic inhibin peptides did not affect the oestrus response in Malpura ewes but relatively higher ovulatory response was observed by administering anti-sera generated against 30-mer peptide as compared to 17-mer peptide.(Naqvi *et al.*, 2009).

Multiple ovulation and embryo transfer (MOET) technique

Embryo transfer is one of the most exciting developments in the reproduction of farm animals, the so called second generation reproductive biotechnology, after AI. Technique has been proved to be an effective means of increasing the contribution of superior females to the gene pool of the population. Consequently, multi-ovulation embryo transfer (MOET) is used to accelerate genetic progress in terms of milk, meat and fiber production. In India, specific applications of this technique relate to greater number of progenies from genetically superior goats, *ex situ* conservation of endangered breeds, increasing prolificacy of less prolific breeds (Goel and Agrawal, 2003) in both species, opportunity of pregnancy testing besides catering needs for various reproductive biotechnologies (cloning, transgenesis, embryo splitting to produce identified twins, stem cell research, and sexing by *in vivo* and *in vitro* embryo production). Embryo transfer is a composite technology encompassing synchronization of oestrus, induction of super ovulation, embryo collection and transfer with ultimate production of kids of superior genetic merit. Individual variability in superovulatory response after treatment with exogenous gonadotropins, asynchrony in ovulation, fertilization failure in females with high ovulation rate, post surgical adhesions and formation of antibodies to exogenous gonadotropins have been the major problems associated with ETT in small ruminants (Naqvi *et al.*, 2007). There has been relatively less commercial embryo transfer activity in small ruminants as compared to cattle world over. As per the statistical report published by International Embryo Transfer Society, USA in the year 2005, about 25000 sheep and 7000 goat *in vivo* derived embryos were transferred world wide, amounting to be 2.8 and 0.8% of total bovine embryo (both *in vivo* and *in vitro* produced) i.e. about 8.8 lakhs. The possibility of disease transmission through *in vivo* derived embryos is extremely rare (String fellow *et al.*, 2004) due to development of technical expertise and procedure of ETT. Effective protocols (Efficacy - 70 to 90%) for synchronization of oestrus in donors and recipients are available either by using luteolytic agents or progestagens (Mohmood *et al.*, 1991; Goel and Agrawal, 1998a), intra-vaginal sponges (Mani *et al.*, 1994; Goel and Agrawal, 2000). Use of progesterone in the form of subcutaneous ear implants proved more effective particularly during anoestrus period (Akinlosotu and Wilder, 1993; Kharche *et al.*, 2005a). Intra vaginal sponges patented by CSWRI, Avikanagar, are quite effective and cheaper for synchronization of oestrus in ewes.

a) *Multiple ovulation in donors:* The variation in response to super ovulation and relatively low embryo survival rates after transfer are major factors limiting the efficient use of MOET programme in goats and other farm animals. Highly variable results have been reported by different laboratories due to numerous extrinsic and extrinsic factors including breed, age, body condition of donor and recipients, season and nutrition etc. It is evident that follicular population present at the time gonadotropin treatment for super ovulation determines the superovulatory response (Gonzalez-Bulnes *et al.*, 2003). Different approaches have been attempted to increase the number of small ovarian follicles at the time of superovulatory treatment and to avoid the presence of large dominant follicles (Manchaca *et al.*, 2002; Cognie *et al.*, 2003) through synchronization of follicular wave emergence. Pre-treatment over a 2-week period with an agonist (Buserelin) or 10 days with antagonist (Antarelix) suppresses large follicle, double the number of small ones and improves the response to FSH by 50% (Cognie, 1999). Sheep with high fecundity have been shown to be more responsive to gonadotropins for super ovulation than sheep with low fecundity due to availability of more number of growing follicles (Cahill and Dufour, 1979; Piper *et al.*, 1982; Kelly *et al.*, 1983). A major and unresolved problem of super ovulation in goats is the extreme variability in ovulatory response to exogenous gonadotropins. Therefore, there is no real optimal superovulatory protocol established for goats (Greyling *et al.*, 2002). To induce super ovulation eCG and FSH of porcine, ovine, equine sources are widely used near the end of the luteal phase. The evidence favours the FSH in terms of response and embryo yield (Naqvi and Gulyani, 1999; Pendleton *et al.*, 1992; Rosnina *et al.*, 1992; Goel and Agrawal 1998d; Goel and Agrawal, 2005). A varying but acceptable response and embryo yield by using super ovulatory protocols has been achieved (Noshari and Holtz, 1995; Goel and Agrawal, 1998b,c,d; Bijurkar *et al.*, 2004; Mishra *et al.*, 2004; Goel and Agrawal, 2005) in goats. To overcome the unreliable superovulatory response in conventional techniques, newer approaches such as immunization against inhibin á sub-unit alone or in combination with eCG or FSH has been found useful (Dietrich *et al.*, 1995; Wang *et al.*, 2000). In ewes the combination of both PMSG (eCG) and FSH (Naqvi and Gulyani, 1999; Jabbour *et al.*, 1991) is used to evoke superovulatory response in Indian conditions. The superovulatory response (ovulation rate, number of corpora lutea/ewe) in prolific sheep Garole ranged from 4-25 with a mean of 13.6±3.1 (Naqvi *et al.*, 2006a). The mean ovulation rate was 6.6 in Rambouillet (Naqvi and Gulyani, 1999), 7.4 in Bharat Merino (Naqvi *et al.*, 2002) and 8.4 in Malpura ewes (Naqvi *et al.*, 2006b).

b) *Embryo transfer and pregnancy rate:* During early phase of ETT, conventional surgical techniques resulted in embryo recovery limiting to 40-50%. Presently, with the perfection in technique considerable improvement has been possible (Goel and Agrawal, 1998b; Greyling and Van der Nest, 2000; Greyling *et al.*, 2002; Goel and Agrawal, 2005). Surgical technique though simple and results in consistent higher recovery in relation to the number of corpora lutea, post-surgical adhesions seriously limit repeated collections and transfers. On the contrary respectable recovery (60.7 to 63.2%) under endoscopy could be repeated successfully on the same goat (Baril *et al.*, 1988; Tervit *et al.*, 1992). Laparoscopy is more perfected in ewe than doe, though applications are identical for both species. Sizable numbers of ewe lambs through laparoscopic transfer have been produced at CSWRI, Avikanagar (Naqvi and Gulyani, 1995; Naqvi *et al.*, 2001). Further improvement in collection techniques resulted in development of intra-cervical catheterization of reproductive tract of small ruminants. Trans-cervical approach (non-surgical technique) is competitive to conventional surgical and laparoscopic techniques. Repeated collections from the same animal with varying recovery (2 to12 embryos) are possible (Agrawal *et al.*, 1991; Grupp, 1991, Oliveira *et al.*, 1992; Pereira *et al.*, 1998; Holtz *et al.*, 2000). In India, Goel *et al.* (1995, 2002) after suitable modifications in the technique could collect uterine stage embryo from Indigenous goats. There are certain factors viz. difficulty in catheterization of tortuous cervical folds (3 to 6 in number), non-availability of flexible catheters equipped with ballooning devices, pre mature regression of corpora lutea in 25-30% super ovulated donors often result in in-consistent to nil recovery. To overcome above problems further improvement in the technique would be necessary for consistent embryo recovery. The pregnancy rates following transfer of goat embryos range from 40 to 80% mainly depending upon the quality of embryos, number of embryos per recipient and transfer expertise (Agrawal and Goel, 1991; Grupp, 1991; Mahmood *et al.*, 1991; Goel *et al.*, 1993, 1994a; Mani *et al.*,1994; Greyling *et al.*, 2002; Goel *et al.*, 2006).

Small ruminant production is constrained by the inadequate superior males affecting overall productivity of both species. A large number of superior bucks/rams are required to cover the existing non-descript population of small ruminants in the country to accelerate reproduction rate. The production of large number of animals of superior genetic merit within a short period through conventional breeding techniques is not possible. Therefore for production of sufficient males MOET can be used. Extensive use of superior males over the period of time through natural mating, use of fresh/frozen semen for artificial insemination and wider distribution of breeding sires to innovative/progressive farmers and entrepreneurs is likely to result progenies with enhanced kidding/lambing rates.

Technique of *in vitro* embryo production through *in vitro* fertilization

In vitro fertilization (IVF) was started as early as in early 1950 in the form of assisted reproductive technique by Brittan's Noble laureate Robert Edwards. Relatively efficient techniques for *in vitro* maturation and fertilization of oocytes in small ruminants are more important than in large ruminants due to their short generation interval, prolificacy (particularly in goats), economical rearing, better visibility and large size of pronucleus for biotechnological manipulations viz. during gene transfer, cloning and stem cell research (Kharche *et al.*, 2009, 2011). Therefore, laboratory production of embryos, rather than harvested from living animals using conventional ET and laparoscopic techniques has definite advantages. Progress in cellular and molecular embryology in farm animals has been difficult in the past due to limited availability of suitable experimental material at a reasonable cost. For such reasons, *in vitro* embryo production (IVEP) techniques, particularly based on ovaries of abattoir origin have received greater attention in past two decades (Galli and Lazzari, 2003). Besides the efficiency of *in vitro* derived embryo production using conventional technique of MOET is not optional, rather it is inconsistent due to variable superovulatory response and flushing procedures (Cognie *et al.*, 2003). Alternatively *in vitro* production of embryos provides cheaper and consistent source for supply of specific developmental stages for biomedical research and emerging biotechnologies viz. cloning , transgenesis through somatic cell nuclear transfer (SCNT), intracytoplasmic sperm injection (ICSI) and embryo sexing (Baldassarre *et al.*, 2004; O' Brien *et al.*, 2004; Wang *et al.*, 2003). *In vitro* embryo production technology has been established for goats (De Smedt *et al.*, 1992; Keskintepe *et al.*, 1994; O'Brein *et al.*, 2004). *In vitro* embryo production in small ruminants is a rapidly advancing area of research for producing valuable transgenic goats, capable of producing substances of pharmaceutical value in their milk (Koeman *et al.*, 2003). The use of prepubertal animals would be regarded as particularly helpful; collection of oocytes at an earlier age would reduce generation interval and accelerate the propagation of the genetically valuable livestock. For such reasons major research is currently focused to factors involved in determining the developmental competence of oocytes from prepubertal and adult goats. During the past two decades, considerable advancement has been made in the laboratory production of embryos since the birth of kids following the transfer of IVP embryos (Hanada, 1985; Younis *et al.*, 1991; Keskintepe *et al.*, 1994; Pereira *et al.*, 1995; Han *et al.*, 1996; Kharche *et al.*, 2008a). Substantial research work on various facets of IVEP has been carried out in India, resulting in perfection of technique in sheep (Naqvi *et al.*, 1992; Naqvi and Madan, 1997; Chauhan *et al.*, 1997) and goats (Pawshe *et al.*, 1993; Kharche *et al.*, 2005b, 2006, 2008b, c, 2009; Yadav *et al.*, 2007, 2008). In this context research laboratories in India could succeed in establishment of pregnancies and production of live kids following transfer of *in vitro* produced embryos (Malakar *et al.*, 2005; Kharche *et al.*, 2008a). More recently same group succeeded in establishing pregnancy and production of twin IVF kids (Kharche *et al.*, 2011). These laboratories are engaged in optimizing the *in vitro* embryo development potential in caprine for better results. In India, considering the perspective of this technology, further refinement in IVEP technology, minimization of import of expensive culture media and hormones etc. *vis a vis* improvement in recovery of culturable oocytes by non-invasive trans-vaginal ultrasound guided follicle aspiration (OPU) would be required for optimization of small ruminant production.

Techniques of early pregnancy diagnosis

The diagnosis of early pregnancy is not only a managerial tool in terms of determining the reproductive efficiency of the flock but also in determining the flow of nutrients in terms of animals carrying singletons, twins, triplets or those are barren. The purpose of early scanning lies in identification of non-pregnant flock to minimize unproductive period. Additional interest is to determine foetal numbers (Dhoble *et al.*, 2005a,b) so that special management is provided for higher economic gains and assessing embryonic foetal viability. With the advancement in technologies, we can now rely upon new technologies i.e. micro-quantitation of pregnancy related hormones

(Progesterone) / factors (Pregnancy specific protein B) at 19-21 post-mating by RIA and ELISA (Humblot *et al.*, 1990; Restall *et al.*, 1990; Carmenate *et al.*, 1992, Kaushik *et al.*, 1992; Boscos *et al.*, 2003; Ganaie *et al.*, 2009a) and B-mode real time ultrasonography (Medan *et al.*, 2004; Chandolia *et al.*, 2005; Hoque *et al.*, 2005; Jeoujong *et al.*, 2005; Kumar *et al.*, 2005; Padilla Rivas *et al.*, 2005; Vathsala *et al.*, 2005; Goel *et al.*, 2009b). In recent years a number of pregnancy associated glycoproteins have been characterized in the ruminant species. The assay of these pregnancy associated glycoproteins (PAGs) can constitute an efficient technique to confirm early pregnancy (day 21 or 22) to indicate a feto-placental distress accompanying or preceding an embryonic or foetal mortality in goats (Gonzalez *et al.*, 2000). Hormone assay based tests (Fleming *et al.*, 1990) detected non-pregnancy more accurately (EIA-100%, RIA-80%) than pregnancy (EIA-66%, RIA-75%). The diagnosis of pregnancy at 30 days of gestation has been possible by trans-rectal ultrasonography (Goel *et al.*, 2009b; Ganaie *et al.*, 2009b). In our laboratory pregnancy diagnosis was carried at 28 -35 days of gestation by employing trans-rectal transducer of variable frequency (5, 7, 8 MHz) with 80% accuracy.

a) *Early pregnancy diagnosis at 28 days of gestation:* During ultrasonographic scanning of pregnant uterus at day 28 post-mating, anechoic foetal fluid pocket (black) with while elongated streak extending more than half of foetal fluid in the centre was scanned with 7mHz intra-rectal transducer. In twin foetuses, two anechoic (black) fluid pockets were identified.

b) *Early pregnancy diagnosis at 35-38 days of gestation:* During ultrasonographic scanning of pregnant uterus at day 35 post-mating using 5, 7 MHz intra-rectal transducer, echo dense foetuses were captured on a single ultrasonic image. Foetal body was distinctly imaged into regions (head and trunk). Foetal heart beat was visible in trunk region of developing foetus. At day 38 of pregnancy, amniotic membrane encircled the developing conceptus in the form of distinct hyper echoic dotted line. Developing placentomes in half moon shape (saggital view) or ring shape (horizontal view) were also scanned.

Technique of real time (B–mode) ultrasound scanning

In recent years, the real time B-mode ultrasonography has emerged an important non-invasive and non-disruptive diagnostic tool in veterinary science. Currently the sonography of reproductive organs is the standard practice for determining pregnancy, foetal viability and multiple births in small ruminant production. In particular, ultrasonic imaging of internal organs and soft tissues is one of the most revolutionary advances in animal reproduction (clinical and research). In animal reproduction, besides early pregnancy diagnosis, foetal number counts, sexing and foetal viability (Chandolia *et al.*, 2005; Dhoble *et al.*, 2005a, b; Kumar *et al.*, 2005; Goel *et al.*, 2009b), it has tremendous other applications (Kahn, 1994) to appreciate follicular were pattern during oestrous cycle, ovulation profile, ovulatory response in hormonally induced does, ovarian pathological conditions and as an aid to aspirate follicular oocytes from live animals for increased goat production.

Genetic resource banking for conservation by utilizing reproductive biotools

Conservation is defined as the analysis and protection of the earth's biological diversity. Endangerment of goat breeds may include habitat loss, breed replacement, natural calamities, and loss of genes within individuals. Genetic diversity in goat population has potential merit as an important resource for the future. A number of livestock species in the world deemed at risk of extinction has been estimated at 27% in goats, 22% in sheep, 13% in buffaloes, 29% in cattle, 40% in pigs, 42% in horses, 23% in asses and 8% in camels (Galal, 2005). The FAO (1998, 2000) defines "breeds at risk" (critical and endangered) at those with fewer than 1000 females, with fewer than 20 males or with a total population size approximately 1200. This risk increases as the proportion of females declines below 80%. In India, Jamunapari, Jakhrana, Beetal and Surti are considered to be endangered. The kinds of conservation that will be needed, depends upon the nature and status of the threats. A coherent strategy includes a suitable mix of three basic kinds of conservation: *In situ, Ex situ in vivo* and *Ex situ in vitro*.

In situ conservation is community based conservation and management under its normal habitat and will be the preferred method where the maintenance of a particular breed / breeds represents as a source of livelihood option for the people who rear the animals. *Ex situ in vivo* conservation is an option to support the conservation of institutional or community owned flocks / NGOs that may be differ from native environment. This needs revitalization of the in situ on farm conservation traditions of local communities rearing them. *Ex situ in vitro* conservation is needed as a secure back up for any disasters for livestock populations that might driven to extinction faster than the other approaches can respond. Cryo-preservation of sperms, egg and body cells are all potential options. In fact both *in situ* and *ex situ* approach of conservation of invaluable genetic heritage should be complementary rather competitive to each other. There is a need to improve the technologies and reduce costs of cryopreservation of gametes, embryos and somatic cells of most animal species of human use.

In addition to above techniques, the technique of Somatic Cells Nuclear Transfer (SCNT) leading to cloning is a much flexible technique of breed conservation. FAO as early as in 1997 identified SCNT as a viable option for emergency conservation actions where other more established techniques may be difficult to implement. More recently in addition to cloning, Intra Cytoplasmic Sperm Injection (ICSI) and Stem Cell Technologies are also emerging for conservation of endangered / extinct animal species. These techniques need to be systematically integrated into breeding programmes and care would be needed to preserve genetic diversity. National Bureau of Animal Genetic Resources (NBAGR), Karnal is actively engaged to work on this aspect, besides both species specific (goat and sheep) institutes.

Reproductive cloning

It is a reproductive technique of production of an exact genotypic replica of the organisms, indistinguishable from the donor that contributes the diploid cell nucleus. Splitting or bisection of embryos has been utilized to produce monozygotic twins (clones), which are genetically identical both in their nuclear and mitochondrial genes. Embryo splitting is done in late morulae or blastocysts (day 6-10). This procedure enables an increase in the number of off springs from parents of outstanding genotype in an MOET programme. Alternatively animal clones have also been produced by electro fusion of the diploid nucleus of individual blastomeres or somatic cells into enucleated undivided cytoplasm of a recipient oocyte (Wilmut *et al.,* 1997). Cloned progeny derived from transfer of nuclei either from blastomeres or adult somatic cells are not exact replica due to cytoplasmic inheritance of mitochondrial DNA of enucleated oocytes. Cytoplasmic factors present in the oocytes may influence reprogramming of genome of the transferred nucleus and subsequent development (Cummins, 2001).

Recently, zona free nuclear transfer with mechanical aspiration of the metaphase plate as a means of enucleation was also reported to increase the cell fusion success as compared to zona enclosed procedure (Lagutina *et al.*, 2007). In cloned progeny due to cytoplasmic inheritance, behavioural aspect is lacking. In cytoplasmic inheritance, the amount of cytoplasm contributed by egg (mother) is always much greater than that in the sperms (viz. plasmids in plants, viruses, mitochondria, microsomes and kappa particles in paramecium. It is because her genes that impress upon the cytoplasm of all her eggs, phenomenon is called 'maternal determination'.

Research efforts are being concentrated to explore the mechanism of reprogramming gene expression in the transferred nucleus and reasons of failures. Congenital abnormalities, large off spring syndrome and high rates of foetal prenatal and neonatal mortality are associated factors for low success rate of full term development and survival of cloned progeny. Neonates often experience respiratory distress and cardiovascular abnormalities. These losses are assumed to occur due to inappropriate expression of genes during various stages of development (Bazer and Spencer, 2005). Embryonic Stem Cells in suitable culture conditions are potential and inexhaustible source of genetic material for nuclear transfer. Clone formation requires good technique for maturation and enucleation of oocytes, fusion of nuclei with enucleated oocytes and *in vitro* culture of the resulting embryos to the late morale / blastocysts stage. 'Electro fusion' is used to activate the oocytes during nuclear transfer. The birth of Dolly sheep in 1997, following the fusion of an adult mammary gland cell nucleus from a pregnant sheep with an enucleated metaphase II oocytes of an ewe and the blastocysts so derived grown in the womb of yet another recipient ewe, aroused the possibility of cloning pet and farm animals, and for infertile couples to have babies of their own genetic make up. Initial success in animal cloning (transferring nucleus from adult tissue cells to enucleated oocytes of same species) has opened up the possibility of producing more useful animals. The genetically cloned animal can yield higher quantities of products of human use, manifest heritable genes transcribing human products, help in understanding the process of embryonic development and aging and serve good 'animal model' for human diseases. The procedure can also help in enhancing the biodiversity ensuring, continuation of rare breeds and endangered species. Exciting work is ongoing in animals models e.g. the use of adult stem cells cured diabetes in mice and acute liver failure in rats.

Cloning technology offers the potential for the exponential reproduction of a population of embryos derived from donors of outstanding genetic merit.

Scientists of National Dairy Research Institute (NDRI), Karnal in 2009 succeeded in creating the World's first cloned buffalo calf 'Samrupa', which succumbed to a lung infection, five days after birth. Second cloned buffalo calf was born on 6th June 2009. NDRI scientists developed an indigenous cloned method i.e. Hand Guided Cloning Technology, which was much simpler and an advanced modification of conventional cloning method used to create Dolly. In this technique, the oocytes isolated from abattoir ovaries were matured *in vitro* and treated with enzymes to clear zona pellucida and then isolated with the help of a hand held fine blade. Then somatic cells derived from the ear of the donor buffalo were electro fused with the oocytes grown in vitro for a week. Resultant embryos were transferred to a recipient buffalo for the production of a calf of derived sex. One of the biggest advantages of this technique is that sexed calf can be produced and so breed is conserved.

Parthenogenesis

Parthenogenesis is a form of reproduction in which the ovum develops into a new individual without fertilization (absence of contribution from male gametes). The process of parthenogenesis is more frequent in aphids, daphnia and some other invertebrates including insects and many plant species, where offspring identical to mother is produced. Although, parthenogenesis is not a common mode of reproduction in vertebrates, but there have been incidences of viable births through parthenogenesis such as Komodo dragon and Bony head shark etc. In higher vertebrates (including poultry) parthnogenetic embryo development and conception has been observed without birth. However, pregnancy in bovine parthenote sustained upto day 67 of gestation period.

Parthenogenesis essentially a biological process was discovered in 18th century by Charles Bonnet. In next century, Jacques Loeb incidentally produced artificial parthenogenesis when he picked unfertilized eggs with a needle and found normal embryonic development in some eggs. In 1936, Gregory Pinus induced parthenogenesis in mammalian eggs (Rabbit) by temperature change and chemical agents. Kano *et al.* (2004) produced the first parthenogenetic mice. Parthengenetic embryos are essentially uni parental and uni parental embryos are either androgenetic or gynogenetic origin. Recently in 2007, Hwang Woosuk of South Korea succeeded in production of human embryos through parthenogenesis. This success opened vista for creating stem cells that were genetically matched to particular woman for treatment of degenerative disease. Turkey is a common parthenogenetic poultry bird. At present several problems of developmental arrest in parthenogenetic embryos have been identified because of lack of full genomic complement unlike in vivo derived embryos. It is assumed, if the full genetic component of oocytes can be brought forward to parthenogenetic embryos then a viable animal can be produced through it. The reasons for developmental defect in diploid parthenogenetic and somatic cell nuclear transfer (SCNT) embryos are being studied in laboratory animals as well as higher mammals like goat ,sheep, cattle etc. It has been observed that several developmental related gene expressions are lacking in different types of parthnogenetic and SCNT embryos during different stages of embryo development. However limited approach has been made to study the comparison on genomic expression in parthenogenetic as well as SCNT derived embryos *vis a vis in vitro* and *in vivo* derived embryos which are supposed to have normal developmental related genes. Presently knowledge on molecular mechanism of parthenogenesis in mammals is lacking. Several higher vertebrates viz. reptiles and birds (turkey) express spontaneous parthenogenesis. Once the reasons for such spontaneous parthenogenesis are known, then it may lead to induce parthenogenesis in higher mammals (goat, sheep, cattle and buffalo).

The ongoing multi-dimensional NAIP funded mega research project at different locations in India ((IVRI Izatnagar, NDRI Karnal, CARI Izatnagar, CIRG Makhdoom, JNKVV Jabalpur) is mandated to establish procedures for generation of parthenogenetic embryos by studying the molecular mechanism of parthenogenesis in livestock species with the aim to propagate valuable female germplasm in the country thereby increasing the productive efficiency of animals. Its applications are:

- Parthenogenetic embryos with two sets of equivalently imprinted chromosomes are very useful models for studying genomic imprinting and its role in ontogenesis.
- Mammalian parthenotes serve as ideal models for studying the function of the maternal centrosome.

- Parthenogenesis will help in multiplying superior germplasm without involvement of male counterpart.
- Cryo-preservation of parthenogenetic embryos will be an alternative method for conservation of endangered farm animal species.

Transgenesis

Genetic engineering of livestock to produce animal with altered traits such as disease resistance, wool growth, body growth, prolificacy and reproductive efficiency and milk composition is being researched in laboratories globally (Niemann and Kues, 2003; Paterson *et al.*, 2003; Wheeler *et al.*, 2003; Baldassare *et al.*, 2004). During the past two decades, research aimed at the production of transgenic farm animals has been steadily progressing. The term 'transgenic' was coined in early 1980's to describe mammals that had new genes incorporated into their genome (Gordon *et al.*,1980). Transgenesis operates in a Mendalian fashion. Relatively with cattle and buffalo, sheep and goat have the advantage of a much shorter generation internal and a greater number of offspring. Numerous methods have been used to produce transgenic progeny (Niemann and Kues, 2003) with varying success. These techniques are DNA transfer by retroviruses, microinjection of genes into pronuclei of fertilized ova, injection of embryonic stem cells, embryonic germ cells pre exposed to foreign DNA into the cavity of blastocysts, sperm mediated gene transfer (SMGT) during IVF, liposome mediated DNA transfer into cells and embryos, electroporation of DNA into sperm, ova or embryos and nuclear transfer of somatic cells, ES or EG cells. Among them pronuclear microinjection and somatic cell nuclear transfer (SCNT) have been suggested as the methods of choice to produce transgenic goats and sheep. Microinjection of cloned DNA into pronucleus of a zygote has been most widely used and successful method for producing transgenic mice. This method encompasses microinjection of several thousand copies of DNA into pronuclei of zygote. Offspring produced on transfer of such embryos are screened for integration and expression of foreign gene. One offspring of transgenic sheep and cow cost around US$ 60,000 and 46,000, respectively when microinjection zygotes were used (Wall *et al.*, 1992; Wall, 1996). During the present decade substantial advancement in livestock transgenesis has been made through application SCNT. The merger of Nuclear Transfer with molecular tools such as targeted genetic modification and conditioned gene expression will be boosting the technology of transgenesis (Niemann and Kues, 2003). Nuclear transfer from embryonic and somatic cell can be used to produce transgenic animals with the gene inserted at specific sites. The main advantages of nuclear transfer from cultured cells in comparison to microinjection method are: it can be confirmed by gene sequencing that desired genetic change has been introduced in cultured cells before nuclear transfer, genetic targeting techniques can be utilized to switch off or for different function through precise genetic change in endogenous gene and several copies of modified offspring can be obtained.

With the advancement of this technology, a new industry is emerging for the production of pharmaceuticals in transgenic animals such as goat, which is more effective than production by any conventional means. Researchers in USA have produced transgenic goats carrying the genes for a larger active form of tissue plasminogen activator (tPA), with some goats producing this clot dispersing factor of about 3 gm per liter of milk (Ebert *et al.*, 1991). It is favoured by outstanding protein synthesis capacity of the mammary gland. Transgenic animals have the ability to produce recombinant proteins in a more efficient way than traditional systems based on microorganisms or animal cells like Chinese Hamster ovary (bioreactors). Genetically engineered animals are a better alternative for producing proteins, which forms the basis of all biological drugs. More recently in 2010, a new era in genetic engineering began by the invention of J. Craig Venter in Rockville, Maryland (USA) and Venter's team in San Diego by creating self replicating microbial cell of *Mycoplasma* series with synthetic DNA in the enduring quest to create 'Artificial Life' (World's First Synthetic Cell). They produced a living cell powered with man made DNA. Group identified two species of *Mycoplasma* of goat species. First they chemically synthesized the genome of *M. mycoides* having 1.1 million copies of DNA and then transferred it into a living cell from a different *Mycoplasma* species. With initial delay, the recipient cell started out with synthetic DNA and its original cytoplasm. The new genome booted up the recipient cell to start producing only proteins that normally would be found in the copied goat *Mycoplasma*. The modified cell reproduced to confirm that new cells really looked and behaved like *M. mycoides*. The research paves the way for the ultimate goal; designing organisms that worked differently from the way nature intended for a wide range of uses i.e.

new fuels, better way to clean water and faster vaccine production etc.

Important applications of transgenic technology

Bio steel from goats: Nexia Biotechnologies Inc, Canada has developed transgenic goats to produce 'Bio steel' in their milk, which is spider silk protein, stronger and more flexible than steel. It can be used for manufacturing bullet proof vests and in aerospace industry. Company has developed an approach to goat transgenics designed to enable rapid progress to be made from construct design to produce recombinant protein in milk; product manufactured by it is 'BELE' (bred early, lactate early) transgenic goat system. It has short generation interval, early sexual maturity, multiple offspring, lack of seasonality and good milk yields.

Xenogenic cells and tissues: Production of xenogenic cells and tissues are other areas of application of this technology. Xenogenic cells, in particular from the pig and goat hold great promise for successful cell therapies for human patients because these cells can be implanted at the optimum therapeutic location (Edge *et al.*, 1998).

Production of a new class of antibiotics and other pharmaceuticals: With the increasing antibiotic resistance to bacteria, there is a growing need to develop new classes of anti-microbial agents - cationic and antimicrobial peptides (AMPs) have many of such desired peptides belonging to the innate immune defense, which acts as a first barrier ahead of humoral and cellular immune systems and neutralizes bacteria by interacting specifically with their cell membranes. Goat, sheep and other farm animals can be exploited for the production of new class of antibiotics by using transgenic approach. GTC Bio therapeutics Inc, USA in 2009 has claimed to come out with genetically engineered goats to make a human protein in their milk that prevents dangerous blood clots formation. The drug produced 'Atryn' is under clearance with FDA- the first drug from a genetically engineered animal to be approved in the USA.

Stem cell technology

In recent years stem cells have acquired tremendous interest in the area of biological research for investigating how an organism develops from single cell zygote and damaged cells are replaced by healthy cells. These cells are increasingly being seen as the promise of a cure for all known diseases. Stem cells are the blank cells (master cells, miracle cells) that can modify into any types of body tissue. The sit on the top of the lineage hierarchy and have the ability to regenerate tissues over a lifetime, therefore can herald a new era in regenerative medicine. The stem cell research is mainly focused on (i) to understand the process of development to learn how specific tissue and organs are formed, (ii) to understand what disturbances occur in cells to cause disease and (iii) to study therapeutic value of stem cells. This uniqueness makes stem cells most promising to treat a number of debiliting diseases of human nature. Stem cells also have the potential for developing organs and tissues which are used for organ replacement that are diseased or destroyed.

Contrary to popular perception, stem cells can be sourced from more than on site of the human body. These two broad categories of mammalian stem cells are embryonic stem cells derived from the blastocyst and the adult stem cells, which are sourced from the adult tissues (cord blood, placenta, liver, bone marrow, pulp of milk teeth and endometrial linings etc.). Embryonic stem cells are pluripotent cells that can be maintained in an undifferentiated state. In non adherent culture they aggregate to form embryoid bodies (EBs) that differentiate into primordial ectoderm, mesoderm and endoderm that can further differentiate into progenitors of organ-specific cell types.

Application of stem cell research in animal production: The stem cell technology in animal science also has the potential to improve the quality of life by producing genetically manoeuvred animals and food products by cloning to maintain animal biodiversity and continuation of endangered breeds of livestock, drug testing, animal models for male infertility and iron deficient anaemia and enhancing better understanding of human body functions. Important applications of stem cells technology in animal production are:

- Transgenic animal models for male infertility and animal models for iron deficient anaemia.
- Faster multiplication of animals with rare production potential by using totipotent stem cells.
- Use in veterinary therapeutics (production of pharmaceuticals proteins).

Realizing the potential of stem cell research the Department of Biotechnology (DBT) has allocated substantial funds over the last five years towards basic and applied research in stem cell technology. Premier institutes in India carry out stem cell research in collaboration with DBT and various medical and veterinary institutions. They include Centre for Stem Cell Research (CSCR), Vellore and National Centre for Cell Sciences (NCCS), Pune. Other institutes where research work on stem cells is actively progressing include Reliance Life Sciences, Navi Mumbai and hospitals such as All India Institute of Medical Sciences (AIIMS), New Delhi, Jaslok Hospital, Mumbai and L.V. Prasad Eye Institute, Hyderabad. In India Professionals and general public have conflicting thoughts concerning embryonic stem cells as far as its research, medical, societal, ethical and religious implications are concerned. Research on embryonic stem cell research is a controversial issue globally because of the differing views on when a human life begins. Internationally, there are many universities such as Harvard Stem Cell Institute, McGowan Institute for Regenerative Medicine at University of Pittsburgh, Stanford University School of Medicine, and University of Maryland, USA which have separate divisions focusing on stem cell research. In a major breakthrough, recently Swedish scientists have cultured human embryonic stem cells (ESC) completely under chemically defined environment without using other cells or substances from animals. Instead they are cultured on a matrix of a single human protein Laminin 511.

Technique to control kiddings

The induction and synchronization of kidding is an effective and promising reproductive management tool for programming of parturition within a close time interval. Technique is useful in reducing neonatal mortality, handling problems related to gestation where it is desirable to induce parturition for clinical reasons. Furthermore in commercial flocks for profitable goat production, technique is much more relevant in terms of use of farm personnel's, economize time where parturitions are normally spread over a time period (Bosu *et al.*, 1979; Ott *et al.*, 1980; Thakur and Verma, 1990). Prostaglandins or its analogues alone or in combinations with other hormones (dexamethasone, oxytocin) have been successfully employed to control parturition in goats (Ott *et al.*, 1980; Jain and Madan, 1989; Thakur and Verma, 1990; Goel *et al.*, 1994 b; Giri *et al.*, 2004, 2005) with varying success of acceptable degree. Most of these combinations did not affect various parturition related traits (placental expulsion time, kid survival and birth weight) or post-partum fertility. Prostaglandins responded better than other combinations and peak kiddings occurred between 30 and 35 hr following administration of hormone therapy.

Training of subject matter specialists and livestock owners

The ultimate role of smail ruminant production in providing mankind with protein of animal origin is well known in the society. Meat is one of the ready sources of protein of high biological value. It is a fact that research efforts alone are of limited significance unless scientific knowledge percolates to its ultimate beneficiaries. In this context, it is imperative to further disseminate scientific knowledge and impart trainings to professionals, veterinarians, technicians, progressive farmers as well as farmers engaged in goat rearing activities. It will prevent wastage of technical knowledge/expertise and know-how emerging from research efforts. Knowledge of basic biology of species used to produce meat, milk, fiber, skin and hair is a prerequisite for the development of any production or reproduction programme.

Acknowledgement

The author wish to thank Dr. D. Swarup, Director, CIRG, Makhdoom for permitting to present this paper. Author is also thankful to the organizing committee of National Seminar on "Prospects and Retrospect of Small Ruminant and Rabbit Production: Contribution to Socio-economic Security", Jaipur for inviting me to present this paper.

References

Agrawal, K.P. and Goel, A.K. 1991. Production of elite Jamunapari kids by embryo transfer technology. Indian Journal of Animal Reproduction 12: 78-80.

Agrawal, K.P., Goel, A.K. and Tyagi, S. 1991. Successful non-surgical embryo recovery from a goat. Indian Journal of Experimental Biology 29: 1144.

Akinlosotu, B.A. and Wilder, C.D. 1993. Fertility and blood progesterone levels following LHRH - induced super ovulation in FSH treated anoestrous goats. Theriogenology 40: 895-904.

Avdi, M., Alifakiotis, T. and Driancourt, M.A. 1991. Effect of active immunization against androsterodione on reproductive and productive performance of dairy goats. Livestock Production Science 29: 87-92.

Baldassarre, H., Wang, B., Keefer, C.L., Lazaris, A. and Karatzas, C.N. 2004. State of the art in the production of transgenic goats. Reproduction Fertility and Development 16: 465-470.

Baril, G. and Saumande, J. 2000. Hormonal treatments to control time of ovulation and fertility of goats. In: Proc. 7th International Conference on Goats, France 15-21 May, pp 400-402.

Baril, G., Casamitjana, P., Perrin, J. and Vallet, J.C. 1988. Embryo production, freezing and transfer in Angora, Alpine and Saanen goats. In: Proc. 4th Meeting of European Embryo Transfer Association, Lyon, pp 67-93.

Bazer, F.W. and Spencer, T.E. 2005. Reproductive biology in the era of genomics biology. Theriogenology 64: 442-446.

Bijurkar, R.G., Tandle, M.K., Sonwane, S.D. and Honnappagol, S.S. 2004. Effect of eCG on reproductive performance of Bidri goats. In: Proc. XX Annual Convention of ISSAR and National Symposium on Advanced Reproductive Technologies for Management of Fertility in Livestock, Anjora, Drug 14-16 December, p.150.

Boscos, C.M., Samartizi, F.C., Lymberopolous, A.G., Stefanakis, A. and Belibaski, S. 2003. Assessment of progesterone concentration using Enzyme Immuno Assay for early pregnancy diagnosis in sheep and goats. Reproduction in Domestic Animals 38: 170-174.

Bosu, W.T.K., Serna, J. and Barker, A.W. 1979. Peripheral plasma levels of progesterone in pregnant goats and non - pregnant goats treated with prostaglandin F2 alpha. Theriogenology 11: 131-148.

Cahil, L.P. and Dufour, J. 1979. Follicular population in ewe under different gonadotropin levels. Annals de Biologie Animale Biochimie Biophysique 19:1475-1481.

Carmenate, C., Pedroso, R., Gonzalez, N., Arencibia, J. and Alvarez, T. 1992. Pregnancy diagnosis in goats on the basis of blood progesterone concentration using radio immuno assay. Revista Cabana de Reproduction Animal 17-18: 93-100.

Chandolia, R.K., Pradeep, S.V., Kumar Jitendra and Tayal, R. 2005. Comparative ultra sonographic foetal studies in goats and dog. Indian Journal of Animal Sciences 75: 1054-1056.

Chauhan, M.S., Katiyar, P.K. and Madan, M.L. 1997. In vitro production of blastocyst of goat, sheep and buffaloes. Indian Journal of Animal Sciences 67: 394-396.

Cognie, Y. 1999. State of the art in sheep goat embryo transfer. Theriogenology 51: 105-116.

Cognie, Y., Baril, G., Paulin, N. and Marimillod, P. 2003. Current status of embryo technologies in sheep and goat. Theriogenology 59: 171-188.

Cummins, J.M. 2001.Cytoplasmic inheritance and its implications for animal biotechnology. Theriogenology 55: 1381-1399.

Daroliya, R.K., Verma, S.K. and Chandolia, R.K. 1990. Increasing lambing performance of ewes by active immunization with poly andro albumin. Theriogenology 33: 1143-1150.

De Smedt, V., Crozet, N., Ahmed Ali, M., Martino, A, and Cognie, Y. 1992. In vitro maturation and fertilization of goat oocytes. Theriogenology 37: 1049-1060.

Dhoble, R.L., Deokate, K.R., Gaikwad, S.M. and Sawale, A.G. 2005a. Ultrasonic examination for confirmation of twins in goats. In: Proc. XXI Annual Convention of ISSAR and National Symposium on Recent Trends and Innovations in Animal Reproduction, 23-25 November, Jammu, p. 208.

Dhoble, R.L., Gaikwad, S.M. and Sawale, A.G. 2005b. B–mode real time ultrasonography for early pregnancy diagnosis in goats. In: Proc. XXI Annual Convention of ISSAR and National Symposium on Recent Trends and Innovations in Animal Reproduction, 23-25 November, Jammu, pp. 234-237.

Dietrich, E., Hennies, M., Holtz, W. and Voglmayr, J.K. 1995. Immunization of goats against human inhibin alpha subunit: effects on inhibin binding, mating behavior ovarian activity and embryo yield. Animal Reproduction Science 39: 119-128.

Driancourt, M.A., Philipon, P., Terqui, M., Molenat, G., Mirman, B., Louault, C., Avdi, M., Folch, J., and Cognie, Y. 1990. Possibilities for immunization against steroids to improve ovulation rate and litter size in sheep and goats. Production Animals 3: 31-37.

Ebert, K.M., Selgrath, J.P., Ditullio, P., Denman, J., Smith, T.E., Memon, M.A., Schiendler, J.E., Monastersky, G.M., Vitale, J.E. and Gordan, K. 1991. Transgenic production of a variant of human tissue type plasminogen activator in goat milk: generation of transgenic goats and analysis of expression. Biotechnology 9: 835-838.

Edge, A.S.B., Gosse, M.E. and Dinsmore, J. 1998. Xenogenic cell therapy: developments in porcine cell implantation. Cell Transplant 7: 525-539.

FAO. 1998. Secondary Guidelines: management of small population at risk. Food and Agriculture Organization of the United Nations, Rome, Italy, p. 215.

FAO. 2000. World Watch List of Domestic Animal Diversity. Third Edition, Rome, Italy, p. 726.

Flemming, S.A., Camp, S.D. Van and Chapin, H M. 1990. Serum progesterone determination as an aid for pregnancy diagnosis in goats bred out of the season. Canadian Veterinary Journal 31: 104-107.

Galal, S. 2005. Biodiversity in goats. Small Ruminant Research 60: 75-81.

Galli, C. and Lazzari, G. 2003. In vitro production of embryos in farm animals. In. Proc. 19th Meeting of Embryo Transfer Association (Rostok), p. 93.

Ganaie, B.A., Khan, M.Z., Makhdoomi, D.M., Islam, R. and Wani, G.M. 2009a. Plasma progesterone profile during gestation and peri-partum period in Corriedale sheep. Indian Journal of Animal Reproduction 30: 18-21.

Ganaie, B.A., Khan, M.Z., Qureshi, S., Islam, R. and Wani, G.M. 2009. Early pregnancy diagnosis in Corriedale sheep by real time B-mode ultrasonography. Indian Journal of Animal Reproduction 30: 45-49.

Giri, S., Singh, M.P., Sinha, N.K. and Sinha, M.P. 2004. Induction of parturition with prostaglandin in Black Bengal goats. In: Proc. 20th Annual Convention of ISSAR and National Symposium on Advanced Reproductive Technologies for Management of Fertility in Livestock, 14-16 December, Anjora, Durg p. 156.

Giri, S., Singh, M.P., Sinha, A.K. and Sinha, M.P. 2005. Induction of parturition in goat with prostaglandin, corticosteroid and oxytocin. In: Proc. XXI Annual Convention of ISSAR and National Symposium on Recent Trends and Innovations in Animal Reproduction, 23-25 November, Jammu p 230.

Goel, A.K. and Agrawal, K.P.1998a. Oestrus synchronization in cyclic goats following lutalyse administration. Indian Journal of Animal Sciences 68: 155-156.

Goel, A.K. and Agrawal, K.P. 1998b. Efficacy of different gonadotrophins on super ovulation and embryo recovery in Jamunapari goats. Indian Journal of Animal Reproduction 19: 102-105.

Goel, A.K. and Agrawal, K.P. 1998c. Super ovulatory responses and embryo recovery rate in Sirohi goats treated twice with Super - Ov. Indian Veterinary Journal 75: 1092-1094.

Goel, A.K. and Agrawal, K.P. 1998d. Super ovulation and embryo collection in Sirohi goats treated with super - Ov. Indian Journal of Animal Sciences 68: 153-154.

Goel, A.K. and Agrawal, K.P. 2000. Oestrus synchronization in Jakhrana goats following administration of prostaglandin and intra - vaginal sponges. Indian Journal of Animal Sciences 70: 714-175.

Goel, A.K. and Agrawal, K.P. 2002. Intra-cervical recovery of caprine embryos. In: Proc. 9th International Congress on Biotechnology in Animal Reproduction, 2-4 December, Chennai p 215.

Goel, A.K. and Agrawal, K.P. 2003. Ovulation in Jakhrana goats native to tropical climates. Small Ruminant Research 50: 209-212.

Goel, A.K. and Agrawal, K.P. 2005. Ovulatory response and embryo yield in Jakhrana goats following treatments with PMSG and FSH. Tropical Animal Health and Production 37: 549-558.

Goel, A.K., Agrawal, K.P. and Sinha, N.K. 1993. Application of MOET in production of elite goats. Indian Journal of Animal Sciences 64: 281-282.

Goel, A.K., Agrawal, K.P. and Sinha, N.K. 1994a. Production of elite kids using low milk producing does as foster mothers. In: Proc. International Symposium Cell Signaling and on implantation AIIMS, New Delhi, 21-23 November, pp. 39-40.

Goel, A.K., Tyagi, S., Sinha, N.K. and Agrawal, K.P. 1994b. Induction and synchronization of parturition in goats. Indian Journal of Animal Physiology 2: 56-59.

Goel, A.K., Tyagi, S. and Agrawal, K.P. 1995. Non - surgical collection of embryos from goats. Indian Journal of Animal Sciences 65: 293-296.

Goel, A.K., Kharche, S.D., Jindal, S.K. and Sinha, N.K. 2006. Embryo production and kids born through embryo transfer in Jakhrana goats treated with pFSH. Indian Journal of Animal Reproduction 27: 75-76.

Goel, A.K., Kharche, S.D. and Jindal. S.K. 2009a. Efficacy of progestin implant - eCG to increase kidding rate in post -partum anoestrus Jakhrana goats. Indian Journal of Animal Sciences 79: 473-476.

Goel, A.K., Kharche, S.D. and Jindal, S.K. 2009b. Determination of early pregnancy and embryonic development by trans rectal ultrasonography in goats. Indian Journal of Animal Sciences 79: 476-478.

Gonzalez, F., Calero, P., Quesada, E., Garbayo, J.M. and Beckers, J.F. 2000. The Pregnancy Associated Glycoproteins (Pags): fundamental and clinical approach. In: Proc. 7th International Conference on Goats, France 15-21 May, pp. 413-415.

Gonzalez-Bulnes, A., Garcia-Garcia, R.M., Castellanous, V., Santiago-Moreno, J., Dominguez, V., Lopez-Sebastian, A., Tregurres, J.A.F. and Cocero, M.J. 2003. Influence of maternal environment on the number of transferable embryos obtained in response to superovulatory FSH treatment in ewes. Reproduction Nutrition and Development 43: 17-28.

Gordon, J.W., Scangos, G.A., Plotkin, D.J., Barbosa, J.A. and Ruddle, F.H. 1980. Genetic transformation of mouse embryos by microinjection of purified DNA. In: Proc. National Academy of Science, USA 77: 7380-7384.

Greyling, J.P.C and Van Der Nest, M. 2000. Multiovulation and embryo transfer (MOET) in South African Boer and Indigenous goats. In: Proc. 7th International Conference on Goats, France, 15-21 May, pp. 411-412.

Greyling, J.P.C., Van Der Nest, M., Schwallbach, L.M.J. and Muller, T. 2002. Super ovulation and embryo transfer in South African Boer and Indigenous Feral goats. Small Ruminant Research 43: 45-51.

Grupp, T. 1991. Investigations on dilation of the cervix and transcervical embryo recovery in ewes and goats. Thesis, Ludwig Maximilians Universitat Munchen, Germany, p 144.

Han, Y., Meintjes, M., Graff, K.J., Denniston, R.S., Ebert, K.M., Ziomek, C. and Godke, R.A. 1996. Offspring born from the transfer of caprine blastocysts after IVM/IVF and IVC of transvaginal ultrasound-guided aspirated oocytes. Theriogenology 45: 357.

Hanada, A. 1985. In vitro fertilization in goats. Japanese Journal of Animal Reproduction 31: 21-26.

Holtz, W., Pereira, R.J.T.A., Suyadi Wang, X.L., Padilla, G. and Sohnrey, B. 2000. Collection of goat embryo via trans- cervical route. In: Proc. 7th InternationalConference on Goats, France, 15-21 May pp 490-491.

Hoque, M., Mehrotra, S., Agarwal, S.K. and Shankar Uma. 2005. Comparative evaluation of pregnancy by trans-rectal and trans-abdominal ultra sonographic scanning in Black Bengal goats. In: Proc. XXI Annual Convention of ISSAR and National Symposium on Recent Trends and Innovations in Animal Reproduction, 23-25 November, Jammu, p 183.

Humblot, P., Montigny, G. De, Jeanguyot, N., Tetedoie, F., Payen, B., Thibier, M. and Sasser, R.G. 1990. Pregnancy specific protein B and progesterone concentration in French Alpine goats throughout gestation. Journal Reproduction and Fertility 89: 205-212.

Jabbour, H.N., Ryan, J.P., Evans, G. and Maxwell, W.M.C. 1991. Effects of season, GnRH administration and lupin supplementation on the ovarian and endocrine responses of Merino ewes treated with PMSG and FSH-p to induce super ovulation. Reproduction Fertility and Development 3: 699-707.

Jain, G.C. and Madan, M. 1989. Plasma prostaglandin F, oestradiol 17 ß, Cortisol and progesterone in induced parturient goats. International Journal of Animal Sciences 4: 152-156.

Jeoujong Shyu, Chiung, H., Cheng, Ying-Ling W.U., Chau Hwo, Chi. 2005. The application of ultra sonography in pregnancy diagnosis of goat in Taiwan. Animal Breeding Abstracts 73: p 401.

Kahn, W. 1994. Veterinary Reproductive Ultrasonography. English translation by Volkmann and R.M. Kenny. Mosby – Wolfe, London.

Kano, T., Obata, Y., Wu, Q., Niwa, K., Ono, Y., Yamamoto, Y., Park, E.S., Seo, J.S. and Ogawa, H. 2004. Birth of parthenogenetic mice that can develop to adulthood. Nature 428: 860-864.

Kaushik, H.K., Bugalia, N.S., Khar, S.K. and Rana, Z.S. 1992. Plasma progesterone and oestradiol 17-Beta profiles during pregnancy in goats. In: Recent Advances in Goat Production. In: Proc. 5th International Conference on Goats (R.R. Lokeshwar, Ed.), 2-8 March, New Delhi, pp. 1298-1308.

Kelly, R.W., Owens, J.L., Crosbie, S.F., Mc Natty, K.P. and Judson, N. 1983. Influence of Booroola Merino genotype on responsiveness of ewe to pregnant mare serum gonadotropin, luteal tissue weight and peripheral progesterone concentration. Animal Reproduction Science 6: 199-207.

Keskintepe, L., Luvoni, G.C., Bassiony, M.M. and Brackett, B.G. 1994. In vitro caprine blastocyst development from immature oocytes. Biology of Reproduction 50(suppl. I): 189.

Kharche, S.D., Goel, A.K., Jindal, S.K. and Sinha, N.K. 2005a. Efficacy of Crestar ear implant for oestrus synchronization and super ovulation with PMSG and FSH-P in goats. In: Proc. XXI Annual Convention of ISSAR and National Symposium on Recent Trends and Innovations in Animal Reproduction, 23-25 November, Jammu, p 95.

Kharche, S.D., Sharma, G.T. and Majumdar, A.C. 2005b. In vitro maturation and fertilization of goat oocytes vitrified at germinal vesicle stage. Small Ruminant Research 57: 81-84.

Kharche, S.D., Goel, A.K., Jindal, S.K. and Sinha, N.K. 2006. In vitro maturation of caprine oocytes in different concentrations of oestrous goat serum. Small Ruminant Research 64: 186-189.

Kharche, S.D., Goel, A.K., Jindal, S.K. and Sinha, N.K. 2008a. Birth of a female kid from *in-vitro* matured and fertilized caprine oocytes. Indian Journal of Animal Sciences 78: 680-685.

Kharche, S.D., Goel, A.K., Jindal, S.K., Sinha, N.K. and Yadav, P. 2008b. Effect of somatic cell co-culture on cleavage and development of *in-vitro* fertilized caprine embryos. Indian Journal of Animal Sciences 78: 686-692.

Kharche, S.D., Yadav, E.N., Goel, A.K., Jindal, S.K. and Sinha, N.K. 2008c. Influence of culture media on *in-vitro* fertilization of goat oocytes. Indian Journal of Animal Sciences 78: 1075-1077.

Kharche, S.D., Goel, A.K., Jindal, S.K., Yadav, E.N., Yadav, P. and Sinha, N.K. 2009. Effect of serum albumin supplementation on *in-vitro* capacitation and fertilization of caprine oocytes. Small Ruminant Research 81: 85-89.

Kharche, S.D., Goel, P., Jha, B.K., Goel, A.K. and Jindal, S.K. 2011. Factors influencing in vitro embryo production efficiency of caprine oocytes: A Review. Indian Journal of Animal Sciences 81: 344-361.

Koeman, J., Keefer, C.L., Baldassarre, H. and Downey, B.R. 2003. Developmental competence of prepubertal and adult goat oocytes cultured in semi-defined media following laparoscopic recovery. Theriogenology 60: 879-889.

Kumar Jitendra, Chandolia, R.K. and Verma, S.K. 2005. Ultra sonographic imaging of early fetal development in Black Bengal goats. Indian Journal of Animal Reproduction 26: 39-42.

Lagutina, I., Lazzari, G., Duchi, R., Turini, P., Tessaro, I., Brunetti, D., Colleoni, S., Crotti, G. and Galli, C. 2007. Comparative aspects of somatic cell nuclear transfer with conventional and zona free method in cattle, horse, pig and sheep. Theriogenology 67: 90-98.

Leboeuf, B., Nercy, C. and De Ruyter, T. 1994. L'insémination artificielle caprine au Rwanda. Adaptation à la chèvre rwandaise de la méthode utilisée pour les races laitières européennes. Revue d'Elevage et de Médecine Vétérinaire des Pays Tropicaux 47: 240-243.

Mahmood, S., Kaul, G.L. and Biswas, J.C. 1991. Comparative efficacy of FSH-p and PMSG on super ovulation in Patina goats. Theriogenology 35: 1191-1196.

Malakar, D., Das, S.K. and Goswami, S. 2005. IVF born male kid and surrogate marker produced normal offspring after natural service. In: Proc. International Symposium Stem Cells, Premises and Promises for Research and Therapeutics at NIRRH, Parel, Mumbai p. 43.

Manchaca, A., Pinczak, A. and Rubianes, E. 2002. Follicular recruitment and ovulatory response to FSH treatment initiated on day 0 day 3 post ovulation in goats. Theriogenology 58: 1713-1721.

Mani, A.U., Watson, E.D. and Mckelvey, W.A.C. 1994. The effects of sub nutrition before or after embryo transfer on pregnancy rate and embryo survival in does. Theriogenology 41: 1673 -1678.

Medan, M., Watanabe, G., Absy, G., Sasaki, K., Sharawy, S. and Taya, K. 2004. Early pregnancy diagnosis by means of ultrasonography as a method of improving reproductive efficiency in goats. Journal of Reproduction and Development 50: 391-397.

Mishra, O.P., Gawande, P.G., Nema, R.K. and Tiwari, S.K. 2004. Oestrus behavior and super ovulatory response in Black Bengal goats (*Capra hircus*) following administration of prostaglandin and gonadotropins. Asian - Australasian Journal of Animal Sciences 17: 1374-1377.

Naqvi, S.M.K. and Gulyani, R. 1995. Recent advances in ovine embryo transfer technology In: Proc. III National Seminar on Sheep and Goat Production and Utilization, CSWRI, Avikanagar pp. 193-202.

Naqvi, S.M.K. and Gulyani, R. 1999. Ovarian response and embryo recovery to different superovulatory regimens in Rambouillet ewes under semi-arid conditions. Small Ruminant Research 34: 127-131.

Naqvi, S.M.K. and Madan, M.L.1997. Influence of caffeine on heparin treated spermatozoa for in vitro fertilization of in vitro matured ovine oocytes. International Journal of Animal Sciences 12: 65-67.

Naqvi, S.M.K, Madan, M.L., Manik, R.S., Chauhan, M.S. and Singla, S.K. 1992. In vitro development of ovine oocytes matured and fertilized in vitro to compact morula in co-culture system of oviductal cells and conditioned medium. In: Proc. 12th International Conference on Animal Reproduction 3: 1327-1329.

Naqvi, S.M.K., Joshi Anil, Das, G.K. and Mittal, J.P. 2001. Development and application of ovine reproductive technologies: An Indian Experience. Small Ruminant Research 39: 199-208.

Naqvi, S.M.K., Gulyani, R., Joshi, A., Das, G.K. and Mittal, J.P. 2002. Effect of dietary regimens on ovarian response and embryo production of sheep in tropics. Small Ruminant Research 46: 167-171.

Naqvi, S.M.K., Gulyani, R., Joshi, A., Maurya, V.P., Kumar, D., Mittal, J.P. and Singh, V.K. 2006a. Production of 24 transferable embryos in one flush by a Garole micro sheep. Veterinary Record 158: 414-415.

Naqvi, S.M.K., Joshi, A., Gulyani, R., Kumar, D., Kolte, A.P., Kumar, S., Maurya, V.P., Saha, S., Mittal, J.P. and Singh, V.K. 2006b. Production of prolific micro sheep by embryo transfer into large non-prolific sheep. Veterinary Record 159: 522-526.

Naqvi, S.M.K., Joshi, A. and Maurya, V.P. 2007. Application of reproductive technologies for improving reproductive efficiency of sheep. A review. Indian Journal of Small Ruminants 13: 115-143.

Naqvi, S.M.K., Joshi, A., Gulyani, R. and Kumar, D. 2009. Effect of passive immunization against synthetic inhibin peptides on estrus response and ovulation rate in Malpura owes. Indian Journal of Small Ruminants 15: 194-199.

Niemann, H. and Kues, W.A. 2003. Application of transgenesis in livestock for agriculture and biomedicine. Animal Reproduction Science 79: 291-317.

Noshari, M.A. and Holtz, W. 1995. Super ovulation of goats with purified pFSH supplemented with defined amounts of pLH. Theriogenology 43: 979-802.

O'Brien, J.K., Hollinshead and Maxwell, W.M.C. 2004. In vitro development capacity of in vitro produced embryos derived from sex-sorted and re-cryopreserved frozen-thawed ram sperm. Reproduction Fertility and Development 16: 286.

Oliveira, V.S., Visintin, J.A. and Gonzalez, C.I.M.1992. Non-surgical collection of embryos in goats. In: Pre Conference Proc. (Vol. I), V International Conference on Goats, New Delhi, 2-8 March p 362.

Ott, R.S., Nelson, D.R., Memon, M.A., Lock, T.F. and Hixon, J.E. 1980. Dexamethasone and Prostaglandin F_2 alpha for induction of parturition in goats. In: Proc. IX International Conference on Goat Production and AI, Madrid (Spain), 16-20 June, pp. 492-495.

Padilla Rivas, G.R., Sohnrey, B. and Holtz, W. 2005. Early pregnancy detection by real time ultra sonography in Boer goats. Small Ruminants Research 58: 87-92.

Paterson, L., DeSouza, P., Ritchie, W., King, T. and Wilmut, I. 2003. Application of reproductive biotechnologies in animals: implication and potentials. Animal Reproduction Science 79: 137-143.

Patil, A.D., Raughuwanshi, D.S., Kumbhar, U.B. and Maini, S. 2009. Efficacy of herbal heat inducers and mineral supplementations for inducing fertility in postpartum anoestrus Deccani sheep. Indian Journal of Animal Reproduction 30: 67-69.

Pawshe, C.H., Jain, S.K. and Totey, S.M. 1993. Effect of commercially available follicle stimulating hormone on in vitro maturation of goat oocytes. Indian Journal of Animal Reproduction 14: 69-71.

Pendleton, R.J., Youngs, C.R., Rorie, R.W., Memon, M.A. and Godke, R.A. 1992. Follicle stimulating hormone versus pregnant mare serum gonadotrophin for super ovulation of dairy goats. Small Ruminant Research 8: 217-224.

Pereira, R.J.T.A., Agoub, M. and Holtz, W. 1995. Birth of live kids after transfer of in vitro matured and fertilized embryos. In: Proc. 11th Meeting of European Embyro Transfer Association (Hanover), p. 224.

Pereira, R.J.T.A., Sohnrey, B. and Holtz, W. 1998. Non-surgical embryo collection in goats treated with prostaglandin F2Ü and oxytocin. Journal of Animal Science 76: 360-363.

Piper, L.R., Bindon, B.M., Curtis, Y.M., Cheers, M.A. and Nethery, R.D. 1982. Response to PMSG in Merino and Booroola Merino sheep. In: Proc. Australian Society of Reproductive Biology 14: 82.

Restall, B.J., Milton, J.T.B., Klong-yutti, P. and Kochapakdee, S. 1990. Pregnancy diagnosis in Thai native goats. Theriogenology 34: 313-317.

Ritar, A.J., Salamon, S., Ball, P.D. and O'May, P.J. 1989. Ovulation and fertility in goats after intravaginal device-PMSG treatment. Small Ruminant Research 2: 323-331.

Rosnina, Y., Jainudeen, M.R. and Nihayah, M. 1992. Super ovulation and egg recovery in goats in tropics. Veterinary Record 130: 97-99.

String fellow, D.A., Givens, M.D. and Waldrop, J.G. 2004. Biosecurity issues associated with current and emerging technologies. Reproduction Fertility and Development 16: 93-120.

Tervit, H.R., Thompson, J.G.E., James, R.W., Gowers, L.T. and Parton, G.A.J. 1992. Development of improved surgical uterine embryo recovery techniques in sheep. In: Proc. 12th International Congress on Animal Reproduction, The Hague, Netherlands, pp. 820-822.

Thakur, M.S. and Verma, S.K. 1990. Induction of parturition in goats with prostaglandin F2 alpha. Indian Journal of Animal Reproduction 11: 148-152.

Vathsala, M., Sathesh Kumar, S. and Palanisamy, A. 2005. Pregnancy diagnosis in goats using ultra sonography. In: Proc. XXI Annual Convention of ISSAR and National Symposium on Recent Trends and Innovations in Animal Reproduction, Jammu, 23-25 November, p 184.

Wall, R.J. 1996. Transgenic livestock: progress and prospects in the future. Theriogenology 45: 57-68.

Wall, R.J., Hawk, H.W. and Nel, N. 1992. Making transgenic livestock: genetic engineering on large scale. Journal of Cellular Biochemistry 49: 113-120.

Wang, X.L., Beckers, J.F., Brown, R. and Holtz, W. 2000. Ovarian response to exogenous gonadotropins in goats immunized against inhibin. In: Proc. 7th International Conference on Goats, France, 15-21 May, p. 470.

Wang, B., Baldassarre, H., Pierson, J., Cote, F., Gauthier, M. and Naveu, N. 2003. Transgenic goat produced by DNA pronuclear microinjection of in vitro derived zygotes. Molecular Reproduction and Development 63: 437-443.

Wheeler, M.B., Walters, E.M. and Clark, S.G. 2003. Transgenic animals in biomedicine and agriculture: outlook for the future. Animal Reproduction Science 79: 265-289.

Wilmut, I., Schnieke, A.E., McWhir, J., Kind, A.J. and Campbell, K.H. 1997. Viable offspring derived from foetal and adult mammalian cells. Nature 385: 810-813.

Yadav, E.N., Kharche, S.D., Goel, A.K., Jindal, S.K. and Johri, D.K. 2007. Comparative efficacy of different techniques for oocyte recovery from prepubertal goat ovaries. Indian Journal of Animal Sciences 77: 988-990.

Yadav, E.N., Kharche, S.D., Goel, A.K., Jindal, S.K., Sinha, N.K. and Johri, D.K. 2008. Effect of serum source on *in vitro* maturation and fertilization of pre pubertal goat oocytes. Indian Journal of Animal Sciences 78:146-149.

Younis, A.I., Zuelke, K.A., Harper, K.M., Oliveira, M.A.L. and Brackett, B.G. 1991. In vitro fertilization of goat embryos. Biology of Reproduction 44: 1177-1182.

❑❑❑

Chapter 7

The State of the Art in the Artificial Insemination of Sheep

S.M.K. Naqvi and Davendra Kumar
Division of Physiology and Biochemistry, Central Sheep and Wool Research Institute, Avikanagar- 304 501 (Rajasthan)

Artificial insemination (AI) is not only one of the oldest but also the most widely applied reproductive technology worldwide in livestock improvement programmes (Thibier and Guerin, 2000). The AI in farm animals is the first generation of reproductive biotechnologies, which has developed over the last six decades and being applied in a variety of means to increase the genetic merit of animals and efficiency of progeny testing schemes. The AI in sheep on a major scale was started in Russia during the fourth decade of last century with the establishment of AI facilities and programme involving a group of flocks. Extensive AI programme in sheep were also adopted in China which later spread to central Europe. It was then widely applied commercially in France and Brazil (Gordon, 1997). The techniques for AI in sheep have been developed, simplified and improved during the last few decades. Nevertheless, AI has not yet received universal acceptance in sheep industry due to several technical and economical reasons. However, with the advent of recent advances in reproductive technologies, the efficiency of AI in terms of conception and lambing rate has improved. The success of AI in sheep is dependent on many intrinsic and extrinsic factors (Anel *et al.*, 2006). The most potent intrinsic factors are related to reproductive activity and genital morphology of female and production of quality semen by male. Extrinsic factors include environmental conditions, sanitary status, handling and management of animals, and the technique of AI used (Shackell *et al.*, 1990; Donovan *et al.*, 2004; Paulenz *et al.*, 2004).

The ideal technique for AI, in any species, is transcervical intrauterine deposition of sperm. Although, in sheep efforts are still going on worldwide but till date, no perfect technique has been developed to deposit sperm inside the uterus through the cervix. Therefore, in sheep, the semen is deposited into the vagina or at the os of cervix. As far as AI with fresh semen is concerned there is no problem and acceptable fertility results have been achieved. But, inspite of good post-thaw sperm motility of frozen ram semen compared to other species, the vaginal or cervical insemination with frozen-thawed semen usually results in unacceptably low fertility. On the basis of site of semen deposition and instruments used, methods of AI in sheep are broadly classified as: i) vaginal insemination, ii) cervical insemination, iii) laparoscopic intrauterine insemination (IUAI) and iv) transcervical intrauterine insemination (TCAI). These methods differ with each other in their effectiveness, cost and complexity and have been tried with varying success by different workers. The first two methods involve the use of fresh diluted or short-term preserved semen whereas the next two are complex and generally used for frozen-thawed semen.

Artificial insemination with liquid semen

To date the success of AI in sheep is limited to liquid semen (Maxwell and Salamon, 1993). The main methods of short-term preservation of ram semen in a liquid state are based on storage at reduced temperature (0-5 or 10-15°C) by reversible inactivation of spermatozoa. The spermatozoa deteriorate on storage irrespective of the diluents composition, dilution rate and temperature leading to reduce motility, a decline in viability and consequent decrease in fertility after 24 hr of preservation (Maxwell and Salamon, 1993). Gillen *et al.* (2004) summarized the critical studies on liquid semen for AI in sheep and concluded that fertility decreased at the rate of 10-35% per day of storage. The lambing rate following use of liquid semen stored for one, two and three days were 45-50, 25-30 and 15-20%, respectively. For achieving good fertility with liquid semen, a diluent - Egg yolk

McIllvaine glucose (EYMG) has been developed at CSWRI (Srivastava *et al.*, 1987; Mathur *et al.*, 1993).

Vaginal insemination: Vaginal insemination is deposition of semen into anterior vagina without an attempt to locate the cervix. The ewes in heat are restrained in head down position by lifting the hind legs. A plastic or glass pipette connected to a 1.0 ml syringe is loaded with semen and carefully introduced into vagina. This method is simplest and quickest but gives variable and poor results of lambing and hence generally not recommended.

Cervical insemination: In sheep, cervical penetration with the catheter is generally not possible due to the anatomical structure of the cervix. Semen is generally deposited at os-cervix or slightly anterior. Ewes are presented in head down position over the rail. Vulva and external genitalia are washed and cleaned. A glass speculum is introduced into vagina and cervix is viewed with the aid of headlight / daylight. The cervix can be located by gentle manipulation of speculum into the anterior vagina. Attempt is made to introduce pipette as deep as possible without using force. This is relatively easy, economic and most commonly used technique of AI in sheep and involves deposition of semen into the first fold of the os-cervix.

Artificial insemination at farmer's flock: CSWRI, Avikanagar launched an AI programme for improving rural sheep of semi-arid region of the country using liquid semen of exotic Awassi and native Patanwadi rams. Awassi is a triple purpose sheep suitable for mutton, milk and wool production of South West Asia (Epstein, 1985). The climatic features of its natural habitat are similar to semi-arid regions of India. Thus there seems to be good scope for introducing productive and adaptive merits of Awassi breed into native sheep for enhancing their productive performance. Semen was obtained daily in the morning from adult rams. Ejaculates having good semen quality were diluted 1:1 with EYMG diluent and stored in ice containing semen shipper. AI was done daily in estrus ewes for one cycle by depositing 0.1 ml containing 100 million sperm per os. AI with Awassi ram semen was performed in ewes exhibiting natural estrus while with Patanwadi ram semen in ewes exhibiting estrus after induction and synchronization. The results are summarized in table 1.

Table 1 : AI at farmer flocks using fresh diluted ram semen

Breed	Year	No. of ewes inseminated	No. (%) of ewes lambed
Awassi	1995	112	65 (67.7)*
	1996	84	58 (69.0)
	1997	37	14 (46.7)*
	Overall	233	137(65.2)
Patanwadi	2005	63	32 (50.8)**
	2007	23	20 (91)
	2008	33	28 (85)
	2009	65	38 (58.5)
	2010	44	29 (65.9)
	Overall	228	147 (64.5)
Malpura	2009	70	38 (54.3)
Overall		**531**	**322 (60.6)**

* Out of ewes available at the time of lambing; **AI after induction of estrus in anoestrus ewes

Artificial insemination at organized farms: AI with fresh diluted semen has also been conducted by our institute at organized sheep farms. At institute farm a total of 466 inseminations were done in Malpura ewes at natural estrus with Garole semen between the year 1997 and 2006, which resulted in 52.4 per cent lambing (244 out of 466). At Asad Farm located in the Anantpur district of Andhra Pradesh, a fertility trial was conducted under the participatory research approach during autumn 2007 using fresh diluted semen of Dorper rams. Semen samples collected from Dorper rams were evaluated and diluted 1:1 with Egg yolk citrate glucose (EYCG) extender. Fixed time AI was performed in 586 ewes of Nellore Zodpi breed after synchronization of estrus using 0.1 ml (100 million sperm) of fresh diluted semen, which resulted in 67.2 per cent lambing (394 out of 586).

Artificial insemination with frozen ram semen

AI with frozen semen can have a significant impact on genetic improvement by allowing faster multiplication of superior germ plasm. A data based on conservative estimate made by Australian worker had shown that the potential numbers of lambs sired by a ram each year using AI with liquid semen and AI by laparoscopy with frozen semen are 23 and 545 times higher respectively, than natural mating (Maxwell, 1984). Other advantages of frozen storage of ram semen are conservation of superior or endangered germ plasm for future use, insurance against loss of elite sire, transport of semen over long distances etc. However, unlike cattle, AI in sheep using frozen semen has not progressed much (Salamon and Maxwell, 1995; Maxwell and Watson, 1996). Cervical insemination using frozen-thawed semen usually results in unacceptably low (10-40%) fertilization rate (Maxwell and Hewitt, 1986; El-Gaafary *et al.*, 2001; Donovan, *et al.*, 2004; King *et al.*, 2004; Anel *et al.*, 2005; O'Meara *et al.*, 2007). Exceptionally, in Norway, Olesen (1993), Paulenz *et al.* (2004, 2005) and Nordstoga *et al.* (2009) have reported high fertility results (58 and 70%, respectively) after inseminating ewes with frozen semen into either the cervical orifice or deep vagina. It is surprising that, considering the advantages of using frozen semen and the encouraging results found in these studies, there are currently no commercial programmes applying frozen semen for intra-cervical AI, all of them restoring to AI by laparoscopy.

The major factors limiting the successful conception in ewes with the conventional AI technique i.e. os-cervical is the inability of frozen-thawed ram sperm to transit the cervical canal, short duration of sperm survival (Eppleston and Maxwell, 1993) and the complex anatomy of cervix (Halbert *et al.*, 1990a; Eppleston and Maxwell 1993, Naqvi *et al.*, 1998, 2001). The other factors, which also affect the fertility, are composition of diluent, sperm dose, site of insemination and time of insemination. The diluents commonly used for freezing ram semen are egg yolk tris glycerol (EYTG) and egg yolk test glycerol (EYTESTG). In some species, especially the cattle, the interior of the cervix is sufficiently wide to allow passage of an insemination catheter into the uterus. The ewe has an extremely narrow cervix so that semen is deposited at the point where the cervix joins the vagina. The inability to manipulate the ewe cervix per rectum, in the same way as in the cow, is a further difficulty. As a result of cryo-damage, only a small proportion of frozen-thawed spermatozoa are able to establish themselves within the cervix and fewer still traverse its full 5 to 6 cm length to reach the uterus. Sheep cervix also contributes to two major barriers for sperm (i) shape and size of external cervical os and (ii) inner surface of the cervix which has 4-5 annular and non-aligned folds. These barriers also limit the intrusion of the catheter. The problem of the cervical barrier in the ewe can be overcome by deposition of frozen-thawed semen directly into the uterus by laparoscopic IUAI or via the cervix through TCAI.

Laparoscopic intrauterine artificial insemination

With the aid of laparoscope, the semen is directly deposited into the lumen of uterine horn and thus circumventing or by-passing the cervical barrier. This method has invariably improved the fertilization rate over cervical insemination using fresh diluted or frozen-thawed semen. Killen and Caffery (1982) were the first to report intrauterine insemination in sheep with the aid of laparoscope. There has been vast refinement in the instruments in last two decades with greater visualization. The technique has been refined and standardized for use with native sheep at the institute. Conception rate in sheep using IUAI with frozen-thawed semen ranged from 45-80% (Halbert *et al.*, 1990c; Fukui *et al.*, 1993a, b, 1994, 2002, 2007, 2008; Windsor *et al.*, 1994; El-Gaafary *et al.*, 2001; Wulster-Radcliffe *et al.*, 2004; Hill *et al.*, 1998; King *et al.*, 2004; Anel *et al.*, 2005; Hiwasa *et al.*, 2009). The IUAI procedures for frozen semen have also been adopted for use with frozen-thawed sexed semen in sheep (Hollinshead *et al.*, 2002; De Graaf *et al.*, 2007). The results of a study conducted at the institute in a flock of adult Malpura ewes after IUAI with frozen-thawed ram semen in two consecutive cycles are presented in the table 2.

Table 2 : Pregnancy and lambing rates of ewes inseminated with frozen semen using IUAI

Insemination cycle		No. of ewes inseminated	No. (%) of ewes pregnant *	No. (%) of ewes lambed
Trial-1	1	39	25 (64.1)	14 (35.8)
Trial-2	1	63	35 (55.5)	21 (33.3)
	2	28	17 (60.7)	7 (25.0)
Overall		63	52 (82.5)	28 (44.4)

* On the basis of non-return to heat (Source: Naqvi *et al.*, 1997)

Use of frozen–thawed semen, which requires deposition within the uterus for successful fertilisation, still relies on laparoscopic penetration of the abdomen in ewes (Fukui *et al.*, 2010). One of the major advantages of the IUAI has been in obtaining a high rate of fertilization in superovulated ewes for embryo transfer programme. Hormonal treatment of female for superovulation is known to effect sperm transport and viability following natural mating and cervical AI. Number of motile sperm requirement in IUAI is minimal (70-100 Million) as compared to TC AI (500 Million). This could possibly allow more widespread utilization of potential germ plasm of superior merit. It is also possible to perform IUAI in postpartum ewes during weaning and lactating period and bypassing the sperm from hostile environment of involuting uterus. This allows use of early postpartum ewes for embryo collection. The IUAI has been used in sheep only in few countries like Australia, New Zealand, France, U.K. Canada, USA and Argentina. Abbott (1994) estimated that the cost of each AI produced lamb in Australia is between $50 and $80. The cost of per AI in sheep varies depending upon technique, germ plasm demand and condition and location of farm etc.

Transcervical intrauterine artificial insemination

Although, direct deposition of semen in uterus with the aid of laparoscope has resulted in acceptable lambing, but the cost, skill, complicacy and minor surgery involved in the procedure limits its greater utilization. Alternatively, a non-invasive AI technique known as Guelph system of TCAI (GS-TCAI) has been developed in Canada (Halbert *et al.*, 1990a; Buckrell *et al.*, 1992). Despite of chances of the added complication of invasion of the peritoneal cavity from accidental puncturing of the reproductive tract with the inseminating pipette as well as damage to the epithelial lining over the entire length of the cervix in ewes for which penetration is complete, concerted efforts are going on in major sheep rearing countries to develop a simple, cost-effective and non-invasive TCAI technique in order to penetrate the cervix and achieve the acceptable lambing with frozen semen.

Complete penetration of the cervix at insemination increase the numbers and the quality of spermatozoa reaching the oviducts (Fukui and Roberts, 1977). In the Halbert *et al.* (1990c) study, complete cervical penetration was achieved in 49 of 90 ewes (54%) and 40 of the 49 ewes (82%) lambed. In the much larger Buckrell *et al.* (1994) study, the corresponding percentages for 2060 ewes were 88 and 33, with significant effects of the time of year (breeding vs. non-breeding season) and interval from previous lambing, on lambing outcome. Complete penetration rates increased from 76% for the first 500 ewes inseminated in the study to 98% for the last 500 and the corresponding mean times to achieve complete penetration decreased from 8.6 to 3.6 min, reflecting the importance of operator experience. In the separate New Zealand study of Smith *et al.* (1995), complete penetration of the cervix, using the Guelph inseminating pipette, was also much lower than that achieved by Buckrell *et al.* (1994), however, conception rates for those ewes that were completely penetrated were similar to those achieved by Buckrell *et al.* (1994) using laparoscopy. The same is true for the observations of Windsor *et al.* (1994). Thus, not surprisingly, Smith *et al.* (1995) concluded that research should concentrate on ways of increasing the incidence and ease of cervical penetration.

Anatomical features of sheep cervix

The anatomical features of sheep cervix are unique and have been described by many using classical morphometric techniques, indirect studies with silicon moulds, tridimensional reconstruction from histological preparations or nuclear magnetic resonance (Halbert *et al.*, 1990a; Naqvi *et al.*, 2005, Kaabi *et al.*, 2006). The cervix of ewe is a highly tortuous with complex fibrous structure and with many non-aligned folds (Halbert *et al.*, 1990a; Kershaw *et al.*, 2005). The numbers of cervical folds are variable ranging from 3 to 7 and are conical / funnel shape placed eccentrically on each other (Halbert *et al.* 1990a). It is important to understand the anatomy of cervix and cervical canal of sheep in order to improve the technique of TCAI (Bunch and Ellsworth, 1981; More, 1984; Halbert *et al.*, 1990b). Halbert *et al.* (1990a) studied the anatomy of cervix of crossbreds raised in temperate environment of Canada and reported that the length of cervical canal was 6-7 cm and that cervix had 4-5 asymmetrical accentric funnel shaped folds. There exists a large difference in the morphology and anatomical features among different breeds of sheep (Halbert *et al.*, 1990a; Kaabi *et al.*, 2006).

The complex anatomy of the cervix does not facilitate easy transcervical passage for an insemination catheter. Detail anatomical features of Indian native Malpura and Kheri breeds raised under semi-arid tropical environment were studied by casting silicone moulds of the reproductive tracts for measuring the dimensions of the cervix (Naqvi *et al.*, 2005). The cervical canal of each tract was filled with a silicone sealant for casting the mould. The mean lengths of the cervical mould of ewe lambs and adult ewes were 3.8±0.12 and 5.3±0.15 cm, respectively. The average number of funnel shaped folds in the cervical mould of ewe lambs and adult ewes were 3.2±0.19 and 3.4±0.22, respectively. However, the second and third folds from the os were observed to be accentric in both ewe lambs and adult ewes. Other parameters of cervix of ewe lambs and adult ewes are given in table 3. There is also a vaginal tissue at the opening of the cervix that makes entry through the first two cervical folds difficult. On the basis of the shape of the vaginal tissue the cervix are classified as duckbill, flap, rosette and spiral (Halbert *et al.*, 1990b).

Table 3 : Internal diameter and length of cervical folds of ewe lambs and adult ewes

	Internal diameter of fold (cm)					Distance from os to fold (cm)				
	1st fold	2nd fold	3rd fold	4th fold	5th fold	1st fold	2nd fold	3rd fold	4th fold	5th fold
Ewe lambs	0.18 ±0.01	0.16 ±0.00	0.14 ±0.00	0.17 ±0.01	0.13 ±0.00	0.21 ±0.01	0.19* ±0.01	0.17 ±0.01	0.18 ±0.03	0.18 ±0.01
Adult ewes	0.29 ±0.01	0.26 ±0.01	0.25 ±0.01	0.22 ±0.02	0.20 ±0.03	0.39** ±0.01	0.41** ±0.01	0.38 ±0.01	0.39 ±0.02	0.32 ±0.02

Values with different superscripts within rows are significantly different, (*P<0.05), (**P<0.01) (Source: Naqvi *et al.*, 2005)

Endocrine stimulation of cervical relaxation at estrus

All the evidence suggests that the hyaluronan content of the cervix is enhanced by the high-oestrogen, low progesterone status of the ewe during the pre-LH surge phase. An accompanying feature at this time is the abundant expression of the hyaluronan receptor, CD44, in the epithelial layer (Perry *et al.*, 2010). In view of the central role that peri-oestrous endocrine changes play in the collagen and elastin remodelling processes that promote cervical relaxation, the research emphasis in ewes in recent years has been on improving understanding of their mechanistic pathways (Mitchell *et al.*, 2002, 2005; Kershaw *et al.*, 2007; Leethongdee *et al.*, 2007, 2010; Kershaw-Young *et al.*, 2009, 2010). An overview of the findings from these studies is illustrated below in Fig. 1.

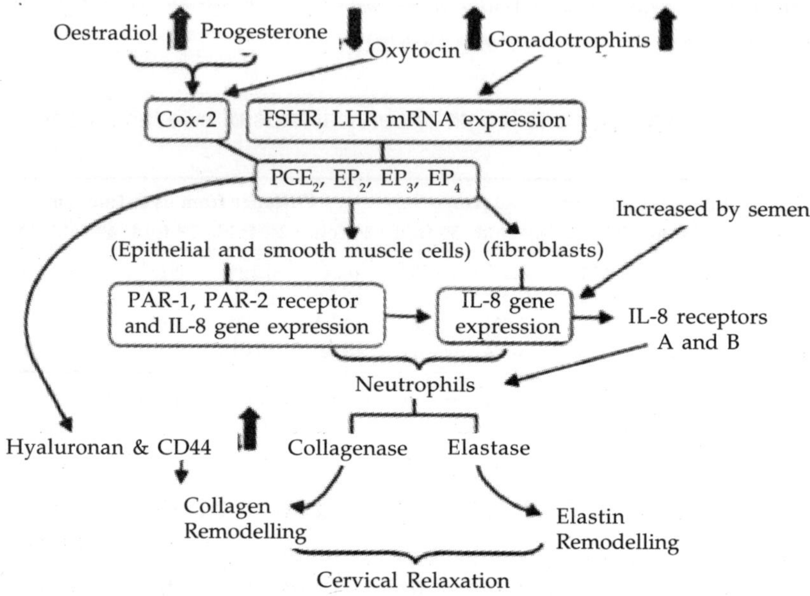

Fig.1 : Overview of recent findings, in the ewe, on endocrine stimulation of cervical relaxation at oestrus. Cox-25cyclooxygenase-2; FSHR5follicle-stimulating hormone receptor; LHR5luteinizing hormone receptor; PGE25prostaglandin; EP5prostaglandin E receptors; PAR5 proteinase-activated receptor; IL5interleukin; CD445hyaluronan receptor (cited from Robinson *et al.*, 2011).

Development of equipments for TCAI

Based on the anatomical features of cervix, the Institute has developed simple equipments and cradle ideally suited for TCAI in native sheep breeds. The equipments fabricated for this purpose were made up of the following components: (a) Spinal needle with a screw end that was suitably modified to fit to the AI gun. Figure 2 and 3 describes the three different types of needles fabricated for TCAI. The other end of the needle was soldered, made blunt and bent at an angle of 45°, (b) An AI gun utilizing 0.5 ml straws (similar to that used in cattle) was shortened and suitably modified to a length of 28 cm. A screw was soldered to the anterior end to adapt the needle head, (c) vaginal speculum, fabricated using a hard plastic cylinder, with an outer diameter of 2.5 cm and length 15 cm with a slit (1 cm) at one end and provision for a battery operated light source on the opposite end, (d) cradle was fabricated using a piece of tractor tyre of 1.2 m length, 0.26 m width and 0.22 m height. Provisions were made in the cradle to contract and relax the tyre with the aid of two screw rods fitted on the lateral sides of the tyre. The tyre can also be moved up and down at the rear end to restrain the ewes in dorsal position at a desired angle. Figure 4 describes the side view of the TCAI cradle while figure 5 describes the procedure of TCAI.

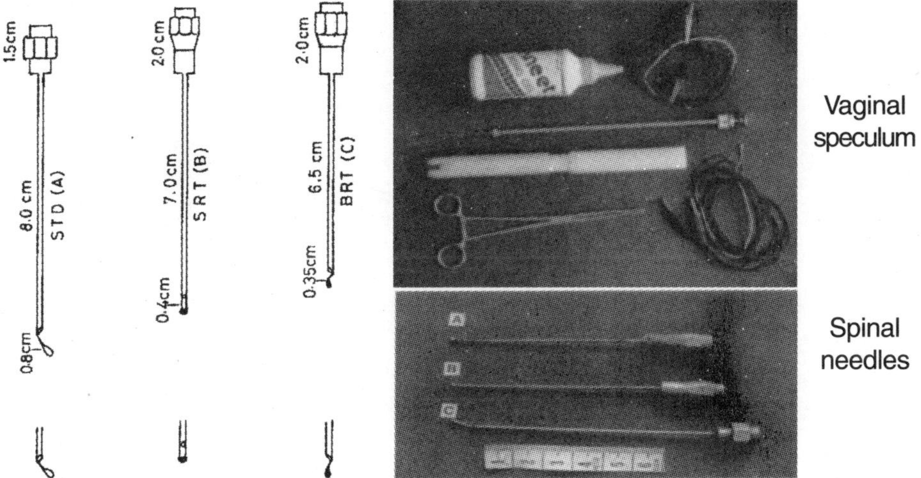

Fig. 2 : Fabrication of modified needles for TCAI

Fig. 3 : Vaginal Speculum and Spinal needles used in TCAI

Method of TCAI: For TCAI the ewes exhibiting estrus are restrained in the cradle with the hindquarter elevated so that the vulva is positioned at an angle of 80 to 90° from the ground. The speculum with plunger is lubricated with small amount of medical gel and introduced into the vagina. The external os is located after removal of the plunger with the aid of the light. The needle is gently introduced into cervix by grasping the external cervical os and sometimes stretching the cervix whilst manipulating the insemination catheter past the folds of the cervix (McKelvey and Simm, 1996). Once the cervical folds are penetrated, the semen is deposited in the body of the uterus. The scoring of depth of cervical penetration is done as: (i) os to second fold: partial, (ii) third to last fold: mid and (iii) needle inserted to its full length: uterine deposition. The depth from the os to the first 2 folds of the cervix has been shown to be the major factor limiting the cervical penetrability (Eppleston and Maxwell, 1993; Eppleston *et al.*, 1994). Higher doses of sperm are required for TCAI with frozen semen as compared to IUAI, because the semen has farther to travel to the point of fertilization. Out of 47 cervical penetrations performed, partial, mid and full depositions were achieved in 14.8, 40.4 and 44.7% ewes, respectively. Following TCAI with frozen semen, success has been achieved for the first time in the country in terms of 22.7% lambing rate (Naqvi *et al.*, 1998), which later on improved to 38.2% (Naqvi *et al.*, 2001). Lambing rates on the basis of depth of insemination is given in table 4.

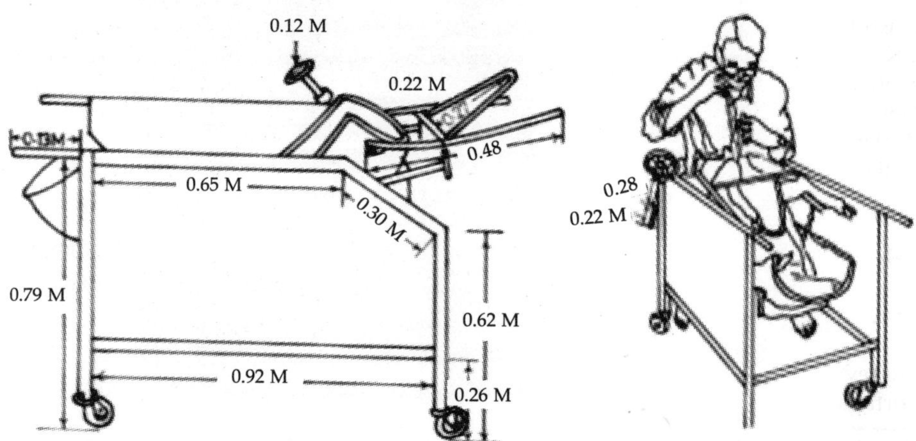

Fig. 4 : Side view of TCAI cradle

Fig. 5 : Description of TCAI

Table 4 : Effect of depth of insemination on lambing rates (Source: Naqvi *et al.*, 1998)

Depth of insemination	No. of ewes inseminated	No. (%) of ewes lambed
Os	4	0 (0)
Mid	7	2 (28.5)
Full	11	3 (27.2)
Overall	22	5(22.7)

Pregnancy and lambing rates obtained worldwide in different sheep breeds after TCAI with frozen semen is summarized in table 5. Although the pregnancy rate ranging from 26 to 64%, confirmed on the basis of ultrasonography between 60-75 days, have been reported but the available reports on lambing rate using frozen semen range from 4 to 42%. It is generally recommended that maiden ewes not to be inseminated trans-cervically due to smaller size of their reproductive organs and less predictable in their responses to hormonal manipulation of the reproductive cycle.

Table 5 : Pregnancy / lambing rate obtained after TCAI of sheep with frozen semen

Country	Breed	No of ewes attempted	Pregnancy / lambing	Reference
Canada	-	38	40*	Halbert *et al.*, 1990c
	Mixed	1809	32.5*	Buckrell *et al.*, 1994
Australia	Merino	264	26**	Windsor *et al.*, 1994
UK	Grey face/ black face	200	18*	Mylne *et al.*, 1993
Scotland	Crossbred	100***	42*	King *et al.*, 2004
New Zealand	Romney	39	64**	Smith *et al.*, 1995
India	Malpura	22	22.7*	Naqvi *et al.*, 1998
	Malpura	21	38.8*	Naqvi *et al.*, 2001
	Bharat Merino	140	26.4**, 9.3*	Kumar *et al.*, 2009
Italy	-	99	22*	Falaschi *et al.*, 1998
	Sarda	-	7*	Cappai *et al.*,1998
USA	Rambouillet x Targhee x Polypay	99	4*	Wulster-Radcliffe *et al.*, 2004
Turkey	Kivircik	120	40*	Gunduz *et al.*, 2010
Portugal	Portugese sheep	-	3.8 - 20.5	Valente *et al.*, 2010

*Lambing; **Pregnancy (confirmed by ultrasonography); *** Multiple insemination

Cervical dilation

The sheep cervix is hard, tortuous and composed of fibrous connective tissue (Kershaw *et al.*, 2005). The relaxation of the cervix at estrus and/or parturition involves enzymatic breakdown of the connective tissues and, to a lesser extent, relaxation of its smooth muscle fibers. With the knowledge of cervical relaxation, cervical dilation has been attempted with the use of hormones (relaxin, oxytocin, PGE2, PGE1) and other chemicals with the aim to facilitate catheter penetration in the cervical canal or to increase contractility of genital tract to improve sperm transport in the lumen.

Oxytocin injection in ewes induces cervical dilation and permits transcervical passage of catheter to the uterus (Khalifa *et al.*, 1992; Sayre and Lewis, 1996) but cervical traumas are still evident (Khalifa *et al.*, 1992; Sayre and Lewis, 1997). Variable and equivocal results were presented on the effect of oxytocin on subsequent fertility of the inseminated ewes with frozen semen. Sayer and Lewis (1997) did not observe adverse effect but Stellflug *et al.* (2001) showed detrimental effect of oxytocin on the fertility. King *et al.* (2004) concluded that oxytocin injection prior to TCAI resulted in reduction in lambing rates and suggested that, when using oxytocin for enhancing cervical dilation and os cervix activity, it may be advantageous to replace a single relatively large bolus dose of oxytocin, which results in an extended period of elevated oxytocin concentrations, with a series of smaller doses that more closely mimic, in number, amplitude and duration, the pulses in plasma concentrations that occur during natural estrus. Therefore, It is evident from these studies that exogenous oxytocin may improve the cervical dilation but may also decrease fertility, pregnancy, and lambing rates.

The secretion of prostaglandins from the cervix of the ewe increases significantly at the time of labour and has been shown to play a role in the cervical dilation (Ellwood, 1980) by inducing the release of collagenase which promote the softening of the collagen (Sayre and Lewis, 1997) and stimulating myometrium contraction (Katz *et al.*, 2000). A synthetic analogue of PGE1, Misoprostol, has been shown to be effective in cervical dilation, stimulating the activity of myometrium contraction (Katz *et al.*, 2000; DeRossi *et al.*, 2009). Recently, Candappa *et al.* (2009) have used a constant-release PGE2 (0.3 mg/hr) vaginal insert (Cervidil^R) developed for use in women for inducing cervical ripening and enhancing the ease of TCAI in anoestrous ewes. Transcervical deposition was possible in four out of six ewes treated with Cervidil^R and showed a possibility of developing a technique to improve TCAI in sheep.

Administration of Valethamate bromide (Epidosin) prior to TCAI facilitates the penetration of the AI catheter through the cervix but have adverse effect on conception and lambing rates (Naqvi *et al.*, 2004). Human interleukin 8 (huIL-8) is a cytokine involves in softening of cervix by increased secretion / activities of collagenases in the cervix during the periparturient period in mammals. Croy *et al.* (1999) used huIL-8 to induce the cervical dilation process but did not have much success in inducing cervical softening in ewes. Carazolol (l-[carbazol4-yloxy]-3-isopropylamino-2-propanol), a beta-adrenergic blocking agent has also been tried for cervical dilation. Bademkiran *et al.* (2007) reported that intravenous administration of carazolol @ 0.01 mg/kg prior to insemination improves fertility of AI in Awassi sheep. Whereas Gunduz *et al.* (2010) reported that intramuscular injection of 0.5mg of carazolol half-an-hour before insemination did not permit complete penetration, and despite deep cervical penetration being increased in carazolol-treated ewes (48% vs. 33%), there was no overall statistically significant improvement in lambing rate or litter size. Recently, DeRossi *et al.* (2009) evaluated the sub-arachnoid administration of ketamine as a tool to be used in cervical dilation of the ewe and showed easy, fast and less stressful transcervical penetration of a stainless steel rod into the uterus. However, this anaesthetic technique may interfere with fertility, pregnancy or lambing rate in ewes after AI.

Conclusions and Perspectives

The technology for AI with liquid semen is viable and gives good results under field conditions and is being used in breed improvement programmes of sheep. However, for AI with frozen semen further research efforts are still needed for conducting large scale sheep breed improvement programmes and making this technology acceptable in field. Advances have been made in the science of ovine cervical relaxation and its pharmacological stimulation with associated improvements in physical penetration that have facilitated TCAI. At the same time, progress is being made in improving semen processing and in reducing the damaging effects of freezing and thawing on sperm viability and membrane integrity. There has also been success in producing pre-sexed offspring, albeit following IUAI rather than deposition in the os cervix. The goal now is to achieve this through TCAI by creative science, which builds on the advances in stimulating cervical relaxation and in improving semen quality that have accrued from applied through to molecular research.

The identification of production and other trait genes will allow Artificial Breeding companies to capture these benefits by targeted selection of sires through specific markers. The common theme is to use cloning, IVF or large scale embryo transfer to establish the base population for these unique genotypes. However, AI will remain the most cost effective method to disseminate these genes. It is more than likely that the combination of AI with new and emerging biotechnologies will form a strong base on which various selection or breeding policies will be based. It is also very likely that all these biotechnologies will use sperm dispersal in some form to establish the required genes. The future for AI continues to be promising. Critical discoveries in the next decade or so in assisted reproductive technologies will challenge the pre-eminent position of AI as the low cost option to disseminate alleles of choice. In all such cases, the main driver will continue to remain simplicity of application, probability of success and the level of economy of the technology adopted.

References

Abbott, K.A. 1994. Cost-benefit evaluation of artificial insemination for genetic improvement of wool-producing sheep, Australian Veterinary Journal 71: 353-360.

Anel, L., Kaabi, M., Abroug, B., Alvarez, M., Anel, E. Boixo, J.C., Fuente, P.P. and de Paz, P. 2005. Factors influencing the success of vaginal and laparoscopic artificial insemination in Churra ewes: a field assay. Theriogenology 63: 1235-1247.

Anel, L., Alvarez, M., Martinez-Pastor, F., Garcia-Macias, V., Anel, E. and de Paz, P. 2006. Improvement strategies in ovine artificial insemination. Reproduction in Domestic Animals 41: 30-42.

Bademkiran, S., Celik, R., Gurbulak, K., Yokus, B. and Ozdemir, N. 2007. Blocade of the â-adrenoceptors with carazolol improves fertility of artificial insemination in Awassi sheep. Medycyna Vet. 63: 298-300.

Buckrell, B.C., Buschbeck, C., Gartlet, C.J., Kroetsch, T., McCutcheon, W., Martin, J., Penner, W.K. and Walton, J.S. 1992. A breeding trial using a transcervical technique for artificial insemination in sheep. In: Proc. 12th International Congress of Animal Reproduction, The Hague, 3: 1531-1533.

Buckrell, B.C., Buschbeck, C., Gartley, C.J., Kroetsch, T., McCutcheon, W., Martin, J., Penner, W.K. and Walton, J.S. 1994. Further development of a transcervical technique for artificial insemination in sheep using previously frozen semen. Theriogenology 42: 601-611.

Bunch, T.D. and Ellsworth, H.S. 1981. Gross anatomy of the ovine cervix. International Goat Sheep Research 1: 282-285.

Candappa, I.B.R., Bainbridge, H.C., Price, N.T., Hourigan, K.R. and Bartlewski, P.M. 2009. A preliminary study on the suitability of Cervidil[R] to induce cervical dilation for artificial insemination in ewes. Research in Veterinary Science 87: 204-206.

Cappai, P., Sanna, S.R., Branca, A., Fraghi, A. and Bomboi, G. 1998. Comparison of laparoscopic and transcervical insemination with frozen semen. Animal Science 66: 369-373.

Croy, B.A., Prudencio, J., Minhas, K., Ashkar, A.A., Galligan, C., Foster, R.A., Buckrell, B. and Coomber, B.L. 1999. A preliminary study on the usefulness of huIL-8 in cervical relaxation of the ewe for artificial insemination and for embryo transfer. Theriogenology 52: 271-287.

De Graaf, S.P., Beilby, K., O'Brien, J.K., Osborn, D., Downing, J.A., Maxwell, W.M.C. and Evans, G. 2007. Embryo production from superovulated sheep inseminated with sex-sorted ram spermatozoa. Theriogenology 67: 550–555.

DeRossi, R., Carneiro, R.P.B., Ossuna, M.R., Zanenga, N.F., Alves, O.D., Jorge, T.P., Costa-e-Silva, E.V. and Vasconcelos, J. 2009. Sub-arachnoid ketamine administration combined with or without misoprostol / oxytocin to facilitate cervical dilation in ewes: a case study. Small Ruminant Research 83: 74-78.

Donavan, A., Hanrahan, J.P., Kummen, E., Duffy, P. and Boland, M.P. 2004. Fertility in ewes following cervical insemination with fresh or frozen thawed semen at natural and synchronized oestrus. Animal Reproductive Science 84: 359-368.

El-Gaafary, M.N., Chemberlain, A.G., Axford, R.F.E. and Owen, J.B. 2001. Fertility of the frozen ram semen. Indian Journal of Animal Science 71: 328-330.

Ellwood, D.A. 1980. The hormonal control of connective tissue changes in the ovine cervix in pregnancy and at parturition. Biochemical Society Transaction 8: 662-667.

Eppleston, J. and Maxwell, W.M.C. 1993. Recent attempts to improve the fertility of frozen ram semen inseminated into the cervix. Wool Technology and Sheep Breeding 41: 291-302.

Eppleston, J., Salamon, S., Moore, N.W. and Evans, G. 1994. The depth of cervical insemination and site of intrauterine insemination and their relationship to the fertility of frozen-thawed ram semen. Animal Reproductive Science 36: 211-225.

Epstein, H. 1985. The Awassi sheep with special reference to the improved dairy type. FAO Animal Production and Health, Paper 57, Rome.

Falaschi, U., Rassu, P.G. and Enne, G. 1998. Transcervical artificial insemination in sheep. Summa 15: 21-27.

Fukui, Y. and Roberts, E.M. 1977. Sperm transport after non-surgical intrauterine insemination with frozen semen in ewes treated with prostaglandin F2a. Journal of Reproduction and Fertility 51: 141-143.

Fukui, Y., Hirai, H., Honda, K. and Hayashi, K. 1993a. Lambing rates by fixed-time intrauterine insemination with frozen semen in seasonally anestrous ewes treated with two different progestogen-impregnated sponge or CIDR devices. Journal of Reproductive Development 39: 1-5.

Fukui, Y., Fujii, M. and Tashiro, Y. 1993b. Insemination doses of frozen-thawed semen in seasonally anestrous ewes treated with two different progesterone-impregnated intravaginal devices Journal of Reproductive Development 39: 269–273.

Fukui, Y., Tabuchi, K., Yamada, A., Hayashi, N. and Tanaka, K. 1994. Effect of insertion periods of controlled internal drug release device (CIDR) on conception rate by fixed-time intrauterine insemination with frozen semen in seasonally anestrous ewes. Journal of Reproductive Development 40: 221–226.

Fukui, Y., Iida, K., Okada, A., Zyouzyou, Y., Wach, S. and Togawa, M. 2002. Fertility of estrusinduced ewes during the non-breeding season and artificially inseminated with frozen semen imported from New Zealand. Journal of Reproductive Development 48: 485–488.

Fukui, Y., Kohno, H., Togari, T. and Hiwasa, M. 2007. Fertility of ewes inseminated intrauterinally with frozen semen using extender containing bovine serum albumin. Journal of Reproductive Development 53: 959–962.

Fukui, Y., Kohno, H., Togari, T., Hiwasa, M. and Okabe, K. 2008. Fertility after artificial insemination using a soybean-based semen extender in sheep. Journal of Reproductive Development 54: 286-289.

Fukui, Y., Kohno, H., Okabe, K., Katsuki, S., Yoshizawa, M., Togari, T. and Watanabe, H. 2010. Factors affecting the fertility of ewes after intrauterine insemination with frozen–thawed semen during the non-breeding season. Journal of Reproductive Development 56: 460-466.

Gillan, L., Maxwell, W.M.C. and Evans, G. 2004. Preservation and evaluation of semen for artificial insemination. Reproduction Fertillity and Development 16: 447-454.

Gordon, I. 1997. In: Controlled reproduction in sheep and goats. CAB International Wallingford, Oxon, U.K.

Gunduz, M.C., Turna, O., Cirit, U., Ucmak, M., Cagatay, T., Sabuncu, A. and Bacinoglu, S. 2010. Lambing rates and litter size following carazolol administration prior to insemination in Kivircik ewes. Animal Reproduction Science 118: 32-36.

Halbert, G.W., Dobson, H., Walton, J.S. and Buckrell, B.C. 1990a. The structure of the cervical canal of ewe. Theriogenology 33: 977-992.

Halbert, G.W., Dobson, H., Walton, J.S. and Buckrell, B.C. 1990b. A technique for transcervical intrauterine insemination of ewes. Theriogenology 33: 993-1010.

Halbert, G.W., Dobson, H., Walton, J.S., Sharpe, P. and Buckrell, B.C. 1990c. Field evaluation of a technique for transcervical intrauterine insemination of ewes. Theriogenology 33: 1231-1243.

Hill, J.R, Thompson, J.A. and Perkins, N.R. 1998. Factors affecting pregnancy rates following laparoscopic insemination of 28,447 Merino ewes under commercial conditions: a survey. Theriogenology 49: 697-709.

Hiwasa, M., Kohno, H., Togari, T., Okabe, K. and Fukui, Y. 2009. Fertility after different artificial insemination methods using a synthetic semen extender in sheep. Journal of Reproductive Developmenr 55: 50-54.

Hollinshead, F.K., O'Brien, J.K., Maxwell, W.M.C. and Evans, G. 2002. Production of lambs of pre-determined sex after the insemination of ewes with low numbers of X- or Y- chromosome bearing spermatozoa. Reproduction and Fertility Development 14: 503-508.

Kaabi, M., Alvarez, M., Anel, E., Chamorro, C.A., Boixo, J.C., de Paz, P. and Anel, L. 2006. Influence of breed and age on morphometry and depth of insemination catheter penetration in the ewe cervix: A postmortem study. Theriogenology 66: 1876-1883.

Katz, V.L., Farmer, R.M., Dean, C.A. and Carpenter, M.G. 2000. Use of mesoprostol for cervical ripening. South Medical Journal 93: 881-884.

Kershaw, C.M., Khalid, M., McGowan, M.R., Ingram, K., Leethongdee, S., Wax, G. and Scaramuzzi, R.J. 2005. The anatomy of the sheep cervix and its influence on the transcervical passage of an inseminating pipette into the uterine lumen. Theriogenology 64: 1225-1235.

Kershaw, C.M., Scaramuzzi, R.J., McGowan, M.R., Wheeler-Jones, C.P.D. and Khalid, M. 2007. The expression of prostaglandin endoperoxide synthase 2 messenger RNA and the proportion of smooth muscle and collagen in the sheep cervix. Biology of Reproduction 76: 124-129.

Kershaw-Young, C.M., Khalid, M., McGowan, M.R., Pitsillides, A.A. and Scaramuzzi, R.J. 2009. The mRNA expression of prostaglandin E receptors EP2 and EP4 and the changes in glycosaminoglycans in the sheep cervix during the estrous cycle. Theriogenology 72: 251-261.

Kershaw-Young, C.M., Scaramuzzi, R.J., McGowan, M.R., Pitsillides, A.A., Wheeler- Jones, C.P.D. and Khalid, M. 2010. The effect of estradiol on Cox-2, EP2 and EP4 mRNA expression and the extracellular matrix in the cervix of the hypogonadotrophic, ovariectomised ewe. Theriogenology 73: 620-628.

Khalifa, R.M., Sayre, B.L. and Lewis, G.S. 1992. Exogenous oxytocin dialates the cervix in ewes. Journal of Animal Science 70: 38-42.

Killen, I.D. and Caffery, G.J. 1982. Uterine insemination of ewe with the aid of a laproscope. Australian Veterinary Journal 59: 95.

King, M.E., McKelvey, W.A.C., Dingwall, W.S., Matthews, K.P., Gebbie, F.E., Mylne, M.J.A., Stewart, E. and Robinson, J.J. 2004. Lambing rate and litter sizes following intrauterine or cervical insemination of frozen/thawed semen with or without oxytocin administration. Theriogenology 62: 1236-1244.

Kumar, D, Naqvi, SMK, Joshi, A. and Maurya, V.P. 2009. Effect of single or double inseminations on conception and lambing rates of Bharat Merino ewes following transcervical artificial insemination with frozen semen. In: Proc. 96th Indian Science Congress, Shilong, Jan 3-7, p 162.

Leethongdee, S., Khalid, M., Bhatti, A., Ponglowhapan, S., Kershaw, C. and Scaramuzzi, R.J. 2007. The effects of the prostaglandin E analogue Misoprostol and folliclestimulating hormone on cervical penetrability in ewes during the peri-ovulatory period. Theriogenology 67: 767-777.

Leethongdee, S., Kershaw-Young, C.M., Scaramuzzi, R.J. and Khalid, M. 2010. Intracervical application of Misprostol at estrus alters the content of cervical hyaluronan and the mRNA expression of follicle stimulating hormone receptor (FSHR), luteinizing hormone receptor (LHR) and cyclo-oxygenase-2 in the ewe. Theriogenology 73: 1257-1266.

Mathur, A.K., Srivastava, R.S. and Joshi, A. 1993. Effect of cortisol incorporation on preservability of ram spermatozoa extended in EYMG extender. Indian Journal of Animal Production 14: 39-40.

Maxwell, W.M.C. 1984. Current problems and future potential of artificial insemination programmes. In: Reproduction in Sheep. (D.R. Lindsay and D.R. Pearce, Eds.), Cambridge University Press, Cambridge. pp 291-298.

Maxwell, W.M.C. and Hewitt, L.J. 1986. A comparison of vaginal, cervical and intrauterine insemination of sheep. Journal of Agricultural Science (Cambridge) 106: 191-193.

Maxwell, W.M.C. and Salamon, S. 1993. Liquid storage of ram semen: a review. Reproduction, Fertility and Development 5: 613-638.

Maxwell, W.M.C. and Watson, P.F. 1996. Recent progress in the preservation of ram semen. Animal Reproductive Science 42: 55-65.

McKelvey, W.A.C. and Simm, G. 1996. Intrauterine insemination, transcervical insemination and embryo transfer for practical breed improvement in small ruminants. Stocarstvo 50: 185-198.

Mitchell, S.E., Robinson, J.J., King, M.E., McKelvey, W.A.C. and Williams, L.M. 2002. Interleukin 8 in the cervix of non-pregnant ewes. Reproduction 124: 409-416.

Mitchell, S.E., Robinson, J.J., King, M.E. and Williams, L.M. 2005. Proteinase-activated receptors in ovine cervical function. Reproduction, Fertility and Development 17: 693–699.

More, J., 1984. Anatomy and histology of the cervix uteri of the ewe: new insights. Acta. Anat. INRA Toulouse, 120: 156-159.

Mylne, M.J.A., Buschbeck, C., Dingwall, W.S., Buckrell, B.C. and McKelvey, W.A.C. 1993. Results from a comparative trial using laparoscopic intrauterine insemination and the Guelph transcervical method for the insemination of frozen semen in sheep. In: Proc. 3rd International Veterinary Science Conference, Edinburgh, p130.

Naqvi, S.M.K, Joshi, A., Mathur, A.K., Bag, S. and Mittal, J.P. 1997. Intrauterine artificial insemination of Malpura ewes in natural estrus with frozen ram semen. Indian Journal of Animal Sciences 67: 982-983.

Naqvi, S.M.K., Joshi, A., Bag, S., Pareek, S.R. and Mittal, J.P. 1998. Cervical penetration and transcervical AI of tropical sheep (Malpura) at natural estrus using frozen-thawed semen. Small Ruminant Research 29: 329-333.

Naqvi, S.M.K., Joshi, A., Das, G.K. and Mittal, J.P. 2001. Development and application of ovine reproductive technologies: an Indian experience. Small Ruminant Research 39: 199-208.

Naqvi, S.M.K., Pandey, G.K., Gautam, K.K., Joshi, A. and Mittal J.P. 2004. Effect of epidosin on catheter penetration in cervix and fertility in ewes inseminated with frozen semen. In: Proc. National Seminar on Opportunities and Challenges in Nutrition and Feeding Management of Sheep, Goat and Rabbit for Sustainable Production, Feb 10-12, Avikanagar, pp 366.

Naqvi, S.M.K., Pandey, G.K., Gautam, K.K., Joshi, A., Geethalakshmi, V. and Mittal J.P. 2005. Evaluation of gross anatomical features of cervix of tropical sheep using cervical silicone moulds. Animal Reproduction Science 85: 337-344.

Nordstoga, A.B., Soderquist, L., Adnoy, T. and Paulenz, H. 2009. Effect of different packages and freezing/ thawing protocols on fertility of ram semen. Reproduction in Domestic Animals 44: 527-531.

Olesen, I. 1993. Effects of cervical insemination with frozen semen on fertility and litter size of Norwegian sheep. Livestock Production Science 37: 169-184.

O'Meara, C.M., Donovan, A., Hanrahan, J.P., Duffy, P., Fair, S., Evans, A.C.O. and Lonergan, P. 2007. Resuspending ram spermatozoa in seminal plasma after cryopreservation does not improve pregnancy rate in cervically inseminated ewes. Theriogenology 67: 1262-1268.

Paulenz, H., S¨derquist, L., A dnoy, T., Nordstoga, A., Gulbrandsen, B. and Berg, K.A. 2004. Fertility results after different thawing procedures for ram semen frozen in minitubes and mini straws. Theriogenology 61: 1719-1727.

Paulenz, H., Soderquist, L., Adnoy, T., Nordsroga, A. and Berg, K.A. 2005. Effect of vaginal and cervical deposition of semen on the fertility of sheep inseminated with frozen-thawed semen. Veterinary Record 156: 372-375.

Perry, K., Haresign, W., Wathes, D.C. and Khalid, M. 2010. Hyaluronan (HA) content, the ratio of HA fragments and the expression of CD44 in the ovine cervix vary with the stage of the oestrous cycle. Reproduction 140: 133–141.

Robinson, J.J, McKelvey, W.A.C., King, M.E., Mitchell, S.E., Mylne, M.J.A., McEvoy, T.G., Dingwall, W.S. and Williams, L.M. 2011. Traversing the ovine cervix - a challenge for cryopreserved semen and creative science. Animal 5: 1791-1804.

Salamon, S. and Maxwell, W.M.C. 1995. Frozen storage of ram semen.II. Causes of low fertility after cervical insemination and methods of improvement. Animal Reproductive Science 38: 1-36.

Sayre, B.L. and Lewis, G.S. 1996. Cervical dilation with exogenous oxytocin does not affect sperm movement into the oviducts in ewes. Theriogenology 45: 1523-1533.

Sayre, B.L. and Lewis, G.S. 1997. Fertility and ovum fertilization rate after laparoscopic or transcervical intrauterine artificial insemination of oxytocin-treated ewes. Theriogenology 48: 267-275.

Shackell, G.H., Kyle, B. and Littlejohn, R.P. 1990. Factors influencing the success of a large scale artificial insemination programme in sheep. In: Proc. New Zealand Society of Animal Production 50: 427-430.

Smith, J.F., Aspinall, J.E., Oliver, M.G., Smith, J.K. and Upreti, G.C. 1995. Field scale evaluation of semen diluent for cervical AI in sheep. An attempt at technology transfer. In: Proc. New Zealand Society of Animal Production 55: 232-235.

Srivastava, R.S., Mathur, A.K. and Kalra, D.B. 1987. Effect of alpha tocopherol on preservability of ram semen. Indian Journal of Animal Sciences 57: 553-554.

Stellflug, J.N., Wulster-Radcliffe, M.C., Hensley, E.L., Cowardin, E.A., Seals, R.C. and Lewis, G.S. 2001. Oxytocin induced cervical dilation and cervical manipulation in sheep: effects of laparoscopic artificial insemination. Journal of Animal Science 79: 568-573.

Thibier,M. and Guerin, B., 2000. Hygienic aspects of storage and use of semen for artificial insemination. Animal Reproductive Science 62: 233-251.

Valente, S.S., Pereira,R.M., Baptista, M.C. , Marques, C.C., Vasques, M.I. , Silva, Pereira, M.V.C., Horta, A.E.M. and Barbas, J.P. 2010. In vitro and in vivo fertility of ram semen cryopreserved in different extenders. Animal Reproductive Science 117: 74–77.

Windsor, D.P., Szell, A.Z., Buschbeck. C., Edward, A.Y., Milton, J.T.B. and Buckrell, B.C., 1994. Transcervical artificial insemination of Australian Merino ewes with frozen-thawed semen. Theriogenology 42: 147-157.

Wulster-Radcliffe, M.C., Wang, S. and Lewis, G.S. 2004. Transcervical artificial insemination in sheep: effect of new transcervical artificial insemination instrument and traversing the cervix on pregnancy and lambing rates. Theriogenology 62: 990-1002.

□□□

Chapter 8

Climate Change and Sheep Production : Concept of Multiple Stresses, Adaption and Mitigation Strategies to Sustain Production

V. Sejian* and S.M.K. Naqvi
Division of Physiology and Biochemistry, Central Sheep and Wool research Institute, Avikanagar-304 501 (Rajasthan)

Livestock production is thought to be adversely affected by detrimental effects of extreme climatic conditions. Consequently, adaptation and mitigation of detrimental effects of extreme climates have played a major role in combating the climatic impact in livestock production (Khalifa, 2003). Among the environmental variables affecting animals, heat stress seems to be one of the more intriguing factors making animal production difficult in many areas of the world (Koubková *et al.*, 2002). In fact, the animals can adapt to the hot climate, nevertheless the response mechanisms helpful for survival are detrimental to performance (Rivington *et al.*, 2009).

Heat stress is considered to be the most challenging factors negatively affecting animal production in several regions of the world. The animals tend to adapt to adverse climate, nonetheless the mechanisms obliging survival have damaging effects on productivity. During stress, various endocrine responses are involved in improving the fitness of an individual. The front-line hormones to surmount stressful situations are the glucocorticoids and catecholamines. The secretion of glucocorticoids is an archetypal endocrine response to stress (Kannan *et al.*, 2000). Currently it appears that glucocorticosteroids provide an initial integrating signal, which in conjunction with other hormones and paracrine secretions, may determine specific behavioral, physiological and biochemical responses to adapt to different environmental conditions (Wingfield and Kitaysky, 2002; Sejian *et al.*, 2010). Thyroid gland is one of the most sensitive organs to the ambient heat variation (Rasooli *et al.*, 2004). Appropriate thyroid gland function and activity of thyroid hormones are considered crucial to sustain the productive performance in domestic animals (Todini, 2007). When the animals are suffering due to heat, feed intake is reduced and metabolism slows down causing a hypo-function of the thyroid gland (McManus *et al.*, 2009). One of the principal functions of glucocorticoid under thermal stress is to control hepatic gluconeogenesis and insulin concentration in such conditions directly depicts the energy status of animal to sustain production under extreme environmental conditions (Sejian *et al.*, 2008a; Sejian and Srivastava, 2010). Hence measuring the metabolic hormones such as thyroid hormones and insulin will give a clue about how an animal adapts itself to the changing environments by altering its metabolic activity.

Sheep grazing in hot semi-arid environment face extreme fluctuations in the quantity and quality of feed on offer throughout the year (Martin *et al.*, 2004). It has been postulated that nutrition is one of the main factors affecting ovulation rate and sexual activity in sheep (Vinoles *et al.*, 2005; Forcada and Abecia, 2006). It is generally accepted that nutrition modulates reproductive endocrine functions in many species including sheep (Martin *et al.*, 2004; Sejian *et al.*, 2011a). Further, under-nutrition affects reproductive function in ruminants at different levels of the hypothalamus-pituitary-gonadal axis (Chadio *et al.*, 2007).

Thermal stress and feed scarcity are the major predisposing factor for the low productivity of sheep under hot semi arid environment (Martin *et al.*, 2004). High ambient temperature augments the effort by sheep to dissipate body heat, resulting in increased rate of respiration, body temperature, heart beat and water consumption (Marai *et al.*, 2000). Increased body temperature and respiration rate are the most important signs of heat stress in sheep (Al-Haidary, 2004). Further, increase in body temperature is associated with marked reduction in feed intake, redistribution in blood flow and changes in endocrine functions that negatively affect the productive and reproductive performance of sheep (Averos *et al.*, 2008). In addition, exposure of sheep to elevated temperature results in a decrease of body weight, growth rate and body total solids (Marai *et al.*, 2007). It has been reported that depleted body condition during periods of energy deficiency also reduces heat tolerance (Minka and Ayo, 2009). This paper covers, in detail, information on climate change and concept of multiple stresses and sheep adaptation to such multiple stresses in terms of their physiological responses, blood biochemical responses and endocrine responses. Additionally this paper will also address the various management strategies available to counter the environmental stresses arising due to climate change.

Climate change and its consequences on livestock production

Global climate change is expected to alter temperature, precipitation, atmospheric carbon dioxide levels and water availability in ways that will affect the productivity of crop and livestock systems (Hatfield, *et al.*, 2008). For livestock systems, climate change could affect the costs and returns of production by altering the thermal environment of animals thereby affecting animal health, reproduction and the efficiency by which livestock convert feed into retained products (especially meat and milk). Climatic changes could increase thermal stress for animals and thereby reduce animal production and profitability by lowering feed efficiency, milk production, and reproduction rates.

Climate changes, could impact the economic viability of livestock production systems worldwide. Surrounding environmental conditions directly affect mechanisms and rates of heat gain or loss by all animals (NRC, 1981). Environmental stress reduces the productivity and health of livestock resulting in significant economic losses. Heat stress affects animal performance and productivity of dairy cows in all phases of production. The outcomes include decreased growth, reduced reproduction, increased susceptibility to diseases and ultimately delayed initiation of lactation. Heat stress also negatively affects reproductive function (Amundson *et al.*, 2006). Normal oestrus activity and fertility are disrupted in livestock during summer months. Economic losses are incurred by the livestock industries because farm animals are generally raised in locations and/or seasons where temperature conditions go beyond their thermal comfort zone. The livelihood of the rural poor in developing countries depends critically on local natural resource-based activities such as crop and livestock production. As a result of negative weather impact on livestock rearing, the poor shepherds/farmers whose principal livelihood security depends on these animal performances is directly on stake. Housing and management technologies are available through which climatic impacts on livestock can be reduced, but the rational use of such technologies is crucial for the survival and profitability of the livestock enterprise (Gaughan *et al.,* 2002).

Climate change and concept of multiple stresses

Livestock researchers aiming at improving livestock production under changing climatic scenario must aim at counteracting multiple stresses as these stresses are common occurrences in most ecological zones where livestock are reared. Under the changing climatic scenario, the concept of multiple stresses emerges as a potential threat to livestock production and its survival. Hence, research needs to be prioritized to tackle multiple stresses simultaneously to improve the economy of the livestock farms.

Generally when animals are exposed to one stress at a time, they can effectively counter them based on their stored body reserves without altering the normal body functions. However, if they are exposed to more than one stress at a time, the summated effects of the different stressors might prove detrimental to these animals. This is because of their inability to cope with the combined effects of different stressors simultaneously. In such a case, the animal's body reserves are not sufficient to effectively counter such environmental extremes. As a result their adaptive capability are hampered and the animals struggle to maintain normal homeothermy. Moberg (1999) explained that when animals are exposed to only one stress, they may not require the diversion of biological resources needed for other functions. If, however, two of these stressors occur simultaneously, the total cost may have a severe impact on other biological functions. As a result their normal basal functions are drastically affected leading to lowering of production.

Multiple stresses impact on sheep production and reproduction

(i) *Feed intake and growth*: It is known that sheep that are exposed to high ambient temperatures, augments the efforts to dissipate body heat, resulting in the increase of respiration rate, body temperature and consumption of water and a decline in feed intake (Marai *et al.*, 2007). This finding of reduced feed intake after thermal exposure was in agreement to the findings of Pereira *et al.* (2008). They reported that the rate of feed intake by sheep tended to decrease after the heat exposure. Further, Padua *et al.* (1997) reported that apart from feed intake, feed conversion also significantly decreased under hot condition in climatic chamber as compared to shelter during spring. Marai *et al.* (2007) had postulated a reason for this reduced feed intake in sheep after thermal exposure. They explained that exposure of the animal to a high environmental temperature, stimulates the peripheral thermal receptors to transmit suppressive nerve impulses to the appetite centre in the hypothalamus and thereby causing a decrease in feed intake. The decrease in feed intake could be due to the adaptive mechanism of sheep to produce less body heat. The water intake of combined stress group was significantly higher as compared to *ad libitum* fed groups. This shows that the high water intake which is utilized to combat heat stress may be indicating that restricted fed animals are under more stress (Minka and Ayo, 2009). Further, it is an established fact in small ruminants that lack of food and particularly the potassium content, impedes the sodium uptake from the reticulum-rumen causing hyponatraemia and hypo-osmolality (Holtenius and Dahlborn, 1990). The average body weight of thermal, nutritional, combined and multiple stresses groups significantly decreased as compared to control group (Table 1). Growth, the increase in the live body mass or cell multiplication, is controlled genetically and environmentally (Marai *et al.*, 2007). Habeeb *et al.* (1992) reported that elevated ambient temperature is considered to be one of the environmental factors influencing average daily gain. Similar findings of impaired body weight and growth rate following exposure to elevated temperatures were reported by Marai *et al.* (1991) and Ismail *et al.* (1995). The reason for the effects of elevated ambient temperature on growth reduction could be due to decrease in anabolic activity and the increase in tissue catabolism (Marai *et al.*, 1999). They attributed this increase in tissue catabolism due to increase in catecholamines and glucocorticoids after exposure to heat stress in sheep.

Table 1 : Effect of thermal, nutritional, combined and multiple stresses on growth and reproductive parameters of Malpura ewes (Source: Sejian *et al.*, 2011a)

Parameters	Control	Thermal stress	Nutritional stress	Combined stresses	Multiple stresses
Initial body weight (Kg)	33.75±2.56[a]	33.52±1.85[a]	34.68±1.70[a]	34.87±1.46[a]	32.63±0.98[a]
Final body weight (Kg)	39.67±2.65[a]	35.19±1.46[ab]	30.39±1.50[b]	30.04±1.35[b]	29.55±1.22[b]
ADG (g)	169.14±0.01[a]	47.71±0.07[b]	-122.57±0.06[c]	-138.00±0.07[c]	-88.00
Ewes in heat (%)	85.71[a]	57.14[b]	85.71[a]	71.43[ab]	41.7[c]
Estrus duration (hr)	38.00±2.41[a]	23.40±3.34[b]	28.50±5.68[bc]	18.75±3.75[bd]	14.4±2.78[c]
Estrus cycle length (days)	18.17±0.31[b]	20.28±0.74[ab]	18.00 ±0.27[b]	22.25±1.67[a]	23.56±1.45[a]
Conception rate (%)	71.43[a]	42.86[ab]	57.14[ab]	28.57[b]	-
Lambing rate (%)	71.43[a]	42.86[ab]	57.14[ab]	28.57[b]	-
Estradiol (pg/mL)	14.58±0.96[a]	12.06±0.73[b]	12.80±0.91[b]	10.04±0.74[c]	7.19±0.23[d]
Progesterone (ng/mL)	3.31±0.56[c]	4.48±0.32[ab]	3.98±0.26[bc]	5.19±0.27[a]	7.34±0.28[d]

Combined stresses-thermal and nutritional stress; Multiple stresses- thermal, nutritional and walking stress; Means(±SE) within a row having different superscripts differ significantly (P<0.05)

(ii) *Reproduction*: Multiple stresses showed highly significant influence on estrus duration and estrus cycle length (Table 1). This could be related to the high plasma progesterone concentration in multiple stressed ewes. Presumably, therefore, the longer estrus cycles were due to a slower rate of follicular maturation after corpus luteum (CL) regression. There are evidences proving the influence of nutrition on folliculogenesis and ovulation rate (Kiyma *et al.*, 2004; Scaramuzzi *et al.*, 2006). Another hypothesis put forward by Downing *et al.* (1995) states that ovarian responses are influenced by availability of nutrients. Nutrient deficiency potentially acts on the reproductive process and affects estrus behavior and ovulation rate. Nutritional influences on reproduction may be linked through variations in the insulin-like growth factor-1 (IGF-1) system (Roberts *et al.*, 2001). Acute nutrient restriction to the point of decreasing IGF-1 secretion may affect the ability of developing follicles to respond to FSH through a reduction in FSH receptor expression (Kiyma *et al.*, 2004).

Combined stress had relatively more detrimental effect on the conception rate (Table 1). The probable reason for this could be reduced sex steroid receptor and altered sex steroids concentration. This view is supported by the fact that there is evidence for inhibitory effect of under-nutrition on the number of uterine sex steroid receptors which will in turn affect conception rate (Sosa *et al.*, 2006). It has been established that sheep embryo is most susceptible to maternal heat stress (Thwaites, 1971). In addition, Lawson and Cahill (1983) postulated that variations in the physiological range of peripheral progesterone concentration due to management factors such as nutrition may induce asynchrony between the embryo and uterus resulting in failure of pregnancy to be established. Lambing rate also showed results similar to conception rate in combined stress group. The probable reason for low conception rate in combined stress group could be the insufficient progesterone concentration to maintain pregnancy as the thermal and nutritional stress were withdrawn after mating at the end of the experimental period. Higher level of nutrition has been found to be associated with lower circulating progesterone concentrations in ewes (O'Callaghan *et al.*, 2000). Ample evidence supports that under-nutrition of ewes before and after mating increases embryonic mortality which in turn reduces the lambing rate (Abecia *et al.*, 2006).

Plasma estrogen and progesterone showed reverse trend in individual, combined as well as multiple stresses groups (Table 1). The effect of thermal stress is more severe than nutritional stress on plasma estradiol 17-â level (Sejian *et al.*, 2011a). It is generally accepted that nutrition modulates reproductive endocrine function in many species including sheep. Kiyma *et al.* (2004) reported that serum concentrations of estradiol were lower in undernourished ewes. Decreased concentration of estrogen may result from diminished ovarian follicular development caused by suppressed peripheral concentration of gonadotrophins (Gougeon, 1996). The level of nutrition and peripheral progesterone concentrations are inversely related (Parr, 1992) in ewes. This inverse relationship between level of feed intake and plasma progesterone concentration was attributed to difference in metabolic clearance rate of progesterone (Parr *et al.*, 1993). This view was further strengthened by the finding of Abecia *et al.* (2006) which states that difference in the rate of clearance rather than differences in secretion levels can explain the apparent inverse relationship between nutrition and peripheral progesterone concentrations in ewes. The increased plasma progesterone concentration in undernourished ewes in these studies might be due to the limited extravascular pool in such animals with low body fat content (Lamond *et al.*, 1972).

Adaptation of sheep to environmental stresses

(i) *Behavioral and Morphological adaptability*: An adaptation is referred to means by which an animal makes it possible for it to live in a particular place and in a particular way. It may be a phenotype adaptation, like the size or shape of the animal's body or the way in which its body works i.e. physiological adaptation or it may be the way the animal behaves. Each adaptation has been produced by evolution. A novel study by a team of scientists in Britain reported that average body size of a wild Soay sheep of Hirta (Scottish island) in the St Kilda archipelago has decreased by approximately 5% over the last 24 years. This is in contradiction to evolutionary theory which suggests that average size of wild sheep increases during process of evolution in colder environment and tend to be more likely to survive and reproduce than smaller ones. The reason for bringing down the size of Soay sheep was attributed to shorter and milder winters caused by global climate change. In the changing climate conditions, the weight gain by the lambs during early months of life was diminished as compared to few decades back when winters were colder. The lambs had to put more weight to survive under extreme cold for survival.

The advantage of dark coloured coat of animals over lighter counterparts in colder environment is linked to conservation of solar energy and saving food energy for maintenance of homeothermy. The change in climate (warmer cold season) has been associated with the change in the proportion of light coloured Soay sheep in total population. A study has revealed that dark coloured Soay sheep have decreased over the past 20 years as the ambient temperature was increased.

(ii) *Physiological adaptability*: Normal fluctuations in physiological responses, i.e. respiration rate, pulse rate, rectal temperature and sweating rate vary with the changes in season in an effort to maintain normal body temperature independent of the fluctuation in environmental temperature. Hence, these are considered important indices for comparative adaptability of different genotypes. Increased respiration rate is the first reaction when animals are exposed to environmental temperatures above the thermoneutral zone (Maurya *et al.,* 2007). This response ensures direct heat stimulation of the peripheral receptors, which transmit nervous impulses to the heat centre in the hypothalamus. With the increasing environmental temperature, the respiration rate continues to rise linearly until a certain temperature afterwards rate of respiration slows down and depth of breathing increases (Kaushish *et al.,* 1989). At this level, the respiratory muscle reach a threshold of maximum activity and thus the respiration rate cannot increase further. Respiration rate can be used as an indicator of heat stress (Habeeb *et al.,* 1992) when activity of respiratory muscle is not suppressed due to fatigue.

Heat tolerance of non-pregnant adult ewes of Chokla, Nali and their crosses with Merino and Rambouillet were studied under solar exposure during summer. Native had lower rectal temperature and pulse than exotic breeds, while crossbred had intermediate values. The magnitude of physiological responses evoked by thermal stress and time required for their subsequent return to normalcy after removing the stress were considered useful indices for assessing the thermal ability of animals. Rai *et al.* (1983) showed that Rambouillet x Chokla experienced more stress at 40°C than Chokla when exposed for short duration (2 hr) and both breed attained normalcy within 2 hr after removing from the hot chamber and exposure to 20°C. The physiological response under hot semi-arid environment varied enormously during forenoon and afternoon. This is because the animals maintained under semi-arid condition are usually exposed to high ambient temperatures during hot summer months. The increase in ambient temperature through the morning and towards the afternoon may explain the reason for rise in the physiological responses in the afternoon when compared to morning values (Maurya *et al.,* 2004). The nutrition and body condition score (BCS) also seem to affect the respiration rate under heat stress conditions (Sejian *et al.,* 2010a).

Sweating in sheep is considered to be important in heat dissipation than respiratory evaporative cooling. The native animals were found to utilize cutaneous evaporative cooling relatively more than exotic animals during thermal stress at high ambient temperature (Ghosal *et al.,* 1981). Rai *et al.* (1979) observed no breed difference among

Rambouillet, Chokla, Malpura and their half-breed in response of increase in sweating rate from 20°C to 35°C, but at 42°C Chokla showed a considerable rise. It might reflect that stimulation for increasing the sweating activity is dependent on the temperature. Rai *et al.* (1979) also found a linear increase in the sweating from birth to adult age and ram had high sweating rate than ewes at high temperature (41-43°C). Significant differences were observed between sweating rate at different regions of body of sheep at high ambient temperature (43-44.5°C). The sweat samples collected from Malpura, Chokla, Rambouillet and their crosses at 38-40°C did not show difference in sodium, potassium and protein contents, but chloride content was higher in Rambouillet samples (Rai *et al.*, 1982). At high ambient temperature (41°C) sodium and potassium increased in Rambouillet and decreased or remain unchanged in Malpura and Chokla. The sweating rate of nutritionally depleted sheep under summer condition and under hot chamber maintained at 40°C/6 hr/day was reduced similarly (Naqvi and Rai., 1987). The environmental variables viz., ambient temperature, relative humidity and wind velocity have been found to influence sweat gland structural dimensions and coat characteristics in sheep. Further, apart from heat stress and nutritional stress, walking stress also significantly influences the physiological responses in sheep (Sejian *et al.*, 2011b). This shows that physiological responses serve as a good indicator of stress in sheep.

Adaptation based on biochemical and endocrine responses

The effect of multiple stresses on the biochemical and endocrine responses are depicted in table 2. Biochemical response pays an important role in the attempt of animals to counteract heat stress. There are enough literatures to support this statement. Seasonal variations in the haemoglobin concentration and PCV in blood of Corriedale rams were reported by Chahal and Rattan (1981). The plasma and blood volume of Chokla and Malpura in terms of percent body weight was found to be significantly higher than that of Rambouillet during summer. During thermal stress there is a decrease in the haemoglobin concentration (Maurya *et al.*, 2007), which could be attributed to haemodilution and increase in the blood volume of these animals. The packed cell volume also decreases in heat stressed animals either due to red cell destruction or haemodilution (Marai *et al.*, 2007). However, Srikandakumar *et al.* (2003) reported that there was no effect of heat stress on haemoglobin in Omani sheep but was decreased in Merino.

Table 2 : Effect of thermal, nutritional, combined and multiple stresses on blood biochemical parameters of Malpura ewes (Source: Sejian *et al.*, 2010a, b).

Parameters	Control	Thermal stress	Nutritional stress	Combined stresses	Multiple stresses
Hb (g/dl)	11.91±0.35^{a}	9.48±0.26^{c}	10.75±0.32^{b}	8.59±0.17^{d}	10.91±0.12^{b}
PCV (%)	41.33±1.46^{a}	31.31±1.64^{b}	35.80±1.73^{b}	26.54±2.05^{c}	35.80±0.75^{b}
Glucose (mg/dl)	52.08±2.43^{a}	47.80±1.61^{ab}	44.19±1.91^{b}	42.99±2.52^{b}	39.39±0.53^{c}
Total Protein (g/dl)	8.88±0.33^{a}	7.95±0.41^{ab}	7.91±0.26^{ab}	7.08±0.33^{b}	6.37±0.08^{c}
Total Cholesterol (mg/dl)	52.31±1.86^{a}	42.96±2.29^{b}	42.65±2.21^{b}	35.62±2.33^{c}	30.58±1.78^{d}
ACP (KA Units)	2.14±0.12^{a}	1.48±0.14^{bc}	1.78±0.09^{ab}	1.16±0.18^{c}	-
ALP (KA Units)	5.89±0.25^{a}	5.10±0.37^{b}	5.57±0.25^{ab}	4.10±0.33^{c}	-
T_3 (nmol/L)	1.71±0.01^{a}	1.33±0.00^{b}	1.42±0.00^{b}	1.14±0.01^{c}	1.39±0.05^{b}
T_4 (nmol/L)	76.24±4.17^{a}	58.90±3.22^{b}	62.97±3.64^{b}	45.94±5.14^{c}	24.41±0.10^{d}
Cortisol (nmol/L)	18.63±1.30^{d}	76.98±5.18^{a}	8.50±1.06^{e}	46.44±3.64^{b}	31.03±1.08^{c}
Insulin (MicroIU/mL)	47.44±2.92^{a}	39.79±3.20^{ab}	35.15±1.39^{bc}	26.41±2.84^{c}	-

Combined stresses-thermal and nutritional stress; Multiple stresses- thermal, nutritional and walking stress; Means(±SE) within a row having different superscripts differ significantly (P<0.05).

Blood glucose concentration was found to decrease during short-term exposure of sheep to 35°C ambient temperature for 24 hr and as well as during 5 days. However, when exposed to 40°C there was either small decline in native Nali sheep or no decline in half breds Soviet Merino x Nali sheep. Several researchers have studied the effect of thermal stress on the blood glucose concentrations but the results reported by them were conflicting. The decrease in glucose level during heat exposure relates to decrease in concentration of insulin and thyroxin, which are closely associated to energy metabolism during heat exposure. Decrease in plasma glucose could also be due to the marked dilution of blood. Serum proteins, particularly albumin concentration, usually decrease in heat exposed cattle (Habeeb, 1987). The decrease in the plasma protein may be due to dilution of plasma proteins and decrease in protein synthesis as a result of depression of anabolic hormone secretion. In addition to this, there is also increase in glucocorticoids concentration. The reduced feed intake in heat stressed animals also leads to decrease in nitrogen concentration in the body, which leads to low protein level. The serum total lipid concentration was also decreased in the animals exposed to prolonged thermal stress, which might be due to increase in utilization of fatty acids for energy production as a consequence of decrease in glucose concentration (Kamal *et al.*, 1989). Plasma free fatty acids, total lipids and cholesterol concentration were decreased during prolonged exposure of hot environment. Lower levels of ruminal ammonia and blood urea nitrogen were also reported in Merino sheep maintained at high temperature (35°C) than those of same animals when kept at low temperature (15°C).

Heat stress causes an increase in the activities of serum glutamic oxaloacetic transaminase (SGOT) and serum glutamic pyruvic transaminase (SGPT) due to increased stimulation of gluconeogenesis by corticoids (Kamal *et al.*, 1989). Singh *et al.* (1983) reported increased alkaline phosphatase activity in Nali and Nali x Soviet Merino sheep exposed to heat stress. Serum protein concentrations were increased at 35°C and 40°C exposure. Blood plasma vitamin A level was decreased as the ambient temperature increased while atmospheric pressure was decreased in rams and no show specific trend in ewes. Further the activity of plasma acid phosphates and lactatic acid dehydrogenase (LDH) were comparatively higher during summer than spring season in ewes while SGOT, SGPT and alkaline phosphates did not change much.

Hormones play a critical and important role in the thermoregulation of animal's body. On prolonged heat exposure, hypothalamic releasing hormones is suppressed which in turn drastically affects the release of pituitary hormones (Magiakou *et al.*, 1997) During stress various endocrine responses are involved to improve the fitness of the individual animals. Endocrine responses to stress in general work towards suppressing productive functions such as growth and reproduction, in favour of maintenance and survival. The front-line hormones overcoming stressful situations are the glucocorticoids and catecholamines. The secretion of glucocorticoids is a classic endocrine response to stress (Kannan *et al.*, 2000). The association between thermal stress and increased secretion of cortisol, the principal glucocorticoid hormone in small ruminants is well documented (Ali and Hayder, 2008; Sejian *et al.*, 2008a). Currently it appears that glucocorticoids provide an initial integrating signal, which in conjunction with other hormones and paracrine secretions may determine specific behavioural and physiological responses to adapt to different environmental conditions (Wingfield and Kitaysky, 2002). Heat stress is associated with significant depression in thyroid gland activity resulting in lowering of thyroid hormones level (Nazifi *et al.*, 2003). However, other investigators did not detect any significant changes in thyroid hormones (Al-Haidary, 2004). In a study conducted at CSWRI on Malpura rams, it has been established that BCS of sheep under hot semi-arid environment had significant influence on plasma cortisol, T_3, T_4 and testosterone concentrations. A recent report suggests the involvement of melatonin to counteract heat stress in farm animals (Sejian *et al.*, 2008a). Further there is evidence for the role of melatonin and prolactin to up regulate heat shock protein (HSP) 70 gene expression during heat stress (Collier *et al.*, 2008).

Ameliorative measures to counter environmental stresses

Reducing environmental stresses on livestock requires a multi-disciplinary approach with emphasis on animal nutrition, housing and animal health (Collier *et al.*, 2008). Some of the biotechnological options may also be used to reduce thermal stress. It is importance to understand the livestock responses to environment, analyse them, in order to design modifications of nutritional and environmental management thereby improving animal comfort and performance. So a range of technologies are needed, to match the different economic and other needs of smallholders. Figure 1 describes the various approaches for ameliorating adverse effects of thermal stress on livestock.

(i) Physical modification

Significance of animal housing: Animal housing has been a matter of concern since domestication of livestock. Its basic aim is to moderate the range of animal's micro-climate and to optimize their production by protecting them from climate extremes. Consequently, a house should provide 5 freedoms (eating, resting, moving, voiding and respiring and also the comfort to all type of stresses (climate, social, nutritional and disease). With the changing climate construction of animal housing needs thorough review of site selection, housing design and future requirements for the livestock species to be reared at a particular locality (Sharma and Singh, 2008).

Ambient temperature is the most important climatic variable that affects design of the house. Its effect can be ameliorated by providing shade, shelters and planting trees. Roofing materials and their painting (outside/ inside with black/white) can help in providing desired effects within the house. Roof and wall made of wood, thatch, bamboo and mud radiate least heat in comparison to stone, concrete, asbestos, tin and steel (Sharma and Singh, 2008). The effects of humidity, both low (rapid evaporation, skin irritation and general dehydration) and high (heat stagnation in confinement) are harmful to animals. In humid areas, house should be open having high roof (spacious), airy and well ventilated. Rainfall has direct and indirect effects on livestock production. Heavy rains increase humidity, lowers down forage quality, grazing and feed intake. Heavy rainfall areas are not suitable for animals having heavy coat. In such areas, the stilted, loose, airy and ventilated and protective (from ecto-parasites) house should be constructed at raised platform.

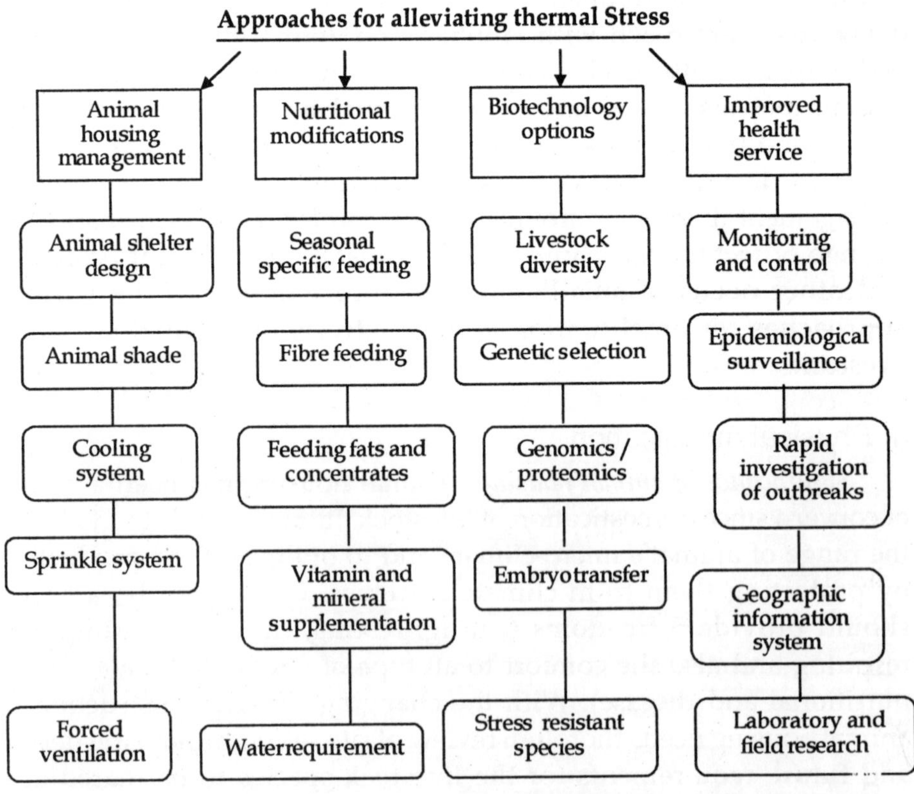

Fig. 1 : Different approaches for alleviating thermal stress in livestock

Animal shelter design for comfort: Physical modification of the environment is based on two basic concept of protecting the livestock from the factors contributing to heat stress, and enhancing evaporative heat loss by the animal. The different environmental modification systems have been classified according to the different impact they can have on animals' productive performance (Hahn, 1981). The first are those that help decrease heat gain by radiation interception. Among the latter there is a range that covers from the forced ventilation and sprinkling of water, each separately, to combinations of both systems, including evaporative cooling, and even air conditioning.

Ensuring proper ventilation: Ventilation systems in livestock housing serve an important function, maintaining a comfortable animal environment. Ventilation systems continuously remove the heat, moisture, and odours created by livestock, and replenish the oxygen supply by bringing in drier and cooler outside air. Adequate air exchange also removes gases such as ammonia (NH_4), hydrogen sulfide (H_2S), and methane (CH_4) which can be harmful to both animal and operator health. The components of the ventilation system should provide the following basic features.

- *Air exchange*: Sufficient air exchange is accomplished by the natural driving forces of wind and buoyancy.
- *Control*: Ventilation rates require adjustment based on inside and outside conditions. This is typically achieved with manually opened and closed curtains, doors or ventilation panels.
- *Flexibility*: Ventilation needs based on different seasons require different operating conditions. At least following three operating conditions must be provided.

i. Continuous minimum air exchange is required to remove moisture constantly produced by the animals. This minimum air exchange is vital during sub-freezing weather.

ii. Temperature control which is needed during cool and mild weather conditions to remove excess heat from the building.

iii. High air exchange rates and air velocity past the animals is needed during hot weather to help remove heat from the cow's body.

- *Proper barn construction*: Naturally ventilated barns must have sufficient and properly located openings that can be adjusted to take advantage of buoyancy effects, as well as wind forces and direction.

Using shades: The most obvious environmental modification to reduce the thermal stress of livestock during hot climate condition is the use of proper shade (Blackshaw and Blackshaw, 1994). So shelter management is one of the key techniques to reduce heat stress. Shade against direct solar radiation can be provided by either trees like banana or house made of straw and other locally available materials. Animals kept in or outside during summer are comfortable under tree shade and protect them from direct sun light during peak hours of the day (Buffington *et al.*, 1983).

A properly designed shading structure provides the most adequate protection to the livestock not only in hot summer but also in winter (Armstrong, 1994). For tropical climate condition loose housing system is considered most appropriate (Hahn, 1981). The longer side of the animal shelter should have an east-west orientation. This reduces the amount of direct sunlight shining on side walls or entering the house (Ugurlu and Uzal, 2010). In addition to this roof can be extended with shading material and the vertical shading moved to the outside of the roof. Such devices give much better protection from the direct solar radiation and sun. The west side of the shed can also be protected similarly and fitted with side covers and gunny bags or curtains. The height of the shed structure should be greater than 2.4 meters to allow sufficient air movement under shade. However, tall structures (> 3.05 meters high) are not economically viable.

There are other ways of removing the hot air trapped under the roof, inside the shed. Outer coverings and shading, perhaps combined with a roof-spray, are popular greenhouse technologies which can be applied in the structural design of shed to reduce the height of the shed. There are also various roof systems which gives improved natural ventilation by means of roof openings, enhanced solar chimney effect, etc. In addition to this, painting the roof with white colour may increase the level of sunlight reflected, thus reducing the amount of absorbed solar energy. Increasing air flow is another important component for effective ventilation in animal shelters.

Increasing air flow: In an animal shed, air movement should be free and in all area of shed (Bryant *et al.*, 2007). To increase air flow, two main approaches may be used: one is to install large fans so that air movement is increased and the second is to open the side of the shed. In many cases, walls of the shed may be made partially of concrete. In such situation, opening the lower level of the barn to increase air flow is not an option, so the addition of fans is essential to increase air circulation. In shed, where sheet metal is used for the walls, it may be practical to remove the side and install netting over these areas. The netting can be raised to increase air flow during the summer and lowered during the winter. Increasing the roof venting is yet another option that may be used for animal sheds. Another approach which can be used, similar to housing used for human, is the double wall approach. In this, extra wall layer at either end of shed is constructed and the outer layer is kept 10 cm away from the inside wall, with vertical openings at both ends. The bottom opening allows cold air to enter, and the upper opening allows hot air to exit. The 10 cm of air between the two walls provides a thermal barrier to prevent conductive thermal energy from entering the animal house. Double wall approach is an effective and proven technology in structural design for increasing or reducing temperature.

Using sprinklers: Some studies reported beneficial effects of wetting the animals through sprinklers during periods of high temperature. In Mexico, a region of sub-humid tropical climate, there was a 7% increase in milk production in cows sprinkled between 12:00 and 13:00 hr under the shade. Also, positive results were reported in few studies conducted in Missouri when animals were sprinkled between 11:00 and 17:30hr during moderate summer. In Israel, when cows were sprinkled for one hour, four times a day, it relieved the stress. In Australia when the cows were watered every time at the temperature exceeded 26 °C, similar effect was seen (Davison *et al.*, 1996). Sprinkling maximizes the amount of heat removed from the animal through evaporative cooling at a reduced water cost. In addition, the ambient air temperature is lowered in the area immediately surrounding the animal, increasing the heat gradient and increasing the effectiveness of non-evaporative cooling mechanism (Morrison *et al.*, 1973). To achieve adequate heat loss when sprinkling, droplets must wet the hides of the animal as accumulation of water in the hair may increase the humidity around the animal and reduce effective heat loss (Means *et al.*, 1992). High pressure irrigation-type sprinklers can improve inexpensive wetting of animals, especially when coupled with fans, to increase air movement (Nienaber *et al.*, 1999). However, cooled animal have limited ability to adapt to warm condition and may become reliant on sprinkling to keep cool even in milder condition. Cessation of sprinkling during the day on hot days may increase the heat load in cattle, even though ambient temperature and humidity may be decreasing (Gaughan *et al.*, 2008; Mader *et al.*, 2002). Altering the microclimate of the sprinkled area helps in improving the wellbeing of feedlot cattle under extreme environment condition by reducing body temperature. Therefore, one point which should be kept in mind while using evaporative cooling system in hot and humid subtropical region is that cooling requires the use of forced ventilation.

Forced ventilation using fans: When there is no sufficient natural ventilation, layer of air close to the animal, gets warmer. This slows down the processes of heat dissipation from the surface of the animals to surrounding. The role of fans is to increase heat loss by convection. Fans can reduce the body temperature by 0.3 to 0.4 ° C, provided that the temperature of the provided air is lower than the surface temperature of the animal. However, fan is not enough to reduce conditions of heat stress in high producing dairy cows in hot weather. However, when working in areas where the humidity is high, consideration should be given that any system that introduces water into the environment may be negative because water will evaporate further increasing the humidity and saturating the air. It is for this reason that systems are designed to combine the forced ventilation with wetting.

(ii) Nutritional modification to combat heat stress

Feed requirement: During hot dry summer, there is decreased dietary feed intake which is responsible for the reduced productivity. In this situation, the efficient practical approaches like frequent feeding, improved forage quality, use of palatable feeds, good nutrition balance and greater nutrient density are required. However, feeding excessive quantities of nutrients, like crude protein, can contribute to reduced efficiency of energy utilization, potentially adding to stress levels. Likewise, if less forage is consumed, and the forage is high in quality, the cows' rumination activity may decrease. So, a through understating of dietary manipulation to minimize heat stress is necessary (NRC, 2001). Heat production from feed intake peaks 4 to 6 hr after feeding. Therefore heat production in animal feed in the morning will peak in the middle of the day when environmental temperature is also elevated. Consequently, it has been suggested that feeding animals later in the day prevents the coincidal occurrence of peak metabolic and environmental heat load (Brosh *et al.*, 1998). Furthermore, limiting energy intake can effectively decrease basal metabolic heat production (Carstens *et al.*, 1989) and therefore decrease total metabolic heat load of animals subjected to high environmental temperature.

Concept of cold diet: A cold diet is one that generates a high proportion of net nutrients for the synthesis and decreases heat generated during fermentation and metabolism. The salient features of a cold diet are: higher energy content per unit volume, more digestible fibre, effective fibre, lower protein degradability and more by-pass nutrients.

Antioxidant supplementation: Nutritional tools, such as antioxidant feeding (vitamin A, selenium, zinc etc.) and ruminant specific live yeast can help. Studies have shown that addition of antioxidant in diets of cows is able to reduce stress and is a good strategy to prevent mastitis, optimize feed intake and reduce the negative impact of heat stress on milk production. Moreover, the use of antioxidant such as vitamin E, A, selenium and selenium enriched yeast help reducing the impact of heat stress on the oxidant balance, resulting in improved milk quality and cow health. A recent study in cattle showed that the supplementation of vitamin E help in reducing the heat stress and improves the antioxidant status and lowers the incidence of mastitis, metritis, and retention of placenta. During period of heat stress, the risks of rumen acidosis are increased particularly in high producing cows maintained on high concentrate diets. Factors that contribute to rumen acidosis problems in cow are related to decrease DM intake particularly lower forage intake and higher levels of fermentable carbohydrates. A decreased rumination and decreased salivary activity reduce buffering power of rumen. A low rumen pH impairs fibre digestion efficiency due to effect on rumen fibrolytic bacteria.

Fibre feeding: Because there is greater heat production associated with metabolism of acetate compared with propionate, there is a logical rationale for the practice of feeding low fibre rations during hot weather. Feeding more concentrate at the expense of fibrous ingredients increases ration energy density and reduces heat increment. Altered proportions of ruminal volatile fatty acids (VFA) may explain a part of the differences in heat increment with fibre feeding during heat stress. VFA constitute a large proportion of the energy available to the cow, and declining intake during heat stress reduces the quantity of VFA in the rumen because fermentable carbohydrate is reduced. Increased feeding of concentrates is a common practice during conditions conducive to heat stress, but maximal benefit from concentrates appears to be approximately 60 to 65% of the diet (Coppock, 1985). Excessive concentrate feeding leads to acidosis and the associated production, health, and metabolic difficulties. The large amount of highly fermentable carbohydrate fed in typical high-concentrate diets should minimize the heat production observed in the very high fibre diets, which were used in research settings. Although high fibre diets contribute to heat stress, the level of intake is far more critical to the total amount of metabolic heat produced. Growing heifers fed pellet rations containing 75% alfalfa or 25% alfalfa produced 48.8 and 45.5 MJ/d of heat (Reynolds *et al.*, 1991). However, when the low and high intake (4.2 and 7.1 kg DMI /d) in heifers were compared, heat production was 38.2 and 56.1 MJ/d. Therefore, intake effects have a substantial effect on heat production and must be considered in designing an effective nutritional and environmental management program. Research suggests that lower fibre, high grain diets may indeed reduce metabolic heat production and contribute to lower heat load in the animal. Further, the low fibre, high grain diets provide more efficiently used end products, which contribute to lower dietary heat increment. However, low fibre, high grain diets must be balanced with the need for adequate fibre to promote chewing and rumination to maintain ruminal pH and cow health.

Feeding fats and concentrates: The addition of fat to the diet of lactating dairy cows is a common practice, and the greater energy density and the potential to reduce heat increment of high-fat diets may be particularly beneficial during hot weather. There is reference which shows that fat can be added to the ration to the level pf 3 to 5% without any adverse effects to ruminal microflora. Improved efficiency and lower heat increment should make fat especially beneficial during hot weather. Ruminally protected fats allow the inclusion of a substantial quantity of fat in the diet, which could lower heat increment significantly.

Water balance and water requirements: Water is the most essential element for the survival of animals. Water requirements for livestock can be met in three ways:

i. Metabolic water, derived from the oxidation of organic substrates and tissue
ii. Water contained in food
iii. Drinking water

In any event the first route is the most important in quantitative terms and in summer it is by far the largest source. During the summer, any factor that limits access to water, directly affects the production of sheep. Sheep with water restrictions manifest higher body temperature, with a degree of heat stress higher than normal. Furthermore, water consumption and dry matter intake are closely related (NRC, 2001).Under intense heat, ingestion of large volumes of water provides comfort to the animals by reducing the temperature of the rumen reticulum.

(iii) Physiological modification

Diaphoretics administration: These compounds are used to increase sweat production for increasing the evaporative cooling of the heat stressed animals (Marai *et al.*, 2008). However, such treatments cause significant increases in each of rectal temperature and respiration rate.

Diuretics administration: These compounds are used to increase water excretion to increase the heat loss by excreting water in urine with the same body temperature and then followed by drinking water which is also of lower temperature than that of the body.

Goitrogens administration: These compounds block thyroidal iodine uptake and consequently depress thyroid gland activity. It depresses the secretion of T_4 in the heat stressed animals to decrease heat production. However, this technique is not favoured under heat stress conditions, since the treated animals under such conditions may be affected seriously due to their need to more energy for greater muscular activity for the high respiratory activity, O_2 consumption and energy metabolism (Marai *et al.*, 2008).

Hormonal substances administration: Administration or injection of hormones can be used as a technique for alleviation of heat load on animal, since secretion of most of the hormones is depressed under heat stress conditions. However, injection of T_4 for this purpose was found to be associated with the increase of body temperature of the animals (Marai *et al.*, 2008). Similarly, insulin injection in the udder was found to show the same effect, besides it increases milk production. Injection by BST also minimized the negative effects of moderately high environmental temperatures on milk yield by increasing heat loss and minimizing the endogenous heat production and related physiological functions without any significant increase in rectal temperature and respiratory rates. However, such techniques require some specific precautions and are expensive at the same time.

(iv) Improved health service

Increase in temperature and humidity due to climate change is strongly associated with emerging and re-emerging animal diseases by (i) increasing the diffusion of insects (*Culicoides imicola*) that are the main vectors of several arboviruses (e.g. Bluetongue and African sickness); (ii) increasing the survival of viruses from one year to the next, (iii) improving conditions for new insect vectors that are now limited by colder temperatures (Mellor and Wittmann, 2002; Gould *et al.*, 2006). This will lead to production losses. Thus, improved diseases control strategies and health service at a big scale is required.

For prevention, monitoring and control of livestock diseases good data exchange mechanism are required at both state and national level. These should cover the distribution of animal diseases, ecological conditions including climate, and associated drugs and chemo-therapeutants. In this contest, epidemiological surveillance is a critical component and it not only involves the early identification of emerging diseases and trends but also for resource planning and measuring the impact of control strategies (Upadhyay *et al.*, 2011). A global approach to epidemiological surveillance should be taken and should involve collaboration between professionals involved human, animal and environmental health. Such surveillance programmes are essential in allowing us to recognize and respond to emerging risk to climate change. We can also use the geographic information system (GIS) by which we can both monitor the level of stress and how our climate is changing and monitor the spread of diseases. We can use it to look for periods or heavy rainfall using a spatial analyst and illustrate it using GIS. This system tells us which pathogens will flourish, under their preferred condition. This tool can also help to pinpoint period of continually high minimum temperature. Likewise predictive modeling system can also be used to predict the probability of an outcome. It has potential to predict the probability of global climate change on ecological system and emerging hazards. Furthermore, laboratory and field research will also help in illuminating how climate changes influence pathogen characteristics, and models will help researchers and producers predict and plan for pathogen threats.

Conclusion

Livestock researchers aiming at improving livestock production under changing climatic scenario must aim at counteracting multiple stresses as these stresses are common occurrences in most ecological zones where livestock are reared. On individual basis, sheep were better able to adapt to nutritional stress than thermal stress. However, when both these stresses were coupled, it had severe impact on productive and reproductive performance of sheep. Hence, it is very pertinent to conclude that when two or more than two stressors occur simultaneously, the total impact may be severe on biological functions. Further, these studies reveal the importance of providing optimum nutrition to sheep to counteract thermal stress during summer. It is also evident from the experiments that when nutrition is not a limiting factor then ewes were able to cope with thermal stress. This chapter also elaborates on ameliorative strategies that need to be given due consideration to prevent huge economical losses incurred due to environmental stresses on sheep productivity. Further, this chapter details the issues of less-than-perfect information on climate impacts and vulnerabilities, and need for better informed decisions on "resilient adaptation" by merging adaptation, mitigation and prevention strategies. It offers new perspectives for policy-makers, institutions, societies and individuals on improved ways of identifying most at-risk communities and "best practices" of coping with current climate variability and extreme climate events.

References

Abecia, A.J., Sosa, C., Forcada, F. and Meikle, A. 2006. The effect of undernutrition on the establishment of pregnancy in the ewe. Reproduction Nutrition Development 46: 367-378.

Al-Haidary, A.A. 2004. Physiological responses of Naimey Sheep to heat stress challenge under semi-arid environments. International Journal of Agriculture and Biology 2: 307-309.

Ali, A. and Hayder, M. 2008. Seasonal variation of reproductive performance, Foetal development and progesterone concentrations of sheep in the subtropics. Reproduction in Domestic Animal Doi: 10.1111/j.1439-0531.2007.00980.x.

Amundson, J.L., Mader, T.L., Rasby, R.J. and Hu, Q.S. 2006. Environmental effects on pregnancy rate in beef cattle. Journal of Animal Science 84: 3415-3420.

Armstrong, D.V. 1994. Heat stress interaction with shade and cooling. Journal of Dairy Science 77: 2044-2050.

Averos, A., Martin, S., Riu, M., Serratosa, J. and Gosalvez, L.F. 2008. Stress response of extensively reared young bulls being transported to growing-finishing farm under Spanish summer commercial conditions. Life Sciences 119: 174-182.

Blackshaw, J.K. and Blackshaw, A.W. 1994. Heat stress in cattle and the effect of shade on production and ffects: a review. Australian Journal of Experimental Agriculture 34: 285-295.

Brosh, A., Aharoni, Y., Degen, A.A., Wright, D. and Young, B.A. 1998. Effects of solar radiation, dietary energy, and time of feeding on thermoregulatory responses and energy balance in cattle in a hot environment. Journal of Animal Science 76: 2671-2677.

Bryant, J.R., Lo´ pez-Villalobos, N., Pryce, J.E., Holmes, C.W., Johnson, D.L. and Garrick, D.J. 2007. Environmental sensitivity in New Zealand dairy cattle. Journal of Dairy Science 90:1538–1547.

Buffington, D.E., Collier, R.J. and Canton, G.H. 1983. Shade management systems to reduce heat stress for dairy cows in hot, humid climates. Transactions of the ASAE. 26: 1798-1802.

Carstens, G.E., Johnson, D.E., and Ellenberger, M.A. 1989. Energy metabolism and composition of gain in beef steers exhibiting normal and compensatory growth. Energy Metabolism of Farm Animals. European Association for Animal Production Publication 43:131.

Chadio, S.E., Kotsampasi, B., Papadomichelakis, G., Deligeorgis, S., Kalogiannis, D., Menegatos, D. and Zerwas, G. 2007. Impact of maternal undernutrition on the hypothalamic-pitutary-adrenal axis responsiveness in the sheep at different ages postnatal. Journal of Endocrinology 192: 495-503.

Chahal, A.S. and Rattan, P.J.S. 1981. Seasonal variation in the contents of haemoglobin and the packed cell volume in the blood of coriedale rams. Journal of Research (PAU, Ludhiana, India), 18: 341-344.

Collier, R.J., Collier, J.L., Rhoads, R.P. and Baumgard, L.H. 2008. Genes involved in the bovine heat stress response. Journal of Dairy Science 91: 445-454.

Coppock, C.E. 1985. Energy nutrition and metabolism of the lactating dairy cow. Journal of Dairy Science 68: 3403-3410.

Davison, T., McGowan, M., Mayer, D., Young, B., Jonsson, N., Hall, A., Matschoss, A., Goodwin, P., Gaughan, J. and Lake, M. 1996. Managing hot cows in Australia. Queensland Department of Primary Industry, Brisbane, Australia.

Downing, J.A., Joss, J. and Scarmuzzi, R. J. 1995. Ovulation rate and the concentration of gonadotrophins and metabolic hormones in ewes infused with glucose during the late luteal phase of the oestrous cycle. Journal of Endocrinology 146: 403-410.

Forcada, F. and Abecia, A.J. 2006. The effect of nutrition on the seasonality of reproduction in ewes. Reproduction Nutrition Development 46: 355-365.

Gaughan, J.B., Holt, S.M., Mader, T.L. and Lisle, A. 2008. A new heat load index for feedlot cattle. Journal of Animal Sciences 86: 226-234.

Gaughan, J.G., Goopy, J. and Spark, J. 2002. Excessive heat load index for feedlot cattle. In: Meat and Livestock-Australia Project Report, FLOT.316. MLA Ltd, Sydney, NSW.

Ghosal, A.K., Purohit, S.K., Goswami, A.K., Singh, L.B. and Jatkar, P.R. 1981. Rate on physiological responses and coat characteristics of Nali and Corriedale sheep during canary season in India. Indian Journal of Animal Sciences 51: 243-245.

Gougeon, A. 1996. Regulation of ovarian follicular development in primates: facts and hypotheses. Endocrine Reviews 17: 121-155.

Gould, T.W., Buss, R.R., Vinsant, .S., Prevette, D., Sun, W., Knudson, C.M., Milligan, C.E. and Oppenheim, R.W. 2006. Complete dissociation of motor neuron death from motor dysfunction by Bax deletion in a mouse model of ALS. Journal of Neuroscience 26: 8774-8786.

Habeeb, A.A. 1987. The role of insulin in improving productivity of heat-stressed farm animals with different techniques. Ph.D. thesis. Faculty of Agriculture, Zagazig University, Zagazig, Egypt.

Habeeb, A.A., Marai, I.F.M. and Kamal, T.H. 1992. Heat stress. In: Farm Animals and the Environment (C. Philips and D. Piggens, Eds.), CAB International, 27-47.

Hahn, G.L. 1981. Housing and management to reduce climatic impacts on livestock. Journal of Animal Science 52: 175-186.

Hatfield, J., Boote, K., Fay, P., Hahn, L.C., Izaurralde, B.A., Kimball, T., Mader, J., Morgan, D., Ort, W., Polley, A., Thomson, and Wolfe, D. 2008. Agriculture. In: The effects of climate change on agriculture, land resources, water resources, and biodiversity in the United States. A Report by the U.S. Climate Change Science Program and the Subcommittee on Global Change Research. Washington, DC, USA, 362.

Holtenius, K. and Dahlborn, K. 1990. Water and sodium movements across the ruminal epithelium in fed and food deprived sheep. Experimental Physiology 75: 57-67.

Ismail, E., Abdel-Latif, H., Hassan, G.A. and Salem, M.H. 1995. Water metabolism and requirement of sheep as affected by breed and season. World Review on Animal Production 30: 95-105.

Kamal, T.H., Habeeb, A.A., Abdel-Samee, A.M. and Abdel-Razik, M.A. 1989. Supplementation of heat-stressed Friesian cows with urea and mineral mixture and its effect on milk production in subtropics. In: Proc. International Symposium on the Constraints and Possibilities of Ruminant Production in the Dry Subtropics. Cairo, Egypt, pp. 183-185.

Kannan, G., Terrill, T.H., Kouakou, B., Gazal, O.S., Gelaye, S., Amoah, E.A. and Samake, S. 2000.Transportation of goats: Effects on physiological stress responses and live weight loss. Journal of Animal Science 78:1450-1457.

Kaushish, S.K., Karim, S.A. and Rawat, P.S. 1989. Responses of native and crossbred sheep to solar exposure during summer in semi-arid region. Indian Veterinary Journal 66: 852-856.

Khalifa, H.H. 2003. Bioclimatology and adaptation of farm animals in a changing climate. In: Interactions between climate and animal production, EAAP Technical Series 7: 15-29.

Kiyma, Z., Alexander, B.M., Van Kirk, E.A., Murdoch, W.J., Hallford, D.M. and Moss, G.E. 2004. Effect of feed restriction on reproductive and metabolic hormones in ewes. Journal of Animal Science 82: 2548-2557.

Koubková, M., Knížková, I., Kunc, P., Härtlová, H., Flusser, J. and Doležal, O. 2002. Influence of high environmental temperatures and evaporative cooling on some physiological, hematological and biochemical parameters in high-yielding dairy cows. Czech Journal of Animal Science 47: 309-318.

Lamond, R.D., Gaddy, G.R. and Kennedy, W.S. 1972. Influence of season and nutrition on luteal plasma progesterone in Rambuillet Ewes. Journal of Animal Science 34: 626-629.

Lawson, R.A.S. and Cahill, L.P. 1983. Modification of the embryo-maternal relationship in ewes by progesterone treatment early in the oestrous cycle. Journal of Reproduction and Fertility 67: 473-475.

Mader, T.L., Holt, S.M., Hahn, G.L., Davis, M.S. and Spiers, D.E. 2002. Feeding strategies for managing heat load in feedlot cattle. Journal of Animal Science 80: 2373-2382.

Magiakou, M.A., Mastorakos, G., Webster, E. and Chrousos, G.P. 1997. The hypothalamic-pituitary-adrenal axis and the female reproductive system. Annals of the Newyork Academy of Sciences 816: 42-56.

Marai, I.F.M., Abdel-Samee, A.M. and El-gafaary, M.N. 1991.Criteria of responses and adaptation to high temperature for reproductive and growth traits in rabbits. Options Mediterraneennes Series A 17: 127-134.

Marai, I.F.M., Habeeb, A.A.M. and Farghaly, H.M. 1999. Productive, physiological and biochemical changes in imported and locally born Friesian and Holstein lactating cows under hot summer conditions of Egypt. Tropical Animal Health and Production 31: 233-243.

Marai, I.F.M., Bhagat, L.B., Shalaby, T.H. and Abdel-Hafez, M.A. 2000. Fattening performances, some behavioral traits and physiological reactions of male lambs fed concentrates mixture alone with or without natural clay, under hot summer of Egypt. Annals of Arid Zone 39: 449-460.

Marai, I.F.M., El-Darawany, A.A., Fadiel, A. and Abdel-Hafez, M.A.M. 2007. Physiological traits as affected by heat stress in sheep – A review. Small Ruminant Research 71: 1-12.

Marai, I.F.M., El-Darawany, A.A., Fadiel, A. and Abdel-Hafez, M.A.M. 2008. Reproductive performance traits as affected by heat stress and its alleviation in sheep. Tropical and Subtropical Agro ecosystems 8: 209-234.

Martin, G.B., Rogar, J. and Blache, D. 2004. Nutritional and environmental effects on reproduction in small ruminants. Reproduction Fertility Development 16: 491-501.

Maurya, V.P., Naqvi, S.M.K. and Mittal, J.P. 2004. Effect of dietary energy level on physiological responses and reproductive performance in Malpura sheep in hot semi-arid region of India. Small Ruminant Research 55: 117-122.

Maurya, V.P., Naqvi, S.M.K., Joshi, A.. and Mittal, J.P. 2007. Effect of high temperature stress on physiological responses of Malpura sheep. Indian Journal of Animal Sciences 77: 1244-1247.

McManus, C., Paludo, G.R., Louvandini, H., Gugel, R., Sasaki, L.C.B. and Paiva, S.R. 2009. Heat tolerance in Brazilian sheep: physiological and blood parameters. Tropical Animal Health and Production 41: 95-101.

Means, S.L., Bucklin, R.A., Nordstedt, R.A., Beede, D.K., Bray, D.R., Wilcox, C.J. and Sanchez, W.K. 1992. Water application rates for a sprinkler and fan dairy cooling system in hot, humid climates. Applied Engineering in Agriculture 8: 375-379.

Mellor, P.S. and Wittmann, E.J. 2002. Bluetongue virus in the Mediterranean Basin 1998–2001. Veterinary Journal 164: 20-37.

Minka, N.S. and Ayo, J.O. 2009. Physiological responses of food animals to road transportation tress. African Journal of Biotechnology 8: 7415-7427.

Moberg, G.P. 1999. When does stress become distress? Lab Animals 28: 422-426.

Morrison, S.R., Givens, R.L. and Lofgreen, G.P. 1973. Sprinkling cattle for relief from heat stress. Journal of Animal Sciences 36: 428-431.

Naqvi, S.M.K. and Rai, A.K. 1987. Heat tolerance of nutritionally depleted Avivastra and Chokla sheep. In: Proc. National Seminar on Small Ruminant Production, CSWRI, Avikanagar (Rajasthan). 5-7 January,

Nazifi, S., Saeb, M., Rowghani, E. and Kaveh, K. 2003. The influence of thermal stress on serum biochemical parameters of Iranian fat-tailed sheep and their correlation with triiodothyronine (T_3), thyroxine (T_4) and cortisol concentrations. Comparative Clinical Pathology 12: 135-139.

Nienaber, J.A., Hahn, G.L. and Eigenberg, R.A. 1999. Quantifying livestock responses for heat stress management: a review. International Journal of Biometeorology 42: 183-188.

NRC (National Research Council). 1981. Effect of Environment on Nutrient Requirements of Domestic Animals. Committee on Animal Nutrition. Subcommittee on Environmental Stress. National Academy Press, Washington DC.

NRC (National Research Council). 2001. Pages 318-319 in Nutrient Requirements of Dairy Cattle. 7th ed. National Academy of Science, Washington, D.C.

O'Callaghan, D., Yaakub, H., Hyttel, P., Spicer, L.J. and Boland, M.P. 2000. Effect of nutrition and superovulation on oocyte morphology, follicular fluid composition and systemic hormone concentrations in ewes. Journal of Reproduction and Fertility 18: 303-313.

Padua, J.T., Dasilva, R.G., Bottcher, R.W. and Hoff, S.J. 1997. Effect of high environmental temperature on weight gain and food intake of Suffolk lambs reared in a tropical environment. In: Proc 5th International Symposium, Bloomington, Minnesota, USA, 809-815.

Parr, R.A. 1992. Nutrition-progesterone interactions during early pregnancy in sheep. Reproduction, Fertility and Development 4: 297-300.

Parr, R.A., Davis, I.F., Miles, M.A. and Squires, T.J. 1993. Feed intake affects metabolic clearance rate of progesterone in sheep. Research in Veterinary Science 55: 306-310.

Pereira, A.M.F., Baccari Jr,F., Titto, E.A.L. and Almeida, J.A.A. 2008. Effect of thermal stress on physiological parameters, feed intake and plasma thyroid hormones concentration in Alentejana, Mertolenga, Frisian and Limousine cattle breeds. International Journal of Biometeorology 52: 199-208.

Rai, A.K., Mehta, B.S. and Singh, M. 1979. Thermal sweating in different body regions of sheep. Journal of Agricultural Sciences (Cambridge) 92: 511-512.

Rai, A.K., More, T. and Singh, M. 1982. Composition of sweat in sheep exposed to high ambient temperatures. Indian Journal of Animal Sciences 52: 1056-1059.

Rai, A.K., More, T., and Singh, M. 1983. Certain blood attributes in different genetic groups of sheep on feed lot ration. Indian Veterinary Journal 60: 839-841.

Rasooli, A., Nouri M., Khadjeh, G.H. and Rasekh, A. 2004. The influence of seasonal variations on thyroid activity and some biochemical parameters of cattle. Iranian Journal of Veterinary Research 5: 1383-1391.

Reynolds, C.K., Tyrrell, H.F. and Reynolds, P.J. 1991. Effects of diet forage-to-concentrate ratio and intake on energy metabolism in growing beef heifers: Whole body energy and nitrogen balance and visceral heat production. Journal of Nutrition 121: 994-1003.

Rivington, M., Matthews, K.B., Buchan, K., Miller, D. and Russell, G. 2009. Investigating climate change impacts and adaptation options using integrated assessment methods. Aspects of Applied Biology 93: 85-92.

Roberts, A.J., Funston, R.N. and Moss, G.E. 2001. Insulin-like growth factor binding proteins in the bovine anterior pituitary. Endocrine Journal 14: 399-406.

Scaramuzzi, R.J., Cambel, B.K., Downing, J.A., Kendall, N.R., Khalid, M., Gutierrez, M. and Somchit, A. 2006. A review of the effect of supplementary nutrition in the ewe on the concentration of reproductive and metabolic hormones and the mechanism that regulate folliculogenesis and ovulation rate. Reproduction Nutrition Development 46: 339-354.

Sejian, V. and Srivastava, R.S. 2009. Effects of melatonin on adrenal cortical functions of Indian goats under thermal stress. Veterinary Medical International doi:10.4061/2010/348919.

Sejian, V. and Srivastava, R.S. 2010. Pineal-adrenal-immune system relationship under thermal stress: effect on physiological, endocrine and non-specific immune response in goats. Journal of Physiology and Biochemistry 66: 339-349.

Sejian, V., Srivastava, R.S. and Varshney, V.P. 2008a. Pineal-adrenal relationship: Modulating effects of glucocorticoids on pineal function to ameliorate thermal-stress in Goats. Asian-Australian Journal of Animal Science 21: 988-994.

Sejian, V., Sanyal, S., Das, P.K., Ghosh, P.R., Sivakumar, B. and Pandiyan, G.D.V. 2008b. Effect of unilateral adrenalectomy on the blood biochemistry of Black Bengal goats (Capra hircus). Turkish Journal of Veterinary and Animal Science 32: 249-254.

Sejian, V., Srivastava, R.S. and Varshney, V.P. 2010. Effect of thermal stress on endocrine profile and phagocytosis index in Marwari goats. Indian Veterinary Journal 87: 1156-1157.

Sejian, V., Maurya, V.P. and Naqvi, S.M.K. 2010a. Adaptability and growth of Malpura ewes subjected to thermal and nutritional stress. Tropical Animal Health and Production 42:1763-1770.

Sejian, V., Maurya V.P. and Naqvi, S.M.K. 2010b. Adaptive capability as indicated by endocrine and biochemical responses of Malpura ewes subjected to combined stresses (thermal and nutritional) under semi-arid tropical environment. International Journal of Biometeorology 54: 653-661.

Sejian, V., Maurya V.P. and Naqvi, S.M.K. 2011a. Effect of thermal, nutritional and combined (thermal and nutritional) stresses on growth and reproductive performance of Malpura ewes under semi-arid tropical environment. Journal of Animal Physiology and Animal Nutrition 95: 252-258.

Sejian, V., Maurya V.P. and Naqvi, S.M.K. 2011b. Effect of walking stress on growth, physiological adaptability and endocrine responses in Malpura ewes under semi-arid tropical environment. International Journal of Biometeorology DOI: 10.1007/s00484-011-0420-y

Sharma, R.J. and Singh, D.V. 2008. Climate stress and its amelioration for improved production in dairy animals. In: Proc. 17th Annual Conference of Society of Animal Physiologist of India and National Symposium on Current Concepts in Productivity Management in Livestock and Poultry Environment, Nutrition and Stress, Pantnagar, Uttarakhand, India, 137-148.

Singh, M., Rai, A.K. and Karim, S.A. 1983. Relative heat tolerance of Indian Nali and Soviet Merino x Nali halfbred sheep to continuous 35°C and 40°C temperature conditions. Journal of Animal Physiology and Animal Nutrition 49: 18-23.

Sosa, C., Albecia, J.A., Forcada, F., Vinoles, C., Tasende, C., Valares, J.A., Palacin, I., Martin, G.B. and Meikle, A. 2006. Effect of undernutrition on uterine progesterone and oestrogen receptors and on endocrine profiles during the ovine oestrous cycle. Reproduction, Fertility and Development 18: 447-458.

Srikandakumar, A., Johnson, E.H. and Mahgoub, O. 2003. Effect of heat stress on respiratory rate, rectal temperature and blood chemistry in Omani and Australian Merino Sheep. Small Ruminant Research 49: 193-198.

Thwaites, C.J. 1971. Short term heat stress and embryo mortality in sheep. Australian Journal of Experimental Agriculture and Animal Husbandry 11: 265-267.

Todini, I. 2007. Thyroid hormones in small ruminants: Effects of endogenous, environmental and nutritional factors. Animal 1: 997-1008.

Ugurlu, N. and Uzal, S. 2010. The effect of new designed micro animal housing on the air speed distribution in the barn for providing of climatic comfort to the cattles. Journal of Animal and Veterinary Advances 9: 169-172.

Upadhyay, R.C., Singh, S.V., Ashutosh, Hooda, O.K., Asharaf, S., Banerjee, D., Kumar, A., Rani, R., Bhan, C., Narwade, B.M., Wakchaure, R., Suresh, S. and Gupta, P. 2011. Vulnerability of Indian cattle to climate change and coping strategies. In: Proc. XX Annual conference of Society of Animal Physiologists of India and International Symposium on Advances in

Physiologic Research for Sustainable Development of Livestock and Poultry Production, Kolkata, 2-4 November, pp 108-117.

Vinoles, C., Forsberg, M., Martin, G.B., Cajarville, C., Repetto, J. and Meikle, A. 2005. Short term nutritional supplementation of ewes in low condition affects follicle development due to an increase in glucose and metabolic hormones. Reproduction 129: 299-309.

Wingfield, A.S. and Kitaysky, J.C. 2002. Endocrine responses to unpredictable environmental events: Stress or anti-stress hormone. Integrative and Comparative Biology 42: 600-609.

□□□

Chapter 9

Male Reproductive Biotechnology of Goats - Advances and Constraints

S.K. Jindal and Priyadharshini Raju
Division of Physiology, Reproduction and Shelter Management
Central Institute for Research on Goats, Makhdoom- 281 112, Farah
Mathura (UP)

Considering the rapidly changing patterns of demand for livestock and their products, sheep and goat farming has emerged as one of the most promising livestock enterprise with immense opportunities to enhance their productivity. Effective management of male reproduction is desirable for enhancing profitability of livestock enterprises utilizing small ruminants. The reproductive efficiency of farm animals has been substantially enhanced by using a vast array of reproductive biotechnologies. Among the various biotechnologies, semen cryopreservation, artificial insemination, sex-sorting of sperm, sperm mediated gene transfer and male germ cells are discussed here.

Semen cryopreservation

Long-term storage of semen in ultra low temperatures facilitates semen transport over distances, permits the quarantine of semen and enables extended use of superior germplasm, even after the sire's death. For agriculturally important animals, semen cryopreservation is established industry worldwide, particularly for dairy cattle. Genome resource banking to preserve the biodiversity of endangered species or valuable transgenic lines also would benefit from sperm cryopreservation. For many mammals however, effective semen cryopreservation is not a reality because a large number of sperm are apparently infertile following freezing and thawing. The cryopreservation process involves the steps of temperature reduction, cellular rehydration, freezing and thawing. Mammalian sperms are not adapted to endure low temperatures. Therefore, cryopreservation of these cells happens at the expense of cellular viability and normal function. Thus, to insure even minimal success, not only proper diluents, dilution freezing, cooling and thawing are required but also an intricate knowledge of the sperm physiology for the species is essential to maximize post-thaw recovery of sperm and consequently the fertility.

Diluents/extenders: The main purpose of the diluents is to extend fresh semen to increase total volume of the semen ejaculated from a particular animal at a time and its extended use over large number of females. Diluents should possess similar properties of fresh semen in terms of hydrogen ion concentration (pH), tonicity and energy source. Immediately after collection and physical evaluation, semen samples should be diluted in a suitable diluent. Various diluents with citrate buffer have been advocated to dilute the semen before cryopreservation. An ideal extender has to meet certain requirements like

i) Increases the volume of the semen to perform multiple inseminations
ii) Provide a buffer to combat the changes in pH as lactic acid is formed
iii) Maintains proper osmotic pressure and electrolyte balance
iv) Provide nutrients as a source of energy
v) Helps in maintaining metabolic activities of the sperm
vi) Provide protection against the effects of freezing
vii) Contains antimicrobial agents to inhibit microbial growth

The earlier diluents were significantly influenced by the discovery of egg yolk as a useful non penetrating cryoprotectant and the phosphate as a primary buffering component, but subsequent use of citrate enhanced the survivability of sperm at low temperatures. Egg yolk has been a more common used but reconstituted skim milk and coconut milk have also been used to preserve fertility of spermatozoa. Various diluents available for cryopreservation of semen are milk dilutor, citric acid whey, egg yolk citrate, Tris citric acid fructose dilutor, laciphos, milk glycine dilutor, Cornell university extender, spermasol with or without egg yolk, dilopten with egg yolk and coconut milk with sodium citrate.

Cryoprotectant: The era of cryobiology began in 1949 when Polge and his colleagues discovered glycerol as an effective cryoprotectant to cryopreserve sperm. Cryoprotective agents that diminish cell damage are usually divided into two general classes related to their ability to move across the cell membrane: permeable and impermeable.

Cryoprotectants are added in the cryopreservation medium to reduce the physical and chemical stresses derived from cooling, freezing and thawing of sperm cells. Permeable cryoprotectants lower the temperature at which cells are exposed to a critical salt concentration. They cause membrane fluidity, faster dehydration at lower temperatures, reduced intracellular ice formation and increased survival and examples are Glycerol, dimethyl sulfoxide, ethylene glycol, propylene glycol (Holt, 2000). Impermeable agents dehydrate the cells allowing them to be cooled rapidly before lethal injury due to solution effects takes place and examples are trehalose, aminoacids, dextrans, sucrose. Though glycerol or dimethyl sulfoxide can induce osmotic stress and toxic effects to spermatozoa glycerol is commonly used in cryopreservation of semen. In semen frozen by the slow conventional method and using mainly hypertonic extenders glycerol is frequently used within the range of 6-8%.

Besides glycerol and the other penetrating cryoprotectants, sugars such as raffinose and lactose, polymers such as polyvinyl pyrollidone (PVP) and the amphipathic compounds like glycine, betaine, glutamine and proline have been identified as potentially cryoprotective. Raffinose has been used with and without glycerol, for the preservation of mouse spermatozoa; 11% lactose in combination with glycerol has been found useful in combination with pellet freezing methods, where it has been used for carnivore e.g. Ferret, Giant panda, as well as for ram and boar spermatozoa. Sugars are thought to act by increasing the percentage of unfrozen water at any given temperature or reducing the concentration of salts in the unfrozen aqueous solution. Glycine, betaine, proline and trehalose are thought to interact directly with membrane lipids and proteins, altering their phase transition behaviour and hydration state. Experimentally, however, these amphiphatic substances have only proved effective in the presence of glycerol and egg yolk when tested with ram and stallion spermatozoa. In addition to these various cryoprotective compounds, egg yolk is routinely included in cryopreservation protocols for semen from domestic animals and many exotic species. Egg yolk is regarded as protecting against cold-shock, a lipid-phase transition cryoprotective effect. Cryoprotectants can also be used in combination with one or more cryoprotectants (eg. Propylene glycol and glycerol, dimethyl sulfoxide and glycerol and dextran).

Semen freezing

Evaluation of semen for freezing: The fresh semen immediately after collection is observed macroscopically for its volume, colour, consistency and presence of foreign material and dust. Volume in ml is recorded from the calibrated collection cup/tube itself. The colour varies from white to milky or creamy white. Yellow colour indicates more riboflavin content while brown colour indicates more dead cells. Consistency of semen varies from thick to thin, where thick consistency is associated with high concentration. Then a drop of it is kept on a microscopic slide and the mass activity is noted under lower power objective of microscope. The collective and comprehensive movement of spermatozoa or their wave motion is called mass activity. The samples with rapid waves and swirls are graded as 5, less rapid waves and eddies as 4, slow swirls scattered in the field as 3, no swirls and individual motility is evident then 2, no wave motion as 1 and no motility as 0. According to the mass motility samples are graded between five and zero and samples falling under three and above grading usually selected for further processing.

The neat semen immediately after macroscopic evaluation is to be kept in water bath at 37°C and then diluted with an equal volume of suitable extender promptly (initial dilution); a drop(5-10μl) of it is spread on a clean, grease free, warm microscopic slide by a cover slip and observed under high power objective (40X) of microscope. The sperm with progressive movement from one point to another in a straight line is an important characteristic to be noted and the total number of motile sperms in three different random fields is to be counted subjectively. The concentration of spermatozoa in a given semen sample is determined by using Spancer's bright line haemocytometer, colorimeter or spectrophotometer. This is very time consuming but accurate. This can be replaced by a spectrophotometer or colorimeter that has been calibrated to a haemocytometer they have the advantage of being precise and fast. A spectrophotometer is preferred and is set at 550nm.

Addition of extender and equilibration: Seminal plasma alone provides only limited protection for sperms against changes in temperature. For storage at reduced temperature, it is necessary to extend semen in appropriate diluents. Glycerol and egg yolk are the most commonly used permeable and impermeable cryoprotectants, respectively. It is a commonly known fact, that the time spermatozoa exposed to the cryoprotectant prior to freezing has effects on its post-thaw characteristics. Glycerol equilibration times that exceed 4 h are considered harmful to post-thaw sperm motility. Equilibration time is necessary for preservation of motility and integrity of sperm membranes. Equilibration for 4 h resulted in the greatest preservation of total and progressive motility, as well as the integrity of plasma and acrosomal membranes during cryopreservation. Furthermore, there were some significant interactions between equilibration time and extender which lead to greater sperm survival.

Dilution rate: The objective of extending semen is to provide an appropriate volume or to inseminate with a sufficient number of sperm to give optimum fertility without any loss. Sperm motility appears to be maintained best at an extension rate of 1:5 to 1:10 and poorest at 1:1.

Methods of semen freezing

Conventional method: The neat semen samples after evaluation are finally diluted to achieve a desired a concentration per dose, are filled by manual method or automated filler machines and sealed in French mini (0.25ml) or medium (0.5ml) straws inside a cold handling cabinet and equilibrated for 2-4h at 5°C. The straws were then spread in the freezing rack and ramp inside the cold handling cabinet and are kept in liquid nitrogen vapour 2-4cm above the surface of liquid nitrogen in a thermo cool box for 10-20 min before plunged and finally dipped into the liquid nitrogen.

Automatic bio-freezer: In bio-freezer, there is no scope for double step/multi-step addition of glycerol hence single addition is to be followed. The samples should be processed similar to the conventional method till final dilution. Then the samples are filled and sealed before the straws are loaded in the bio-freezer. Before loading, the bio-freezer should be started using the already set programme having the desired cooling, equilibration and freezing rate. The straws are then loaded into bio-freezer and preserved according to the programme prescribed to the species.

Pellet freezing of semen: Nagase *et al.* (1964) reported the methods to prepare pellets of frozen semen. Semen is extended in egg yolk-glucose-glycerol and is cooled to 5°C. After equilibration for 5-10 hrs, semen is sprayed with micro syringe on solid carbon dioxide (-79°C). These pellets are stored in dry containers on dry ice. Thawing of semen is done in suitable buffer solution viz. glucose, milk, 3% sodium citrate, 0.9% sodium chloride, Tris-buffer, 3% glycine, 10.5% lactose. The survival of spermatozoa in pellets increases when sugars of high molecular weight are used. The pelleted semen gives better post thaw motility and conception rate but due to the increase in chances of contamination during thawing and difficult in inventory management, it has not been accepted for routine use.

Freeze drying of semen

Freeze drying of semen have been attempted by several workers but it's very discouraging. However the usefulness of freeze dried semen may lie in reducing the difficulties experienced in transport, otherwise no better gains may be expected with its use in artificial insemination. Most commonly used method is the conventional method of freezing and storing. Once the freezing is over one or two straws are taken out of the liquid nitrogen to examine the effect of freezing on sperm motility (post thaw motility). This is important to be assured to have straws of good quality spermatozoa available for fertilization once inseminated into the female reproductive tract.

Thawing of semen

To revive back the frozen spermatozoa thawing is done. Thawing means to melt or become liquid from frozen solid state. Thawing of frozen semen should be done before use and as quickly as possible to prevent recrystallization of water into big crystals. The survivability of frozen thawed spermatozoa is very short and they do not withstand refreezing for further long term storage. Hence thawing should be done for immediate use for post thaw seminal assessment/artificial insemination. The time and temperature to be allowed for thawing depends on the size of the packaging used. The most widely practiced thawing temperature of 37-40°C for 30 sec is suitable to get optimum post thaw survival of spermatozoa. Thawing at temperatures higher than 40°C and also below 37°C has been tried. But higher temperature demands lesser exposure time while lower temperature demands longer exposure time. In case of frozen semen, fast thawing is required to prevent recrystallization of any intracellular ice present in the spermatozoa. Spermatozoa thawed at faster rate are exposed less time to the concentrated solute and cryoprotectant, and the restoration of the intra and extracellular equilibrium is more rapid than with slower thawing (Fisher *et al.*, 1987).

Cryopreservation of buck and ram semen

The first attempts to freeze ram semen were made by Bernstein and Petropaclovsky in 1937 that used glycerol solution for storage. The cryopreservation extenders used for buck and ram semen have either egg yolk or non fat dried skimmed milk. Buck and ram semen may be diluted using one or two step method. Glycerol is commonly added at the rate of 6%. Normally, diluted buck semen is cooled to 4-5°C during 1.5-3.0 hr and then filled in mini straws, frozen in liquid nitrogen vapour at 4-5cm height for 10-20min before plunged into liquid nitrogen. In buck semen, there are some differences in the cryopreservation method from other domestic species, because sometimes there are negative interactions between the phospholipids of the egg yolk or the milk based extenders and the bulbourethral gland secretions in seminal plasma. The enzyme responsible is named egg yolk coagulating enzyme (EYCE). EYCE was identified as phospholipase-A acting as a catalyst that hydrolyses egg yolk lecithin into fatty acids and lysolecithin which are toxic to sperm cells. This hydrolyses stimulates the acrosome reaction, and chromatin decondensation. To overtake this problem if encountered, the goat semen is diluted in a physiologic saline serum 2-3 times during 10-15 min at 550-600g to remove supernatant. This step increases post thaw motility and acrosomal integrity. But not all the samples require this treatment as the coagulation effect is not consistent.

Artificial insemination in small ruminants

Artificial insemination (AI) is a powerful tool to achieve faster genetic improvement through its formidable ability to produce many progeny per male in multiple environments over time. The success of AI depends upon the inherent fertility of the sperm, proper handling of the semen prior to insemination, insemination at the right time during oestrus and proper semen deposition. There are three main techniques of AI in small ruminants which are described in brief here.

Blind AI: Deposition of semen in to the anterior vagina of the female without any attempt to locate the cervix is termed blind AI. Very low conception rate was observed even with neat semen in this technique so practically not applicable if frozen semen is used.

Cervical AI: In this method the cervix is located with the help of a speculum and a light source. The tip of the AI gun is fixed in the external os and then it is gently pushed into the cervix before releasing the semen. Thought this method yields better conception rate, only in 30-40% females passing of the AI gun into deep cervix/uterus is possible.

Laparoscopic insemination: This technique demands a skilled person in handling the equipments. However, if properly used, conception rates up to 90% can be achieved since semen is deposited directly in to the uterus. Animals have to be kept on fasting for 24-48 hrs prior to this insemination. A proper restraint is essential either mere physical restraint or chemical restraint using some drugs like acepromazine (@ 0.5-1mg/kg body weight, i/m). The laparoscopy in small ruminants is usually performed under general anaesthesia or sedation with local infiltration. The animals are positioned with their hind quarters raised to 45 degrees. While performing laparoscopy the selection of a midline, right or let lateral abdominal approach depends on the organs to be examined or manipulated. The abdominal area is clipped surgically scrubbed, disinfected and draped. Pnemoperitoneum is established first and a Veress needle is inserted in the lower right abdominal quadrant, 4-8 cm lateral to the midline. After ascertaining the position of the needle is the gas hose from the laparoflator is attached to the luer lock and a moderate pnemoperitoneum is established using a flow rate of approximately 1litre per min to a final intra abdominal pressure approximately 10-15 mmHg. The site for trocar insertion and the number of ports depends on the organs of interest and the type of procedure. Once the insemination is done in to the uterine horn it is important to evacuate the gas. Generally a single suture for each skin incision should be sufficient, wound dressing and parental antibiotics depend on the measures of sterility maintained.

Sex-sorting of mammalian sperm

In mammals, sex is determined by which spermatozoon fertilizes the ovum, the X- or Y-chromosome–bearing gamete. The flow cytometric method was immediately applied to the sperm of domestic animals (Garner *et al.*, 1983). The DNA content differences in the bimodal populations of sperm from bulls, boars, rams, and rabbits were 3.9, 3.7, 4.0 and 3.9%, respectively (Garner *et al.*, 1983). The method of preparing sperm for flow cytometric analysis was destructive because the tails and most of the membranes and cytoplasm were removed, leaving the sperm biologically unusable (Gledhill, 1988).

Flow cytometry was also used to test validity of claims that semen had been enriched in either the X or Y sperm by other methods. Using a variety of separation techniques for enrichment, including sedimentation, electrophoresis, Sephadex G-50 filtration, centrifugation, albumin gradients, convection-counter streaming galvanization and galvanic and electrical charge differences, semen samples were analyzed to determine if either the X or Y sperm populations had been enhanced.

Sorting sperm: The analytical flow cytometric system could identify the X and Y sperm populations, but this technology could not separate living sperm. The analytical system developed at Lawrence Livermore National Laboratory measurement system did not effectively separate intact X and Y sperm. To attain this goal, a Coulter EPICS V laser-based orthogonal flow cytometer /cell sorter at USDA in Beltsville,Maryland, was modified by bevelling the sample injection tube tip and substituting a forward angle fluorescence detector and an optical fibre bundle for the light scatter detector so that fluorescence could be measured accurately. Analysis of the sorted sperm sample predicted that 80% would be male. Samples sorted for X sperm with a purity of 80% were inseminated, resulting in 74% females. This is the first demonstration in large farm animals that the sex ratio of offspring could be significantly altered.

Use of sex-sorted sperm with in vitro fertilization: Sex-sorted bovine sperm were used for *in vitro* fertilization (IVF) to generate embryos from *in vitro*-matured oocytes (Cran *et al.*, 1993). Sperm were sorted using a modified Becton Dickinson FAC Star Plus flow cytometer / cell sorter. The sperm were stained with Hoechst 33342 and sorted at the rate of 100 cells to obtain an X and Y sperm populations of 79 and 70% purity, respectively (Cran *et al.*, 1993). Twin transfers of 9 sex-selected embryos produced 4 pregnancies, resulting in 3 males and 3 female calves (Cran *et al.*, 1993), all of the projected sex. These births demonstrated that sex-sorted bovine sperm could result in living offspring. Further studies revealed that a sex ratio of 90% male could be achieved (Cran *et al.*, 1995). The skewed sex ratio of the calves born from these transfers was consistent with the predetermined sex as determined by the polymerase chain reaction assay of excised cells from similarly selected blastocysts (Cran *et al.*, 1993). These findings set in motion the potential commercialization of the sorting and IVF technology when the USDA issued a license to Mastercalf, Ltd of the United Kingdom.

Sperm mediated gene transfer

Recent developments in studies of sperm-mediated gene transfer (SMGT) now provide solid ground for the notion that sperm cells can act as vectors for exogenous genetic sequences. A substantive body of evidence indicates that SMGT is potentially useable in animal transgenesis, but also suggests that the final fate of the exogenous sequences transferred by sperm is not always predictable. The analysis of SMGT-derived offspring has shown the existence of integrated foreign sequences in some cases, while in others stable modifications of the genome are difficult to detect. The appearance of SMGT-derived modified offspring on the one hand and, on the other hand, the rarity of actual modification of the genome, suggest inheritance as extrachromosomal structures. Several specific factors have been identified that mediate distinct steps in SMGT. Among those, a prominent role is played by an endogenous reverse transcriptase of retrotransposon origin. Mature spermatozoa are naturally protected against the intrusion of foreign nucleic acid molecules; however, particular environmental conditions, such as those occurring during human assisted reproduction, can abolish this protection. The possibility that sperm cells under these conditions carry genetic sequences affecting the integrity or identity of the host genome should be critically considered. These considerations further suggest the possibility that SMGT events may occasionally take place in nature, with profound implications for evolutionary processes (Smith and Spadofora, 2005).

Male germ cells

Recent studies by Brinster and colleagues from University of Pennsylvania have shown that the injection of spermatogonial stem cells into the testes of sterile recipient mice gives rise to functional sperm in the recipients. These results provide a new technique for the investigation of the physiological of the spermatogonial stem cells and more importantly lead to new approaches for the construction of transgenic animals. Spermatogenesis, the process by which the type A spermatogonial stem cell divide and differentiate to produce the mature spermatids.

Spermatogenesis is a highly productive and tightly regulated process. Spermatogonial stem cells (SSCs) are responsible for maintaining spermatogenesis throughout life in males by continuously producing type A spermatogonia that are committed to differentiate into spermatozoa, which transmit genes to subsequent generations. This characteristic of SSCs relies on their ability to self-renew as well as to produce daughter cells that differentiate. Although normal spermatogenesis depends on strict control of the self-renewal and differentiation decision of SSCs, the mechanism of this regulation has remained elusive. Progress in understanding the mechanism involved is hampered largely because the concentration of SSCs in the testis is extremely low, presumably as few as 1 in 3000-4000 cells in adult mouse testis, and no unique phenotypic markers to identify and isolate SSCs have been described. Stem cells of all types are defined by their biological function. Therefore, identification depends on the availability of a functional assay, which usually entails transplantation of putative stem cells and assessment of their ability to generate the differentiated tissue. Unequivocal identification of SSCs is possible by transplanting stem cell populations into the seminiferous tubules of a recipient testis, in which only a SSC can generate a colony of donor cell-derived spermatogenesis. With the transplantation assay as a functional endpoint, enrichment of murine SSCs by multiparametric separation using fluorescence activated cell sorting (FACS) and monoclonal antibodies for specific surface markers has been developed.

Cryopreservation of spermatogonial stem cells

Spermatozoa from a number of species can be cryopreserved and then subsequently used to fertilize eggs. However, this technique has several limitations. First, the freezing protocol varies for each species and must be determined empirically, and for some species appropriate methods have not yet been identified. Second, because these cells are fully differentiated, they will not undergo replication when thawed, and recombination of genetic information cannot occur. We now demonstrate, by using the recently developed spermatogonial transplantation technique, that male germline stem cells can be successfully cryopreserved. Donor testis cells isolated from prepubertal or adult mice and frozen from 4 to 156 days at -196 °C were able to generate spermatogenesis in recipient seminiferous tubules. Relatively standard preservation techniques were used, suggesting that male germ cells from other species can also be stored for long periods. Because transplanted testis stem cells will ultimately undergo replication and meiotic recombination during spermatogenesis, one might consider these preserved male germ lines as biologically immortal.

Male germ cell transplantation

Spermatogonial stem cell transplantation was first reported by Ralph Brinster's laboratory in 1994. It has proven to be a technological breakthrough in the study of both stem cells and Sertoli cell–germ cell interactions. This technique can be used to transfer testicular stem cells successfully from one animal to another of the same species (referred to as syngeneic transplants) and sometimes to an animal of a different species (xenogeneic transplants). This transfer technique, combined with developments in cryopreservation, long-term culture, and the enrichment of stem cell populations makes more significant breakthroughs likely in the near future. Ultimately, the application of spermatogonial stem cell transfer will allow transplantation of cultured stem cells manipulated genetically *in vitro* to give rise to functional male gametes with an altered genotype. This achievement will have applications in basic science, human medicine, and domestic and wild animal reproduction. Although progress toward this goal has been swift, potentially significant barriers, such as the stable incorporation of genetic material into stem cells and immunological responses to the introduced germ cells, remain to be overcome.

Future impact

The biological activities of spermatogonial stem cells (SSCs) are the foundation for spermatogenesis and thus sustained male fertility. Therefore, understanding the mechanisms governing their ability to both self-renew and differentiate is essential. Moreover, because SSCs are the only adult stem cell to contribute genetic information to the next generation, they are an excellent target for genetic modification. Investigating the niche environment and transplantation of the stem cells can be used to enhance our understanding of SSC biology as well as to produce genetically modified animals.

The ability to derive multipotential stem cells from the neonatal testis has important implications for germ cell biology and opens the possibility of using these cells for biotechnology and medicine and also new opportunity for understanding the regulatory mechanism that governs spermatogonial stem cells. Combining germ cell transplantation with culture and cryopreservation of spermatogonia opens new pathways for genetic engineering and conservation of livestock. In addition, autologous transfer of spermatogonia might be used as an approach for fertility preservation in oncological patients.

Genetic manipulation of isolated germ line stem cells and subsequent transplantation will result in the production of transgenic sperm. Transgenesis through the male germ line has tremendous potential in domestic animal species where embryonic stem cell technology is not available and current options to generate transgenic animals are inefficient. As an alternative to transplantation of isolated germ cells to a recipient testis, ectopic grafting of testis tissue from diverse mammalian donor species, including horses and primates, into a mouse host represents a novel possibility to study spermatogenesis, to investigate the effects of drugs with the potential to enhance or suppress male fertility, and to produce fertile sperm from immature donors. Therefore, transplantation of germ cells or xenografting of testis tissue are uniquely valuable approaches for the study, preservation and manipulation of male fertility in domestic animals.

References

Cran, D.G., Johnson, L.A. and Polge, C. 1995. Sex pre selection in cattle: a field trial. Veterinary Record 136: 495-496.

Cran, D.G., Johnson, L.A., Miller, N.G.A., Cochrane, D. and Polge, C. 1993. Production of bovine calves following separation of X- and Y-chromosome bearing sperm and in vitro fertilization. Veterinary Record 132: 40-41.

Fisher, P.S., Ainsworth, L. and Fairull, R.W. 1987. Evaluation of a new diluent and different processing procedures for the cryopreservation of ram semen. Theriogenology 28: 599-607.

Garner, D.L., Gledhill, B.L., Pinkel, D., Lake, S., Stephenson, D., Van Dilla, M.A. and Johnson, L.A. 1983. Quantification of the X- and Y-chromosome-bearing spermatozoa of domestic animals by flow cytometry. Biology of Reproduction 28: 312-321.

Gledhill, B.L. 1988. Gender pre selection: historical, technical and ethical perspectives. Semin Reprod Endocrinol 6: 385-376.

Holt, W.V. 2000. Basic aspects of frozen storage of semen. Animal Reproduction Science 62: 3-22.

Nagase, H., Niwa, T., Yamashita, S. and Irie, S. 1964. Deep freezing of bull semen in concentrated pellet form. II. Protective action of sugars. Proceeding of V International Congress on Animal Reproduction & A. L, Trento 4: 498-502.

Smith K and Spadafora, C. 2005. Sperm mediated gene transfer: application and implication. Bioessay 27: 551-562.

□□□

Chapter 10

Understanding Stress Pathways Involved in Modulation of GnRH/LH release in the Ewe

J.B. Phogat[1] and S.P.S. Ghuman[2]
[1]North Temperate Regional Station, (CSWRI), Garsa, Kullu- 175 141 (HP) [2]Department of Veterinary Gynaecology and Obstetrics, College of Veterinary Science, Guru Angad Dev University of Veterinary and Animal Sciences, Ludhiana-141 004 (Punjab)

'Stress' is responsible for sub-fertility in ruminants. Environmental and management stressors have a major impact on profitability of small ruminant production. In fact, tightly regulated communications between ovary and brain ensure the occurrence of appropriately timed neural signal for ovulation (Ghuman *et al.,* 2011). At the brainstem and hypothalamic level, estradiol-dependent regulation of GnRH secretion is a critical component of this communication system (Ghuman *et al.,* 2006). To delineate the mechanisms involved in the late follicular phase, various experimental models have been used viz. transport, insulin or endotoxin administration. These stressors might reduce luteinizing hormone (LH) pulse frequency and amplitude leading to a delayed or absent LH surge (Scherzer *et al.,* 2009). The disruptions in LH release could affect follicular function and have negative consequences on oocyte quality. We will focus on central pathways involved in regulation of GnRH release under normal and stressful conditions.

Hypothalamic and brainstem areas involved in GnRH release

Major population of GnRH neuron cell bodies (~60-65%) is located in the medial preoptic area (mPOA) and in the mediobasal hypothalamus {MBH, consisting of ventromedial nucleus (VMN) and the arcuate nucleus (ARC)}, with their axons terminating near the external zone of median eminence (ME) as depicted in Fig. 1 (Lehman *et al.,* 1986). It is proposed that GnRH surge depends upon the coordinated activity of widespread GnRH neurones whereas a subset of GnRH neurones located in the MBH is sufficient for tonic release. However, the pathway through which this scattered network of GnRH neurons is affected by stress and affects the final GnRH output remains under scrutiny (Ghuman *et al.,* 2010).

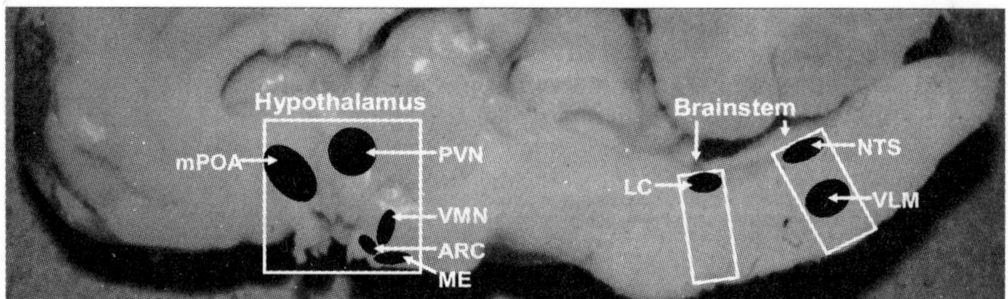

Fig. 1 : Saggital section of ewe hypothalamus showing important hypothalamic and brainstem areas

Steroid responsive neurons associated with GnRH release

In the hypothalamus, the effects of progesterone (P) and estrogen (E) are not exerted directly on GnRH neurones because GnRH neurones do not express steroid-receptors (Herbison, 1998). Therefore, intermediary neurones containing steroid receptors should transmit the message of steroids on to GnRH neurones through synapses particularly in the mPOA. High density of estrogen receptor (ER)-a containing neurones exist in the hypothalamic areas viz., mPOA and MBH and in the brainstem in the nucleus of solitary tract (NTS) and the ventrolateral medulla (VLM). The identity of these ERa-expressing neurones is γ-amino butyric acid (GABA) in the mPOA, b-endorphin (opioid) in the ARC and noradrenergic (NA) in the VLM and NTS (Herbison *et al.,* 1993). On the other hand, progesterone receptor (PR)-containing neurones are also detected with highest density in the mPOA, VMN and the ARC (Skinner *et al.,* 2001). The neurochemical identity of these neurones is not clear though GABA in the mPOA and b-endorphin in the ARC are the candidates.

Organized interactions between neurons leading to GnRH surge

In an ovariectomized (OVX) ewe model, the pattern of GnRH secretion is similar to the normal estrous cycle and is produced by exogenous treatment with E and P. To elucidate the steps by which E induces the GnRH surge, a three stage surge-induction/generation model was developed (Fig 2). First stage of this model is E-dependent whereas second and third stages are E-independent. Starting from E-implant insertion, the first stage is an E message-reading or activation stage (5-10 hr), during which E message for the onset of GnRH surge activates E-sensitive neurones. The second stage is for message processing or transmission (11-16 hr), when the message is processed and transmitted to GnRH neurones by E-responsive neurones or via one or more interneurones. The third stage involves initiation of GnRH surge release (beginning at 21 hr), the time of actual discharge of GnRH that stimulates the LH surge (Evans *et al.*, 1997; Battaglia *et al.*, 1999; Harris *et al.*, 1999).

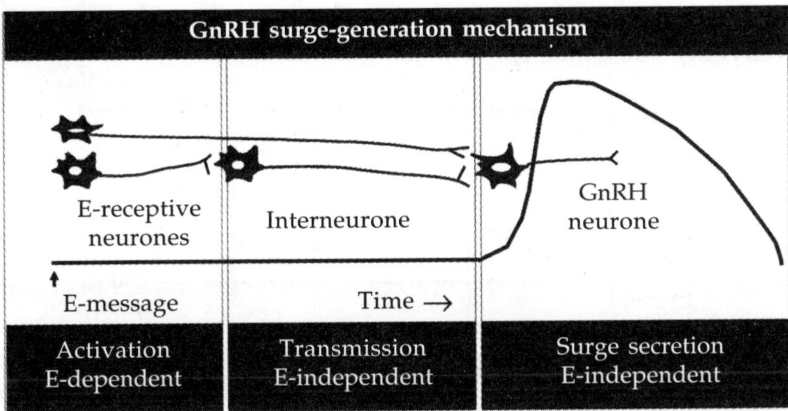

Fig. 2 : Diagram showing estradiol (E)-induced GnRH surge-generation mechanism (Evans *et al.*, 1997; Battaglia *et al.*, 1999)

Low GnRH pulse frequency during luteal phase is maintained by P-induced activation of GABA and opioid neurones which inhibit the activation of GnRH neurones (Herbison, 1998) (Fig. 3). During the early follicular phase, suppression of GnRH secretion is still maintained as the increasing E stimulates GABA. It can be speculated that with E trigger, besides the increase in surge-stimulatory NA activity, elevated surge-inhibitory GABA and opioid activity prevents the premature activation of GnRH neurones. After the reading of E message during early follicular stage, prolong message-processing phase corresponds to sequential communication between multiple neurones within the GnRH network which ultimately generate surge-stimulating message. Neurones directly as well as through activation of NA neurones which synapse to, and activate GABA neurones (Robinson *et al.*, 1991). During the mid-follicular phase, immediately before surge onset, under the continuous E stimulation, there is suppression of GABA and opioid neurones which activate NA neurones thus causing switch from tonic to the GnRH surge release (Robinson *et al.*, 1991; Herbison, 1997).

Stress-induced interruption of neuroendocrine mechanisms leading to GnRH surge

Stressors such as endotoxins, transport, undernutrition as well as presence of P during the follicular phase may act as surge-disrupters during any stage of GnRH surge-generation pathway. The stress induced decrease in GnRH release ultimately deprives the ovarian follicle of adequate LH support. This will lead to reduced estradiol production by slower growing follicles. A marked decrease in estradiol secretion was observed after reducing the frequency of exogenous LH pulses driving follicular growth (Dobson *et al.*, 1999).

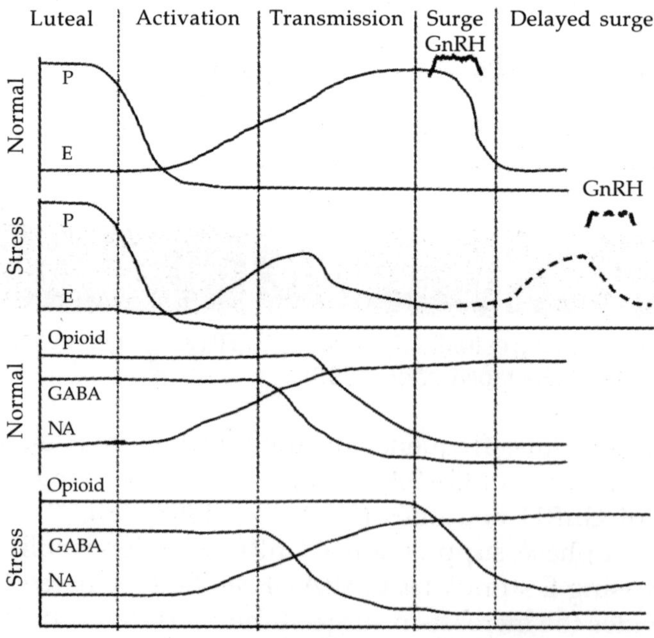

Fig. 3 : Normal and stress-induced alterations in ovarian hormone and neurotransmitter release during luteal and follicular (activation, transmission and surge) phases of estrous cycle in ewe.

The identity of stress (immunological, physical or metabolic)-activated neurones or the pathways through which they act to disrupt the normal onset of GnRH surge is not fully understood in the ewe. Interestingly, neurones involved in GnRH surge-generation also control the stress-induced GnRH surge-suppression. Noradrenergic neurones are stimulatory both to surge-generation and surge-suppression processes (Ghuman *et al.,* 2008 a, c), however different functional subsets are involved in two processes as origin of NA neurones involved in surge-generation or suppression is from different functional subsets may be involved in two processes as the origin of NA neurones involved in surge-generation or suppression is from different brainstem regions (Fig 4, Rawson *et al.,* 2001). For the disruption of GnRH surge, NA neurones act by projecting either directly to mPOA, or indirectly via the hypothalamic paraventricular nucleus (PVN) by releasing corticotrophin releasing hormone (CRH) and arginine vasopressin (AVP) (Fig 4, Smith *et al.,* 2003). Activation of CRH neurones stimulates GABA and opioid neurones in mPOA which ultimately reduce GnRH neurone activation thus leading to interruption in timely and normal onset of GnRH surge. Following hypoglycaemic stress near the end of follicular phase, both brainstem and hypothalamic nuclei appear to have a major role in GnRH surge-interruption. Noradrenergic neurones in the caudal brainstem and CRH and AVP neurones in the PVN were found active; however the activity of ARC beta-endorphin neurones was suppressed (Fig 4, Ghuman *et al.,* 2010, 2011).

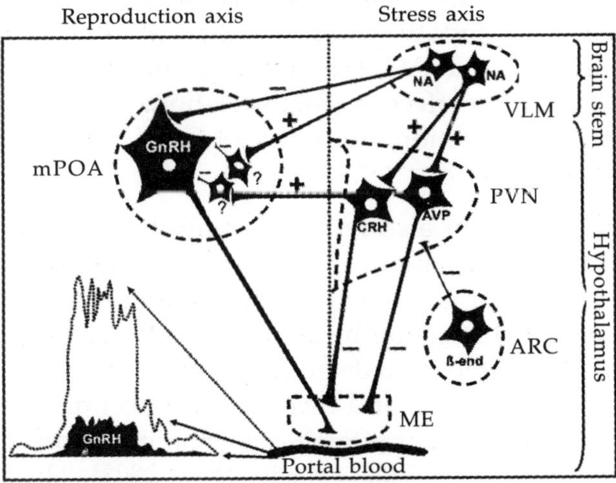

Fig. 4: Stress-induced neuronal interactions leading to disruption of GnRH surge onset (Ghuman *et al.,* 2007, 2008a,b,c, 2010, 2011).

Progesterone inhibits tonic LH release during the luteal phase as well as blocks the LH surge. Progesterone blocks the surge-generating E message during the activation stage, indicating that P has no direct action on GnRH neurones (Harris *et al.*, 1999). In acute stressors, the beta-adrenergic involvement and the activation of endogenous opioid system is evident in the cortisol response which mitigates adrenal response (Phogat and Parvizi, 2007).

Impact of adrenal stimulation during the late follicular phase on fertility

The relation between stressors, rise in cortisol and suppression of reproductive activity suggest the role of cortisol as an important mediator of inhibitory effects of stress on reproduction (Tilbrook *et al.*, 2000).

At hypothalamus: Cortisol can influence reproduction by inhibiting LH secretion through action at the hypothalamus whereby it can interact with gonadal steroids to suppress GnRH secretion (Tilbrook *et al.*, 2000; Ghuman *et al.*, 2011).

At pituitary: Cortisol can act at the pituitary to reduce gonadotroph sensitivity to GnRH (Breen and Karsch, 2004) and lastly at the ovarian level by altering androgen synthesis (Spicer and Chamberlain, 1998). Exogenous ACTH replicates the effects of stressors to delay the pre-ovulatory LH surge in sheep. Actually, ACTH reduces the GnRH self-priming effect *in vivo* and delays the LH surge, at least partially by direct effects at the pituitary gland (Phogat *et al.*, 1999a). However, *in vitro* studies revealed that ACTH1-24 did not affect tonic LH secretion, the GnRH self-priming effect or E-sensitisation. The entire ACTH1-39 increased tonic LH secretion, but reduced GnRH self-priming and E-sensitisation (Phogat *et al.*, 1997).

At Ovary: Stress can also reduce fertility by negatively affecting corpus luteum (CL) formation. LH pulses after the pre-ovulatory LH surge are necessary for CL development (Quintal-Franco *et al.*, 1999). Suppression of luteal function by short-term (10 days) glucocorticoid treatment was associated with decreased concentrations of cholesterol, IGF-I and IGF-II in plasma, and increase in concentrations of plasma glucose and insulin without affecting plasma gonadotropin levels or growth of the dominant follicle (Maciel *et al.*, 2001). Thus, short-term increases in glucocorticoids have little impact on follicular function but may have a negative impact on luteal function (Maciel *et al.*, 2001).

Cortisol elevation may also prolong the lifespan of the CL. In general, ACTH administration to the diestrous animals resulted in a delayed plasma progesterone decline.

Mechanism of gonadotropin release disruption by various stressors

Transport stress: Transport of ewes in a vehicle for short duration (2 hr) produces an immediate and constant increase in AVP and CRH concentrations in hypophyseal-portal blood of ewes, both of these are ultimately responsible for increase in plasma cortisol (Smith *et al.*, 1997). Transport for 4-8 hr reduces LH pulsatile release in the late follicular phase (Dobson *et al.*, 1999). Transport affected the E-induced LH surge by causing a 50% reduction in the self-priming effect of exogenous GnRH, but hypothalamic effects were also revealed by a two-fold decrease in spontaneous LH pulse frequency in saline-treated ewes (Phogat *et al.*, 1999b). Transport stress just before the LH surge delays surge onset suggesting disruption of the later phase of transmission pathway of surge -generating mechanism. Moreover, transient painful stress was not able to affect the LH values although it altered the opioidergic and catecholaminergic-modulation of LH secretion. The interference with opioid system is possibly mediated by ACTH (Phogat and Parvizi, 2010).

Hypoglycemic stress: After an insulin injection, the HPA axis response occurs after the blood glucose concentrations decreases below a threshold (Scherzer *et al.*, 2009; Ghuman *et al.*, 2011). The reduction in LH pulse frequency suggests an effect of these stressors on GnRH pulsatile secretion mediated through effects at the hypothalamus, whereas effects on the LH pulse amplitude could either be mediated by the hypothalamus, or at the pituitary. In fact, hypoglycaemic stress disrupts the surge at any time before actual onset (Ghuman *et al.*, 2010, 2011).

Under nutrition stress: Fasting during the luteal phase may influence fertility by perturbing gonadotropin secretion, delaying ovarian follicle development, and decreasing follicular secretion of estradiol (Kiyma *et al.*, 2004). Chronic undernourishment of ewes also reduced serum and hypophyseal concentrations of LH (Snyder *et al.*, 1999) and FSH (Kile *et al.*, 1991) due to a suppressed release of GnRH from the hypothalamus (Dunn and Moss, 1992).

Endotoxin stress: Bacterial endotoxin may potently suppress gonadotropin secretion and disrupt the ovulatory cycle. Endotoxin stress suppresses both tonic and surge GnRH/LH release as well as delays the onset of the E-induced LH surge, without any effect on surge amplitude or duration (Battaglia *et al.*, 2000). Direct evidence of the suppressive effects of an acute stressor on GnRH secretion has been provided after endotoxin administration (Battaglia *et al.*, 1997). Endotoxin disrupts both hypothalamic and pituitary function, inhibiting pulsatile GnRH secretion and pituitary responsiveness to GnRH (Battaglia *et al.*, 1997, Williams *et al.*, 2001). Furthermore, endotoxin appears to suppress pulsatile GnRH and LH secretion indirectly, via a cascade of intermediates that include cytokines, such as IL-1 and TNF-α, as well as prostaglandins (Rivest and Rivier, 1993).

Conclusion

Stressors can reduce fertility by interfering with the mechanisms that regulate the precise timing of events leading to ovulation and CL formation. It is beneficial to understand how and which neurones of GnRH surge-generating network are modulated by various stressors. Cortisol release after adrenal stimulation mediates the effects of stress on reproduction and hence delays follicular development and ovulation through impaired LH release. Ultimately, poor pre-ovulatory follicle may influence the triggering of events responsible for onset of luteal regression. The farmers and veterinarians need to understand the consequences of increased production under lower costs and thus require a deeper understanding about the impact of stress on fertility. Unraveling the neuroendocrine mechanisms involved in stress-induced suppression of fertility will help to improve treatments and develop strategies for optimization of fertility in various stress-associated reproductive dysfunctions.

References

Battaglia, D.F., Krasa, H.B., Viguie, C. and Karsch, F.J. 1997. Immune stress disrupts the estrogen-induced LH surge: Interference with estrogen signal processing or surge generation? Biology of Reproduction 56: 43-43.

Battaglia, D.F., Beaver, A.B., Harris, T.G., Tanhehco, E., Viguie, C. and Karsch, F.J. 1999. Endotoxin disrupts the estradiol-induced luteinizing hormone surge: interference with estradiol signal reading, not surge release. Endocrinology 140: 2471-2479.

Battaglia, D.F., Krasa, H.B., Padmanabhan, V., Viguie, C. and Karsch, F.J. 2000. Endocrine alterations that underlie endotoxin-induced disruption of the follicular phase in ewes. Biology of Reproduction 62: 45-53.

Breen, K.M. and Kersch, F.J. 2004. Does cortisol inhibit pulsatile luteinizing hormone secretion at the hypothalamic or pituitary level? Endocrinology 145: 692-698.

Dobson, H., Campbell, B.K., Scaramuzzi, R,J. and Baird, D.T. 1999. Effect of reducing LH pulse frequency and amplitude on ovarian oestradiol production in the ewe. In: 5th International Symposium on Reproduction in Domestic Ruminants. Journal of Reproduction and Fertility (Suppl), 54.

Dunn, T.G. and Moss, G.E. 1992. Effects of nutrient deficiencies and excesses on reproductive efficiency of livestock. Journal of Animal Science 70: 1580-1593.

Evans, N.P., Dahl, G.E., Padmanabhan, V., Thrun, L.A. and Karsch, F.J. 1997. Estradiol requirements for induction and maintenance of the gonadotropin-releasing hormone surge: Implications for neuroendocrine processing of the estradiol signal. Endocrinology 138: 5408-5414.

Ghuman, S.P.S., Prabhakar, S., Smith, R.F. and Dobson, H. 2006. Oestradiol stimulates the release of AVP and GnRH from the ewe hypothalamus in vitro. Reproduction in Domestic Animals 41: 514-521.

Ghuman, S.P.S., Prabhakar, S., Smith, R.F and Dobson, H. 2007. Gamma amino butyric acid control of AVP release from ewe hypothalamic slices in vitro: sensitivity to oestradiol. Reproduction in Domestic Animals 42: 527-535.

Ghuman, S.P.S., Prabhakar, S., Smith, R.F and Dobson, H. 2008a. Noradrenergic control of AVP release from ewe hypothalamic slices in vitro: sensitivity to oestradiol. Reproduction in Domestic Animals 43: 137-143.

Ghuman, S.P.S., Jones, D.N., Smith, R.F. and Dobson, H. 2008b. Gamma amino butyric acid control of GnRH release from ewe hypothalamic slices in vitro: sensitivity to oestradiol. Reproduction in Domestic Animals 43: 531-541.

Ghuman, S.P.S., Jones, D.N., Prabhakar, S., Smith, R.F. and Dobson, H. 2008c Noradrenergic control of GnRH release from ewe hypothalamic slices in vitro: sensitivity to oestradiol. Reproduction in Domestic Animals 43: 753-759.

Ghuman, S.P.S., Morris, R., Spiller, D.G., Smith, R.F. and Dobson, H. 2010 Integration Between Different Hypothalamic Nuclei Involved in Stress and GnRH Secretion in the Ewe. Reproduction in Domestic Animals 45: 1065-1073.

Ghuman, S.P.S., Morris, R., Scherzer, J., Routly, J.E., Mobasheri, A., Smith, R.F. and Dobson, H. 2011. Neuronal responses in the brainstem and hypothelemic nuclei following insulin treatment during the late follicular phase in the ewe. Reproduction in Domestic Animals 46: 121-129.

Harris, T.G., Dye, S., Robinson, J.E., Skinner, D.C. and Evans, N.P. 1999. Progesterone can block transmission of the estradiol-induced signal for luteinizing hormone surge generation during a specific period of time immediately after activation of the gonadotropin-releasing hormone surge-generating system. Endocrinology 140: 827-834.

Herbison, A.E. 1997. Noradrenergic regulation of cyclic GnRH secretion. Reviews of Reproduction 2: 1-6.

Herbison, A.E. 1998. Multimodal influence of estrogen upon gonadotropin-releasing hormone neurons. Endocrinology Reviews 19: 302-330.

Herbison, A.E., Robinson, J.E. and Skinner, D.C. 1993. Distribution of estrogen receptor-immunoreactive cells in the preoptic area of the ewe: co-localization with glutamic acid decarboxylase but not luteinizing hormone-releasing hormone. Neuroendocrinology 57: 751-759.

Kile, J.P., Alexander, B.M., Moss, G.E., Hallford, D.M. and Nett, T.M. 1991. Gonadotropin-releasing hormone overrides the negative effect of reduced dietary energy on gonadotropin synthesis and secretion in ewes. Endocrinology 128: 843–849.

Kiyma, Z., Alexander, B.M., Van Kirk, E.A., Murdoch, W.J., Hafford, D.M. and Moss, G.E. 2004. Effects of reed restricition on reproductive and metabolic hormones in ewes. Journal of Animal Science 82: 2548-2557.

Lehman, M.N., Robinson, J.E., Karsch, F.J. and Silverman, A.J. 1986. Immunocytochemical localization of luteinizing hormone-releasing hormone (LHRH) pathways in the sheep brain during anestrus and the mid-luteal phase of the estrous cycle. Journal of Comparative Neurology 244: 19-35.

Maciel, S.M., Chamberlain, C.S., Wettemann, R.P. and Spicer, L.J. 2001. Dexamethasone influences endocrine and ovarian function in dairy cattle. Journal of Dairy Science 84: 1998-2009.

Phogat, J.B. and Parvizi, N. 2007. Beta-adrenergic and opioidergic modulation of cortisol secretion in response to acute stress. Experimental and Clinical Endocrinology and Diabetes 115:354-359.

Phogat, J.B. and Parvizi, N. 2010. Involvement of opioids and catecholamines in stress modulation of LH secretion in the male pig. Animal Reproduction Science 121: 152-158.

Phogat, J.B., Smith, R.F. and Dobson, H. 1997. Effect of adrenocorticotrophic hormone on gonadotrophin releasing hormone-induced luteinizing hormone secretion in vitro. Animal Reproduction Science 48: 53-65.

Phogat, J.B., Smith, R.F. and Dobson, H. 1999a. Effect of adrenocorticotrophic hormone(ACTH1-24) on ovine pituitary gland responsiveness to exogenous pulsatile GnRH and oestradiol-induced LH release in vivo. Animal Reproduction Science 55: 193-203.

Phogat, J.B., Smith, R.F. and Dobson, H. 1999b. Effect of transport on pituitary responsiveness to exogenous pulsatile GnRH and oestradiol-induced LH release in intact ewes. Journal of Reproduction and Fertility 116: 9-18.

Quintal-Franco, J.A., Kojima, F.N., Melvin, E.J., Lindsey, B.R., Zanella, E., Fike, K.E., Wehrman, M.E., Clopton, D.T. and Kinder, J.E. 1999. Corpus luteum development and function in cattle with episodic release of luteinizing hormone pulses inhibited the follicular and early luteal phases of the estrous cycle. Biology of Reproduction 61: 921-926.

Rawson, J.A., Scott, C.J., Pereira, A., Jakubowska, A. and Clarke, I.J. 2001. Noradrenergic projections from the A1 field to the preoptic area in the brain of the ewe and Fos responses to oestrogen in the A1 cells. Journal of Neuroendocrinology 13: 129-138.

Rivest, S. and Rivier, C. 1993. Centrally injected interleukin-1 inhibits hypothalamic LHRH secretion and circulating LH levels via prostaglandins in rats. Journal of Neuroendocrinology 5: 445-450.

Robinson, J.E., Kendrick, K.M. and Lambart, C.E. 1991. Changes in the release of gamma-aminobutyric-acid and catecholamines in the preoptic septal area prior to and during the preovulatory surge of luteinizing-hormone in the ewe. Journal of Neuroendocrinology 3: 393-399.

Scherzer, J., Ghuman, S.P.S., Pope, M., Routly, J.E., Walter, I., Smith, R.F. and Dobson, H. 2009. Follicle and oocyte morphology in ewes after treatment with insulin in the late follicular phase. Theriogenology 71: 817-828.

Skinner, D.C., Caraty, A. and Allingham, R. 2001. Unmasking the progesterone receptor in the preoptic area and hypothalamus of the ewe: no colocalization with gonadotropin-releasing neurons. Endocrinology 142: 573-579.

Smith, R.F., Gore, S.W., Phogat, J.B. and Dobson, H. 1997. The psychological stress of transport stimulates both CRF and AVP secretion into hypophysial portal blood. Journal of Endocrinology 152: 172.

Smith, R.F., Ghuman, S.P., Evans, N.P., Karsch, F.J. and Dobson, H. 2003. Stress and the control of LH secretion in the ewe. Reproduction Suppl 61: 267-282.

Snyder, J.L., Clapper, J.A., Roberts, A.J., Sanson, D.W., Hamernik, D.L. and Moss, G.E. 1999. Insulin-like growth factor-I, insulin-like growth factor-binding proteins, and gonadotropins in the hypothalamic-pituitary axis and serum of nutrient restricted ewes. Biology of Reproduction 61: 219-224.

Spicer, L.J. and Chamberlain, C.S. 1998. Influence of cortisol on insulin- and insulin-like growth factor 1 (IGF-1)-induced steroid production and on IGF-1 receptors in cultured bovine granulosa cells and thecal cells. Endocrine 9: 153-161.

Tilbrook, A.J., Turner, A.I. and Clarke, I.J. 2000. Effects of stress on reproduction in non-rodent mammals: the role of glucocorticoids and sex differences. Reviews of Reproduction 5: 105-113.

Williams, C.Y., Harris, T.G., Battaglia, D.F, Viguie,´C. and Karsch, F.J. 2001. Endotoxin inhibits pituitary responsiveness to gonadotropin-releasing hormone. Endocrinology 142: 1915-1922.

□□□

Chapter 11

Stem Cells : Advances and Prospects in Farm Animals

Satish Kumar
Animal Biotechnology Section, Central Sheep and Wool Research Institute Avikanagar- 304 501 (Rajasthan)

Stem cells are unspecialized cells which can transform into any cell types (i.e. specialized or differentiated cells). Stem cells having capability of long-term self-renewal (proliferation) and differentiation into specialized cells. Embryonic stem (ES) cells represent a promising research tool for genetic engineering, developmental biology, nuclear reprogramming and disease models. At the same time, these cells may provide an unlimited source of clinically important adult cells/tissues such as bone, muscle, liver, heart or blood cells in regenerative medicine. ES cells can be maintained indefinitely in culture and yet to show competence to produce all the cells of fetus and adult. In mouse and primate, purely competent ES cell lines have been established, however in farm animals ES like cells or putative ES cells have been isolated, but these cell lines have to be further validated as pluripotent using an appropriate model. Several cell surface markers and pluripotency associated markers have been studied in farm animals, but identification of species specific stem cell markers, signaling pathways and transcription factors involved in maintaining the pluripotency needs to be further studied for production of the proven ES cell lines. The mouse model has been used, but it is not appropriate when long term effects of cell replacement need to be evaluated. Thus, farm animal has been considered the best model for preclinical development of therapeutic treatment in human. Several ES cell line has been developed in livestock animals like sheep, goat, pig, cattle and buffalo. However, establishment of the proven ES cells in livestock species is urgently required for their use in human medicine as well as for improving the livestock traits (milk, meat and disease resistance) in the near future.

Stem cells can be derived from various sources like adult, fetal and embryonic cells

Adult stem cells are cells found in the post-natal tissues that can yield only the specialized cell types of the tissue from which they originated. For e.g. hematopoietic stem cells that can give rise to blood cells and mesenchymal stem cells that give rise to cells of connective tissues, bones, neural, skin, skeletal muscle cells, fat, endothelial progenitors cells (EPCs). Fetal stem cells are placental, umblical cord, and amniotic fluid cells. Stem cells that can derive from the placenta are called placental stem cells. Umbilical cord stem cells are rich source of hematopoietic stem cells, whereas amniotic fluid stem cells are more flexible than adult stem cells. ES cells are derived from ICM (inner cell mass) of the blastocyst, they are pluripotent and have an ability to differentiate into various cell types. ES cells can be self-renew indefinitely in culture medium. Embryonic germ (EG) cells are derived from the fetal tissue of 5 to 10-weeks of the fetus of human. These cells are also derived from primordial germ cells (PGCs) of post-implantation embryos. Embryonal carcinoma (EC) cells are derived from PGCs in the embryonic gonad, which are usually detected as components of the testicular tumors in the adult. In this paper, the advances and prospects of the embryonic stem cells particularly in livestock species will be described.

Embryonic stem cells were first isolated from ICM of *in vivo* produced mouse blastocysts. After a few years, ES cell lines were established from mice by culturing ICM in presence of leukemia inhibitory factor (LIF) (Williams *et al.*, 1988). Human ES cell lines were first isolated from *in vitro* produced blastocysts (Thomson *et al.*, 1998), which possesses the remarkable property of pluripotent, giving rise to all cells of an organism. Over the past 15 years, porcine, caprine, ovine and equine ES cell lines have been isolated, and these lines are often presented as 'ES like' cells. Bovine ES like cells have been isolated from *in vivo* and *in vitro* produced blastocysts (Evans *et al.*, 1990; Saito *et al.*, 2002, 2003; Pant and Keefer, 2006). Subsequently, ES cell lines have been isolated from several other domesticated species. ES cells can be maintained in the culture indefinitely. Thus, these cells have been used for studying the embryogenesis, particularly the genes involved in the embryonic development. In animals, ES cells may be used in genetic modification of the farm animals for improving the production traits and products, for disease resistance and for bio-pharming (Keefer *et al.*, 2007). For example, ES cells can be used for production of the transgenic animals and spermatogonial stem cells (SSC) for the semen production of elite bulls. These goals can be achieved either through the chimeric technology or by improving the efficiency of SCNT (somatic cell nuclear transfer) technology (Wall *et al.*, 2005). In addition, ES cells may provide powerful tool for studying gene targeting, disease model, and cloning etc. Thus, the availability of ES cells could facilitate the development of efficient methods for SCNT, transgenesis, and gene regulation in farm animal species.

Main properties of the embryonic stem cells

Pluripotency can be defined as the ability of cells to give rise to all of the cells of an embryo and adult (Solter, 2006). The main properties of the pluripotent embryonic stem cells are the self-renewal through proliferation and differentiation into specialized cells. These unique properties make them exceptionally valuable for cell replacement therapies, drug discovery and regenerative medicine.

ES cell proliferation (*Self-renewal*): Maintenance of pluripotency is an essential requirement for proper embryonic development. In fact, ES cells can be self-renew continuously for the years, if they are cultured under conditions that prevent their differentiation. For example, leukemia inhibitory factor (LIF) is a growth factor that prevents the differentiation and maintains ES cells in a proliferative and undifferentiated manner (Suda *et al.*, 1987). LIF belongs to the interleukin-6 cytokine family, which binds to a heterodimeric receptor consisting of the LIF-receptor and gp130. This binding results in the activation of the canonical Jak/Stat (Janus kinase-signal transducer and activator of transcription) pathway. It has been found that Stat3 activation maintained the pluripotency of mouse ES cells (Niwa *et al.*, 1998; Matsuda *et al.*, 1999). While, human ES cells do not require gp130 signalling and Stat3 activation for their maintenance (Humphrey *et al.*, 2004; Sumi *et al.*, 2004). Although, the precise mechanism that regulates self-renewal and pluripotency in stem cells remains largely unknown. Several genetic regulators play an important role in maintaining the self-renewal and pluripotency including extracellular signaling factors, transcription factors, cell cycle regulators, microRNA, genes implicated in chromosomal stability, and DNA methylation (Liu *et al.*, 2007).

ES cell differentiation: ES cells are described as pluripotent and they can differentiate directly into three cell types: the primitive ectoderm, the primitive endoderm and trophectoderm cells, analogous to the differentiation ability of ICM cells. The differentiation of mouse ES cells can be induced by the ectopic expression of certain transcription factors. For example, the expression of transcription factor Gata6 in ES cells can results in their differentiation into primitive endoderm (Fujikura *et al.*, 2002). Similarly, the expression of caudal-type homeobox transcription factor 2 (Cdx2) induces ES cells to differentiate into trophectoderm (Niwa *et al.*, 2005). Therefore, both factors have to be tightly repressed for ES cell self-renewal. Differentiation of ES cells is accompanied by the downregulation of whole series of transcription factors and signaling molecules that maintain the pluripotent state, such as Oct4 and NANOG, and upregulation of transcription factors involved in the differentiation.

Characterization of the embryonic stem cells

For ES cell line, the phenotypic definition of the ES cell is that of pluripotency, i.e. most of the cells should be capable of giving rise to somatic cells representative of the three primary embryonic germ layers. Furthermore, they should be able to differentiate into germ cell, i.e. oocytes and spermatozoa. Thus, ES cells should be competent to contribute to all cells of the developing fetus. ES cell lines must be able to self renew as stem cells, thereby maintaining their ability to differentiate into all cell types. A limitation to the establishment of ES cells in domestic species is to identify truly pluripotent cells. The most criteria used to define ES cells are the distinctive morphological features. Most colonies are considered as "ES like", when cells are small and rounded and have a large nucleus with one or two prominent nucleoli are said to be ES like cells (Piedrahita *et al.*, 1990a). It seems that ungulate ES cell lines are the most similar to primate ES cells in colony and cell morphology. Future studies need to be focus more intensely on the critical characteristics that define true ES cell lines. The essential criteria include proof of continuous self-renewal, clear description of morphology, use of cell specific markers and demonstration of truly pluripotency. However, morphological criteria are not appropriately linked to the parameters of self-renewal and pluripotency, therefore cellular and molecular markers are used to define the state of cell lines. A common proof of the pluripotency of primate and mouse ES cell lines is that of teratoma formation in immunocompromised mice. This *in vivo* demonstration of pluripotency is lacking in putative ungulate ES cell lines with some exception. Andersson *et al.* (1996) demonstrated that bovine and porcine teratomas in mice can be obtained using ICM cells. These studies do demonstrate some degree of ES like pluripotency of an ungulate ES like cells. Characterization of ES cell lines is done on the basis of their pluripotent nature (expression of surface i.e., extracellular and transcription-based i.e., intracellular markers), morphology (shape of ES cell colonies), longevity (indefinite passages), genetic stability (karyotyping, telomeric length assay), differentiating capacity (ability to form all 3 germ layer cells) and epigenetic status (methylation pattern).

Cell surface markers: Several workers have used alkaline phosphatase (AP) and stage-specific embryonic antigens (SSEA) as ES cell characteristics markers. Talbot *et al.* (1993) first demonstrated AP as a reliable cell surface marker for undifferentiated ES cells in pig and sheep. The SSEA-1 and SSEA-4 genes were expressed in both ICM and trophectoderm of caprine embryos (He *et al.*, 2006). Similarly, equine ES like cells expressed the AP, SSEA-1, SSEA-3, SSEA-4, TRA-1-60 and TRA-1-81 (Guest and Allen, 2007). Alkaline phosphatase, SSEA-1, SSEA-3, SSEA-4, has been used as markers in buffaloes (Verma *et al.*, 2007; Huang *et al.*, 2007). Thus, these markers have been used and considered as ES cell characteristics markers, but these may not be used as definite markers.

Intracellular markers (*transcription factors*): Oct4 (also known as POU5F1) is a useful marker for pluripotency after the activation of embryonic genome (Mitalipov *et al.*, 2003). Oct4 has been expressed in ICM and trophectoderm cells of pig, cattle and goat embryos (Van Eijk *et al.*, 1999; Kirchhof *et al.*, 2000; He *et al.*, 2004; Yadav *et al.*, 2005). POU5F1 mRNA has been detected in immature oocytes and in *in vitro* produced preattachment-stage embryos of bovine (van Eijk *et al.*, 1999). Oct4 has been confined to ICM of hatched pig blastocysts, but it was observed in the epiblast after the formation of embryonic disk (Vejlsted *et al.,* 2006). It has been found that bovine Oct4 protein is not restricted to the ICM of the blastocyst-stage; therefore Oct4 may not be a key regulator of pluripotency (Kurosaka *et al.,* 2004). Wuensch *et al.* (2007) monitored the quantitative expression of POU5F1-EGFP reporter gene construct and endogenous POU5F1 mRNA in SCNT bovine embryos. Magnani and Cabot (2008) used the quantitative real time PCR to assess the relative expression of Oct4, NANOG, and Sox2 in cleaved pig embryos. They also showed that Oct4, NANOG, and Sox2 possess similar, but not identical patterns of expression between *in vitro* and *in vivo* derived pig embryos. Expression of NANOG has been detected in bovine and caprine embryos (He *et al.,* 2004; 2006; Pant and Keefer, 2006). It has been found that NANOG appear to be specific marker for pluripotency because NANOG m-RNA and protein are found in the ICM and strongly downregulated in the trophectoderm of caprine blastocysts (He *et al.,* 2005, 2006). NANOG expression was not only expressed in the pluripotent cells, but also detected in the adult pig somatic tissues (ovary, heart and muscle) (Brevini *et al.,* 2005). NANOG expression has been studied in pig oocytes and preimplantation embryos, it was found similar to the mouse, bovine and goat (Hart *et al.,* 2004; Brevini *et al.,* 2005; He *et al.,* 2006; Gandolfi *et al.,* 2006).

Isolation and establishment of ES cells from farm animals

After the isolation of the mouse ES cell, human and primate ES cell lines were established, that possesses the remarkable property of pluripotent giving rise to all cells of an organism. Further, ES cell lines were isolated from rodents viz. hamster (Doetschman *et al.,* 1988), rat (Iannaccone *et al.,* 1994; Vassilieva *et al.,* 2000) and rabbit (Schoonjans *et al.,* 1996), however, none of these cell lines proven to be purely ES cells, as similar to human, monkey and mouse.

During the past years, the porcine, bovine, caprine, ovine and equine ES cell lines have been isolated, and these cell lines are often presented as 'ES like' cells. Isolation of porcine ES cells was first established in 1990 (Notarianni *et al.,* 1990; Evans *et al.,* 1990; Strojek *et al.,* 1990; Piedrahita *et al.,* 1990). These cell lines were obtained from *in vivo* produced hatched blastocysts and *in vitro* produced pig embryos. These cell lines were seeded and propagated on STO cells (the murine embryonic fibroblast) commonly used as a feeder layer for mouse ES cells. It is interesting to note that pig ES cell lines do not express LIF receptor indicating that the addition of LIF to the culture medium is not essential for the maintenance of pluripotency (Brevini *et al.*, 2007). The ovine, equine and caprine ES like cells have been isolated from *in vivo* derived blastocysts (Notarianni *et al.*, 1991; Keefer *et al.*, 1996; Saito *et al.*, 2002). However, *in vitro* produced (IVP) embryos are commonly used for making ES cells in cattle. Early blastocysts are the most frequently used in cattle ES cell lines. The bovine ES or ES like cell lines have been isolated from IVP early blastocyst embryos (Evans *et al.*, 1990; Strelchenko, 1996; Cibelli *et al.*, 1998; Iwasaki, *et al.*, 2000; Mitalipova *et al.*, 2001; Saito *et al.*, 2002, 2003). Mitalipova *et al.* (2001) reported that the bovine ES cells can remain as pluripotent in culture for more than 150 passages. Several reports of similar ES like cell lines from pig, goat and bovine were appeared from the primordial germ (PG) cells, referred to as embryonic germ (EG) cell lines (Piedrahita *et al.*, 1997; Shim *et al.*, 1997; Mueller *et al.*, 1999; Tsung *et al.*, 2003; Rui *et al.*, 2004).

Recently, another type of pluripotent stem cells, known as induced pluripotent stem cells (iPSCs), have been successfully generated from mouse, human, monkey, rat and pig. Sheep fibroblasts can be reprogrammed to pluripotency by defined factors (Li *et al.*, 2011). In the recent year, sheep iPSC (induced pluripotent stem cells) is an alternative to pluripotent cell type to ESCs, have been generated using fibroblasts by ectopic expression of transcription factors OCT4, SOX2, KLF4, and cMYC (Liu *et al.*, 2011). These reprogrammed sheep iPSCs may constitute a robust pluripotent alternative to elusive sheep ESCs, with great potential for use in agriculture and pharmaceutical biotechnology.

Future prospects

The establishment of ungulate ES cell lines, either derived from *in vivo* or IVP blastocysts, carries many known and unknown challenges. It involves innovative genetic manipulation technique for targeted cell ablation, ectopic gene expression (Chambers *et al.*, 2003) or gene expression knockdown. Few strains of mice have been used in establishment of germ line competent ES cell lines (McWhir *et al.*, 1996). Chambers *et al.* (2003) demonstrated that the over expression of the NANOG gene in mouse ES cells encouraged undifferentiated proliferation even in absence of LIF. Over expression of telomerase gene has also aided in the maintenance of ES cells by conferring resistance to apoptosis (Lee *et al.*, 2005). These schemes (like over expression of pluripotency associated genes) should also prove suitable for application in farm animal species. Uses of ES like cell lines to produce chimeric animals by injection of the ES like cells into blastocyst stage of ungulate embryos. These efforts produce animals displaying minor chimera contribution from the ungulate ES like cells. Some ungulate ES cell lines were used as nuclear donor cells to create cloned animals by nuclear transfer (Saito *et al.,* 2003). The use of the cells in nuclear cloning in no way proves their ES cell character since numerous types of fully differentiated somatic cells nuclei have proven competent for the creation of cloned animals (Kato *et al.,* 2000; Wakayama and Yanagimachi, 2001). Efforts should be taken to use the ungulate ES like cells to transfect the fibroblast using the somatic cell reprogramming technique.

Researchers working with farm animals now have new resources (gene bank, BAC libraries, microarrays and quantitative PCR), which will aid in identifying specific marker of the pluripotency. Several studies have been published in which sequential analysis of gene expression (SAGE), EST and microarrays have been used to compare and identify the unique expression pattern of transcripts found in human and mouse. Though such studies, a list of several 'stemness related genes' have been identified. These genes and pathways that appear to be related to stemness in mouse and primate ES cell lines may be good candidates for study in embryo derived from farm animal species.

References

Andersson, G.B., BonDurant, R.H., Goff, L., Groff, J. and Moyer A.L. 1996. Development of bovine and porcine embryonic teratomas in athymic mice. Animal Reproduction Science 45: 231-240.

Brevini, T.A.L., Cillo, F., Antonini, S. and Gandolfi, F. 2005. Expression pattern of NANOG gene in porcine tissue and parthenogenetic embryos. Reproduction in Domestic Animals 40: 384.

Brevini, T.A.L., Tosetti, V., Crestan, M., Antonini, S. and Gandolfi, F. 2007. Derivation and characterization of pluripotent cell lines from pig embryos of different origins. Theriogenology 67: 54-63.

Chambers, I., Colby, D., Robertson, M., Nichols, J., Lee, S., Tweedie, S. and Smith, A. 2003. Functional expression cloning of Nanog, a pluripotency sustaining factor in embryonic stem cells. Cell 113: 643-655.

Cibelli, J.B., Stice, S.L., Golueke, P.J., Kane, J.J., Jerry, J., Blackwell, C., Ponce de Leon, F.A. and Robl, J.M. 1998. Transgenic bovine chimeric offspring produced from somatic cell derived stem like cells. Nature Biotechnology 16: 642-646.

Doetschman, T., Williams, P. and Maeda, N. 1988. Establishment of hamster blastocyst derived embryonic stem (ES) cells. Developmental Biology 127: 224-227.

Evans, M.J., Notarianni, E., Laurie, S. and Moor, R.M. 1990. Derivation and preliminary characterization of pluripotent cell lines from porcine and bovine blastocysts. Theriogenology 33: 125-128.

Fujikura, J., Yamato, E., Yonemura, S., Hosoda, K., Masui, S., Nakao, K., Miyazaki, J.J. and Niwa, H. 2002. Differentiation of embryonic stem cells is induced by GATA factors. Genes Development 16: 784-789.

Gandolfi, F., Cillo, F., Antonini, S., Colleoni, S., Lagutina, I., Lazzari, G., Galli, C. and Brevini, T. 2006. Expression pattern of Nanog and Par3 genes in *in vitro* derived bovine embryos. Reproduction, Fertility and Development 18: 231.

Guest, D.J. and Allen, W.R. 2007. Expression of cell surface antigens and embryonic stem cell pluripotency genes in equine blastocysts. Stem Cells Development 16: 789-795.

Hart, A.H., Hartley, L., Ibrahim, M. and Robb, L. 2004. Identification, cloning and expression analysis of the pluripotency promoting NANOG genes in mouse and human. Developmental Dynamics 230: 187-198.

He. S., Pant, D., Bischoff, S., Melican, D., Gavin, W. and Keefer, C.L. 2004. Expression of embryonic stem cell (ESC) markers in preimplantation goat embryo. Biology of Reproduction (Suppl.) 1: 212.

He, S., Pant, D., Bischoff, S., Gavin, W., Melican, D. and Keefer, C.L. 2005. Expression of pluripotency determining factors Oct4 and Nanog in preimplantation goat embryos. Reproduction, Fertility and Development 17: 203.

He, S., Pant, D., Schiffmacher, A., Bischoff, S., Melican, D., Gavin, W. and Keefer, C.L. 2006. Developmental expression of pluripotency determining factors in caprine embryos: novel pattern of Nanog protein localization in the nucleolus. Molecular Reproduction and Development 73: 1512-1522.

Huang, B., Xie, T.S., Shi, D.S., Li, T., Wang, X.L., Mo, Y., Wang, Z.Q. and Li, M.M. 2007. Isolation and characterization of EG-like cells from Chinese swamp buffalo (*Bubalus bubalis*). Cell Biology International 31: 1079-1088.

Humphrey, R.K., Beattie, G.M., Lopez, A.D., Bucay, N., King, C.C., Firpo, M.T., Rose-John, S. and Hayek, A. 2004. Maintenance of pluripotency in human embryonic stem cells is STAT3 independent. Stem Cells 22: 522-530.

Iannaccone, P.M., Taborn, G.U., Garton, R.L., Caplice, M.D. and Brenin, D.R. 1994. Pluripotent embryonic stem cells from the rat are capable of producing chimeras. Developmental Biology 163: 288-292.

Iwasaki, S., Campbell, K.H., Galli, C. and Akiyama, K. 2000. Production of live calves derived from embryonic stem-like cells aggregated with tetraploid embryos. Biology of Reproduction 62: 470-475.

Kato, Y., Tani, T. and Tsunoda, Y. 2000. Cloning of calves from various somatic cell types of male and female adult, newborn and fetal cows. Journal of Reproduction and Fertility 120: 231–237.

Keefer, C.L., Karatzas, C.N., Lazaris-Karatzas, A., Gagnon, I., Poulin, S. and Downey, B.R. 1996. Isolation and maintanance of putative embryonic stem cells derived from Nigerian dwarf goat embryos. Biology of Reproduction 54: 462.

Keefer, C.L., Pant, D., Blomberg, L. and Talbot, N.C. 2007. Challenges and prospects fro the establishment of embryonic stem cell lines of domesticated ungulates. Animal Reproduction Science 98: 147-168.

Kirchoff, N., Carnath, J.W., Lemme, E., Anastassiadis, K., Scholar, H. and Neimann, H. 2000. Expression pattern of Oct-4 in preimplantation embryo of different species. Biology of Reproduction 63: 1698-1705.

Kurosaka, S., Eckardt, S. and McLaughlin, K.J. 2004. Pluripotent lineage definition in bovine embryos by Oct4 transcript localization. Biology of Reproduction 71: 1578-1582.

Lee, J.B., Lee, J.E., Park, J.H., Kim, S.J., Kim, M.K., Roh, S.I. and Yoon, H.S. 2005. Establishment and maintenance of human embryonic stem cell lines on human feeder cells derived from uterine endometrium under serum free condition. Biology of Reproduction 72: 42-49.

Li, Y., Cang, M., Lee, A.S., Zhang, K. and Liu, D. 2011. Reprogramming of sheep fibroblasts into pluripotency under a drug-inducible expression of mouse-derived defined factors. Plos One Jan 6: e15947.

Liu, N., Lu, M., Tian, X. and Han, Z. 2007. Molecular mechanisms involved in self-renewal and pluripotency of embryonic stem cells. Journal of Cellular Physiology 211: 279-286.

Liu, J., Balehosur, D., Murray, B., Kelly, J.M., Sumer, H. and Verma, P.J. 2011. Generation and characterization of reprogrammed sheep induced pluripotent stem cells. Therigenology (In press).

Magnani, L. and Cabot, R.A. 2008. *In vitro* and *in vivo* derived porcine embryos possess similar, but not identical, patterns of Oct4, Nanog, and Sox2 mRNA expression during cleavage development. Molecular Reproduction and Development 75: 1726-1735.

Matsuda, T., Nakamura, T., Nakao, K., Arai, K., Katsuki, M., Heike, T. and Yokota, T. 1999. STAT3 activation is sufficient to maintain an undifferentiated state of mouse embryonic stem cells. The EMBO Journal 18: 4261-4269.

McWhir, J., Schnieke, A.E., Ansell, R., Wallace, H., Colman, A., Scott, A.R. and Kind, A.J. 1996. Selective ablation of differentiated cells permits isolation of embryonic stem cell lines from murine embryos with a non-permissive genetic background. Nature Genetics 14: 223–226.

Mitalipov, S.M., Kuo, H.C., Hennebold, J.D. and Wolf, D.P. 2003. Oct-4 expression in pluripotent cells of the rhesus monkey. Biology of Reproduction 69: 1785-1792.

Mitalipova, M., Beyhan, Z. and First, N.L. 2001. Pluripotency of bovine embryonic cell line derived from precompacting embryos. Cloning 3: 59-67.

Mueller, S., Prelle, K., Rieger, N., Petznek, H., Lassnig, C., Luksch, U., Aigner, B., Baetscher, M., Wolf, E., Mueller, M. and Brem. G. 1999. Chimeric pigs following blastocyst injection of transgenic porcine primordial germ cells. Molecular Reproduction and Development 54: 244-254.

Niwa, H., Burdon, T., Chambers, I. and Smith, A. 1998. Self-renewal of pluripotent embryonic stem cells is mediated *via* activation of STAT3. Genes Development 12: 2048-2060.

Niwa, H., Toyooka, Y., Shimosato, D., Strumpf, D., Takahashi, K., Yagi, R. and Rossant, J. 2005. Interaction between Oct3/4 and Cdx2 determines trophectoderm differentiation. Cell 123: 917-929.

Notarianni, E., Laurie, S., Moor, R.M. and Evans, M.J. 1990. Maintenance and differentiation in culture of pluripotential embryonic cell lines from pig blastocysts. Journal of Reproduction and Fertility 41 (Suppl): 51-56.

Notarianni, E., Galli, C., Laurie, S., Moor, R.M. and Evans, M.J. 1991. Derivation of pluripotent, embryonic cell lines from the pig and sheep. Journal of Reproduction and Fertility 43: 255-260.

Pant, D. and Keefer, C.L. 2006. Gene expression in cultures of inner cell masses isolated from *in vitro* produced and *in vivo* derived bovine blastocysts. Reproduction and Fertility Development 18: 110.

Piedrahita, J.A., Anderson, G.B. and Bondurant, R.H. 1990. On the isolation of embryonic stem cells: Comparative behavior of murine, porcine and ovine embryos. Theriogenology 34: 879-901.

Piedrahita, J.A., Anderson, G.B. and Bondurant, R.H. 1990a. Influence of feeder layer type on the efficiency of isolation of porcine embryo derived cell lines. Theriogenology 34: 865-877.

Piedrahita, J.A., Moore, K., Lee, C., Oetama, B., Weaks, R., Ramsoondar, J., Thomson, J. and Vasquez, J. 1997. Advances in the generation of transgenic pig *via* embryo derived and primordial germ cell derived cells. Journal of Reproduction and Fertility 52 (Suppl.): 245-254.

Rui, R., Shim, H., Moyer, A.L., Anderson, D.L., Penedo, C.T., Rowe, J.D., BonDurant, R.H. and Anderson, G.B. 2004. Attempts to enhance production of porcine chimeras from embryonic germ cells and preimplantation embryos. Theriogenology 61: 1225-1235.

Saito, S., Ugai, H., Sawai, K., Yamamoto, Y., Minamihashi, A., Kurosaka, K., Kobayashi, Y., Murata, T., Obata, Y. and Yokoyama, K. 2002. Isolation of embryonic stem-like cells from equine blastocysts and their differentiation *in vitro*. FEBS Letters 531: 389-396.

Saito, S., Sawai, K., Ugai, H., Moriyasu, S., Minamihashi, A. and Yamamoto, Y. 2003. Generation of cloned calves and transgenic chimeric embryos from bovine embryonic stem-like cells. Biochemical and Biophysical Research Communications 309: 104-113.

Schoonjans, L., Albright, G.M., Li, J.L., Collen, D. and Moreadith, R.W. 1996. Pluripotent rabbit embryonic stem cells are forming overt coat color chimeras following injection into blastocyst. Molecular Reproduction and Development 45: 439-443.

Shim, H., Gutierrez-Adan, A., Chen, L.R., BonDurant, R.H., Behboodi, E. and Anderson, G.B. 1997. Isolation of pluripotent stem cells from cultured porcine primordial germ cells. Biology of Reproduction 57: 1089-1095.

Solter, D. 2006. From teratocarcinomas to embryonic stem cells and beyond: a history of embryonic stem cell research. Nature Review Genetics 7: 319-327.

Strelchenko, N.S. 1996. Bovine pluripotent stem cells. Theriogenology 45: 131-140.

Strojek, R.M., Reed, M.A., Hoover, J.L. and Wagner, T.E. 1990. A method for cultivating morphologically undifferentiated embryonic stem cells from porcine blastocysts. Theriogenology 33: 901-913.

Suda, Y., Suzuki, M., Ikawa, Y. and Aizawa, S. 1987. Mouse embryonic stem cells exhibit indefinite proliferative potential. Journal of Cellular Physiology 133: 197-201.

Sumi, T., Fujimoto, Y., Nakatsuji, N. and Suemori, H. 2004. STAT3 is dispensable for maintenance of self-renewal in nonhuman primate embryonic stem cells. Stem Cells 22: 861-872.

Talbot, N.C., Rexroad, Jr C.E., Pursel, V.G. and Powell, A.M.1993. Alkaline phosphatase staining of pig and sheep epiblast cells in culture. Molecular Reproduction and Development 36:139-147.

Thomson, J.A., Itskovitz-Eldor, J., Shapiro, S.S., Waknitz, M.A., Swiergiel, J.J., Marshall, V.S. and Jones, J.M. 1998. Embryonic stem cell lines derived from human blastocysts. Science 282: 1145-1147.

Tsung, H.C., Du, Z.W., Rui, R., Li, X.L., Bao, L.P., Wu, J., Bao, S.M. and Yao, Z. 2003. The culture and establishment of embryonic germ cell lines from Chinese mini swine. Cell Research 13: 195-202.

van Eijk, M.J.T., van Rooijen, M.A., Modina, S., Scesi, L., Folkers, G., van Tol, H.T.A., Bevers, M.M., Fisher, S.R., Lewin, H.A., Rakacolli, D., Galli, C., de Vaureix, C., Trounson, A.O., Mummery, C.L. and Gandolfi, F. 1999. Molecular cloning, genetic mapping, and developmental expression of Bovine POU5F1. Biology of Reproduction 60: 1093-1103.

Vassilieva, S., Guan, K., Pich, U. and Wobus, A.M. 2000. Establishment of SSEA-1 and Oct-4 expressing rat embryonic stem-like cell lines and effects of cytokines of the IL-6 family on clonal growth. Experimental Cell Research 258: 361-373.

Vejlsted, M., Offenberg, H., Thorup, F. and Maddox-Hyttel, P. 2006a. Confinement and clearance of Oct4 in the porcine embryo at stereomicroscopically defined stages around gastrulation. Molecular Reproduction and Development 73: 709-718.

Verma, V., Gautam, S.K., Singh, B., Manik, R.S., Palta, P., Singla, S.K., Goswami, S.L. and Chauhan, M.S. 2007. Isolation and Characterization of Embryonic Stem Cell-Like Cells From In Vitro-Produced Buffalo (Bubalus bubalis) Embryos. Molecular Reproduction and Development 74: 520-529.

Wakayama, T. and Yanagimachi, R., 2001. Mouse cloning with nucleus donor cells of different age and type. Molecular Reproduction and Development 58: 376–383.

Wall, R.J., Powell, A.M., Paape, M.J., Kerr, D.E., Bannerman, D.D., Pursel, V.G., Wells, K.D., Talbot, N. and Hawk, H.W. 2005. Genetically enhanced cows resist intramammary *Staphylococcus aureus* infection. Nature Biotechnology 23: 445-451.

Williams, R.L., Hilton, D.J., Pease, S., Willson, T.A., Stewart, C.L., Gearing, D.P., Wagner, E.F., Metcalf, D., Nicola, N.A. and Gough, N.M. 1988. Myeloid leukemia inhibitory factor maintains the developmental potential of embryonic stem cells. Nature 336: 684-687.

Wuensch, A., Habermann, F.A., Kurosaka, S., Klose, R., Zakhartchenko, V., Reichenbach, H.D., Sinowatz, F., McLaughlin, K.J. and Wolf, E. 2007. Quantitative monitoring of pluripotency gene activation after somatic cloning in cattle. Biology of Reproduction 76: 983-991.

Yadav, P.S., Kues, W.A., Herrmann, D., Carnath, J.W. and Niemann, H. 2005. Bovine ICM derived cells express the Oct4 ortholog. Molecular Reproduction and Development 72: 182-190.

□□□

Chapter 12

Relevance and Importance of Pasture-Based Production System of Small Ruminants in India

K. Sharma[1]*, A.K. Pattanaik[2] and K.Y. Deshpande[2]
[1]Education Division, Indian Council of Agricultural Research, Krishi Anusandhan Bhawan-II, Pusa, New Delhi- 110 012
[2]Centre of Advanced Faculty Training in Animal Nutrition, Indian Veterinary Research Institute, Izatnagar- 243 122 (UP)

India is endowed with the highest livestock population in the world, a vast majority of which are raised by small and marginal farmers. This valuable animal resource serves as a key source of livelihood by way of providing large-scale self-employment opportunities. As a matter fact, as per a recent estimate, about 6.7% of the work force in rural areas is engaged in animal husbandry sector, with a national average of 5.5% when both rural and urban areas are considered together (NSS, 2005). However, these statistical facts may appear to demean the contribution of livestock sector to the agrarian economy of India, if one takes into account the scope of livestock sector as collateral for enormous indirect employment avenues, which has its own significance in the Indian context. And, this can be best adjudged by the fact that, livestock sector contributes a value output of whopping 24.73% from total agriculture and allied sector (CSO, 2011). The recent graphs of livestock population in India reveal certain striking facts that underscore the rise in adoption of small ruminants to raise livelihood status of marginal farmers. The annual growth rates of sheep and goat populations were 3.87 and 3.10% as compared to

1.83 and 1.84% in that of cattle and buffalo, respectively (DAHDF, 2011). The 18th livestock census in the recent past (2007) witnessed around 16.41 and 13.01% increase in total sheep and goat population of India, respectively, over the previous census in 2003. This huge population of sheep and goats is distributed across several agro-ecological zones of India starting from highly placed pasture lands in northern temperate zone, through semi-arid and arid western zone to Nilgiris in the south. The small ruminant production in the country thus is practiced in diverse climate types and topographies adopting a variety of region-specific feeding systems. However, one thing which holds good throughout the country is that these animals are reared mostly by poor communities like nomads and landless peasants. The small ruminants have been portrayed as socio-economic, cultural and recreational needs of poor farmers with multifarious benefits encompassing stability or asset, supplementary income generation, effective utilization of family labour, food security in form of milk and meat, fertilizer generation through urine and dung, and conversion of crop residue into valued meat, fibre and skin (Devendra, 2001).

The implication of the declined world resources on the livestock production systems is a recognized fact. Oil depletion, pressure to produce bio-fuels, soil fertility decline, the high cost of fertilizers, decreasing water availability and the loss of arable land to erosion and non agricultural purposes, coupled with likely overall decreases in crop production from global warming appear to be interacting such that it will be difficult to produce staples and animal products to meet world demand for an expanding population (Leng, 2009). The quintessential place of small ruminants in the life of rural India notwithstanding, the production system is at the crossroads because of multitude of problems and prospects typical to the present-day changing world scenario involving, (a) environmental concerns of livestock production, (b) skepticism about the relevance of smallholder livestock production system in the era of increasing globalization, (c) emerging market opportunities liked to the projected hike in the demands for animal products, (d) heightened consumer consciousness about quality of animal-origin foods, and above all, (e) the core issue of ensuring animal welfare. Keeping this background truth in mind, an effort has been made in this paper to highlight pertinent issues delineating the relevance of pasture-based production systems of small ruminants in the present day set-up, and suggest a roadmap to make small ruminant production a viable, thriving and sustainable enterprise.

Small ruminant production scenario in India

The widespread expanse of marginal agricultural land ranging from rugged mountainous country and deserts to natural grasslands across the length and breadth of India account for more than 212 million small ruminants. Production systems are largely based on traditional transhumance activities and shepherding small flocks, which graze on different pastures with each season. India, an abode of vast genetic resource, is endowed with 38 and 20 recognized breeds of sheep and goats, respectively (Tantia and Vij, 2000). Most of these breeds demonstrate extensive adaptation to hot and humid tropical clime of their origin, scanty vegetation, scares drinking water and extended migration tracks. This enables sheep and goats to be designated as poor man's cow (especially to later). Certain distinctive merits of small ruminants make them more suitable than large ruminants to be considered as the animals of choice by poor farmers. As mentioned earlier the hardy nature of small ruminants especially goats, their ability to utilize small shrubs, better metabolism of tannin rich or woody plants and better resistance to rain-fed conditions where availability of fodder is low to meager, make them ideal animals to thrive in tropical Indian conditions. The farmers rearing these animals comprise of Gujjars and Bakharwals in northen temperate region and similar underprivileged communities in semi-arid to arid regions of Rajasthan or Deccan plateau and southern peninsular region. The smaller size of these animals helps in many ways like, low initial inputs, easy handling and management, lesser care of feeding and reduced requirement of storage facilities for final perishable products like milk or meat. The concerns about environmental damage are subsided in developing countries of Asia and Africa; as livelihood or food security of migrating population and animals take upper hand (Devendra, 2001). Moreover, the production of dung and urine by these animals helps in improving the fertility of soil in arid and semi-arid regions, which again help to overcome aforesaid concerns.

The prevalent situation in developing world puts forward two urgent needs of food security for bourgeoning human as well as livestock population and raising the livelihood status of poor to very poor, who represent a large portion of population in these countries. The competition for food between humans and animals is ever widening the gap between demand and supply, though the agricultural production is increased in leaps and bounds in last few years. In this scenario the farmer is forced to adopt different production system/

setups to raise different animal species. This is monitored by various factors such as, animal species, size of herd, market demand for type of final product, consumer preference, and availability of feed resources in the vicinity and economical status of farmer. However, the ideal production system must be vibrant, able to address aforesaid factors, sustainable and to help to realize the production potential of goat or sheep breed under consideration.

The small ruminant production in India is carried out adopting two main systems as per prevalence of feeding material/practices and/or season of year viz. semi-intensive/intensive and extensive/migratory. The semi-intensive or intensive system comprises of rearing the animals on crop residues, cut fodder/plants from arable crops, feeding animals on cut and carry basis, tethering on field boundaries, short span exposure to community pastures or even feeding on grasses grown at road side. Whereas, extensive system includes pasture based feeding of animals; in which animal travel long distances at the end of winter and feed on natural pastures, fallow/waste lands, tree fodder/top feeds during migration through forests, residues of seasonal crops and community grazing land. Out of these systems, migratory flocks are widespread practice throughout India. However, profitability of this system is marred by the scarcity of good quality pastures in the country. A generally low level of productivity emerges from substandard nutritional management, where very little or no concentrates, salt, or mineral licks are provided, except in the case of dairy cows. The area cultivated under fodder is about 4.6% of the total cultivable area. Exclusive pastures and grasslands are widespread and are grazed by the domestic animals. Total area under permanent pastures and grasslands is about 12.4 million hectares (NABCONS). An area of 15.6 million ha is classified as wasteland and is also available for grazing. However, majority of these lands have either been degraded or encroached upon restricting their availability for livestock grazing (Annual report 2010-11, DAHDF, GOI, New Delhi). Though, the traditional small ruminant production system in India is extensive or migratory type and is in dire need of research or promotion of schemes to revive the pastures or convert the wastelands into pastures; the efforts are meager to do so. Judging the need of hour, research today is focused on raising the fodder production, tree fodder cultivation and search of futuristic feeds that would supplement the native feedstuffs to meet out requirements of greens, concentrate or dry matter *per se*. Along with this, efforts towards sustainable pasture based small ruminant production are also imminent. Some of few such studies accentuate the role of efficient natural resource production and management to sustain economic small ruminant production in diverse Indian niche.

Pasture-based production system: advantages revisited

A pasture-based system of livestock farming is truly sustainable. Pasture-raised animals roam freely in their natural environment, and eat nutritious grasses and other plants that their bodies are adapted to digest. In addition to dramatically improving the welfare of farm animals, pasturing also helps reduce environmental damage, and yields animal products that are more nutritious than foods produced adopting intensive system.

Pasture-based production typically facilitates an animal's environment and immune system to work together, thereby imparting an acceptable level of production while naturally maintaining the integrity of the ecological connections between the animal, the soil and the pasture plants. When considered *vis-a-vis* intensively reared animals, ruminants on pasture experience fewer health problems due partially to reduced stress, resulting in reduced proneness to diseases such as acidosis, mastitis and respiratory disease etc. The votaries of pasture-based rearing system often criticize the intensive way production as a system that has a singular focus i.e., productivity, and this, in turn, is responsible for more problems than a systems approach. On the other hand, a well-planned and managed pasture-based operation can maintain reasonable production, reduce input costs and achieve a positive economic return, given a well-conceived marketing plan (Reinhart, 2008).

The process of grazing and the resultant impact of animals thriving on it imparts positive inputs into the pasture systems, which contributes to the ecological sustainability of the rangelands through the following mechanisms (Reainhart, 2008): (a) nutrient cycling through feces and urine, (b) timely defoliation and removal of plant material that encourages regrowth, (c) root death through leaf removal, resulting in underground organic matter accumulation and nutrient cycling, (d) increased water-holding capacity through accumulation of soil organic matter and (e) hoof action that breaks soil surface and compacts soil, thereby allowing greater germination of seeds and encouraging regeneration of pasture swards.

Small ruminants have been credited with the unique ability to convert low quality forages into animal products of high value. Owing to this unique reason, sheep and goat rearing have conventionally been related to grazing, thus increasing the usefulness of farmland unsuitable for cultivation such as mountainous areas or semi-arid regions. Small ruminant grazing systems offer a number of environmental, sociological or nutritional advantages (Ruiz *et al.*, 2009). Furthermore, it has been shown that if managed appropriately, grazing systems for small ruminants (goats) show a certain level of sustainability, higher than more intense systems (Nahed *et al.*, 2006).

Sheep and goats offer an alternative to utilizing forage and vegetation which is otherwise *wasted*; when compared *vis-a-vis* the dietary preferences of cattle, goats have a very high preference for browse and sheep are with a higher preference for weeds. In a pasture situation goats are *top down* grazers, consuming only the best parts of a wide range of grasses, legumes, and browse plants including brush, shrubs, trees, and vines with woody stems, which results in uniform grazing. Since goats, cattle, and sheep different forage-preferences, these species do not compete for the same pasture component in a grazing situation. As a result, sheep and goat can be integrated quite profitably in a multispecies grazing system, allowing the land to be used more effectively thereby generating more income per unit grazing area. Some studies have shown that land grazed by both goats and cattle returns 25% more than land grazed only by cattle (Lemus and Brown, 2008). Furthermore, because of their grazing behaviour, adding sheep and goats to a grazing system will have additional benefits in terms of weed-control; goats have a general preference for such weeds, therefore decreasing the need for commercial herbicides or mowing.

Feed is the single largest cost associated with raising small ruminants, typically accounting up to two-thirds of total production costs. With pastures or forages being the cheapest feed sources for both sheep and goat, any system which aims to use these resources to their fullest extent would certainly constitute a pragmatic and more enterprising way for a sustainable and economic small ruminant production.

The products obtained from grazing systems present certain features which differentiate them from other feeding systems, such as the fact that the milk produced in the former is rich with micro-components (fatty acids and vitamins) and volatile compounds (flavours and terpenes) which favour human nutrition and health (Morand-Fehr *et al.,* 2007). Recent research has focused on the nutritional importance of the n-6:n-3 fatty acid ratio in the human diet, and on conjugated linoleic acid (CLA) isomers because of their anticarcinogenic properties. The nutritional value of n-3 PUFAs is well recognized, and increased consumption of these fatty acids has been recommended. Ruminant fats are among the richest natural sources of CLA, in particular the cis-9, trans-11 isomer, which arises from microbial hydrogenation of dietary linoleic acid in the rumen. There are plenty of research reports which have shown that including grass in the diet of ruminants increased CLA concentration in milk and meat. Results from a recent study suggest that the negative image of beef attributed to its highly saturated nature may be overcome by enhancing the fatty acid profile of intramuscular fat in beef through pasture feeding from a human health perspective (Realini *et al.,* 2004).

Animals on pasture are continuously exposed to gastrointestinal nematodes (GIN) infection because eggs shed in faeces hatch into free-living larvae that crawl up grass blades and are eaten along with the forage, thus reinfecting the animal. Most of the larvae are found within six inches of the ground, so animals grazing the most desirable, short, highly nutritious forage will ingest more parasites. Forages can affect GIN control either indirectly or directly. Any forage can impact animal tolerance to GIN through indirect means, simply by providing a superior source of nutrients that strengthen the animals' immune system and enables them to better resist the parasite attack. In addition, some forages directly inhibit some phase of the life cycle of the worms. Direct inhibition can be biochemical or mechanical; biochemical inhibition occurs when the plant contains bioactive compounds that are toxic to the parasitic worm like condensed tannins (CT). Obviously, the ideal forage species for this purpose must have the traditional positive traits of good yield and nutritive value, plus a beneficial effect on animal health and GIN control. Condensed tannins in pasture and hay forages can reduce fecal egg count in sheep and goats and have additional benefits in that they prevent bloat and improve protein utilization by ruminants. However, CTs are not palatable and can have negative effects on intake and performance if present in too great a concentration. The range of 2.5 to 4.5% CT is considered beneficial for GIN control (Min *et al.,* 2003). Strategic provision of tannin-rich forages in the pasture not only helps controlling the gastro-intestinal parasitism, but also could boost the nutritive value of forages by way of enhanced protein bioavailability. This, in turn, not only cut down the costs associated with deworming but also constitute a strategy for eco-friendly and organic way of animal production.

Pasture-based production system: a reality check

For millions of rural population, goat/sheep farming plays a significant social role by helping to maintain traditions and contributing considerably to multi-functionality. Notwithstanding the positive aspects of pasture-based production systems for small ruminants, the grazing systems tend to become rapidly intensified on a global scale, and this holds true for India as well. Several different reasons could be ascribed to this trend, which includes: (a) the intensification of agricultural (crop) production to feed a mushrooming human population, (b) the lack of interest among the newer generations to remain clustered within the impoverished and rugged life typical to a shepherd/nomad, especially in view of the lure of urban life, (c) the trend to eliminate seasonality in meat and milk production in consequence of huge demands for these products coupled with remunerative market prices, (d) the availability of breeds with a highly productive potential and (e) the increasing difficulties in having access to grazing in natural or protected areas and rising land prices.

Pasture-based production system: roadmap ahead

Finding a appropriate solution for the present trend would certainly require a deep knowledge of how these systems work, and it becomes all the more necessary that their weaknesses can be detected and improvement strategies can be proposed on the one hand, and on the other, issues external to the systems themselves such as their environmental and social contributions, can be ascertained.

Understanding the nutritional needs of goats and sheep is important in developing an efficient, remunerative and all-inclusive pasture-based system for them. It has been recognized that sheep and goats usually need a more concentrated diet than cattle because their digestive tract size is smaller relative to their maintenance energy needs. Average goats (weaner kids) reared for mutton production require about 10-14% crude protein and 60-65% TDN, on a dry matter basis, in the total diet which represents a TDN:CP ratio range of 4.9-5.4. While weaned lambs require 75-81.8% TDN and 14.5-16% CP in their diet which represents a TDN:CP ratio range of 5.1-5.2 (Turner *et al.*, 2009). Older, mature does and ewes have lower dietary requirements.

In pasture-based system of production, pasture, weeds, and browse are all small ruminants need to meet their nutritional requirements since they tend to be high in energy and protein especially when in a vegetative state. Thus using vegetative pasture as the primary source of nutrients makes the sheep and goats rearing the most economical. In most cases, rotating the pastures to keep plants in a vegetative state is important since palatability and digestibility decline as the plants mature. During the early part of the grazing season, the pasture tends to be higher in protein and energy than ordinary pasture. Sheep are excellent weed eaters while goats are generally considered a browse-consuming species and have the unique ability to select plants when they are at their most nutritious state.

There is not just one type of pasture than can or even should, be used; it is always preferable to have a diversity of grass/browse/weed-species to minimize need for supplementary feeds. This situation, as a matter of fact, helps to exploit the specific advantages and disadvantages associated with individual plant species in order to derive the maximum benefits.

Silvipastoral system

The lower productivity of small ruminants in rainfed areas, which is typically associated with low quality of native grasses as well as the shortage of good quality forage, especially during the dry season could be improved by developing silvipastoral/hortipastoral systems wherein pasture and foliage component are introduced under trees so as to provide nutritious green forage and foliage to small ruminants for getting higher production from unit of land. Associations of tree crops and animals are established farm practice in many developing countries. New technologies to intensify production and better scientific guidelines for managing the components of silvo-pastoral systems are now available that can lead to higher farm incomes and a more protected environment. However, future development of these integrated systems will require policy support to encourage the introduction of ruminants and to increase their productivity (Devendra, 2011). Lessons can be taken from many such successful systems combining animals and perennial cropping, e.g., coconuts-sheep integration in Philippines, oil palm-cattle integration in Malaysia, and even to some extent cashew/orange-small ruminant in South India. The presence of a range of perennial tree crops in different parts of India provides immense scope for the development of integrated systems involving small ruminants. Such an integrated approach has been successfully demonstrated in many studies done in India. In one such study, Ramana *et al.* (2011) have successfully used mango and sweet orange orchards with suitable understory grass species and boundary plantation of *Leucaena leucocephala* to develop a hortipastoral systems for higher biomass and subsequently higher income through ram lamb production, when lambs were introduced in the middle of rainy season. The concept of silvipastoral system has another powerful application in regeneration of damaged and degraded rangelands. Using appropriate silvipastoral approach, degraded rangelands could be successfully developed into useful reconstituted pasture (Sharma *et al.*, 1995). One such reconstituted three-tier pasture dominated by native plant species such as *Acacia nilotica* and Cenchrus species have been proven to have the potential to sustain the nutrient requirements of goats without adverse seasonal fluctuations in pasture quality (Sharma *et al.*, 1998).

Intensive grazing management

Intensive management generally involves a grazing plan that synchronizes duration of the grazing interval with the growth characteristics of the plant stand, by moving or adjusting the number of grazers on a given land area. Further, this approach takes into consideration the varying nutritive value of the forages with maturity. For example, at the beginning of the green season, the grasses contain on average 9-11% CP with the digestibility of about 60-65%. However, these values decrease rapidly during the dry season; during a prolonged period of the year the protein content could reduce to as low as only 4-5% and the digestibility between 45 and 50% (Kamalzadeh, 2005). In this scenario, intensive grazing management can not only maintain plant persistence and productivity, but also high nutritive value, especially TDN and CP, for improved forage utilization by grazing livestock (Turner *et al.*, 2009). In order to overcome persistent nutritional problems of poor ranges, small ruminants should be taken off the ranges strategically in order to reduce the grazing pressure on the vegetation and to allow regeneration of the range species. In other words, this could mean gradually switching the extensive system of production to a more productive semi-intensive system.

Rotational grazing: It is always advisable to graze sheep and goats with cattle, or in a rotation with cattle. The role of goats and sheep as biological control agents will become increasingly important in pastures in the future due to elevated costs of other control methods such as mechanical cutting and herbicide application, where energy utilization is an issue. Many producers have implemented rotational stocking of livestock on pastures to improve overall forage utilization to achieve more uniform distribution of fecal and urinary nutrients for plant growth. This system helps to maintain forages with high nutritive value for sheep and goats, especially for finishing weaned kids and lambs which have higher nutrient requirements compared to mature animals (Turner *et al.*, 2009).

Rotational grazing is a proven method of increasing the efficiency of pasture systems. Intensively managed rotational grazing systems have the potential of maintaining pastures in a vegetative state for most of the growing season. Rotational grazing coupled with the use of stored forage, it is possible to achieve year-round forage finishing of farm stock. In addition, intensively managed grazing systems make it possible to feed livestock without concentrating wastes in manure pits and lagoons, thereby maintaining nutrients within the pasture ecosystem and preventing them from becoming pollutants (Reinhart, 2008).

If given a choice, livestock will only eat the highest-quality, most palatable plants in a pasture. In order to ensure that plant biodiversity is maintained in the pasture, it is necessary to set up a grazing management system to better control livestock grazing. The elements of grazing to control are the timing and the intensity. This means controlling the number of animals and how long they are in a pasture. Rotational grazing systems take full advantage of the benefits of nutrient cycling as well as the ecological balance that comes from the relationships between pastures and grazing animals. High-density stocking for short periods helps build soil organic matter and develops highly productive, dense, resilient pastures. The basic principles of rotational grazing management include: (a) proper timing of grazing corresponding to plant physiological stage, (b) proper intensity of grazing, or duration on the pasture, (c) residue or plant height after grazing and (d) duration of rest (Reinhart, 2008).

Controlled grazing: Controlled grazing has several positive effects on the environment, as it favours the conservation of the wide variety of vegetation resulting from the different environmental and management conditions, the upkeep of a quality pasture, the conservation of a heterogeneous landscape, the prevention of soil loss due to erosion and the prevention of forest fires, among others (Ruiz *et al.*, 2009).

Stocking rate: Determining the initial stocking rate for a given pasture is relatively simple but more often than not, it is a difficult task to accomplish. There are several key issues to consider when thinking about how many animals a pasture will support. Consideration must be given to forage production potential, utilization patterns by livestock, the nutrient content of the forage and forage growth patterns, the plant species that comprise the pasture, species diversity of the pasture plant community and seasonal variations in temperature and moisture (Reinhart, 2008).

Multispecies grazing: Multispecies grazing refers to the practice of utilizing different livestock species on a single pasture system, and this helps to: (a) diversify farm income, (b) utilize pastures of different ecological types on the farm, (c) manipulate the plant community to meet the production goals of the farm and (d) interrupt parasite life cycles (Reinhart, 2008). Cattle, sheep and goats evolved eating different plant types. Cattle typically consume, in order of preference, grasses, forbs and shrubs. Sheep will consume, also in order of preference, forbs, grasses and shrubs and goats will seek shrubs, forbs and grasses.

Overgrazing: It occurs when the grazing pressure exceeds the carrying capacity of the pasture; this condition is not really a function of how many animals are on a pasture, but how long they remain there. Continuous grazing allows livestock to selectively graze the most palatable plants over and over, and the grazed plant does not get the time to regrow before it is grazed again.

Overgrazing has often blamed for environmental degradation associated with raising livestock on pasture. The issue of managing livestock in degraded environment has been reviewed recently by Masters (2009) and this part of the discussion is based on the concepts presented therein. The very phenomenon of overgrazing could be related to the declined availability of pasturelands, thereby increasing the pressure on the dwindling rangelands beyond the inherent carrying capacity. However, to what extent this damaging effect could be ascribed to livestock alone is open to question. Because, there exists clear evidence that livestock are not inherently damaging to rangelands or farming landscapes, and, in fact, may be required for their sustained health and profitability. Moderate to heavy grazing has, in some cases created highly resilient and ecologically sound systems while under-grazing has resulted in dense woody growth and reduced species diversity (Perevolotsky and Seligman, 1998). Conversion of rangelands into intensive crop/fodder production has also led to progressive loss of diversity, species connectivity and ability to recover (Lambin *et al.*, 2001). More pragmatic approaches involving well-managed livestock in either a grassland or mixed crop/livestock system offer a highly efficient method of increasing the production of high quality food with minimal environmental impact (Tilman *et al.*, 2002).

One of such approach could be demonstrating the potential economic benefit from a well-managed rangeland with the direct involvement of livestock owner, which could be a combination of ensuring responsible grazing by the owner, and revegetation of degraded or partly degraded landscapes through the expenditure of private/public funding. This use of livestock may or may not contribute to the return of the landscape to its original state; in some cases stable vegetation that provides some of the functional benefits of the original landscape, combined with the productive benefits of a profitable livestock system may be the best option available. This then provides an opportunity to design a landscape based on a range of predetermined objectives which include both profit and ecosystem services (Masters, 2009).

Meeting the nutritional and environmental requirements of raising livestock on pasture-based system has been an onerous challenge from the loss-of-diversity point of view. Both over- and under-grazing are likely to result in a loss of species diversity (Oba *et al.*, 2001). As livestock have the ability to select plants with higher digestibility, adequate nitrogen and low or manageable anti-nutritional compounds, loss of diversity will be accompanied by a decline in nutritive value and palatability and reduced ability to deal with toxins (Provenza *et al.*, 2003). In the case of over-grazing the decrease in diversity and nutritive value will be accompanied with a decrease in feed availability. Management of livestock, vegetation and the interaction between the two is critical for productive grazing of such fragile environments (Masters, 2009). The possible strategies to counter the loss of diversity as a consequence of previous over-grazing should centre around three major approaches: (a) complementary feeding, (b) revegetation and (c) grazing management.

Complementary feeding: In general, forages are energy limiting and animals finished on pasture without energy supplementation gain weight slowly and produce leaner carcasses than animal finished in the feedlot on high grain diets (Turner *et al.,* 2009). A mature pasture having high in fiber expectedly would result in slower goat growth rates. On the contrary, ruminants grazing legumes often have higher live weight gains compared to forage grasses. Complementary feeding with appropriate supplements can improve feed intake, feed conversion efficiency and therefore productive potential. Energy supplements can be used, for example, to improve the utilization of plants that contain high levels of non-protein nitrogen. Similarly, supplementation of minerals to take care of deficient availability through low-grade pasture could also be taken up not only to enhance nutrient bioavailability form the pasture but also to ensure better overall health. Likewise, supplementary feeding strategy could also be applied to facilitate the breakdown of anti-nutritional compounds in the forage.

Revegetation: Strategies can be applied for revegetation with selective planting to complement the composition and availability of other feed resources. Where revegetation is an option, there will be additional benefits in assessing the plant options for palatability, nutritive value, anti-nutritional properties, shelter and possible medicinal properties as well as selected ecosystem benefits. These do not need to be long-term and expensive plant breeding projects but may be well designed and localized screening programs based on indigenous plant species with known natural advantages. For reasons described above revegetation should complement rather than replace existing feed resources.

Grazing management: Effective and strategic grazing management is vital to improve the intake and utilization of forages in degraded environments which otherwise have the potential to induce further degradation. Maintenance of low stocking rates helps preventing over-grazing and associated environmental problems in terms of soil erosion, and irreversible damage to the immediate ecosystem.

Periodic review of information on the livestock condition and behavior, as well as forage quality could be used to provide incentive and opportunity for livestock managers to tactically manipulate feeding and production. For example, live weight change may provide information on both available biomass and diversity of feed sources as livestock will begin to lose weight long before feed supply is exhausted. Similarly, animal behaviours, such as time spent walking, grazing and feeding are also equally vital indicators related to feed supply and diversity (Masters, 2009).

Appropriate selection and timely propagation of selective plant species could help extending the period well into the dry season. Likewise, annual forage crops can be an excellent addition to a farm since they extend the grazing season several weeks or even months. To sum up, effective strategies to exploit the benefits from the ever-dwindling rangelands and pasture should aim at the followings as potential intervention points:

- Multispecies grazing
- Pasture renovation and establishment
- Rotational grazing
- Overgrazing prevention
- Diversification of plant species extending the grazing season
- Stockpiling forages (allowing forage growth for deferred grazing during lean period)
- Prescribed grazing on rangeland (a process of developing a grazing system that seeks to integrate the economic and ecological realities)
- Developing a grazing management plan on rangeland: this should focus on creating an inventory, defining goals, determining grazing units, developing a grazing schedule, and developing a monitoring and evaluation plan
- Managing for drought
- Managing plant toxicity

Common property resources management

The International Livestock Research Institute's (ILRI) report on 'Mapping Poverty and Livestock in the Developing World', projects that fifty years from now, existing areas that are within livestock and rangeland based production systems and without any cropping potential, would face a risk of overgrazing and degradation, decreased food security, drought and limited access to local and other markets. Since the last few decades a lot of change have been taken place for traditional pastoralist communities using common lands which ranges from socio-economic and demographic shifts, including pressures arising from population growth, migration and inequalities in assets; loss of grazing and production lands to urbanisation and development activities; conservation politics; and more recently, climate change and its associated impacts (FES, 2011).

In India, permanent pastures for grazing account for less than 4% of the area of the country, and much of this activity is dependent on grazing opportunities in fallow lands, forests and areas that are classified as 'wastelands' that are accessible. There is data to prove that 84 to 100% of poor households derived benefits such as food, fuel, fodder and fibre from common lands (FES, 2011). However, as a result of agricultural expansion, industrialisation and the restrictions imposed on grazing in forests, traditional pastoral institutions are increasingly under threat.

India's 11th Five Year Plan recognised the need to develop government policies and programmes that favour of livestock rearing in arid and semi-arid regions. Grasslands and deserts are the most neglected ecosystems in India. Protection, development and sustainable use of grasslands are very important for the rural economy and livestock. Recognizing the importance of grasslands and deserts for biodiversity conservation, livestock dependency and for poverty alleviation, the Planning Commission constituted a Task Force on Grasslands and Deserts for the Environment and Forests Sector for the Eleventh Five-Year Plan in order to conceptualize a Grassland Development and Grazing Policy in 2006. The Task Force has highlighted the need for: (a) a National Grazing Policy to ensure the sustainable use of grasslands and biodiversity conservation, (b) launching of Integrated Research and Development Programmes in the grasslands and deserts and (c) a countrywide network of grassland ecologists be established (GOI, 2006).

Conclusion

One of the main weaknesses identified with pasture-based system apparently is the inappropriate feeding management, particularly grazing *vis-a-vis* small ruminant productivity. Intensive targeted research on the nutritional utilization of rangelands and pastures coupled with proper feed supplementation could help improve the situation; unfortunately, much of the present day research on small ruminants are targeting intensively-reared animals in our country, which is obviously not helping the situation. Large-scale assessment of the impacts of pastoral grazing on soil quality, land-water interactions and its consequence on the aquatic environment, and socio-economic issues in pasture-based farming are need of the day in order to make the system adaptable to the changing environs of the globe. Accordingly, the impacts of pasture-based production systems on specific areas like impact of livestock grazing on extensively managed grazing lands, environmental effects of pasture-based farming on emission of greenhouse gases, the environmental impacts of pasture-based farming in temperate, irrigated, non-irrigated, semi-arid ecosystems, the e impact of the production system on air, soil and water quality with particular focus on nitrogen and phosphorus cycling, besides biotic and abiotic pressures on animals grazing in mixed production farming are some of the issues which need to be researched in a multi-disciplinary mode involving various stakeholders. Further, meaningful deliberations on the socio-economic factors involved in the adoption of environmental practices would help providing needed insights into the challenges in accounting for environmental impacts at the farm level, the environmental versus financial tradeoffs of change, and the policy and cultural issues that affect producer adoption (McDowell, 2008).

References

CSO, 2011. The Fourth International Joint Conference on Computational Sciences and Optimization (CSO 2011) held at China

DAHDF, 2011. Department of Animal Husbandry, Dairying and Fisheries Report.

Devendra, C. 2001. Small ruminants: Imperatives for productivity enhancement improved livelihoods and rural growth – A review. Asian-Australian Journal of Animal Science 14: 1483-1496.

Devendra, C. 2011. Integrated tree crops-ruminants systems in south-east Asia: advances in productivity enhancement and environmental sustainability. Asian-Australian Journal of Animal Science 24: 587-602.

FES. 2011. Pastoralism and grazing. Common Voices 2: 1-9. Foundation for Ecological Security. (http://iasc2011.fes.org.in/common-voices-2.pdf).

GOI. 2006. Report of the Task Force on Grasslands and Deserts. Planning Commission, Government of India, New Delhi (http://planningcommission.nic.in/aboutus/committee/wrkgrp11/tf11_grass.pdf).

Kamalzadeh, A. 2005. Modeling the productivity of a breeding sheep flock for different production systems. Asian-Australian Journal of Animal Science 18: 606-612.

Lambin, E.F., Turner, B.L., Geist, H.J., Agbola, S.B., Angelsen, A., Bruce, J.W., Coomes, O.T., Dirzo, R., Fischer, G., Folke, C., George, P.S., Homewood, K.,

Imbernon, J., Leemans, R., Li, X., Moran, E. F., Mortimore, M., Ramakrishnan, P. S., Richards, J. F., Skanes, H., Steffen, W., Stone, G.D., Svedin, U., Veldkamp, T.A., Vogel, C. and Xu, J. 2001. The causes of land-use and land-cover change: moving beyond the myths. Global Environmental Change 11: 261-269.

Lemus, R. and Brown, K. 2008. Feeding small ruminants: developing a grazing system for sheep and goats In: Forage News, July, Cooperative Extension Service, Mississippi State University, USA.

Leng, R.A. 2009. Decline in available world resources - implications for livestock production systems. In: Proc. FAO/IAEA International Symposium on Sustainable Improvement of Animal Production and Health, 8–11 June 2009, Vienna, Austria.

Masters, D.G. 2009. Managing livestock in degrading environments. In: Proc. FAO/IAEA International Symposium on Sustainable Improvement of Animal Production and Health, 8–11 June 2009, Vienna, Austria, pp. 133-134.

McDowell, R.W. (Ed.). 2008. Environmental Impacts of Pasture-based Farming. CAB International, Cambridge, MA, p 283.

Min, B.R., Barry, T.N., Attwood, G.T. and McNabb, W.C. 2003. The effect of condensed tannins on the nutrition and health of ruminants fed fresh temperate forages: a review. Animal Feed Science and Technology 106: 3-19.

Morand-Fehr, P., Fedele, V., Decandia, M. and Le Frileux, Y. 2007. Influence of farming and feeding systems on composition and quality of goat and sheep milk. Small Ruminant Research 68: 20-34.

Nahed, J., Castel, J.M., Mena, Y. and Caravaca, F. 2006. Appraisal of the sustainability of dairy goat systems in Southern Spain according to their degree of intensification. Livestock Production Science 101: 10-23.

NSS, 2005. National Sample Survey Annual Reoprt.

Oba, G., Vetaas, O.R. and Stenseth, N.C. 2001. Relationship between biomass and plant species richness in arid-zone grazing lands. Journal of Applied Ecology 38: 836-845.

Perevolotsky, A. and Seligman, N.G. 1998. Role of grazing Mediterranean rangeland ecosystems - Inversion of a paradigm. Bioscience 48: 1007-1017.

Provenza, F.D., Villalba, J.J., Dziba, L.E., Atwood, S.B. and Banner, R.E. 2003. Linking herbivore experience, varied diets, and plant biochemical diversity. Small Ruminant Research 49: 257-274.

Ramana, D.B.V., Reddy, N.N. and Rao, G.R. 2011. Hortipastoral systems for ram lamb production in rain fed areas. Annals of Biological Research 2: 150-158.

Realini, C.E., Duckett, S.K., Brito, G.W., Dalla Rizza, M. and De Mattos, D. 2004. Effect of pasture vs. concentrate feeding with or without antioxidants on carcass characteristics, fatty acid composition and quality of Uruguayan beef. Meat Science 66: 567-577.

Reinhart, L. 2008. Pasture, rangeland and grazing management. National Center for Appropriate Technology. www.attra.ncat.org/attra-pub/PDF/past_range_graze.pdf (retrieved 11/11/2011).

Ruiz, F.A., Mena, Y., Castel, J.M., Guinamard, C., Bossis, N., Caramelle-Holtz, E., Contu, M., Sitzia, M. and Fois, N. 2009. Dairy goat grazing systems in Mediterranean regions: A comparative analysis in Spain, France and Italy. Small Ruminant Research 85: 42-49.

Sharma, K., Saini, A.L., Singh, N. and Dogra, J.L. 1995. Feed selection and nutrient utilization by Jamunapari and Barbari goats on synthesized silvipasture. Indian Journal of Animal Sciences 65: 213-221.

Sharma, K., Saini, A.L., Singh, N. and Dogra, J.L. 1998. Seasonal variations in grazing behaviour and forage nutrient utilization by goats on a semi-arid reconstituted silvipasture. Small Ruminant Research 27: 47-54.

Tantia, M.S. and Vij, P.K. 2000. Population estimates of sheep and goat breeds of India. Indian Journal of Animal Research 34: 60-63.

Tilman, D., Cassman, K. G., Matson, P.A., Naylor, R. and Polasky, S. 2002. Agricultural sustainability and intensive production practices. Nature 418: 671-677.

Turner, K.E. Cassida, K.A. and Belesky, D.P. 2009. Finishing lambs and goat kids on pasture. In: Improving Small Ruminant Grazing Practices (M.R. Morales, Ed.), Mountain State University, Beckley, West Virginia, pp.3-13.

□□□

Chapter 13

Effect of Probiotics (Direct Fed Microbials) on Small Ruminant Production

D.N. Kamra and Neeta Agarwal
Animal Nutrition Division, Indian Veterinary Research Institute
Izatnagar – 243 122 (UP)

Small ruminant sector contributes significantly in the country's agricultural GDP and also livelihood of poor farmers but is the most neglected sector in animal husbandry. The feeds and fodders available for these animals are inadequate and are of poor quality. Their health management is also not taken care of properly. To make this sector profitable, there is a need to achieve maximum production with the available feed and fodder resources. The microbial eco-system of the gastrointestinal tract dictates the performance of animals and any imbalance will results in poor performance. The use of microbial feed additives (probiotics) is a promising tool to improve the production and health of animals by stabilizing the microbial eco-system. These feed additives have been used for improving the feed utilization, control of microbial infection in the gastro-intestinal tract, improving immunity of the animals, detoxification of anti-nutritional factors, methane inhibition and improving the health of animals.

Eleven per cent of world's livestock population lives in India and the country hold second rank in small ruminant population comprising of 61 million sheep and 121 million goats. Small ruminants contribute 10% of total livestock sector's contribution in agriculture GDP of India. Though the small ruminant sector is contributing a lot of country's GDP but it is not being taken care of properly. The goat and sheep farming is mainly done for meat production as it is the main source of animal protein for human consumption. Small ruminant sector is also a source of livelihood for the poor farmers. The low productivity of these animals due to inadequate feed and water resources and poor health care are the main challenges in small ruminant production. In the present Indian scenario because of large human population it is not possible to spare good quality feed for the livestock, therefore there is a need to extract maximum nutrients from the available feed resources to make this sector more profitable. To combat the challenge of getting maximum production with minimum input, the nutritionists and rumen microbiologists have come up with various feeding strategies. The use of feed additives is one of the emerging areas of research and a lot of efforts have been made to explore effective feed additives for various purposes. Feed additives can be defined as "food ingredients (chemicals or microbes) which are not necessarily nutrients and create desirable response in animals when fed to them". The feed additives belong to various categories like antibiotics, ionophores, plant secondary metabolites, microbial cultures etc. Microbial cultures as feed additive are also termed as probiotics or microbial feed additives or direct fed microbials (DFM). The name DFM coined by the US Food and Drug Administration (FDA) in 1989 is widely used. A probiotic is defines as "a live microbial feed supplement that beneficially affects the host animal by improving the intestinal microbial balance"

The newly born young ones of animals including human beings in the womb of the mother have completely sterile gastrointestinal tract (GIT), but after birth it gets colonized by a variety of microorganisms (Savage, 1987). The gut microbial eco-system comprises of both beneficial and harmful microbes but under healthy and non-stressful conditions, the beneficial microbiota overpowers the harmful microbes thus balancing the gut environment. Beneficial rumen and gut microorganisms supply nutrients to the host, aid in digestion of dietary nutrients, compete with potential pathogens and maintain a proper immune system to keep the animal in healthy and productive state. Probiotic feeding improves the performance of animals by directly or indirectly maintaining the beneficial rumen and gut microbiota. Probiotic is an effective and safe alternate of antibiotic feeding as the later is being discouraged in livestock industry because of its side effects on animals as well as on human beings, the ultimate consumers of animal products.

Direct fed microbials (DFM)

DFM broadly belong to two categories; bacteria and fungi. The commonly used fungal cultures are: *Saccharomyces cerevisiae (yeast), Aspergillus oryzae (AO), Candida pintolopesii* and the bacterial cultures are: *Lactobacillus spp., Bacteroides spp., Bifidobacterium spp., Bacillus spp.* (non-antibiotic producing strains only), *Pediococcus spp., Propionibacterium spp., Streptococcus spp.* etc.

Other than the above cited microbes as DFM, the isolates of bacteria and fungi from the rumen have also been successfully used as DFM to improve productivity of the animals and a large number of microbial cultures have been tested in different species of farm animals. For the selection of a culture to be used as a DFM, there are certain criteria which have to be taken into consideration. An effective microbial culture should have large number of viable and metabolically active cells, should survive and proliferate in the rumen, sustain industrial processing and should have a long shelf life. The source of microbe is also very important to get good response of DFM. The microbes isolated from an animal and used as a probiotic for a similar type of animal, the effect of feeding is the most prominent, because such microbes are familiar with the GIT environment and can proliferate enormously, whereas the microbe from other source is a foreigner and has to fight with the wild microbes in the host GIT for its survival.

Effect on livestock productivity

Improved production by feeding fungal DFM through improving rumen fermentation is well documented. Feeding of *S. cerevisiae* provides a very conducive rumen environment for the growth of cellulolytic bacteria by scavenging oxygen entering the rumen along with feed, providing buffering effect by utilizing lactic acid and excreting micro-nutrients (iso-acids) essentially required by the fibre degrading bacteria and thus enabling the rumen microbes to extract more nutrients from feed and resulting in improved productivity. The fungus *Pyromyces* sp. isolated from nilgai when fed to buffaloes increased viable count of total and cellulolytic bacteria and improved nutrient digestibility (Paul *et al.*, 2004a, b). Administration of the rumen fungi isolated from goat with high fibrolytic activity in the sheep rumen, improved feed intake (Lee *et al.*, 2000). The rate of establishment of cellulolytic bacteria increased in gnotobiotic and conventional lambs fed live *S. cerevisiae* cells daily, and this population was more stable than in non-supplemented lambs (Chaucheyras-Durand and Fonty, 2001). Ciliate protozoa, appeared more rapidly in the rumen of conventional lambs fed on dry live yeast (Chaucheyras-Durand and Fonty, 2002). This supports the hypothesis that live yeast supplementation accelerates maturation of the rumen microbial ecosystem. *S. cerevisiae* I-1077 isolated from ruminants was fed to 1000 goats and sheep resulted in 9% increase in milk yield (ranging from 4 to 15%) in goat and 7 to 11% in sheep without any change in the milk composition (Chevaux and Mazzia-Fabre, 2007).

All the strains of *S. cerevisiae* are not efficient DFM and selection of superior strains can be made by *in vitro* screening of different strains (Agarwal *et al.*, 2000). Mode of feeding also affects biological expression of DFM in the host. Live culture gives better response as compared to lyophilized culture. In the authors' laboratory, a very simple method for production of live DFM has been developed. The feed ingredients like crushed maize or wheat bran (common ingredients of animal feed) is mixed with an equal amount of water and inoculated with 24 hr old active culture of either *L. acidophilus* or *S. cerevisiae* at the rate of 10% of feed. The mixture is incubated for 24 hr at room temperature and next day the fermented feed (live DFM) is ready for feeding to the animals. A small portion of fermented feed can be used as inoculum (10% of fresh feed) to ferment new lot of feed for the next day. This process can be continued for 15 days, thereafter a fresh inoculum should be used. The procedure is simple and can be used at the farmer's door. The fermented feed is highly palatable and gives good results.

Improvement in milk yield, milk fat and protein contents by *Bacillus licheniformis* and *B. subtilis* feeding has been reported in sheep (Kritas *et al.*, 2006). Significant improvement in feed intake, feed conversion efficiency and growth performance by oral administration of lactic acid bacteria has been reported in goat (Chiofalo *et al.*, 2004). The feeding of live culture of *S. cerevisiae* or *L. acidophilus* to crossbred calves resulted in improvement in live weight gain (8% higher than the control) from birth to one year of age (Chaudhary *et al.*, 2007). The results of the experiments conducted so far indicate that feed utilization can be improved if proper DFM is included in the diet of animals and livestock production can be made economic.

Effect on health of animals

The lactic acid bacteria are present in normal gut microbiota of animal and human beings (Schneider *et al.*, 2004). The molecular analysis of the strains of lactic acid bacteria isolated from gut and used as DFM, have been identified as pathogen controllers (Soto *et al.*, 2010) such as *Salmonella* spp. and *Escherichia coli* (Shu and Gill, 2002). The lactic acid bacteria control colonization of pathogens by lowering gut pH, secreting antibiotic like substances and competing for nutrients. These microbes are the main cause of diarrhea in young calves which is responsible for high mortality and morbidity (Timmerman *et al.*, 2005). Lactic acid bacteria counteract the negative effects of pathogenic bacteria through stimulation of immune response against these pathogenic bacteria (Frizzo *et al.*, 2010). Chevaux and Mazzia-Fabre (2007) reported an increased faecal *Lactobacilli* and decreased *E. coli* counts by feeding ruminant specific *S. cerevisiae* I-1077 in goat and sheep. Agarwal *et al.* (2002) also observed reduced incidence of diarrhea in buffalo calves fed *L. acidophilus* NCDC-15. Alexopoulos *et al.* (2004) also demonstrated an improvement in health status and fertility by probiotic feeding. During shifting of animal from low to high concentrate diet, use of lactate utilizers like *Megasphaera elsdenii* and *Propionibacterium* as probiotic can protect the animal from acidosis (Kung and Hession, 1995). *Propionibacterium,* a propionate producer can also be used as probiotic for glucose supply. About 67% glucose comes from propionate in growing ruminants and lactating cows. Efficiency of stabilizing pH in rumen of sheep fed on wheat grain diet supplemented with live yeast was also observed by Brossard *et al.* (2006).

Stress amelioration

Stress on the animal is one of the major factors responsible for low productivity and health of animals. There are many types of stresses like; weaning stress, transport stress, production stress, environmental stress, reproductive stress, managemental stress etc. India exports live sheep and goat which takes long days to reach the destination. Research on young calves being weaned and cattle being transported revealed that in both the conditions the gut microbiota get disturbed. In the former case, the animal has immature digestive tract which is prone to pathogen infection and in the later case animal is subjected to restricted feeding and watering for long time during transportation.

At this juncture, feeding of high doses of DFM can restore the normal gut microbiota and can improve animal health.

Effect on methane emission

Methanogenesis in the rumen is a wasteful but essential metabolic process resulting in a significant loss of dietary energy leading to great economic loss to livestock sector and environmental pollution due to its high global warming potential. The small ruminants contribute about 8-10% of total enteric methane emission by the animals. By feeding DFM this dietary energy can be saved upto some extent. In sheep, 10% reduction in methane production was observed by Mwenya *et al.* (2004), but when calculated in terms of dry matter intake the reduction was only 3%. Various strains of *S. cerevisae* were screened for their efficiency to reduce methane production using rumen simulating technique. Methane reduction ranged from 0 to 58% and this variation in the extent of methane inhibition was attributed to different strains of *S. cerevisiae*. A lactate utilizer *Propionibacterium* produced propionate and therefore has been explored to be used as a DFM to reduce methane emission (Kim *et al.*, 2000).

Nitrate might act as an alternate hydrogen sink in the rumen and has a capacity to compete with carbon dioxide. This might result in a reduction in methane emission by the animals. The nitrate reducing bacteria convert nitrate to nitrite and finally to ammonia which is utilized by the microbes for the synthesis of amino acids in the rumen. But the reduction of nitrate to nitrite is 2-3 times faster than the reduction of nitrite to ammonia and therefore, there is an accumulation of nitrite which is toxic to the animal as it is absorbed through rumen wall and enters the blood stream where it combines with hemoglobin converting it into methemoglobin. This hampers oxygen supply to different organs of the body and is fatal in extreme cases. Therefore the reaction of nitrite reduction has to be speeded up so that there is no accumulation of nitrite in the rumen. To achieve this, the number of nitrite reducing bacteria may be enhanced by using them as a probiotic. The normal inhabitant of the goat rumen, which are capable of reducing nitrate and nitrite in the rumen are *Selenomonas ruminantium*, *Veillonella parvula* and *Wollinella succinogenes*. Among the three *S. ruminantium* was the highest in number as compared to the other two, however their population density depends on the type of diet offered to the animals (Asanuma *et al.*, 2002). The *in vitro* studies revealed that inclusion of nitrate in the incubation medium induced significant reduction (up to 60%) in methane emission but there was an accumulation of nitrite in the medium. But when nitrate was included along with nitrate reducing bacteria (NRBB 57) isolated from buffaloes fed on diet supplemented with nitrate, the methane inhibition increased and there was no accumulation of nitrite in the medium (Sakthivel *et al.,* 2010).

Detoxification of anti-nutritional factors

The agricultural by-products which constitute the major components of ruminant feeds in India usually contain a large quantity of anti-nutritional factors like tannins, saponins, lignins, mimosin etc., making these feeds less acceptable and poorly digestible. Rumen microbes do have a capacity to degrade some of these anti-nutritional factors, therefore if these microbes are used as a probiotic, the population of specific microbe can be increased to detoxify the anti-nutritional factors thus improving the digestibility of these poor quality feeds. *Leucaena leucocephala* is a good source of protein but due to presence of mimosin it is toxic for the animals. A microbe capable of hydrolyzing mimosin was identified as *Synergistes jonesii* (Allison *et al.,* 1992). There is a success story of trans-inoculating *Synergistes jonesii* from Hawaiian goat to the Australian goats enabling them to degrade mimosin present in leucaena leaves.

Tannins are widely distributed in plant kingdom including forage trees, shrubs, legumes, cereals and grains. The bacteria with tannin degrading/ tolerating capacity have been isolated from goat and sheep (Nelson *et al.,* 1998; Tjakradidjaja *et al.,* 1999). In the authors' laboratory, tannin degrading bacteria isolated from rumen of goat fed on pakar leaves were able to degrade tannin and by 16S rRNA analysis were identified as *Streptococcus gallolyticus* (Singh *et al.,* 2011; Chaudhary *et al.,* 2011). Feeding of another tannin degrading bacteria TDGB 406 isolated from goat rumen as DFM to the goats, improved digestibility of tannin rich diet. The isolate having high tannase activity was also identified as *S. gallolyticus* by using two primers sets targeting 16S rRNA and the other primer set targeting *SodA* gene (a gene encoding superoxide dismutase enzyme). Presence of lignin is responsible for poor digestibility of lignocellulosic agricultural crop residues because it shields cellulose and hemicellulose from microbial attack. Enzymes like p-coumaryl esterase, feruloyl esterase are the enzymes which break the ester bonds between lignin and cellulose and rumen fungi are the good source of these enzymes (Borneman *et al.,* 1990; Cao and Yang, 2011), hence feeding of fungal isolates as feed additive improves fibre digestibility in buffaloes.

Future research needs

The research conducted so far indicates that there do exist microbial cultures which can be safely used as probiotic and might economize small ruminant production by improving health and production of the animals. Even a slight improvement in feed conversion efficiency will be beneficial for the farmers. Though a lot of successful efforts have been made but still there is a need to develop well defined probiotics for various breeds of animals and production purposes.

References

Agarwal, N., Kamra, D.N., Chaudhary, L.C., Sahoo, A. and Pathak, N.N. 2000. Selection of *Saccharomyces cerevisiae* strains for use as microbial feed additives. Letters Applied Microbiology 31: 270-273.

Agarwal, N., Kamra, D.N., Chaudhary, L.C. Agarwal, I., Sahoo A. and Pathak, N.N. 2002 Microbial status and enzyme profile of crossbred calves fed on different microbial feed additives. Letters Applied Microbiology 34 : 329-336.

Alexopoulos, C., Georgoulakis, I.E., Tzivara, A., Kritas, S.K., Siochu, A. and S.C. Kyriakis, 2004. Field evaluation of the efficacy of a probiotic containing *Bacillus licheniformis* and *Bacillus subtilis* spores, on the health status and performance of sows and their litters. Journal of Animal Physiology and Animal Nutrition 88: 381-392.

Allison, M.J., Maybery. W.R., McSweeney. C.S. and Stahl, D.A. 1992. *Synergistesa Jonesii* Gen. Nov. Sp. Nov. A rumen bacterium that degrades toxic pyridinediols. Syst. Apkll. Microbiol 15: 522-529.

Asanuma, N., Miwa Iwamoto, M., Kawato, M. and Hino T. 2002. Numbers of nitrate-reducing bacteria in the rumen as estimated by competitive polymerase chain reaction. Animal Science Journal 73: 199-205.

Borneman, W.S., Hartley, R.D., Morrison, W. H., Akin, D.E. and Ljungdahl, L.G. 1990 Feruloyl and p-coumaroyl esterase from anaerobic fungi in relation to plant cell wall degradation. Applied Microbiology and Biotechnology 33: 345-351.

Brossard, L., Chaucheyras-Durand, F., Michalet-Doreau, B. and Martin, C. 2006. Dose effect of live yeasts on rumen microbial communities and fermentations during butyric latent acidosis in sheep: new type of interaction. Animal Science 82: 1-8.

Cao, Y.C. and Yang, H.J. 2011. Effect of roughage fibre content on fibrolytic activities and volatile fatty acid profiles of *Neocallimastix* sp. YAK11 isolated from rumen fluids of yak (*Bos grunniens*). Animal Feed Science Technology : www.elsevier.com/locate/anifeedsci.

Chaucheyras-Durand, F. and Fonty, G. 2001. Establishment of cellulolytic bacteria and development of fermentative activities in the rumen of gnotobiotically-reared lambs receiving the microbial additive *Saccharomyces cerevisiae* CNCM I-1077. Reproduction and Nutrition Development 41: 57-68.

Chaucheyras-Durand, F. and Fonty, G. 2002. Influence of a probiotic yeast (*Saccharomyces cerevisiae* CNCMI-1077) on microbial colonization and fermentation in the rumen of newborn lambs. Microbiology and Ecollogy of Health and Diseases. 14: 30-36.

Chaudhary, L.C., Agarwal, N., Sahoo, A., Kamra, D.N. and Pathak, N.N. 2007. Effect of microbial feed additives and replacement of cereal grain with wheat bran on the performance of male crossbred calves. Indian Journal of Animal Sciences 77: 1338-1340.

Chaudhary, L.C., Agarwal, N., Verma, V. and Kamra, D.N. 2011. Effect of feeding superior strain of tannin degrading bacteria (Isolate-6) on growth performance, nutrient utilization and rumen fermentation in goats fed on *Ficus infectoria* leaves. Small Ruminants Research doi:10.1016/j.smallrumres.

Chevaux, Eric and Mazzia-Fabre, M. 2007. Probiotic yeast in small ruminants. Feed Mix 17.

Chiofalo, V., Liotta, L. and Chiofalo, B. 2004. Effects of the administration of *Lactobacilli* on body growth and on the metabolic profile in growing Maltese goat kids. Reproduction and Nutrition Development 44: 449-457.

Frizzo, L.S., Soto, L.P., Zbrun, M.V., Bertozzi, E., Sequeira, G., Rodríguez Armesto R. and Rosmini, M.R. 2010. Lactic acid bacteria to improve growth performance in young calves fed milk replacer and spray-dried whey powder. Animal Feed Science and Technology 157: 159-167.

Kim, S.W., Standorf, D.G., Roman-Rosario, H. Yokoyama, M.T. and Rust, S.R. 2000. Potential use of *Propionibacterium acidipropionici*, strain DH42, as a direct-fed microbial for cattle. Journal of Animal Sciences 78(Suppl. 1): 292.

Kritas, S.K., Govaris, A., Christodoulopouls G. and Burriel, A.R. 2006 Effect of *Bacillus licheniformis* and *Bacillus subtilis* supplementation of ewe's feed on sheep milk production and young lamb mortality. Journal of Veterinary and Medical Ser. 53: 170-173.

Kung, Jr. L. and Hession, A.O. 1995. Preventing *in vitro* lactate accumulation in ruminal fermentation by inoculation with *Megasphaera elsdenii*. Journal of Animal Sciences 73: 250-256.

Lee, S.S., Ha, J.K. and Cheng, K.J. 2000. Influence of an anaerobic fungal culture administration on *in vivo* ruminal fermentation and nutrient digestion. Animal Feed Science Technology 88: 201-217.

Mwenya, B, Santosa, S.C., Gamo, Y., Kobayashi, T. and Takahashi, J. 2004. Effects of including beta 1-4 galacto-oligosaccharides, lactic acid bacteria or yeast culture on methanogenesis as well as energy and nitrogen metabolism in sheep. Animal Feed Science Technology 115: 313-326.

Nelson, K.E., Thonney, M.L., Woolston, T.K., Zinder, S.H. and Pell, A.N. 1998. Phenotypic and phylogenetic characterization of ruminal tannin-tolerant bacteria. Applied Environmental Microbiology 64: 3824-3830.

Paul, S.S., Kamra, D.N., Sastry, V.R.B., Sahu, N.P. and Agarwal, N. 2004a. Effect of administration of an anaerobic gut fungus isolated from wild blue bull (*Boselaphus tragocamelus*) to buffaloes (*Bubalus bubalis*) on *in vivo* ruminal fermentation and digestion of nutrients. Animal Feed Science Technology 115: 143-157.

Paul, S.S., Kamra, D.N., Sastry, V.R.B., Sahu, N.P. and Agarwal, N. 2004b. Effect of anaerobic fungal isolates from wild and domestic ruminants on *in vitro* digestibility, fermentation characteristics and fibrolytic enzyme production on lignocellulosic feed by mixed rumen microflora of buffalo. Nutrition and Reproduction Development 44: 313-319

Sakthivel, P.C., Kamra, D.N., Agarwal N. and Chaudhary, L.C. 2010. Effect of sodium nitrate and nitrate reducing bacteria on *in vitro* methane production and feed fermentation with buffalo rumen liquor. In: Proc. Greenhouse Gases and Animal Agriculture Conference, Banff, Canada, p 178.

Savage, D.C. 1987. Microorganisms associated with epithelial surfaces and the stability of the indigenous gastrointestinal microflora. Die Nahrung 5-6: 383.

Schneider, R., Rosmini, M.R., Ehrmann, M. and Vogel, R. 2004. Identification of lactic acid bacteria form the typical microbiota found in artificial reared calves. FAVE - Ciencias Veterinarias 3: 7-15.

Shu, Q. and Gill, H.S. 2002. Immune protection mediated by the probiotic *Lactobacillus rhamnosus* HN001 (DR20™) against *Escherichia coli* O157:H7 infection in mice. FEMS Immun. Med. Microbiol., 34: 59-64.

Singh, B., Chaudhary, L.C., Agarwal N. and Kamra, D.N. 2011. Isolation and characterization of tannin degrading/ tolerating bacteria from the rumen of goats fed on pakar (*Ficus infectoria*) leaves. Journal of Applied Animal Research 39: 120-124.

Soto, L.P., Frizzo, L.S., Bertozzi, E., Avataneo, E., Sequeira, G. and Rosmini, M. 2010. Molecular microbial analysis of *Lactobacillus* strains isolated from the gut of calves for potential probiotic use. Veterinary Medicine International Article ID 274987, 7.

Timmerman, H.M., Mulder, L., Everts, H., van Espen, D.C., van der Wal, E., Klaassen, G., Rouwers, S.M.G., Hartemink, R., Rombouts, F.M. and Beynen, A.C. 2005. Health and growth of veal calves fed milk replacers with or without probiotics. Journal of Dairy Science, 88: 2154-2165.

Tjakradidjaja, A.S., Brooker, J.D. and Bottema, C.D.K. 1999. Characterization of tannin-resistant bacteria from the rumen fluid of feral goats and camels with restriction analysis of amplified 16S rDNA. In: Tannins in Livestock and Human Nutrition. Proc. International Workshop, Adelaide, Australia, 31 May - 2 June, 151-155.

□□□

Chapter 14

Expanding Feed Resource Base for Nutritional Security of Ruminants

Ramesh C. Jakhmola
Arid Region Campus, Central Sheep and Wool Research Institute
Bikaner, Rajasthan - 334006

Introduction

Agriculture plays a key role in the overall economic and social well being of India. The gross domestic product (GDP) from agriculture and allied sector was Rs. 446,515 crores during 1999-2000 and with a 1.75 fold increase it reached to Rs. 861,753 crores during 2008-09, (GOI, 2009). The share of agriculture, including the allied sectors, in GDP declined from 39 percent in 1983 to 25 percent in 1999-2000 and it further declined to 17.8 percent in 2008-09. However, it was major source of employment in the country. Although its share in total employment declined from 63 percent in 1983 to 57 percent in 1999-2000 indicating that over the period, the share of agriculture in employment has not been reduced. So, the agriculture will continue to support larger population in the years to come and our policies towards this sector need more attention.

Livestock keeping is an integral part of the Indian farming systems since times immemorial. This sector acts as an alternate employment and income opportunity, source of nutritional security, storage of wealth, means of sustaining the soil fertility and source of draught power for agriculture. In order to keep the goal of 4% agricultural growth as laid down in the National Agricultural Policy (2000); the livestock sector is recognized as an important source. Livestock also remain the major source of household income when the crops fail due to natural vagaries. Livestock sector including fisheries contributed nearly 25% to the agricultural sector output, up from 16 % in 1970-71. In absolute terms the contribution of livestock sector including fisheries increased from Rs. 256 billion in 1970-71 to Rs 934 billion in 2002-03 (at 1993-94 prices) at an annual growth rate of 4.3% (Birthal and Taneja, 2006). The globalization of agriculture opens great opportunities for export of processed animal food products. With growing domestic demand for animal based food products and export needs under changing climatic conditions, there is a need to make adjustments in the livestock rearing systems and the production efficiency. A knowledge based, eco-friendly, market oriented, credit supported intensive livestock farming system is needed which is economically rewarding and more resistant to climatic vagaries. This will not only help to attract and retain educated youth in farming, but also achieve productivity improvement that is required to meet the challenges arising from trade liberalisation and globalisation of economies. Among others feed is single factor, that contributes nearly 70% of total recurring cost and in event of deficiency the affect on production, reproduction and health of animals is immense. Thus broadening the feed resource base for ruminant livestock is need of hour. The paper included some of the strategies on this subject.

The Livestock Population Dynamics

India had 185 million cattle, 98 million buffaloes, 124 million goats, 61 million sheep and 14 million pigs and 489 million poultry birds as per 2003 livestock census. The trends of change in population of major livestock species - cattle, buffaloes, sheep and goats indicated that accept of cattle where trend was polynomial and there is a likelihood of reduction of cattle population in the country, other species will show an linear increasing trend. The annual rate of gain (million ACU) in other major ruminants - buffaloes, goats and sheep was 1.590, 0.268 and 0.068 respectively. The rate of gain in total population of livestock in the country was 2.7636 million each year and estimated population in the country that was 392.64 million ACU during year 2009 will however decline to 348.64 million ACU by 2017 (the end of XII plan).

This probably, be due to likely decline in the native cattle population. Therefore, the structure of livestock population seems changing with an increasing trend towards the buffaloes and crossbred cattle as a milch animal, compared to native cattle. With the mechanisation of major agricultural operations and transportation, the importance of cattle as a source of draught power is gradually declining. The high yield of milk and fat content of the milk is giving buffalo an edge over the local cattle as a source of milk production. The buffalo intensification is taking place in the irrigated and well-endowed areas. In the humid regions, the crossbred cattle are also gaining importance. In case of small ruminants, the goat population increased from 68 million in 1972 to 124 million in 2003. However, the increase in sheep population was comparatively low. The decline in the availability of the common grazing land is affecting the production of the small ruminant in India, even though they enjoy high domestic and international demand. The grazing based small ruminant production system is unlikely to sustain for long, unless supplemented by stall-feeding (Birthal and Taneja, 2005). However, native cattle have importance in view of their contribution to nutritional security of millions of families living in difficult terrains where organised milk marketing system not yet reached. Thus, in the ruminant livestock policy there is a need to ensure that the native cattle are not side lined, because they will continue to be of important for rural population as a source of milk and draught.

Feed Requirements

It is tedious to calculate estimated feed requirements of livestock in the country like India, where recording of animals and their productivity is done during periodical census. However, at macro level the requirements calculated on the basis of ACU seems reasonable. The estimated nutrient requirements for ruminant livestock in the country are given in Table 1. These requirements are comparatively lower to the estimates given by Ranjhan (2003).

Ruminant livestock like any other living being need nutrients for their maintenance, production and reproduction. With the strengthening of poultry/ pigs/ captive fisheries enterprises, a competition for concentrate between these enterprises with ruminants is inevitable, wherein ruminants are expected at loss. Thus the ruminant production in India needs to be developed on roughage based. Grazing on pastures is the dominant form of production system adopted traditionally for cattle, camel and goat and sheep production.

Being dependent on rain, large part of the country often encounter drought during which there is severe loss of crop and livestock. During 2002, in Rajasthan only, approximately 40 million people, 50 million livestock were affected from drought and small ruminants were either gone to migration or sold. Due to the non-availability of water and fodder, people had started abandoning their unproductive cattle. There were reports of animals dying of hunger and thirst. Animal carcasses could be seen in the countryside. Many people have started migrating to other states with their animals. There was immense loss to livestock in the region. Such situation leads to leaving the livestock rearing occupation for want of alternate jobs in town/ cities leading to migration. Thus for nutritional security of ruminants there is a need develop plans so that the ruminant production can be continued as sustainable and economically profitable enterprise.

Table 1: Estimated livestock population (ACU) in the country and the nutrient requirements for harvesting optimum production with their welfare.

	Year		
	2003	2009	2017
ACU (Million)	362.62	392.64	348.64
Requirements			
DM (MT)	794.13	859.88	763.52
DCP (MT)	35.36	38.28	33.99
ME (10^9 MJ)	6240.63	6757.31	6000.08
TDN (MT)	410.03	443.98	394.22

MT = Million (10^6) Tonnes

Major Feed and Fodder Resources

Common Property Resources

Community grasslands / pastures are still playing important role in providing nutrients to grazing ruminants are important segment of common property resources (CPRs). CPRs are resources accessible to and collectively owned\ held\ managed by an identifiable community and on which no individual has exclusive property rights. The estimates of per household availability of CPR, given in Table 2, indicated that the CPR land ranged from 1-8% of the geographical area in Gangatic plains, to 38% in western arid areas of the country (GOI, 2009). The common pasture and grazing land is an important constituent of the

CPR land in arid and semi-arid regions. The highest share of the category "common pastures and grazing land" in CPR land was, however, reported in the mountainous western Himalaya. It was relatively high also in the West Coast Plains & Hills, containing the high rainfall regions of Western Ghats and coastal areas. The estimates indicate Fodder accounts for 25% from CPRs. In the agriculturally developed zones (Gangetic plains), the shares of fodder were more than 50%. The estimates also indicated that rural India depends significantly for livestock rearing on CPRs viz., village forests, common grazing land, barren or waste land etc. At the all-India level, while 56% of rural households reported possession of livestock, 20% of the households depended on CPR land for grazing of livestock, 13% of the households collected fodder from CPRs and only a small percentage (2%) of households reported cultivation of fodder on CPR land. States are highly dependent on CPRs for rearing of livestock, in terms of collection of fodder and grazing of livestock on CPR land. States like Rajasthan (84%), Himachal Pradesh (81%), Uttar Pradesh (72%), Madhya Pradesh (68%) and Orissa (58%) reported relatively high percentages (all above the national average of 56%) of possession of livestock. High percentages of households of these States reported use of CPR land for grazing of livestock (34%, 43%, 30%, 62%, 60%). Besides, reported percentages of households possessing livestock in Haryana, Himachal Pradesh, Sikkim and Uttar Pradesh are quite high and relatively high percentages of households (26%, 36%, 33%, 23% respectively) reported collection of fodder from CPR land. Average quantity of fodder collection is also very high in these States. Haryana and Sikkim reported yearly collection of 1743 kg, 1401 kg of fodder respectively indicating dependence on CPR for rearing of livestock. Interestingly, in Punjab, though collection of fodder from CPR is quite high (1095 kg), grazing on CPR land is lowest; only 1% households reported grazing of livestock on CPR land and 18% households reported collection of fodder from CPR land. On the other hand, in States of the north-eastern region, viz., Meghalaya, Mizoram, Nagaland and Tripura, a majority of households (92%,100%, 65% and 69%, respectively) have access to CPR land under forest but are not greatly dependent on CPRs for grazing of livestock or for collection of fodder. Moreover, except for Nagaland where 86% of households reported possession of livestock, percentages of livestock-possessing households in these States are low.

Accessibility to CPR land thus does not imply a high degree of dependence on CPRs for rearing of livestock. In case of Arunachal Pradesh and Orissa, in spite of high accessibility to forest area, collection of fodder reported is unexpectedly low in terms of quantity collected and number of households collecting fodder. In Haryana and Punjab accessibility to forest and non-forest area is not significant, only 35% and 10% of households reported accessibility to CPRs but both the States reported high value in terms of average quantity of fodder collected. Percentages of households possessing livestock and reporting collection of fodder, and average quantity of fodder collected for each category of households. The table reveals that the households possessing less than 0.20 ha land are the lowest placed in terms of possession of livestock (25%), collection of fodder (8%), and average quantity of fodder collected per household (200 kg) from CPRs For all other categories of households, percentage of households reporting possession of livestock increases steadily with the increase in possession of land and the same kind of relation is found in case of percentage of households reporting collection of fodder from CPRs and average quantity of fodder collected from CPRs. But the fifth category of households (possessing 1.00 ha or more land) is an exception, where both the percentage of households (66%) and average quantity of fodder collected from CPRs is relatively low (251 kg). This indicates that large land owning households do not greatly depend on CPR for rearing of livestock. But in general possession of livestock is positively associated with possession of land.

It is observed that rural poor depends to a large extent on the materials available from CPRs for their subsistence. There is a need to involve National Sample Survey organisation for collection of data on regular basis on CPR dependent livestock production systems and its economics.

Green Fodder Production

The area under the fodder crops remained static over last many years. It is reported that out of 55 regions considered for the demand supply scenario of feeds, only 12 showed net surplus (Singh and Majumdar, 1992). However, the condition of green fodder shows a dismal picture as it could increase from 110.43 million tones in 1965-66 to 125.60 million tones in 1996-97 only indicating a meagre growth rate of 0.47 m tonnes (Singh and Ramachandra, 2004). There is possibility to increase legume fodder production through planting leguminous shrubs on the bunds of the cultivated area or cultivation of short duration leguminous fodders in between rationed sugarcane fields. The organised experiments need to be under taken in this area. The preservation technology – silage making, haymaking and briquette making can be applied. At the same time multi-cut grain varieties can be developed. This however, will need a interwoven system where plant breeders and nutritionists work for providing nutritional security to ruminants.

Table 2 : Percentage of CPR land to geographical area and availability of CPR land per household and per capita

Agro-climatic zone	Percentage of CPR land to geo. area	CPR land per house hold (ha)	average household size	CPR land per capita (ha)
Lower Gangetic Plains	1	0.02	5.02	0.00
Upper Gangetic Plains	2	0.03	5.38	0.01
Middle Gangetic Plains	8	0.07	5.69	0.01
Trans-Gangetic Plains	5	0.07	5.61	0.01
all Islands	9	0.12	4.41	0.03
East Coast Plains & Hills	12	0.15	4.28	0.04
Western Coast Plains & Hills	10	0.16	4.57	0.04
Eastern Himalayas & Bramhaputra Valley	5	0.18	5.08	0.04
Southern Plateau & Hills	9	0.18	4.36	0.04
Western Plateau & Hills	10	0.29	5.10	0.06
Eastern Plateau & Hills	19	0.44	4.78	0.09
Western Himalayan	33	0.49	5.00	0.10
Central Plateau & Hills	20	0.65	5.23	0.12
Gujarat Coast Plains & Hills	27	0.71	4.95	0.14
Western Dry Region	38	4.77	5.75	0.83
India	**15**	**0.31**	**5.04**	**0.06**

Crop Residues

Crop residues are important feed resource for ruminants. Owing to the adaptability the Indian livestock – cattle and buffaloes are good converter of the nutrients present in straw into animal products. Table 3 indicates that between year 1997-98 and year 2008-09 there have been sizable increase in production of crop residues and it ranged from 22.5 percent in wheat straw to 89.76 percent in crop residues of oil seeds crops. Sugarcane top is a green by-product available after sugarcane harvesting. At harvesting stage top contain approximately

24 % DM, 3.9 % CP, 46.7% ADF and 6.61 % ash. If the top ensiled with 2 % urea for a month in a silo pit can be fed as sole source of roughage to growing cattle. Ensiling with 10-15 % molasses sizably improve nutrient utilisation and availability. The top if ensiled with urea could have DM 24%, CP 5.14 % and ash 6% and can serve sole roughage source. Feeding of ensiled top can support a growth up to 300g per day in growing bull calves. Other resources like vegetable crop residues also contribute sizeable quantity of feed resource for ruminants. However, there is dire need to conserve, treat and transport these roughages from surplus area to deficit area.

In a few states of the country like UP, Uttarakhand, Haryana, Punjab etc valuable feed resources (Rice and paddy straw, mustard straw, sugarcane leaves, tops and bagasse) are burnt adding environmental pollutions, and on other hand animals die due to hunger in neighbouring states like Rajasthan and Gujrat. Under prevailing circumstances, complete feed block technology seems promising as it provide ease in transportation, storage, feeding and supply of nutrient to animals in a proportionate manner, indeed this technology have future for revolutionary change in our animals production system (Jakhmola, 2003[a]; IFRC, 2004). With the help of a suitable strategy the through development of Feed Banks utilising crop residues livestock productivity in the nation can be enhances by 20-30% from our indigenous cattle/ buffaloes.

Table 3 : Availability (Million Tonnes) of crop residues and other by products for animal feeding.

	1997-98	2008-09	Percent Gain
Crop residues			
Rice	93.366	128.895	38.05
Wheat	65.78	80.58	22.50
Coarse cereals	104.28	157.92	51.44
pulses	44.52	58.64	31.72
Oil seeds	44.52	84.48	89.76
Milling By-products			
Rice bran	5.75	7.93	38.05
Wheat bran	5.26	6.45	22.50
Chunies	0.33	0.44	31.72
Oil cakes/meals	10.39	19.71	89.78

Milling By-Products

There has been tremendous increase in milling by-products production in the country (Table 3). Majority of these by-products are although goes for poultry production. Now a days pig and captive fish production is also becoming major user of these milling by-products especially groundnut cake and soybean meal. The rice bran and chunies, guar korma are major feedstuffs along with mustard cake that are available for ruminant feeding. After preparing a blend of these by-products with leguminous leaf meals and processed in the form of briquette, pallets can increase the nutrient supplies for producing ruminants.

Unconventional Feeds

There are several under utilised feed resources that can be used in ruminant feed. These include Prickly pear (*Opuntia ficus* spp.) cactus, Banana (*Musa paradiosiaca*) leaves and trunks, Amaranthus (*Amaranthus cruentus*) foliage, sugarcane pith and Coir waste (Coconut pith). After suitable processing and enrichment with deficit nutrients these can broaden the feed resource availability to low producing cattle, sheep and goats. Some other explored feed resources are Rubber (*Hevea brasiliensis*) seed cake, Spent Anatto seeds (*Bixa orellana*), Ambadi cake (*Hibiscus cannabinus*), Kokam cake (*Garcinia indica*), Kosum-cake (*Schleichera oleosa*), Cocoa (*Theobroma cacao*) pods, Panewar (*Cassia tora*) seed, etc.

Top Feeds

Leaves and pods are important feed resources that are under utilized. *Prosopis juliflora* (Mesquite) pods, Subabul pod, Rain (*Samanea saman*) tree pods, *Albizia lebback* pods, Babul (Acacia arabica) pods are important from nutrition point of view. In India, 107.57 million ha (19.03 million ha of barren and uncultivated land, 10.91 million ha of permanent pastures and other grazing lands, 3.57 million ha of miscellaneous tree crops and groves, 13.88 million ha of culturable wasteland and 24.12 million ha of total fallow land and 50% of 68.86 million ha of forest land) is available for grazing (Pathak and Gupta, 2003). Thus, rearing livestock with multi purpose tree plantation on grazing lands has scope as well as may gain popularity with increasing general awareness in the masses about climate change. It is in this context of changing life style of the population, the concept of social forestry need to have relevance and the attention of the both planners and animal farmers.

Several of tree leaves have chemicals (plant secondary metabolites, PSM) that appear to be produced for the purpose of deterring invasion or consumption of their leaves by microbes, insects and herbivorous animals. Fodder from trees and shrubs (top feed), in some cases, has poor crude protein digestibility or in other cases death of livestock have been associated with high tannin content of some foliages. While tannins are the best known, there are other secondary plant compounds – saponins, mimosine, cyanogenic glycosides, cyanide, nitrate, fluoroacetate, oxalates, and various sterols are but a few. Alkaloids are generally absent from petioles, ripe fruit and mature seeds. Saponins were found in all types of plant parts. Condensed tannins occurred in almost all plant parts examined (93.6%), while hydrolysable tannins were less ubiquitous (gallotannins in 31.2% of samples, and ellagitannins in 18.9%). These compounds may or may not be modified in the rumen by microbial action or at times the primary compound or its breakdown products in the rumen may be toxic or of no nutritional importance. Some secondary plant compounds are actively detoxified in the liver. For efficient use of top feed they should be included in small proportion depending on the presence of plant secondary metabolites.

Processing and Conservation

Using complete feed block technology several unconventional feed can be used in animal feeding during scarcity or to maintain adult stock even without any treatment. Rumen fermentation of poor quality roughages could be improved by their incorporation in complete diets, this improves nutrient availability to animals when fibrous crop residues fed to ruminants in the form of complete feed block (Jakhmola, 2003[b]). Groundnut straw and mesquite straw 20 and 30 parts can effectively we used in 70 % roughage based feeding in sheep if fed in block form. Sheep had good health and high nitrogen balance on the block feeding which contained groundnut straw 20, mesquite straw 30, de oiled rice bran 20 and groundnut cake 13 parts with mineral and salt supplementation. A restricted quantity of unconventional and unpalatable feeds can be used in animal feeding using feed block technology. The animal responses on block feeding were variable with animal species but favorable, demonstrating the feasibility of the technology. Farmer's perception was favorable and quite interesting for feed block feeding in Nigeria and in India. In block feeding improve milk production as a result of improved intake, dry matter digestion and rumen ecosystem.

Feeding of complete fed block did not reduce forage dry matter intake but an increase organic matter and crude protein digestibility of feed block containing diets has been reported (Raghuvansi, 2004) and the improvement of microbial protein synthesis was also reported. Higher concentration of rumen anaerobic fungi was noticed in goat kids fed complete feed block over mash diet. Therefore, block feeding promotes rumen microbial growth and activity thereby increase in digestion of poor quality roughage. Block feeding synchronizes the supply of nutrients to rumen microorganism, which enhance rumen fermentation. Consumption of hard feed block over the day ensures a synergy between nutrient demand of rumen microorganism to degrade low quality feedstuffs and the provision of adequate level of these nutrient without exceeding the transformation capacity of microbial population. When mash diets are fed concentrate portion of the diet is generally rapidly consumed by animals and degrades early in the rumen, therefore nutrient flux in the rumen peaks in the first few hours of post feeding, great part of which is lost in urine and feces. Consequently, availability of nutrients for rumen microorganism over the rest of the day will be limited and degrading capacity of fibrous feeds will be compromised. Improved intake, nutrient utilization, nitrogen retention and better animal performance are the bright features of block feeding.

Conclusion

The feed resources base is increasing in the country with increasing crop production. There is a need to adapt suitable process technologies for long preservation of feed resources in balanced form and transportation to deficit areas. Author recommend development of feed banks for sustainable livestock production in the country.

References

Birthal, P.S. and Taneja, V. K. 2006. Livestock sector in India: opportunities and challenges for small holders: Workshop on Small holder livestock production in India: Opportunities and challenges 31 Jan – 1 Feb 2006. Delhi.

GOI, 2009. http://india.gov.in/govt/publications/jan09/index.php?id=8

IFRC (International Federation of Red Cross), 2004. Food Security to small holders through live-stock feed banks. Annual Report Senegal, Appeal no. 01.38/ 2004, p 5.

Jakhmola, R.C. 2003a. Forage Conservation. In *Sustainable Livestock Production* (eds. R.C.Jakhmola and R.K.Jain.). Pointer Publishers, Jaipur

Jakhmola, R. C. 2003b. Principle and preparation of complete feed block. Short course on recent advances in Animal Nutrition Research., March 5-25, CAS, IVRI, Izatnagar. Pp139-143.

Pathak P.S. and Gupta J.N. 2003. In *Sustainable Animal Production* (eds. R.C.Jakhmola and R.K.Jain). Pointer Publishers, Jaipur. pp. 25-53.

Raghuvansi, SKS. 2004. Preparation and testing of high roughage based complete feed block in sheep feeding. Ph.D. Thesis, Udai Pratap Autonomus College, Varanasi, UP, India.pp 115.

Ranjhan, S.K. 2003. Livestock and feed situation in India. In *Sustainable Animal Production* (eds. R.C.Jakhmola and R.K.Jain). Pointer Publishers, Jaipur. 1-24.

Singh, K. and Ramachandra, K.S. 2004. Feed and Fodder availability, requirement and strategy fir meeting the shortage in different regions for small ruminants, , National seminar on opportunities and challenges in nutrition and feeding management of sheep, goat and rabbit for sustainable production, February 10-12, CSWRI, Avikanagar

Singh, P. and .Majumdar, A.B. 1992. Current status of feed and forage management of livestock in India, *Agricultural Situation in India*: August: 375-382.

□□□

Chapter 15

Nutritional Augmentation of Consumer Preferred Trait-Specific Quality Enhancement in Meat, Wool and Milk Production

A. Sahoo and R.S. Bhatt
Division of Animal Nutrition, Central Sheep and Wool Research Institute
Avikanagar-304 501 (Rajasthan)

Nutrition of lambs during pre-weaning phase of growth has significant effect on post weaning performance and finishing weight. Higher finishing weights at an early age produce good quantity and quality of carcass. Ewes' nutrition during late pregnancy is critical to meet nutrient requirement of growing foetus, its development, weight at birth and colostrums production, which indeed influence pre-weaning performance of lamb. It also has influence on wool yield and quality form the offspring. Nutritional and genetic manipulation for compositional changes in meat and milk bearing consumer preferred traits has got extra-economic value. In this line, nutrition for designer/ dietetic livestock products (meet, milk and their products) for better health, nutritional intervention to lower saturated fatty acids (SFAs) and raise monounsaturated fatty acids (MUFAs) and poly-unsaturated fatty acids (PUFAs) in meat, milk and their products and use of high forage based diets or oil/oil seed supplements to enhance ù-3 PUFA to support human health and reduce risk of diseases has got immeasurable significance. The aim is to have balanced, varied diets containing even safer and even healthier foods still with a pleasant feel. Meat and its derivatives may be considered functional foods to the extent that they contain numerous compounds thought to be functional. The idea of using food for health purposes rather than for nutrition opens up a whole new field for the meat industry.

Recent evidences of epidemiological linkages between diet and chronic diseases have prompted the search for new clinical insights into the relationship between food and the onset (or prevention) of disease. In this context, the extra-nutritional therapeutic attributes of meat, milk and their products are no longer debated. It is now firmly established that a new generation of value-added products can be harvested from meat, milk and their products. Similarly, augmenting quality wool production from sheep, fiber-bearing goats and rabbits still remains a challenge for the breeder and nutritionist due to less and/or negative economic gain in terms of nutritional input: output ratio while evaluating wool production as the single productive trait. While until recently, emphasis has been on breeding animals to produce more meat, milk, and wool or dual type, the attention is also tuned to adding more value to these attributes and studying its health and user implications. Healthier livestock products or derived functional foods must possess one of the following characteristics: modified composition and/or processing conditions to prevent or limit the presence of certain potentially harmful compounds, and/or the possibility of including certain desirable substances, either naturally or by addition, with the subsequent added benefits to health. The relationship between diet and health, the growing life-expectancy of the population (consumers have a high purchasing power and greater health problems and they are very eager to take part in any initiative to keep healthy), more concern with disease prevention, etc.

Meat as animal protein

The increase in per capita income and urbanization are fuelling the demand for meat and meat products. While the population is expected to double in Asia and Africa by the year 2020, the demand for meat and meat products is expected to triple. Per capita meat consumption in India is relatively low at less than 5 kg/ year as compared to other developing countries such as Pakistan (13.7 kg), China (38.6 kg) and Brazil (58.6 kg). Based on the minimum requirement of 20 g animal protein per capita per day sourced from milk (10 g), meat (4 g), fish (4 g), and eggs (2 g), the estimated demand for meat is 7.7 million metric tonnes as against the present production of 4.6 million metric tonnes. About 1.7% of total meat is processed into meat products and sold through retail network comprising company outlets, supermarkets and high-end grocery shops located in big cities and metropolis.

Meat production systems in the country are very primitive and therefore, the cost of meat production is also comparatively cheaper (basically low/zero input with sustainable output) than the developed countries. To bridge the gap in demand and supply, there is need for augmenting the quantity and quality of meat production through scientific methods of organized livestock production by utilizing various locally available feed resources and by improving meat animal germplasm. Therefore, major goals for the meat industry to grow in India at par with many developed countries would be

- Augmenting the country's meat production
- Harnessing quality and consumer trait-specific meat and value addition with technological manipulation for manufacturing ready-to-eat meat products
- Improving the current status of meat production, handling and marketing
- Developing technologies for value addition to meat by processing into meat products
- Providing research and development and marketing support to the export meat trade
- Launching human resource development programs in teaching, research, training and extension activities of meat science and technology.

Quality enhancement in meat

The term quality means 'achieving sustained customer satisfaction through meeting customer needs and expectations within an organizational environment committed to continued improvement of efficiency and effectiveness'. Research shows that tenderness and flavor are rated as the most important elements of eating quality, while color/ freshness is the most important attributes at point of purchase. Related to the sensory aspects, pH and water holding capacity are important technological factors. All of the sensory traits except colour, are contributing factors to the palatability of meat and meat products.

Quality characteristics of meat are influenced by various intrinsic and extrinsic factors such as muscle structure and its chemical composition, ante-mortem stress as well as postmortem handling and storage conditions.

It is evident from a large body of literature in human as well as in animal models that, w-3 polyunsaturated fatty acids play important role in the development and maintenance of different organs, primarily the brain, and could be useful in the prevention of different pathologies, mainly the cardiovascular diseases, and, as proposed recently, some psychiatric, dermatological or rheumatological disorders. The actual goal is first to identify which foods are naturally rich in w-3 fatty acids, and, second, to determine the true impact of the formulations (enriched in w-3 fatty acids) in the ration of small ruminants and rabbits on the nutritional value of the products and thus their effect on the health of consumers. The nature of fatty acids of reserve triglycerides (found in more or less large amounts depending on the anatomical localisation, that is to say the butcher's cuts) can vary mainly as a function of the food received by the animal. The desired eicosapentaenoic acid (EPA) and docosahexanoic acid (DHA) are mainly present in animal's products. The impact (qualitative and quantitative) of alterations in the lipid composition of animal foods on the nutritional value of derived products (in terms of EPA and DHA content) eaten by humans is more important in single-stomach animals than multi-stomach animals (due to their hydrogenating intestinal bacteria). This is also the case when the diet rich in unsaturated fatty acids are fed to small ruminants, which needs to be protected against ruminal biohydrogenation. Central Sheep and Wool Research Institute, Avikanagar has initiated research on this line and is results obtained so far are promising. The oxidative stability of lamb meat also depends on diet. The pasture-diet presents some advantages over concentrate-diet in term of lipid oxidation and to a lesser extent on protein oxidation (Santé-Lhoutellier, 2007). Moreover, pasture feeding increases polyunsaturated fatty acids (especially ù-3 PUFAs) and conjugated linoleic acid content of the meat, which are beneficial for human health. So considering the meat quality and the dietetic aspect we could recommend this practice.

Carcass composition

Stage of maturity is the main determinant of carcass composition and, at a given live weight, the carcass composition of different mature size breeds will differ, and affect yield. Sanudo *et al.* (2000) stated that carcass composition of: (i) fat tailed and fat rump breeds tend to deposit more subcutaneous fat, especially over the lumbar region, than other breeds, (ii) prolific breeds tend to deposit less fat cover and more internal fat than meat breeds, but produce similar amounts of intramuscular fat and (iii) rustic breeds and hair breeds will tend to deposit more internal fat than meat breeds.

Weaning age and carcass and meat quality

Unweaned lambs raised on a grass-based diet with an *ad libitum* concentrate supplement exhibit greater production efficiency than their weaned counterparts, as they display greater growth, lower concentrate consumption and higher carcass dressing at slaughter (Caneque *et al.*, 2001). Following these same parameters, weaning at 65 days of age is more advantageous in terms of productivity than weaning at 45 days of age. Weaning represents a sudden change for lambs, reducing their growth rate and altering body condition with a drop in fatness and a proportional increase in the quantity of lean muscle. This effect is most pronounced in lambs weaned earliest. The greater fatness of the unweaned lambs, together with their lower total collagen values and the greater lightness of their meat indicates that the consumer may better accept their meat. From the human nutrition standpoint, the higher proportion of SFA in the meat of unweaned lambs is compensated for by its lower ù-6/ù-3 ratio confirming the idea that its consumption is healthier than that of weaned lambs in so far as lowering the risk of suffering cardiovascular disease. With regard to the higher-weight lambs, although their meat is more succulent due to the fact that it displays a higher water holding capacity (WHC), its texture may be affected by the lower solubility of its collagen. The meat of these lambs presents a lower PUFA/SFA ratio, which indicates that it is also inferior from a nutritional standpoint.

Growth of the animal is a major determinant of animal performance and yield of saleable meat from a carcass is of prime importance to meat producers and processors governing profitability. Yield of saleable meat is largely dependent on the rate of development of muscle, bone and fat as an animal matures from birth to maturity. At birth, the skeleton needs to be well developed for an animal to function and therefore bone are an early maturing tissue. During growth, the increase in bone weight is smaller than those for muscle and fat and its proportion decreases as an animal matures. Muscle is considered an average maturing tissue as the increase in muscle weight is similar to the increase in body weight. Fat is mainly a long-term energy store in the body. The relative proportion of fat increases from birth to maturity and therefore, fat is considered a late maturing tissue.

Relationship between body condition score (BCS) and carcass characteristics

Generally the carcass weight and live weight increased as the BCS increased (Gregory *et al.*, 1998). In goats carcass weight increases by 0.43 to 0.54 kg for every one kg increase in live weight (McGregor, 1990). However, carcass length did not showed this trend, suggesting that the increase in weight occurred in the soft tissues rather than in skeletal size. Animals having low condition score had limited body fat reserves. The extent to which the rate of increase in fatness increased as condition score increased. The dressing percentage of slaughter sheep may be influenced by age, weight, sex, body condition, amount of gut fill at slaughter, whether the carcass is weighed hot or cold and, of course, by the number of body components included in the yield calculation (Apple, 1999). Mature adipose tends to be highly saturated, whereas immature or maturing adipose is highly unsaturated when chronologically based, so the degree of non-saturation can be an index of adipose maturity.

Quality attributes of carcass

Tenderness: The most commonly used parameter for measurement of tenderness is the Warner Bratzler shear force value. Shear force is affected by cooking method, dimension of the samples and the shearing blade, speed at which the blade moves, etc. Therefore, it is usually difficult to directly compare results from different laboratories using different protocols or machines (Wheeler *et al.*, 1997).

Breed or genotype or crosses with in the breed hardly affect tenderness and there is little difference in tenderness between breeds. The Merino breed has a poor reputation for eating quality and this is due to the fact that these animals have greater stress sensitivity than other breeds. These animals are more prone to yield high pH meat, which negatively affects eating quality. When fed sufficiently and handled to provide minimal stress before slaughter, the eating quality of meat from Merinos is equal to other breeds (Young *et al.*, 2005). Although differences between breeds are relatively small, variation in tenderness within breeds can be quite considerable (Safari *et al.*, 2001; Hopkins *et al.*, 2005). The age related effects on tenderness are thought to be due to increased cross linking of intramuscular collagen (Kopp and Bonnet, 1987). Given that different muscles contain different amounts of collagen, the effect of animal age on tenderness may be quite variable. Pethick *et al.* (2005) found grilled loin (*Longissimus dorsi*) steak tenderness unaffected up to an age of 20 months. However, the tenderness of grilled silverside (*Biceps femoris*), a high connective tissue cut, decreased beyond 8.5 months of age. In general, the eating quality of lamb is better than hogget, or mutton, but the effect of age on tenderness varies with muscle. There is no evidence that the type of diet affects tenderness (Pethick *et al.*, 2005). However, it is clear that nutrition should be adequate to prevent against high ultimate pH (growth rate in the two weeks prior to slaughter should be a minimum of 100 g/ day; 150 g/day for Merino sheep) and to allow the animals to deposit enough intramuscular fat (4-5%) to achieve optimal palatability for eating (Young *et al.*, 2005).

Juiciness: Juiciness of meat results from release of fluid from the meat upon biting/chewing and the stimulatory effect of fat on salivation. At present, there is no specific parameters that accurately predict juiciness. However, given the importance of water holding capacity of meat for yield of saleable product, many tests have been developed to assess this characteristic. There appear to be little inherent differences in juiciness between breeds and there is no evidence that diet affects juiciness (Pethick *et al.*, 2005). However, the energy content of the diet may affect juiciness in two ways. If the nutritional status of the animals before slaughter is low, glycogen stores may be insufficient to reach a normal ultimate pH of about 5.5. High pH meat, also known as Dark, Firm and Dry (DFD) meat, is less juicy than meat with a normal pH because of its high water holding capacity. Secondly, a low energy diet may result in reduced deposition of intramuscular fat. Fat stimulates salivation and is responsible for the experience of sustained juiciness.

Flavour: Once meat is tender, flavour is the most important determinant of consumer acceptability of meat (Sitz *et al.*, 2005) and flavour is often misconstrued with taste. Taste is one of the five senses and taste sensations include: sweet, salty, sour, bitter, and umami (savoury). Flavour is the perception derived from combining the senses of both taste and smell. At present there are no exact methods to determine meat flavour, and it is unlikely that they will be developed in the near future. One reason for this is that there are over one hundred volatile compounds that influence smell and contribute to meat flavour (Calkins and Hodgen, 2007).

The oxidative deterioration of meat is a major concern for all the stakeholders involved in the production chain. Indeed, the production of unpleasant off-flavours and the deterioration of meat colour consequent to the oxidation of lipids and myoglobin, respectively, are responsible for significant product discards (McKenna *et al.*, 2005). Meat oxidative stability depends on several factors, with one of the most important being the balance between antioxidant and pro-oxidant components in muscle (Descalzo and Sancho, 2008). PUFA in the cell membranes are the preferential substrates where lipid oxidation initiates and propagates (Gray *et al.*, 1996). Therefore, together with metal ions, haem proteins and reactive oxygen species, PUFA can be considered pro-oxidant components, as a high degree of unsaturation of the muscle exposes it to oxidative damages (Morrissey *et al.*, 1998). On the other hand, endogenous antioxidant defences and exogenous antioxidant molecules of dietary origin are able to extend meat shelf life by counteracting the oxidative reactions. The diet of the animals can strongly affect both antioxidants intake and muscle fatty acid composition, with important consequences on meat oxidative stability (Wood and Enser, 1997).

Sheep meat has a distinct flavour and sometimes off-flavour (Jamora and Rhee, 1998; Duckett and Kuber, 2001; Prescott *et al.*, 2001). Several compounds are believed to impact on sheep meat flavour. The flavour associated with mutton is thought to be associated with the concentration of branched chain fatty acids in the fat. Another off-flavour candidate is skatole, which is also associated with the problem of "boar-taint" in pigs. The effect of breed appears to be rather minimal (Shackelford *et al.*, 2003, 2005). Therefore, the main drivers of the intensity of sheep meat flavour and off-flavours, are in the combination of the effects of diet, animal age and the genetic propensity to accumulate flavour compounds in the fat fraction, independent of breed type. Duckett and Kuber (2001) mention that grass feeding and grain feeding generally result in similar flavour intensities but flavour intensity is increased by pastures like white clover and alfalfa. There is an increasing amount of interest in altering omega-3 and omega-6 fatty acid profiles of lamb meat to fulfil niche-marketing opportunities. Most strategies to alter fatty acid profiles involve either grass feeding or long-chain PUFA supplementation in the diet. Regardless of the strategy used, increasing the PUFA ratios may lead to a greater rate of lipid oxidation, which in turn can lead to an increased incidence of off-flavours. Thus, it may be necessary to consider supplementing lambs with additional Vitamin E to help prevent oxidative rancidity and the development of off-flavours for production systems targeting these specialty markets. Compared to diets based on concentrate feeds, dietary strategies based on pasture have been often reported to enhance the concentration of PUFA in muscle and to also provide high levels of antioxidants (such as vitamin E and carotenoids) with a consequent improvement of meat oxidative stability (Faustman *et al.,* 2010). In pigs, it has been reported that feeding restrictions impaired the deposition of vitamin E in muscle and negatively affected meat lipid oxidation over storage (Mason *et al.,* 2005). Furthermore, it has been shown that food restriction in lambs fed a concentrate-based diet consistently lowered the concentration of glutathione in muscle with a consequent reduction of the muscle's overall antioxidant status, although lipid oxidation and colour stability were not measured in that study.

Colour: Consumers base their choice of meat on its appearance and colour is an important aspect of appearance. In red meats, myoglobin (Mb) is primarily responsible for meat colour, but the source (wavelength and intensity) of light illuminating the meat product can also influence its appearance. Color stability attributes of goat meat are different from those of sheep meat, possibly due to species-specific differences in Mb biochemistry. When a freshly cut meat surface is exposed to air, oxygen penetrates into the meat and its binding (oxygenation) to Mb produces cherry-red oxymyoglobin. However, oxidation of Mb during storage results in the formation of grayish brown metmyoglobin. The development of meat colour after the oxygenation of the meat surface (blooming) is believed to be dependent on the final pH of the muscle, with meat lightness (L^* values) being generally lower in meat with high ultimate pH values (Confort and Egbert, 1986; Young *et al.,* 1999). This has been proposed as a possible explanation for the lower lightness (lower L^* values) often observed in meat from pasture-fed animals compared to that from concentrate-fed ones (Priolo *et al.,* 2001). Oxidation, or browning, is fastest at a relatively low oxygen pressure. Therefore browning occurs first at a certain depth below the meat surface, depending on the extent of oxygen penetration. However, after several days of storage the metmyoglobin layer will reach the surface of the muscle, browning will be visible, and the product will be rejected by consumers (Wulf *et al.*, 1995). Colour stability is therefore an economically important aspect of meat quality. Many visual and instrumental methods to evaluate meat colour have been used. One of the most commonly used instrumental methods is the measurement of L*, a* and b* values. In this, L* represents the lightness of the colour (0 = black, 100 = diffuse white), a* represents the position between green and red/magenta, and b* represents the position between blue and yellow.

A greater concentration of Mb produces a darker red colour. The concentration of Mb tends to increase with age, and can be affected by breed (Hopkins *et al.*, 2005; Pethick *et al.*, 2005). Colour can also be influenced by diet; grass fed lambs have slightly darker meat colour (Priolo *et al.*, 2002), presumably associated with a greater intake of carotenoids. However, the most important factor affecting meat colour is its pH, with high pH meat being dark in color and less color stable during display. High pH is generally associated with elevated levels of pre-slaughter stress and / or low glycolytic potential. Since browning of meat during display is due to oxidation of Mb, the most effective way to extend shelf life is increasing the level of antioxidants in the meat. An effective way to achieve this is supplementing the diet with vitamin E. Wulf *et al.* (1995) showed that supplementing lambs in feedlots with 500 IU vitamin E per day for 56 days extended the shelf life of loin retail cuts by about 4 days. Supplementation beyond this amount (1,000 IU) did not result in an increase in vitamin E levels in the muscles and negatively affected growth. Supplementation up to the maximum amount increased vitamin E levels in the muscles and extended shelf life. Thus it appears that the feeding level of vitamin E for lambs in feedlots should be 300-500 IU per day to achieve an optimum effect on shelf life. Plant polyphenols (quebracho tannins) in sheep diets also can improve meat colour stability of fresh lamb during extended refrigerated storage (Luciano *et al.*, 2009). This could be attributed to the positive effects of dietary tannins on haem pigment concentration and metmyoglobin formation. A direct antioxidant effect of tannins in tissue would implicate their absorption and deposition in the muscle; however, to date, the fate of dietary tannins in the organism is not clearly understood. A possible indirect effect of dietary tannins on lamb oxidative stability could involve the modification of muscle fatty acid composition due to the strong effects of tannins on lipid metabolism in ruminants. The improvement in meat colour stability observed in meat from the tannin-supplemented lambs did not involve an improved stability to lipid oxidation.

Restructuring carcass of cull animals

Under Indian condition about 40% of sheep slaughtered are of spent category with low body score, low dressing yield with average carcass fat (Jacob *et al.*, 2005). Meat from such aged sheep is usually tough and fibrous in texture and is not preferred by the consumers (Mendiratta *et al.*, 2008). Aged ewes constitute a considerable proportion of the animal sales and have usually poor body conditions and general appearance due to the burden of repeated pregnancies, lambing and poor nutrition, which reduce their market weights and values. Cull ewes are often sold and slaughtered in unfinished condition having lack of proper body condition and poor lean yield as owners mostly dispose of these ewes at lower value and do not regard them as valuable meat animals. Meat processing by comminution and producing emulsified products has great advantage to augment utilization and add value to meat from cull animals. Due to growing demand of meat in the country, more thrust is given for improving meat yield and quality of growing lambs by better feeding, however, there is ample scope of bridging the demand of meat by improving meat yield and quality of cull sheep by supplementary feeding, which have not been explored at present stage in the country.

Carcass from cull ewes: Generally meat of cull sheep maintained on grazing resources alone contained higher proportion of bone (29.20±2.33%) and lower proportion of fat (5.96±0.55%) and muscles owing to maturity and deteriorating body condition. Beside these limitations, toughness of meat due to higher proportion of connective tissues in spent sheep fetched low sale price in the markets. As such the carcass from these ewes is "tough and sheepy" due to increased cross linking of collagen (Kopp and Bonnet, 1987) and accumulation of volatile branched chain fatty acids (BCFAs) that characterise sheep and goat fats (Wong *et al.*, 1975; Ha and Lindsay, 1991), and from phenols and indoles and the concentration of BCFAs in carcass fats appears to be increased with age (Ha and Lindsay, 1991; Apple, 1999).

Strategies for restructuring of carcass attributes and economization of protocol: Challenge feeding program involving energy rich diet helps the animals to show recuperative changes in intake, metabolism and improvement in body condition. A short duration (45-90 days) feeding strategy with minimum feed input and maximum output in terms of live weight gain may fetch a higher price for the animals, which will compensate the feed and rearing cost and cancel out the recurring expenditure on these animals. Some of possible approaches to prepare energy-dense economic ration for such ewes are:

- Substituting costly protein concentrate with cheaper NPN (urea)
- Substituting a portion of the costly energy concentrate with cheaper molasses or alternate grains (borken wheat/maize)
- Use of bypass fat supplements iv) use of yeast (*Saccharomyces* sp.) as probiotics to enhance feed utilization and animal performance
- Use of alkalizing agents and maintaining acid-base balance during high concentrate feeding
- Use of succulent fodder to enhance voluntary feed intake
- Rumen manipulation with suitable additives (tannins, saponins) for reducing fermentable energy loss
- Optimizing nutrient input (energy: protein ratio) and maximizing microbial protein synthesis for reducing feed wastage and economizing feed input

Realimentation effect on carcass traits: A comparison between responses of growing and mature sheep to starvation and refeeding resulted in faster growth rate, being higher in immature sheep (Hood and Thornton, 1980). Lipogenesis was restored (more quickly in immature sheep) and reached a rate higher than that measured for sheep which were continuously grown on the same diet. The response to realimentation differed between body components, particularly the carcass and viscera (Butler-Hogg, 1984). Above the body weight at which weight loss was imposed the realimented sheep did not differ in chemical composition from the continuously *ad libitum* fed controls when compared at the same weight. Changes in muscle protein degradation affect meat tenderization/ tenderness, changes in muscle protein synthesis are not expected to affect this. Because, muscle growth is determined by hyperplasia and hypertrophy while muscle cell size is determined by the balance between the amount of muscle protein synthesized and the amount of muscle protein degraded. In these type of studies, it is essential to measure as fully as may be the state of the animal at the end of the period of limitation and to compare it with the state of normal animals and that careful attention needs to be given to the choice and the description of the treatment, or preferably treatments, during the rehabilitation period. Several studies have shown that feeding of energy dense diets over short periods to cull cows could be profitable (Sawyer *et al.*, 2004), improve carcass characteristics and meat quality (Stelzleni *et al.*, 2007). Similarly in cull ewes significant improvement in body condition and carcass characteristics was recorded after feeding high energy diet @ 2.5% of body weight for a period of 90 days (Bhatt *et al.*, 2011).

Quality enhancement in wool

Wool is a natural fibre obtained from sheep and has several qualities that distinguish it from hair or fur, namely it is crimped, elastic and grows in staples. The term wool is usually restricted to describing the fibrous protein derived from the specialized skin cells called follicles in sheep. Wool is a protein fibre, composed of more than 20 amino acids. These amino acids form protein polymers. Wool also contains small amounts of fat, calcium and sodium. Nutrition plays an important role on the wool growth of sheep. By nature sheep are grazing animals and nutrients from pasture helps the animals for maintenance and as well as production. During the periods of poor pasture growth or when the quality of pasture is poor, there is a reduction of total fleece yield as well as in the quality of wool per animal and per unit area of grazed land. Proper wool growth requires all the important nutrients like amino acids, carbohydrates, minerals and vitamins. Adequate nutrition increases both the length and diameter of the wool fibre. Though the nutrition of sheep is reported to affect the quantity of wool production and quality (length, diameter, protein composition and strength) of wool fibre, wool growth has also been reported under the condition of negative energy and nitrogen balances. Therefore nutrients requirement for wool production is also included for maintenance requirement. However some of the wool quality parameters like fibre diameter, staple length and fibre strength can be influenced by the supply of nutrients available to wool follicles during the process of fibre growth (Russel, 2002). Nutrition can play a key role in the diameter of a wool fiber. Sheep which have been placed on a high plane of nutrition tend to have coarser diameter than yearling lamb. Although medullation is influenced markedly by genetics and age but a possible effect of nutrition is also to be considered. Protein nutrition is important for wool growth and production, as wool is composed of almost entirely protein with very high level of cysteine and serine compared with other body tissues. Growth of wool requires more protein relative to energy, and draws amino acids, particularly methionine and cysteine, disproportionately from the body pool. This chapter deals in details with the nutrients requirement for wool.

Maternal nutrition and wool production: The maturity of the primary follicle population is completed prior to birth. From about day 85 to the end of pregnancy follicle initiation is confined to the appearance of secondary follicles between the central and primary follicles. The fibre start to grow in secondary follicles 30 days prior to birth and majority of fibre are growing by the time lamb is 35 days old. Hence, it is essential to feed nutritious diet to sheep during later part of pregnancy and first few weeks after lambing. The primary follicles produce the coarse fibre and secondary follicle produce fine fibre. For lifetime wool production, it is essential to strategically manage the nutrition of breeding ewes in a cost effective and sustainable manner. This is expected to benefits not only the lifetime wool production and quality of the progeny but also their survival, growth and parasite resistance.

Nutrition approaches for enhancing wool production: It has been observed that controlled low plane of feeding of fine wool breeds produced superfine wool suitable for processing into worsted yarn (Litherland *et al.*, 1990). The body condition of sheep also influenced wool production when same allowances was offered to fat and heavy weight and thin and light weight ewes, fat ewes gained less and grow more wool than thin and light weight ewes. This indicates differential partitioning of nutrients between wool and other tissue. There is production of sound wool at maintenance level of feeding than restricted feeding. Further, it is reported that restricted feeding reduced the staple length of fibre sizably. This has affected clean fleece yield, 0.41g less on sub-maintenance ration compared to maintenance ration (Kelly *et al.*, 1996). Wool responses were observed when sheep maintained on feed containing 9.6 or 1.5 MJ/kg DM and 10.7 or 21.7 g/kg nitrogen. Voluntary feed intake of sheep increases up to 40% within a week of shearing depending upon environmental conditions and feed quality and reaches to normal level within 6-8 week post shearing. When pasture availability is better, wool growth increased in response to feed intake but when pasture is dried and mature and limited in quantity, wool growth depressed sizably.

Protein supplementation: The use of dietary supplement of sulphur containing amino acid protected from ruminal degradation or analogues which resist degradation in the rumen stimulate wool growth.The deficiency of amino acid particularly supply of cysteine limits the growth of follicle in sheep. The suphur containing amino acid, methionine also increased wool growth.

Energy supplementation: There was a significant interaction between the effects of protein and energy supply on fibre diameter, staple length, growth rate and volume of wool, but it has small relative to the main effect of protein. Extra energy appeared to enhance wool growth at the highest level of protein but reduce it at the lowest level of protein. An optimum ratio of protein to energy absorption is required for maximum wool growth in sheep. If protein is limiting, an increase in protein absorption stimulates wool growth, but an increase in energy absorption reduce it. Conversely, if protein is in excess, an increase in protein absorption reduces wool growth, but it is stimulates by an increase in energy absorption.

Vitamins: The deficiency of folic acid causes loss of crimps and ceases fibre growth. The deficiency of vitamin A causes excessive keratinisation of follicular epithelium, which blocks the opening of follicle and affects wool growth.

Minerals: Copper, zinc, iodine and selenium alter follicle function and wool growth directly. A deficiency of copper causes eases wool growth, lacks crimp, mechanical strength and lustrous appearance. Zn deficiency causes loss of crimp, thin fibre and loose and in some cases shedding of whole fleece Deprivation of Zn also caused thickening, hardening and fissuring of the skin (parakeratosis). Iodine reduces thyroid hormones production and causes poor follicle development, wool growth and quality. The deficiency of dietary S limits ruminal production of sulphur containing amino acids (SAA) and thereby limits rate of fibre growth. The low cost inorganic S sources to enhance SAA supply from ruminal microbes and an additional supply of SAA post-ruminally may enhance wool production.

Designer milk

Nutritional and genetic interventions to alter the milk composition for specific health and/or processing opportunities are gaining importance in dairy biotechnology. Altered fatty acid and amino acid profiles, more protein, less lactose and absence of b-lactoglobulin are some challenges of 'designing' milk for human health benefits. Alteration of primary structure of casein and lipid profile, increased protein recovery, milk containing nutraceuticals and replacement for infant formula are some of the definite processing advantages, which needs to be harnessed for product formulation and development. However, the final acceptability of the newly designed products will depend on animal welfare, safety and enhanced health properties of the products and increased profitability vis-à-vis conventional practices.

By combining the two approaches of nutritional and genetic interventions, researchers are now hoping to develop 'designer milk' tailored to consumer preferences or rich in specific milk components that have implications in health as well as processing. For diet and human health measures, the actions that would be beneficial are:

- Generate a greater proportion of unsaturated fatty acids (USFA) in milk fat,
- Reduce lactose content in milk in order to cater to persons suffering from lactose intolerance
- Remove b-lactoglobulin (b-lg) from milk.

The use of molecular biology to reduce the presence of pathogenic organisms in milk is a potentially advantageous prospect. It might be possible to produce specific antibodies in the mammary gland that are capable of preventing mastitis infection or those that aid in preventing human diseases. Thus, one can foresee antibodies against salmonella, listeria or other pathogens that will produce safer milk products. Research is also underway to manufacture milk through transgenesis for treatment of diseases such as phenylketonuria (PKU), hereditary emphysema, and cystic fibrosis (Sabikhi, 2004). From a technological point of view, there exist vast opportunities in:

- Alteration of primary structure of casein to improve technological properties of milk
- Production of high-protein milk
- Engineering milk meant for cheese manufacturing that leads to accelerated curd clotting time
- Increased yield and/or more protein recovery
- Milk containing nutraceuticals
- Replacement for infant formula

In an interesting combination of sericulture and dairying, goats that produce spider silk in milk have been engineered. When spider genes were introduced into the cells of lactating goats, they secreted silk in tiny strands along with their milk. These polymer strands could be woven into threads after extracting them from the milk and used for applications such as military uniforms, medical microsutures, and tennis racket strings (Anon, 2002).

Conclusion

Without value addition as processed products, the meat wool and milk production sector cannot be fully tapped to its full potential. Ultimate acceptability will depend on the four key factors of animal welfare, demonstrable safety of the product, enhanced health properties of the product and increased profitability compared with conventional practices. Various ethical, legal and social aspects of biotechnological research need to be addressed before we would see designer transgenic herds similar to the organic herds that thrive in the current economic and social climate.

References

Anon. 2002. The Scientific American 50: Celebrating the Year's Top Technology Leaders. Science America 12: 48.

Apple, J.K. 1999. Influence of body condition score on live and carcass value of cull beef cows. Journal of Animal Science 77: 2610-2620.

Bhatt, R.S., Soren, N.M., Sahoo A. and Karim. S.A. 2011. Realimentation strategy to maneuver body condition and carcass characteristics in cull ewes. Animal doi:10.1017/S1751731111001236.

Butler-Hogg, B. W. 1984.The growth of Clun and Southdown sheep: body composition and the partitioning of total body fat. Animal Production 39 : 405-411.

Calkins, C.R. and Hodgen, J.M. 2007. A fresh look at meat flavor. Meat Science 77: 63-80.

Caneque, V., Velasco, S., Diaz, M., Perez, C., Huidobro, F., Lauzurica, S., Manzanares, C and Gonzalez, J. 2001. Effect of weaning age and slaughter weight on carcass and meat quality of Talaverana breed lambs raised at pasture. Animal Science 73: 85-95.

Confort, D.P. and Egbert, W.R. 1985. Effect of rotenone and pH on the color of pre-rigor muscle. Journal of Food Science 50: 34-44.

Descalzo, A.M. and Sancho, A.M. 2008. A review of natural antioxidants and their effects on oxidative status, odor and quality of fresh beef produced in Argentina. Meat Science 79: 423-436.

Duckett S.K. and Kuber P.S. 2001 Genetic and nutritional effects on lamb flavor Journal of Animal Science 79: E249-E259.

Faustman, C., Sun, Q., Mancini, R. and Suman, S.P. 2010. Myoglobin and lipid oxidation 391 interactions: Mechanistic bases and control. Meat Science 86: 86-94.

Gray, J.I., Gomaa, E.A. and Buckley, D.J. 1996. Oxidative quality and shelf life of meats. Meat Science 43: S111-S123.

Gregory, N.B., Robins, J.K., Thomas, D.G. and Purchas, R.W. 1998. Relationship between body condition score and body composition in dairy cows. New Zealand Journal of Agricultural Research 41: 527-532.

Ha, J.K. and Lindsay, R.C. 1991. Volatile alkylphenols and thiophenol in species-related characterizing flavors of red meats. Journal of Food Science 56: 1197-1202.

Hood R.L. and Thornton, R.F. 1980. The effect of compensatory growth on lipogenesis in ovine carcass adipose tissue. Australian Journal of Agricultural Research 31: 155-161.

Hopkins, D.L., Walker, P.J., Thompson, J.M. and Pethick, D.W. 2005. Effect of sheep type on meat quality on meat and eating quality of sheep meat. Australian Journal of Experimental Agriculture 45: 499-507.

Jacob, R.H., Walker, P.J., Skerritt, J.W., Davidson, R.H., Hopkins D.L., Thompson, J.M. and Pethick, D.W. 2005. The effect of lairage time on consumer sensory scores of the *M. longissimus thoracis et lumborum* from lambs and lactating ewes. Australian Journal of Experimental Agriculture 45: 535-542.

Jamora, J.J., and Rhee, K.S. 1998. The uniqueness of lamb: nutritional and sensory properties. Sheep and Goat Research Journal 14: 53-64.

Kelly, R.W., Macleod,I., Hynd,P. and Greeff,J. (1996). Nutrition during fetal life alters annual wool production and quality in young Merino sheep. *Australian Journal of Experimental Agriculture* 36, 259-267.

Kopp, J. and Bonnet, M. 1987. Stress-strain and isometric tension measurement in collagen. In: Advances in meat research. Vol. 4. Collagen as a food (A.M. Pearson, T.R. Dutson van Nostrand Reinhold, Eds.) New York, pp 163-185.

Lee J.H., Yamamoto, I., Jeong J.S., Nade T., Arai T., Kimura N. 2009. Relationship between adipose maturity and fatty acid composition in various adipose tissues of Japanese Black, Holstein and Crossbred (F1) steers. Animal Science Journal 82, 689-697.

Litherland, A., Paterson, D. and Newman, S.A. 1990. The processing potential of superfine wool produced under varying environmental conditions. In: Proc. VIII International Wool Textile Research Conference Christchurch 2: 169-179.

Luciano, G., Monahan F.J., Vasta, V., Biondi L., Lanza, M. and Priolo, A. 2009. Dietary tannins improve lamb meat colour stability. Meat Science 81: 120-125.

Mason, L.M., Hogan, S.A., Lynch, A., O'Sullivan, K., Lawlor, P.G. and Kerry, J.P. 2005. Effects of restricted feeding and antioxidant supplementation on pig performance and quality characteristics of *Longissimus dorsi* muscle from Landrace and Duroc pigs. Meat Science 70: 307-317.

McGregor, B.A. 1990. Boneless meat yields and prediction equations from carcass parameters of Australian cashmere goats. Small Ruminant Research 3: 465-473.

McKenna, D.R., Mies, P.D., Baird, B.E., Pfeiffer, K.D., Ellebracht, J.W. and Savell, J.W. 2005.Biochemical and physical factors affecting discoloration characteristics of 19 bovine muscles. Meat Science 70: 665-682.

Mendiratta, S.K., Kondaiah, N., Anjaneyulu A.S.R. and Sharma, B.D. 2008. Comparisons of handling practices of culled sheep meat for Production of Mutton Curry. Asian-Australian Journal of Animal Science 21: 738-744.

Morrissey, P.A., Sheehy, P.J.A., Galvin, K., Kerry, J.P. and Buckley, D.J. 1998. Lipid stability in meat and meat products. Meat Science 49: S73-S86.

Pethick, D.W., Hopkins, D.L., D'Souza, D.N., Thompson, J.M. and Walker, P.J. 2005. Effects of animal age on the eating quality of sheep meat. Australian Journal of Experimental Agriculture 45: 491-498.

Prescott, J., Young, O. and O'Neill, L. 2001. The impact of variations in flavor compounds on meat acceptability: a comparison of Japanese and New Zealand consumers. Food Quality and Preference 12, 257-264.

Priolo, A., Micol, D. and Agabriel, J. 2001. Effects of grass feeding systems on ruminant meat colour and flavor: A review. Animal Research 50: 185-200.

Priolo, A., Micol, D., Agabriel, J., Parche, S. and Dransfield, E. 2002. 425 Effect of grass or concentrate feeling systems on lamb carcass and meat quality. Meat Science 62: 179-185.

Russel, A.J.F. 2002. Fibre production from sheep and goats. In: Progress in Sheep and Goat Research (A.W. Speedy, Ed.). CAB International, Wallington, UK. p. 235.

Sabikhi, L. 2004. Designer milk – an imminent milestone in dairy biotechnology. Current Science 87: 1530-1535.

Safari, E., Fogarty, N.M., Ferrier, G.R., Hopkins, L.D. and Gilmour, A. 2001. Diverse lamb genotypes. 3. Eating quality and the relationships between its objective measurement and sensory assessment. Meat Science 57: 153-159.

Santé-Lhoutellier, V., Engel, E. and Gatellier, Ph. 2007. Assessment of the influence of diet on lamb meat oxidation. Food Chemistry 109: 573-579.

Sanudo, C., Alfonso, M., Sanchez, A., Delfa, R. and Teixeira, A. 2000. Carcass and meat quality in light lambs from different fat classes in the EU carcass classification system. Meat Science 56: 89-94.

Sawyer, J.E.,C.P. Mathis, and B. Davis. 2004. Effect of feeding strategy and age on live animal performance, carcass characteristics and economics osf short term feeding programs for culled beef cows. Journal of Animal Science 82:3646.

Shackelford, S.D., Leymaster, K.A., Wheeler, T.L. and Koohmaraie, M. 2003. Lamb meat quality progress report number 1.Preliminary results of an evaluation of effects of breed of sire on carcass composition and sensory traits of lamb. Available on line at: http//www.ars.usda.gov (accessed 26 February 2010).

Shackelford, S.D., Leymaster, K.A., Wheeler, T.L. and Koohmaraie, M. 2005. Lamb meat quality progress report number 2. Preliminary results of an evaluation of effects of breed of sire on carcass composition and sensory traits of lamb. Available on line at: http//www.ars.usda.gov (accessed 26 February 2010).

Sitz, B.M., Calkins, C.R., Feuz, D.M., Umberger, W.J. and Eskridge, K. 2005. Consumer sensory acceptance and value of domestic, Canadian, and Australian grass-fed beef steaks. Journal of Animal Science 83: 2863-2868.

Stelzleni, A.M., D.D. Johnson and T.A. Thrift. 2008. Effect of days on concentrate feed and postmortem aging on carcass and palatability characteristics of selected muscles from cull beef cows. The Professional Animal Scientist 24: 334-341.

Wheeler, T.L., Shackelford, S.D., Johnson, L.P., Miller, M.F., Miller, R.K. and Koohmaraie, M. 1997. A comparison of Warner- Bratzler shear force assessment within and among institutions. Journal of Animal Science 75: 2423-2432.

Wong, E., Johnson, C.B. and Nixon, L.N. 1975.The contribution of 4-methylactanoic (hircinoic) acid to mutton and goat meat flavour. New Zealand Journal of Agricultural Research 18: 261-266.

Wood, J.D. and Enser, M. 1997. Factors influencing fatty acids in meat and the role of antioxidants in improving meat quality. British Journal of Nutrition 78: S49-S60.

Wulf, D.M., Morgan, J.B., Sanders, S.K., Tatum, J.D., Smith, G.C. and Williams, S. 1995. Effects of dietary supplementation of vitamin E on storage and case life properties of lamb retail cuts. Journal of Animal Science 73; 399-405.

Young, O.A., Hopkins, D.L. and Pethick, D. 2005. Critical control points for meat quality in the Australian sheep meat supply chain. Australian Journal of Experimental Agriculture 45: 593-601.

Young, O.A., Priolo, A., Simmons, N.J. and West, J. 1999. Effects of rigor attainment temperature on meat blooming and colour on display. Meat Science 52: 47-56.

□□□

Chapter 16

In Vitro Gas Production Technique for Feed Evaluation - An Overview

B. Singh
Retd Principal Scientist, Dairy Cattle Nutrition Division, NDRI
Karnal -132 001

Introduction

Feed evaluation is the use of methods to describe feedstuffs with respect to their ability to sustain different types and levels of animal performance (France *et al.,* 2000). Evaluation of feedstuffs for digestibility, and their ability to supply nutrients, is necessary for provision of a nutritionally balanced ration to the animal. The practical importance of feed evaluation is obvious with respect to optimizing efficiency of feed utilisation, ruminant output and financial return to the producer. The importance of voluntary intake and digestibility in animal nutrition has long been recognized. The determination of intake and digestibility of feedstuffs *in vivo* is time-consuming, laborious, expensive, requires large quantities of feed and is unsuitable for large-scale feed evaluation. Based on quantitative research, feed evaluation methods were developed for various purposes. An efficient laboratory method for feed evaluation should be reproducible and should correlate well with actually measured *in vivo* parameters.

Since feed constitutes a major input to all animal production systems, an understanding of feed quality with reference to its influence on animal production and the environment is a necessity. Although feed quality assessment has been primarily viewed in terms of nutrient composition and digestibility, the accumulated knowledge of gastro-intestinal physiology, and its influence on nutrient utilization, have contributed to orient development of feed evaluation techniques towards those that mimic the fate of feed nutrients in the gut. Such approaches have reduced dependence on animals and created greater flexibility in feed evaluation.

Animal feeding studies are the most accurate method of feed characterization, but require expensive purpose-built facilities, considerable time, expense and labour, and recently have become less attractive due to animal welfare concerns. Tilley and Terry (1963) and Van Soest and co-workers developed in vitro techniques to estimate the digestibility of feeds, which have been instrumental in their characterization for decades. Three major biological digestion techniques are currently available to determine the nutritive value of ruminant feeds: 1) digestion with rumen microorganisms as in Tilley and Terry (1963) or using *in vitro* gas production technique (IVGPT) (Menke *et al.*, 1979), 2) *in situ* incubation of samples in nylon bags in the rumen (Mehrez and Orskov, 1977), and 3) cell-free fungal cellulase (De Boever *et al.*, 1986; Beauchemin *et al.*, 2003). These biological methods are more meaningful since microorganisms and enzymes are more sensitive to factors influencing the rate and extent of digestion than are chemical methods (Van Soest, 1994). As with all laboratory techniques, preparation of the feed sample must consider many factors, which have been discussed for conventional in vitro methods and in situ techniques.

The two-stage technique (conventional *in vitro* or IVDMD) for *in vitro* digestion of forages developed by Tilley and Terry (1963) has been widely used because of its convenience and high degree of correlation to *in vivo* digestibility and accuracy (Tilley and Terry, 1963; De Boever *et al.*, 1986). However, the technique is time-consuming and labor intensive. In sacco rumen degradability techniques measure rate and extent of feed degradation but do not account for digestion of small particulate or soluble feed fractions, and they are more invasive than in vitro digestibility techniques. The *in vitro* and *in situ* techniques now in use have the disadvantage that the contribution of the soluble components of the original feed cannot be assessed, since they rely mainly on the measurement of particle loss. Fermentation, on the other hand, is the anaerobic decomposition of substrates by micro-organisms and can be assessed according to the production of end-products, of which SCFA and gas are the most important.

The gas measuring technique has been widely used for evaluation of nutritive value of feeds. More recently, the increased interest in the efficient utilization of roughage diets has led to an increase in the use of this technique due to the advantage in studying fermentation kinetics. Gas measurement provides a useful data on digestion kinetics of both soluble and insoluble fractions of feedstuffs. The *in vitro* gas production system helps to better quantify nutrient utilization and its accuracy in describing digestibility in animals has been validated in numerous experiments. Based on the strong relationship between measured digestibility and that predicted from gas production, regression equations have been developed and the method has been standardized.

History of development

The idea of measuring gas production as a proxy for ruminal digestion is not new. The principle of determining potential rumen degradability/fermentability of a feed by measuring gas produced from a batch culture was first developed by McBee (1953) who described a manometric method to measure gas production by mixed ruminal bacteria and which was later modified by Hungate (1966). Shibata *et al.* (1961) developed a syringe system while direct displacement of a plunger by fermenting a feedstuff within a glass syringe was developed by Czerkawski and Breckenridge (1975) and this was the basis of the 'Hohenheim Gas Test' (HFT, Hohenheimer Futterwert Test) later developed by Menke *et al.* (1979) in Germany. The syringe technique was originally developed to determine end-point fermentability of feedstuffs, at 24 h, and has been incorporated into the German national feedstuff evaluation system. An earlier technique is by attaching a water displacement manometer to each vessel to measure the gas produced. The main innovation in such method was that the gas production is recorded rather than degradation. Similarly, Beuvink and Spoelstra (1992) used inverted measuring cylinders to determine the volume of water displaced. Beuvink *et al.* (1993) then automated this water displacement technique. The system was based on weighing the amount of fluid replaced by fermentation gas, followed by calculation to gas volume and registration by a data logger.

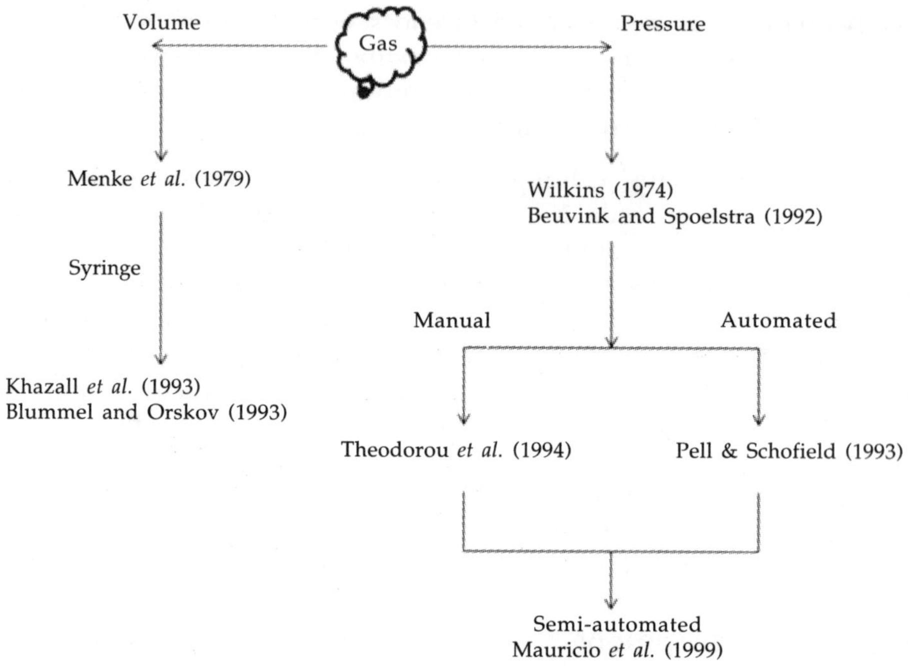

Fig. Development of gas based feed evaluation systems (adapted from Mould, 2003)

The method of Menke *et al.* (1979) was modified by Blümmel and Ørskov (1993) in that feeds were incubated in a thermostatically controlled water bath instead of a rotor in an incubator. Makkar *et al.* (1995) and Blümmel *et al.* (1997) modified the method further by increasing the amount of sample from 200 to 500 mg and increasing the amount of buffer two-fold as a result the incubation volume increase from 30 ml in the method of Menke *et al.* (1979) to 40 ml in the modified method. In the 30 ml system, the linearity between the amount of substrate incubated and the amount of gas produced is lost when the gas volume exceeds 90 ml because of the exhaustion of buffer of the medium; and in 40 ml system, the linearity is lost when the gas volume exceeds 130 ml (Getachew *et al.*, 1998). The exhaustion of the buffer decreases pH of the incubation medium; consequently the fermentation is inhibited.

In the method of Menke *et al.* (1979), fermentations are conducted in 100 ml capacity calibrated glass syringes containing feedstuff and a buffered rumen fluid. The gas produced on incubation of 200 mg feed dry matter after 24 h of incubation together with the levels of other chemical constituents are used to predict digestibility of OM determined *in vivo* and metabolizable energy. Aiple *et al.* (1996) compared three laboratory methods (enzymatic, crude nutrient and gas measuring technique) as predictors of net energy (as estimated by equations based on *in vivo* digestibility) content of feeds and found that for predicting net energy content of individual feeds, the gas method was superior to the other two methods.

The role of the gas production technique to predict nutrient supply in ruminants has also been reviewed. The popularity of *in vitro* gas production stems mainly from (1) the ability to exercise experimental control, (2) the capacity to screen a large number of substrates, (3) the kinetic information which may be derived which, although possible, is a limitation of the end-point techniques such as *in vitro* digestibility (Tilley and Terry, 1963) and (4) the fact that no assumptions need be made on the degradability of the soluble fraction of the substrate, as is required for the *in sacco* technique (Ørskov and McDonald, 1979). Potential use of gas production to approximate *in vivo* kinetics is a major expectation and some studies have been published (Blummel and Ørskov, 1993; Khazaal *et al.* 1993, 1994; Sileshi *et al.* 1996; Lopez *et al.* 1998), where it has been compared with the *in situ* polyester bag method.

Origin of gas

The complex interactions within a mixed rumen microbial population leading to the conversion of plant components to gas and VFA, have been summarized in the form of stoichiometric reaction equations (Wolin, 1960; Van Soest, 1994; Blummel *et al.*, 1997 and Getachew *et al.*, 1998). All of the equations show the relationship between the hexose equivalents fermented, and the proportions of fermentation products produced. Such equations have been used to estimate the extent of digestion of hexose-equivalents on the basis of the fermentation products formed (e.g. Blummel and Orskov, 1993).

Organic matter fermentation can be expressed in glucose equivalents (g) and assuming that the glucose equivalents are fermented to form the end-products: acetic, propionic, and butyric acids and the gases CO_2 and CH_4, as well as being incorporated into microbial biomass.

$$57.5\ C_6H_{12}O_6 \rightarrow 65\ C_2H_4O_2 + 20\ C_3H_6O_2 + 15\ C_4H_8O_2 + 35\ CH_4 + 60\ CO_2 + 25\ H_2O$$

The two major reactions (coupled) of the ruminal fermentation - Degradation of carbohydrates to VFA and ATP generation and production of microbial cells (adapted from Bergen and Yokoyama, 1977).

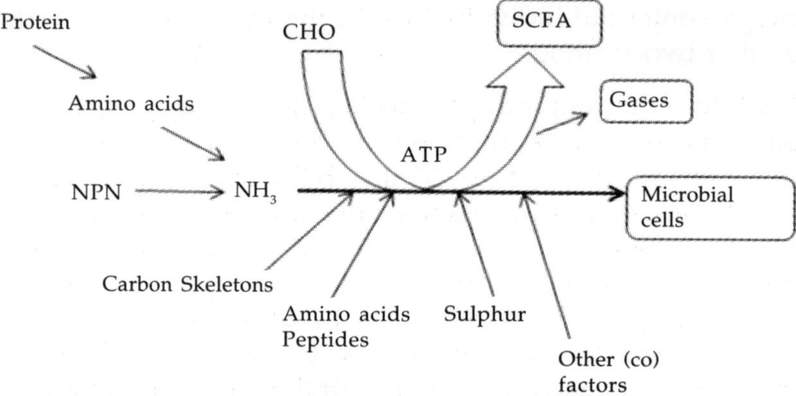

The three reactions giving rise to the main end-products of carbohydrate fermentation in the rumen were summarized by Hungate (1966) as follows:

$$C_6H_{12}O_6 + 2\ H_2O \rightarrow 2\ C_2H_4O_2 + 2\ CO_2 + 4\ H_2$$

$$C_6H_{12}O_6 + 2\ H_2 \rightarrow 2\ C_3H_6O_2 + 2\ H_2O$$

$$C_6H_{12}O_6 \rightarrow C_4H_8O_2 + 2\ CO_2 + 2\ H_2$$

The carbon dioxide produced as an end-product of the above reactions can then be combined with hydrogen to produce methane.

$$CO_2 + 8\ H^+ \rightarrow CH_4 + 2\ H_2O$$

Production of methane does not influence the total amount of gas produced from fermentation because almost all of the hydrogen is incorporated into methane and 1 mol of methane simply replaces 1 mol of carbon dioxide.

The gas produced in the IVGPT is the direct gas produced as a result of fermentation and the indirect gas produced from the buffering of SCFA. For roughages, when bicarbonate buffer is used, about 50% of the total gas is generated from buffering of the SCFA and the rest is evolved directly from fermentation. At very high molar propionate the amount of CO_2 generated from buffering of SCFA is about 60% of total gas production. Each mmol of SCFA produced from fermentation releases 0.8-1.0 mmol of CO_2 from the buffered rumen fluid solution, depending on the amount of phosphate buffer present. Highly significant correlation has been observed between SCFA and gas production. Beuvink and Spoelstra (1992) reported that each mol of VFA produced released 0.87 mol gas from the buffer. Blummel and Ørskov (1993) found that on average 50% of the gas volume consisted of CO_2 and CH_4 arising from fermentation of substrate, the remainder being CO_2 released from the buffer.

Gas is produced mainly when substrate is fermented to acetate and butyrate. The gas that is released with the generation of propionate is only the indirect gas produced from buffering therefore, relatively lower gas production is associated with propionate production. The molar proportion of different SCFA produced is dependent on the type of substrate. Therefore, the molar ratio of acetate to propionate has been used to evaluate substrate related differences. If fermentation of feed leads to a higher proportion of acetate, there will be a concomitant increase in gas production compared with a feed with a higher proportion of propionate. In other words, a shift in the proportion of SCFA will be reflected by changes in gas production.

The gas measurement indicates how much substrate was used for the formation of SCFA and gases, since SCFA and gas production are very closely associated stoichiometrically. The stoichiometric balance also allows calculation of CH_4 and CO_2 expected from the rumen fermentation if the molar proportions and amount of SCFA are known. *In vitro* gas measurements reflect only SCFA production. The relationship between SCFA and microbial mass production is not constant and the explanation for this resides in the variation of biomass production per unit ATP generated. This can impose an inverse relationship between gas volume (or SCFA production) and microbial mass production particularly when both are expressed per unit of substrate truly degraded. Rumen degradability measurements reflect the conversion of feed into essentially three fermentation products Gases, Short chain fatty acids and microbial mass. Based on stoichiometric relationships, the amount of gas is expected to depend on the relative amounts of VFA formed (Hungate, 1966). The chemical composition of the substrate influences the molar proportions of the major VFA formed.

A variable part of the substrate degraded will not be fermented to VFA and gases, but rather incorporated directly into microbial biomass, giving rise to a negative correlation between the amount of gas produced and the microbial biomass yield per unit truly degraded substrate (Blummel *et al.*, 1997). Thus, there are indications that the gas yield (in units of gas produced per unit substrate truly degraded) is not necessarily constant during the course of incubation.

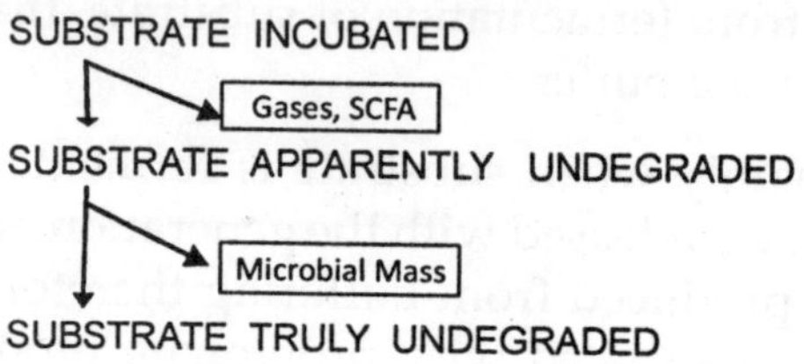

Substrate Incubated – Substrate apparently undegraded = Gases + SCFA
Substrate Incubated – Substrate truly undegraded = Gases + SCFA + Microbial mass
Substrate apparently undegraded - Substrate truly undegraded = Microbial mass

The gas produced on incubation of cereal straws (Blümmel and Ørskov, 1993), a wide range of feeds including many dairy compound feeds and their individual feed components whose protein and fat contents vary greatly (Blümmel *et al.*, 1999a), and tannin containing browses (Getachew *et al.*, 2000a) in absence or presence of polyethylene glycol (a tannin complexing agent) in the buffered rumen fluid was closely related to the production of short chain fatty acids (SCFA) as per Wolin (1960) stoichiometry, which is as follows:

$$\text{Fermentative } CO_2 = \frac{A}{2} + \frac{P}{4} + 1.5 * B$$

where A, P and B are moles of acetate, propionate, and butyrate respectively.

$$\text{Fermentative } CH_4 = (A + 2B) - CO_2 \text{ or } \frac{A}{2} - \frac{P}{4} + \frac{B}{2}$$

$$\text{Total fermentative gas} = (A + 2B)$$

where A and B are moles of acetate and butyrate respectively and CO_2 is moles of CO_2 calculated from previous equation.

Assumption: One mole of SCFA releases one mole of CO_2 from bicarbonate-based buffer described as buffering CO_2 according to:

$$H^+ + HCO^{3-} \rightarrow H_2CO_3 \leftrightarrow CO_2 + H_2O$$

A further assumption is that gas release from neutralisation of VFA is independent of their composition or rate of production.

Gas produced *in vitro* using a bicarbonate buffered system has a dual origin. Firstly, CO_2 and CH_4 that are produced as a result of fermentation (i.e., 'direct' gas production; gas_{direct}) and, secondly, CO_2 is produced upon buffering of short chain fatty acids (SCFA) generated (i.e., 'indirect' gas production; $gas_{indirect}$; Blummel *et al.*, 1997). Molar production of the latter equals molar SCFA production, provided that the incubation medium is saturated with CO_2 and the buffer is entirely based on bicarbonate (Blummel *et al.*, 1997). Moreover, stoichiometric relationships between SCFA, CO_2 and CH_4 (Wolin, 1960), indicated that direct gas production is the result of substrate fermentation to acetate (A) and butyrate (B), but not to propionate (P). Accordingly, the following molar balances could be derived (Blummel *et al.*, 1997):

$$\text{Gas}_{\text{Direct}} = (A + 2B)$$

$$\text{Gas}_{\text{Indirect}} = \text{Total SCFA}$$

$$\text{Total gas} = \text{Gas}_{\text{Direct}} + \text{Gas}_{\text{Indirect}}$$

In IVGP system stoichiometric laws of fermentation can be applied since fermentation products must be derived from the substrate incubated. The stoichiometric balance allows the theoretical calculation of equilibrated amounts of the products (SCFAs and gases). If the molar proportions and amounts of SCFAs are known, the theoretical amounts of CO_2 and CH_4 expected from the rumen fermentation can be calculated. Methane and carbon dioxide production is influenced by the molar proportion of acetate to propionate and also by the partitioning of the truly degraded substrate between SCFA and microbial cells.

Based on fermentation stoichiometry, the distinction between direct and indirect gas production could allow for immediate estimation of the molar productions of SCFA from $\text{Gas}_{indirect}$. As the level of SCFA is an indicator of the energy value of diets, prediction of SCFA from *in vitro* gas measurements might be useful under circumstances where laboratories lack gas chromatographic equipment (Fievez *et al.*, 2005).

Kinetics of gas production

The kinetics of degradation can be determined from differences in the residues after various incubation times e.g., *in sacco* technique.

However, this approach is laborious, expensive and not always accurate enough. Moreover, the course of fermentation of soluble substrate components cannot be quantified (Pell and Schofield, 1993). Alternatively, the kinetics of feedstuff degradation can be determined from the fermentative gas production, which measures the amount of gas released directly as a product of the fermentation and indirectly from buffered rumen fluid (Beuvink and Spoelstra, 1992; Pell and Schofield, 1993; Cone *et al.*, 1994; Theodorou *et al.*, 1994).

The kinetics of gas production is dependent on a sequence of processes. Upon incubation, substrates are partly solubilized. The soluble components are rapidly fermentable after incubation. A gradual shift subsequently occurs towards the fermentation of the insoluble parts, which need to be hydrated and colonized by rumen microorganisms before they can be fermented (Van Milgen *et al.*, 1993). The rates at which these processes can take place depend on the initial concentration and composition of the microbial population, and on the ability of the microorganisms present in the mixture to colonize, ferment and utilize the fermentation products for growth (Demeyer, 1981; Hidayat *et al.*, 1993). Substrates and their components can be resistant to these processes to different extents, resulting in substantially different gas production profiles.

Kinetics of gas production is dependent on the relative proportion of soluble, insoluble but degradable, and undegradable particles of the feed. Mathematical descriptions of gas production profiles allows analysis of data, evaluation of substrate- and media-related differences, and fermentability of soluble and slowly fermentable components of feeds.

Time-related gas production techniques to quantify the kinetics of ruminant feed fermentation have a high resolution. Consequently, fermentation processes with clearly contrasting gas production kinetics can be identified. Parameterization of the separate processes is possible with a suitable multiphasic model and modelling method. Availability of kinetic information from *in vitro* gas production curves of ruminant feeds has created a need for data analysis models in order to estimate nutritionally important variables. In the analysis of gas production data many mathematical functions have been adopted. The use of gas measurements to estimate the rate of forage digestion depends on a close relationship between gas yield and VFA production. Changes in microbial metabolism or yield may alter the relationship between substrate digestion and gas production and could affect the estimation of digestion rate from gas measurements.

Mathematical description of gas production profiles allows analysis of data and comparison of substrates or fermentation environment characteristics, and can provide useful information concerning the substrate composition and the fermentability of soluble and slowly fermentable components of the substrate. Gas production profiles vary in shape, from steep diminishing returns to highly sigmoidal, thereby creating difficulties in choice of an appropriate model. The slope of the profile tends to be zero at early stages of fermentation, as there is little or no gas production, giving rise to a lag phase. Thereafter, a steady increase is generally observed until substrate depletion causes the profile to approach an upper asymptote. Ideally, a function is required that is capable of modelling both a range of shapes with no inflexion point and a range of sigmoidal shapes in which the inflexion point is variable.

The rate of digestion is proportional to the quantity of potentially digestible substrate and decreases continuously. Other factors affecting digestion (e.g. microbes, enzymes, surface area) are therefore assumed to be constant, their effects described by the fractional rate constant. However, it has been shown that the rate of digestion for many feedstuffs initially increases rather than decreases (Mertens, 1973). This has been explained by suggesting that not all potentially digestible substrate is available for digestion immediately upon incubation. This delayed availability of substrate has been represented by discrete (McDonald, 1981) and dynamic lag phases (van Milgen *et al.* 1993).

In first-order kinetics, rate of digestion is a continuous declining function where each subsequent unit of potentially digestible substrate is more difficult to digest. This may be caused by build-up of lignin-carbohydrate complexes (or lack of available potentially digestible substrate) on the surface during the digestion process. Because digestion is a surface phenomenon, rate of digestion is determined by the spatial distribution of potentially digestible substrate (i.e. embedded in tissues or present on the surface), availability of microbes on the surface, and the total surface area.

The inclusion of a discrete lag time finds its origin in the inadequacy of a first-order model to describe digestion during the early hours of incubation. During the lag phase digestion does not occur due to limited hydration and microbial colonization of substrate. During the digestion phase (i.e. when $t > t_{lag}$) digestion is limited only by the quantity of potentially digestible substrate remaining. As a result it is implied that substrate is hydrated and colonized instantaneously at t_{lag}. Although all-or-none processes may exist in biology, this seems an unlikely scenario for hydration and microbial colonization. Gas production is proportional to the amount of metabolic end products produced during bacterial growth. Therefore it is not surprising that gas production curves resemble the sigmoidal growth curves of bacteria grown in batch culture.

Short chain fatty acids

The *in vitro* gas production measured after 24 h incubation of tannin containing browses in the presence or absence of PEG was strongly correlated with gas volume stoichiometrically calculated from SCFA. The relationship between SCFA production (mmol) and gas volume (ml) after 24 h of incubation of browse species with a wide range of CP and phenolic compounds total phenols and total tannins as tannic acid equivalent respectively was (Singh *et al.*, 2005; Makkar, 2005):

SCFA (mmol) = 0.0222* ml Gas at 24 h - 0.00425; $R^2 = 0.94$

These relationships are similar to that obtained for wheat straw (Blümmel *et al.*, 1993). The SCFA production could be predicted from gas values using the above relationship. Since SCFA measurement is important for relating feed composition to production parameters and to net energy values of diets, prediction of SCFA from *in vitro* gas measurement will be increasingly important in developing countries where laboratories are seldom equipped with modern equipments to measure SCFA. The stoichiometric balance also allows calculation of the CH_4 and CO_2 expected from the rumen fermentation if the molar proportions and amount of SCFA are known.

Partitioning factor

Partitioning factor (PF) is defined as the ratio of substrate truly degraded *in vitro* (mg) to the volume of gas (ml) produced by it. The concept of PF analysis demands a close stoichiometrical relationship between SCFA and gas production and a reliable determination of true degradability of the substrate. A feed with higher PF means that proportionally more of the degraded matter is incorporated into microbial mass, i.e., the efficiency of microbial protein synthesis is higher. Roughages with higher PF have been shown to have higher dry matter intake. Different *in vitro* PF values are also reflected by *in vivo* microbial protein synthesis as estimated by purine derivatives (the higher the PF, the higher the excretion of urinary purine derivatives and in methane production by ruminants (the higher the PF, the lower the methane output (Blümmel *et al.*, 1999b). PF calculated *in vitro* provides meaningful information for predicting the DMI, the microbial mass production in the rumen, and the methane emission of the whole ruminant animal. The theoretical range for PF is 2.74 to 4.41. Proportional to the amount of substrate degraded, low gas production (high PF) is indicative of a high efficiency of microbial production (EMP) *in vitro*. For roughages, PF values from 2·75 to 4·45 mg/ml approximately reflecting Y_{ATP} ranges from 10 to 32 (Blummel *et al.*, 1997). High EMP is preferred over high SCFA production. Roughages with higher PF have been shown to have higher dry matter intake. Different *in vitro* PF values are also reflected by *in vivo* microbial protein synthesis as estimated by purine derivatives (the higher the PF, the higher the excretion of urinary purine derivatives and in methane production by ruminants (the higher the PF, the lower the methane output the PF calculated *in vitro* provides meaningful information for predicting the DMI, the microbial mass production in the rumen, and the methane emission of the whole ruminant animal.

Voluntary feed intake prediction

The main constraint to the utilization of roughages by ruminants is voluntary feed intake so prediction of feed intake, particularly of fibrous roughage, is one of the important aspects of ruminant nutrition. Simple and rapid procedures to predict voluntary feed intake are essential to allow correct ration formulation for animals and to adequately predict their performance. Measurements of extents and rates of degradation for prediction of voluntary DMI of forages was advocated by Ørskov *et al.* (1980), who used rumen *in sacco* techniques as the tool to examine degradation characteristics of soluble and insoluble feed fractions. The relationship between voluntary intake and degradation characteristics has been investigated using the nylon bag technique. In *in sacco* technique the extent and rate of digestion are obtained assuming that DM loss equals fermentation, which is not normally the case because considerable substrate is lost from nylon bags. Gas production techniques to study kinetics of rumen digestion has made it possible to overcome this problem, since gas production derives from fermentable fraction of feeds and washing losses are non-existent. The potential of gas production techniques to predict voluntary intake has been investigated by several groups (Blummel and Ørskov, 1993; Blummel *et al.*, 1997; Romney *et al.*, 1998).

The maximum correlation between gas volumes and voluntary intake occurred prior to 12 h of incubation (Rodrigues *et al.*, 2009) which is consistent with earlier observations using either *in vitro* gas production or *in sacco* techniques. Various workers have reported significant correlation between *in vitro* gas production and DMI. Getachew *et al.* (1998) stated that gas volumes in early stages of fermentation best predict the voluntary feed intake. According to Blummel *et al.* (1997a), the gas volumes of 54 forages at 4, 6 or 8 h accounted for approximately 76% of the variation in their DMI while the volume recordings between 12 and 48 h of incubation were statistically less important. It was found that DM degradation after 3 h of incubation *in sacco* and ADF content were the best predictors of DMI, accounting for 68 and 67 %, respectively of the variation observed. In that study, DM degradation after 3 h incubation *in sacco* and NDF content accounted for 84 and 77% of the variation observed in DDMI. Gas production in earlier stages of incubation could be interpreted to represent fermentation of cell contents. This explains the negative correlations observed between *in vitro* gas production and NDF and ADF contents prior to 15 h of incubation.

Blummel and Orskov (1993) have given the following equations for prediction of DMI and digestible DMI (DDMI) from gas production kinetic parameters obtained from the single exponential non sigmoidal model (Orskov and McDonald, 1979).

DM Intake (kg d^{-1}) = 1.529 + 0.455a + 0.0324b

Digestible DM Intake (kg d^{-1}) = - 0.933 + 0.301a + 0.0496b

Further, intake was best predicted from gas volume at 24 h (GV) through the regression equations:

DMI = 19.27 + 0.258* GV

DOMI = - 14.24 + 0.262* GV

Forage cell walls have considerable influence on voluntary feed intake through rumen fill mechanism (Van Soest, 1994). Gas production from extracted NDF was shown to be better correlated to voluntary feed intake than the values obtained from the incubation of whole roughage. The *in vitro* gas production from NDF explained more (82 % vs. 75 %) of the variation in DMI than gas production from whole roughage (Getachew *et al.*, 1998). In the University of California, Davis approach, gas production is recorded at 6, 24 and 72 h and these values are interpreted relative to the carbohydrate fractions. Thus gas produced up to 6 h of incubation is considered to estimate the extent of fermentation of NSC, while gas produced between 6 and 24 h is considered to estimate the amount of NDF that will be digested in cattle at high production levels. Finally, gas produced between 6 and 72 h of fermentation is considered to estimate the amount of NDF that will be digested in cattle fed at maintenance intake levels. The quantities of gas generated at 6, 24 and 72 h of incubation can be used to qualitatively assess intake potential of forages both among and within forage species. They can also be used to assess the extent of short term (through 6 h) fermentation, which may be very important in determining the intake potential of mixed rations, of which forages comprise only a portion.

Blummel *et al.* (1997) showed that the PF value was highly important to accurate prediction of voluntary DMI of forages. Forages with proportionally low gas production per unit substrate degraded had higher voluntary DMI. It is thus recommended to include PF for best prediction of DMI.

Associative effects

Rations formulated for ruminants are generally a mixture of individual feeds, and its net (NE) or metabolizable (ME) energy value is generally calculated by summing the energy values of the individual feeds in it, on the assumption that the NE or ME value of individual feeds will be unchanged when they are fed in combination with other feeds. However this assumption may not be true. Associative effects are seldom taken into account in feed formulation. While the meaning of an associative effect is clear (i.e., the sum of the parts being less, or more, than the combination of the parts), reasons for an associative effect are not clear.

Feeds are commonly evaluated as single entities despite the fact that most of the time an animal is fed a mixture of ingredients. A common approach to study *in vitro* associative effects of feed mixtures has been to look at the differences between single and mixed substrates on the gas production, digestibility, PF. This approach assumes that measured parameters are additive and therefore departures from linearity can be detected. Using this approach, Rosales *et al.* (1998) found significant effects when fodder trees were mixed and incubated *in vitro* as compared with single substrate incubation. Sampath *et al.* (1995), by incubating the basal diet and the supplement, observed a positive interaction in gas production in the early hours of incubation, which according to the authors can be an approach to study the synergetic effects of supplementation.

Evaluation of diets by gas production suggested that associative effects occurred at up to 12 h of incubation (Kiran and Krishnamoorthy, 2007). With a diet that included wheat straw, alfalfa hay and maize gluten feed, replacement of alfalfa hay with wheat straw in the ration depressed DM intake, but had no effect on digestibility of nutrients although wheat straw could replace up to around 200 g/kg of maize gluten feed with no undesirable effects on digestion. The same did not occur when alfalfa hay was added to maize gluten feed and associative effect of alfalfa hay with wheat straw caused a negative effect when no maize gluten feed was added. This suggests that each feed ingredient behaves differently when fed with other ingredients to produce results that differ from those expected from where they are fed as a sole feed.

Evaluation of tannin-containing by-products and forage

Unfortunately, the method based on the gas method and the detergent system of fibre analysis to calculate the microbial mass produced for fibrous feeds did not work for tannin-rich feeds. The PF for tannin-rich feeds ranged from 3.1 to 16.1 (Getachew *et al.*, 2000b), which is well above the theoretical range of PF (2.75 to 4.41). The appearance of tannin-protein complexes as artifacts in the true residue also makes the gravimetric approach of quantification of microbial mass redundant (Makkar *et al.*, 1997).

The system developed for evaluation of tannin-containing feeds depends on incubation of the feed in the presence and absence of polyethylene glycol (PEG MW 4000 or 6000 preferably of 6000; (Makkar *et al.*, 1995) and measurement of gas (or SCFA) and microbial mass using the above mentioned markers. PEG has a high affinity for tannins. Addition of PEG results in the formation of PEG-tannin complexes which inactivates tannins. The changes in gas (or SCFA) and microbial mass as a result of PEG addition represents 'in totality' the tannin effects (biological) as a function of the rumen fermentation parameters. Addition of PEG during the incubation of tannin-rich NDF led to an increase in gas production, suggesting that NDF bound tannins released as a result of NDF degradation by rumen microbes are biologically active and have the potential to influence rumen fermentation (Makkar *et al.*, 1997). Efficiency of microbial protein synthesis is expected to be higher in the presence of tannins. The net microbial mass production would depend on the balance between decreased degradable dry matter and higher microbial mass production per unit of DM digested in presence of tannins.

Estimation of crude protein quality

The need for a rapid, simple, precise and inexpensive method to evaluate forage N is clear. Knowledge of N utilization in the intestines is key to accurate estimation of the true value of tropical forages as CP sources for ruminants, since some of their secondary compounds may impair intestinal digestion. Estimation of available N by subtraction of ADIN is not accurate, since a variable proportion of this fraction is degraded. Although the in situ technique has been widely used for tropical forage evaluation the likelihood that some particles wash out without being fermented by microbes (overestimation) cannot be overcome.

One of the major constraints to accuracy of method of incubation of feeds with rumen fluid is underestimation of N degradation due to microbial synthesis that increases the proportion of N in the incubation residue. Incubation with fungal proteases tends to give higher values than rumen fluid, but the response is substrate dependant.Although the fermentation pattern of forages can be estimated IVGPT (Menke and Steingass, 1988; Theodorou *et al.*, 1994), there are concerns about using this technique to evaluate the CP quality of tropical forages. The widely used rumen in situ technique to measure CP degradation may overestimate its degradability in dried and ground leaves because small particles pass through the bag pores without being degraded. The application of gas production techniques to estimate ruminal CP degradation (Raab *et al.*, 1983) has not received much research attention. Further, the intestinal digestion of CP has also been assessed by incubation of rumen undigested residue with exogenous enzymes Getachew *et al.* (1998) compared estimates of N degradability of cereal straws by the gas/ammonia relationship with those of other *in vitro* methods, and reported a correlation between the gas method and pepsin solubility, but not with the fungal proteases or buffer N solubility, and higher values with fungal proteases versus the gas/ammonia relationship. Pooled residues from IVGPT can be digested *in vitro* with HCl–pepsin at pH 1.9 for 1 h, followed by pancreatin at pH 7.8 for 24 h. The reaction is stopped by adding trichloroacetic acid, and the centrifugation supernatant analysed for N. The N contribution of the pepsin–pancreatin solution blank is subtracted from soluble N. Digestibility is calculated as the proportion of total N that is solubilised.

Digestion kinetics of neutral detergent-soluble fraction

Little is known about the digestion kinetics of this neutral detergent-soluble (NDS) pool because most *in vitro* kinetic studies have followed the disappearance of insoluble cell wall components and the gravimetric techniques used do not measure soluble material. The NDS contain carbohydrates such as starch, sugars, and pectic substances as well as non-carbohydrates, including protein, soluble phenolics, ash, and lipids. The gas measurement method has been used to study digestion kinetics of the neutral detergent soluble fraction of forages, starch-rich feeds and other highly digestible carbohydrate components, which is obtained by subtracting the average gas production curve for the digestible NDF from that of the unfractionated whole feed (Chen *et al.*, 1999). The subtraction procedure might give some useful information relevant to low-NDF fibre feeds, e.g., corn grain (Chen *et al.*, 1999), but it is not suitable for forages rich in NDF (Blümmel *et al.*, 1999b). Blümmel *et al.* (1999b) examined the rate and extent of fermentation of whole roughage and extracted NDF, DM degradability of extracted NDF and the PF for whole roughage and the extracted NDF of 54 roughages. Both the higher degradability and lower PF contributed to higher gas volumes obtained from extracted NDF compared with whole roughage.

Estimation of microbial protein synthesis

Recent advances in ration balancing include manipulation of feed to increase the quantity and quality of protein and energy delivered to the small intestine. This concept of feed evaluation has an extra element of the efficiency of microbial protein synthesis in addition to the more conventional one of the DMD. The limited supply of protein post-ruminally under most feeding systems in developing countries is an important limiting factor which prevents an increase in animal productivity.

It has been proposed that variations in EMP can be detected by a combination of *in vitro* gas volume measurements with a concomitant measure of true substrate degradability (TSD). The degradability measurement accounts for feed conversion into all products of microbial degradation and synthesis, essentially microbial biomass, short chain fatty acids (SCFA) and gases, whereas the gas volume measurement reflects feed conversion into SCFA and gases. The difference between the measures is assumed to be microbial biomass. This allows *in vitro* microbial biomass production (MBP) and EMP to be estimated from concomitant gas volume and TSD measurements (Blummel, 2003) as:

Microbial mass (mg) = mg substrate truly degraded - (ml gas volume x SF)

For roughages, the stoichiometric factor (SF) is 2.20 and 2.34 in case of high (>40%) proportional propionate production.

$$\text{and EMP} = \text{TSD} - \frac{(\text{gas volume} * \text{SP})}{\text{TSD}}$$

Dijkstra *et al.* (2002) have described modelling of microbial protein synthesis *in vivo* from the *in vitro* gas parameters.

Implications for the interpretation of gas production data

Gas production after peak microbial production will be derived from secondary fermentation in addition to direct substrate fermentation. Gas volume would also be contributed by lysed microbial biomass. It is advisable to investigate substrate specific variations in the partitioning of fermentation products at similar microbial growth stages - preferably at the point of inflexion.

Blümmel *et al.* (1998) have highlighted the importance of the fermentation time at which the microbial mass should be measured. In this study, substrate degradation and kinetics of *in vitro* partitioning of three hays, with similar *in vivo* digestibilities, into SCFA, microbial mass yield, and ammonia, carbon dioxide and methane production was examined at 8, 12, 18 and 24 h of incubation in the gas method under both low and adequate nitrogen levels. SCFA and gas production were positively correlated ($P<0.0001$) and cumulative at all times of incubation under both low and adequate nitrogen levels. On the other hand, microbial mass, microbial nitrogen and microbial purine yields declined after 12 h of incubation while ammonia production increased.

For proper characterisation of feed and feed ingredients, approaches need to be developed for measuring the PF at the incubation time at which the lysis of microbes is minimal. Some possible simple approaches worth investigating to identify this incubation time are: i) the time at which half of the maximum gas is produced, and ii) the inflection point at which the rate of gas production is maximum (the rate increases up to a certain incubation time and thereafter decreases as the incubation progresses), both these parameters can be mathematically calculated from the gas profiles. The effect of the nitrogen level in the medium on the PF and the significance *in vivo* of these PFs also need to be investigated.

Further studies are required on: i) the development of simple approaches for identifying the incubation time in the *in vitro* gas system at which the PF is maximum, ii) the effect of N in the incubation medium on the PF iii) the *in vivo* significance of the PF, iv) Models employing gas kinetic parameters and the PF need to be validated for prediction of level of methane emission by ruminants, v) validation of microbial protein supply as derived from digestion kinetic parameters (including PF) *in vitro* with *in vivo* values vi) methods for estimation of kinetic parameters for organic matter constituentsis and their relaton ship with energy and protein synthesis. Very few reports have quantified the extent of hexose utilization for microbial biomass production during gas production experiments. Experiments must be designed to understand the biological significance of the various statistical and functional parameters being calculated using various models.

Research and development efforts are required to establish a data base for feeds evaluated by IVGPT including various kinetic parameters especially for unconventional feedstuffs including information on nutritive values in addition to routine composition analysis.

An important source of variation in methane production, variation in EMP, can be easily quantified by IVGPT that measures gas volume and TSD in the same incubation. IVGPT can improve prediction of methane emission by incorporating microbial efficiency indices obtained from complementing gas measurement with substrate disappearance. Getachew *et al.* (2005) highlights this potential application of IVGPT by determining methane production in a commercial animal production system, potentially adding methane emission as a new criterion in diet formulation.

Conclusion

The gas production approach offers the possibility to generate data that can provide an insight into the ways that cattle will respond to a forage. The IVGPT in which gas production and microbial mass production are concomitantly measured has several major advantages - i) screening a large number of feed resources, ii) be of great value in the development of supplementation strategies using locally available conventional and unconventional feed constituents to achieving maximum microbial efficiency in the rumen, iii) be of immense help in the study of rumen modulators for increasing efficiency of microbial protein synthesis and decreasing methane emission iv) provides a better insight into nutrient-antinutrient and antinutrient-antinutrient interactions, and into the roles of various nutrients with respect to production of fermentative gases, SCFA and microbial mass v) for screening plant-derived rumen modulators, vi) study the effect of tannins on the partitioning of nutrients between microbial protein and SCFAs or gases or to study the efficiency of rumen microbial protein synthesis, vii) as a biological assay to estimate the level of phenolics-related anti-nutritional factors in feed. The approach of incubating tannin containing feeds in the presence and absence of PEG also enables studies to be made on the nutritional significance of both extractable and unextractable (bound) tannins (Makkar, 2004), viii) quantifying feed proteins that have been protected by tannins from degradation in the rumen, ix) determination of fermentation characteristics of starch in feedstuffs without isolating the starch (Chai *et al.*, 2004).

In vitro gas-based feed evaluation systems are extremely powerful research tools and capable of a great deal more than routine analysis of feedstuffs. The ability to strictly control the fermentative environment, coupled with the high capacity of many current systems allows several factors to be examined simultaneously. Nutritional significance of gas production can be enhanced and made clearer through better chemical, biological and mathematical understanding. It may be possible to derive biological quantities important for animal performance from the gas production profiles under controlled conditions, through application of sound models to describe the profiles. These biological quantities include the extent of degradation of substrate and the microbial protein synthesized (Dhanoa *et al.*, 2000). The IVGPT can be used to study the nutritional quality of feed ingredients as well as mixed rations. The technique has been successfully used to assess the impact of grain processing on starch fermentability, the influence of lipids and fatty acids on microbial fermentation, to evaluate empirical equations to estimate the ME content of feeds, and to measure methane production from diets fed to lactating cows. Digestibility is the result of several processes including hydrolysis, absorption, secretion and passage. In order to develop mechanistic models of digestion to be used for feed evaluation, these processes have to be quantified.

The *in vitro* rumen gas technique offers a unique tool for researchers to address a wide range of nutritional issues in ruminants. The IVGPT for feed evaluation will almost certainly play a more important role in future animal production system. With ingenuity and thinking a great deal remains to be achieved with this methodology (Mould *et al.*, 2005).

References

Aiple, K.P., Steingass, H. and Drochner, W. 1996. Prediction of net energy content of raw materials and compound feeds for ruminants by different laboratory methods. Archive of Animal Nutrition. 49, 213-220.

Beauchemin, K.A., Colombatto, D., Morgavi, D.P., Yang, W.Z., 2003. Use of exogenous fibrolytic enzymes to improve feed utilization by ruminants. Journal of Animal Science. 81 (E. Suppl.), E37–E47.

Bergen, W.G. and Yokoyama, M.T. 1977. Productive limits to rumen fermentation. Journal of Animal Science., 46: 573-584.

Beuvink, J., and Spoelstra, S., 1992. Interactions between substrate, fermentation end-products, buffering systems and gas production upon fermentation of different carbohydrates by mixed rumen microorganisms *in vitro*. Applied Microbiology and Biotechnology. 37, 505–509.

Beuvink, J.M.W., De Visser, H., and Klop, A., 1993. In vitro gas production kinetics of different maize products: a comparison to nylon-bag degradation kinetics. In: Beuvink, J.M.W. (Ed.), Measuring and Modelling In Vitro Gas Production Kinetics to Evaluate Ruminal Fermentations of Feedstuffs. DLO-Research Institute for Livestock Feeding and Nutrition (IVVO-DLO) Report. Lelystad, The Netherlands, pp. 31–41.

Blümmel, M., Aiple, K.P., Steingass, H., and Becker, K. 1999a. A note on the stoichiometrical relationship of short chain fatty acid production and gas evolution *in vitro* in feedstuffs of widely differing quality. Jornal of Animal Physiology and Animal Nutrition. 81, 157-167.

Blümmel, M., Makkar, H.P.S. and Becker, K. 1998a. The partitioning kinetics of *in vitro* rumen fermentation products in a gas production test. Journal of Dairy Science. (Suppl. 1), 309.

Blümmel, M., Makkar, H.P.S., and Becker K. 1997. *In vitro* gas production: a technique revisited. Journal of Anima Physiology and Animal Nutrition. 77, 24-34.

Blümmel, M., Mgomezulu, R., Chen, X. B., Makkar H.P.S., Becker K. and Ørskov E. R. 1999b. The modification of in *in vitro* gas production test to detect roughage related differences in *in vivo* microbial protein synthesis as estimated by the excretion of purine derivates. Journal of Agricultural Science. (Camb.) 133, 335-340.

Blümmel, M., Steingass, H., Becker, K. and Soller, H. 1993. Production of SCFA, CO_2, CH_4 and microbial cells *in vitro*. Proceeding of Society of Nutrition and Physiology. 1:9.

Blummel, M., and Ørskov, E. R. 1993. Comparison of in vitro gas production and nylon-bag degradability in predicting feed intake in cattle. Animal Feed Science and Technology. 40:109–119.

Blummel, M., Karsli A. and Russell J.R. 2003. Influence of diet on growth yields of rumen micro-organisms in vitro and in vivo: influence on growth yield of variable carbon fluxes to fermentation products. British Journal of Nutrition. 90, 625-634.

Chai, W.Z., Van Gelder, A.H., and Cone, J.W., 2004. Relationship between gas production and starch degradation in feed samples. Animal Feed Science and Technology 114: 195–204.

Chen, Y-K., Pell, A.N., Chase, L.E., and Schofield, P. 1999. Rate and extent of the ethanol-soluble and neutral detergent-insoluble fractions of corn grain. Journal of Animal Science. 77, 3077-3083.

Cone, J.W., Beuvink, J.M.W. and Rodrigues, M., 1994. Use and applications of an automated time related gas production test for the *in vitro* study of fermentation kinetics in the rumen. Rev. Port. Zootec., 1: 25-37.

Czerkawski, J.W., and Breckenridge, G., 1975. New inhibitors of methane production by rumen micro-organisms. Development and testing of inhibitors *in vitro*. British Journal of Nutrition. 34, 429–444.

De Boever, J.L., Cottyn, B.G., Buysse, F.X., Wainman, F.W., and Vanacker, J.M. 1986. The use of an enzymatic technique to predict digestibility, metabolisable and net energy of compound feedstuffs for ruminants. Animal Feed Science and Technology. 14, 203-214.

Demeyer, D.I., 1981. Rumen microbes and digestion of plant cell walls. Agricultural Environment. 6: 295-337.

Dhanoa, M.S., Lopez, S., Dijkstra, J., Davies, D.R., Sanderson, R., Williams, B.A., Sileshi, Z., and France, J., 2000. Estimating the extent of degradation of ruminant feeds from a description of their gas production profiles observed *in vitro*: comparison of models. British Journal of Nutrition. 83: 131–142.

Dijkstra, J., J. A. N. Mills, and J. France. 2002. The role of modeling in understanding the microbial contribution to rumen functions. Nutrition Research Review. 15: 67–90.

Fievez, V., Babayemi, O.J. and Demeyer, D. 2005. Estimation of direct and indirect gas production in syringes: A tool to estimate short chain fatty acid production that requires minimal laboratory facilities. Animal Feed Science and Technology. 123-124: 197-210.

France, J., Dijkstra, J., Dhanoa, M. S., Lopez, S., and Bannink, A. 2000. Estimating the extent of degradation of ruminant feeds from a description of their gas production profiles observed *in vitro*: derivation of models and other mathematical considerations. British Journal of Nutrition., 83, 143-150.

Getachew, G., Blümmel, M., Makkar H.P.S., and Becker K. 1998. *In vitro* gas measuring techniques for assessment of nutritional quality of feeds: a review. Animal Feed Science and Technology. 72, 261-281.

Getachew, G., Makkar, H.P.S., and Becker, K. 2000a. Stoichiometric relationship between short chain fatty acid and *in vitro* gas production in presence and absence of polyethylene glycol for tannin containing browses, EAAP Satellite Symposium, *Gas production: fermentation kinetics for feed evaluation and to assess microbial activity*, 18-19 August, Wageningen, The Netherlands.

Getachew, G., Makkar, H.P.S., and Becker, K. 2000b. Tannins in tropical browses: effects of tannins on in vitro microbial fermentation and microbial protein synthesis in medium containing different amounts of nitrogen. Journal of Agricultural Food Chemistry. 48, 3581-3588.

Getachew, G., Robinson, P.H., DePeters, E.J., Taylor, S.J., Gisi, D.D., Higginbotham, G.E., Riordan, T.J., 2005. Methane production from commercial dairy rations estimated using an in vitro gas technique. Animal Feed Science and Technology. 123–124, 391–402.

Hidayat, Hillman, K., Newbold, C.J. and Stewart, C.S., 1993. The contributions of bacteria and protozoa to ruminal forage fermentation *in vitro*, as determined by microbial gas production. Animal Feed Science and Technology. 42: 193-208.

Hungate, R.E., 1966. The Rumen and its Microbes. Academic Press, New York, NY, USA.

Khazaal, K. and Orskov, E.R., 1994. The *in vitro* gas production technique: an investigation on its potential use with insoluble polyvinylpolypyrrolidone for the assessment of phenolics-related anti-nutritive factors in browse species. Animal Feed Science and Technology. 47: 305-320.

Khazaal, K., Dentinho, M.T., Ribeiro, J.M., and Orskov, E.R., 1993. A comparison of gas production during incubation with rumen contents in vitro and nylon bag degradability as predictors of the apparent digestibility in vivo and the voluntary feed intake of hays. Animal Production. 57: 105–112.

Kiran, D., Krishnamoorthy, U., 2007. Rumen fermentation and microbial biomass synthesis indices of feedstuffs determined by the in vitro gas production technique. Animal Feed Science and Technology. 134, 170–179.

Lopez, S., Carro, M.D., Gonzales, J.S., and Ovejero, F.J., 1998. Comparison of different in vitro and in situ methods to estimate the extent and rate of degradation of hays in the rumen. Animal Feed Science and Technology. 73: 99–113.

Makkar, H.P.S. 20005. In vitro gas methods for evaluation of feeds containing phytochemicals Animal Feed Science and Technology. *123-124:* 291-302.

Makkar, H.P.S., 2004. Recent advances in the *in vitro* gas method for evaluation of nutritional quality of feed resources. In: Assessing Quality and Safety of Animal Feeds. FAO Animal Production and Health Series 160. FAO, Rome, pp. 55–88.

Makkar, H.P.S., Blümmel, M., and Becker, K. 1995. Formation of complexes between polyvinyl pyrrolidone and polyethylene glycol with tannins and their implications in gas production and true digestibility in *in vitro* techniques. British Journal of Nutrition. 73: 897-913.

Makkar, H.P.S., Blummel, M., and Becker, K., 1997. *In vitro* rumen apparent and true digestibility of tannin-rich forages. Animal Feed Science and Technology. 67: 245–251.

McBee, R.H., 1953. Manometric method for the evaluation of microbial activity in the rumen with application to utilization of cellulose and hemicelluloses. Applied Microbiology. 1: 106–110.

McDonald, I. 1981. A revised model for the estimation of protein degradability in the rumen. Journal of Agricultural Science. (Camb.), 96: 251-252.

Mehrez, A.Z., and Ørskov, E.R. 1977. A study of artificial fibre bag technique for determining the digestibility of feeds in the rumen. Journal of Agricultural Science. (Camb.) 88: 645-650.

Menke, K.H. and Steingass, H. 1988. Estimation of the energetic feed value obtained by chemical analysis and *in vitro* gas production using rumen fluid. Animal Research and Devevelopment. 28: 7-55.

Menke, K.H., Raab, L., Salewski, A., Steingass, H., Fritz, D. and Schneider, W., 1979. The estimation of the digestibility and metabolizable energy content of ruminant feeding stuffs from the gas production when they are incubated with rumen liquor *in vitro*. Journal of Agricultural Science. (Camb.), 93: 217-222.

Mertens, D. R. 1973. Application of theoretical mathematical models to cell wall digestion and forage intake in ruminants. Ph.D. Thesis. Cornell Univ., Ithaca, NY.

Mould, F.L., 2003. Predicting feed quality—chemical analysis and in vitro evaluation. Field Crops Research. 84: 31–44.

Mould, F.L., Morgan, R. Kliem K.E. and Krystallidou E. 2005. A review and simplification of the in vitro incubation medium. Animal Feed Science and Technology. 123–124, 155-172.

Orskov, E.R. and McDonald, I., 1979. The estimation of protein degradability in the rumen from incubation measurements weighted according to the rate of passage. Journal of Agricultural Science. 92: 499-503.

Orskov, E.R., Hovell, F.D.DeB. and Mould, F., 1980. The use of the nylon bag technique for the evaluation of feedstuffs. Tropical Animal Production. 5: 195-213.

Pell, A.N. and Schofield, P., 1993. Computerized monitoring of gas production to measure forage digestion *in vitro*. Journal of Dairy Science.76: 1063-1073.

Raab, L., Cafantaris, B., Jilg, T., and Menke, K.H. 1983. Rumen protein degradation and biosynthesis. 1. A new method for determination of protein degradation in rumen fluid *in vitro*. British Journal of Nutrition. 50: 569-582.

Rodriguez, A.G., Mandaluniz, N., Flores, G., and Oregui, L.M 2005. A gas production technique as a tool to predict organic matter digestibility of grass and maize silage. Animal Feed Science and Technology. 123-124: 267-276.

Romney, D.L., Cadario, F.C., Owen, E., Murray, A.H., 1998. Comparison of parameters from the Theodorou gas production technique using nitrogen-free and nitrogen-rich media as predictors of dry matter intake and digestibility. In: Deaville, E.R., Owen, E., Adesogen, A.T., Rymer, C., Huntington, J.A., Lawrence, T.L.J.

Rosales, M., Gill, M.,Wood, C.D., Speedy, A.W., 1998. Associative effects *in vitro* of mixtures of tropical fodder trees. In: Deaville, E.R., Owen, E., Adesogen, A.T., A.T., Rymer, C., Huntington, J.A., Lawrence, T.L.J.

Sampath, K.T., Wood, C.D. and Prasad, C.S. 1995. Effect of urea and by-products on the *in vitro* fermentation of untreated and urea treated finger millet (Eleusine coracana) straw. Journal of Science Food Agriculture. 67: 323-328.

Sileshi, Z., Owen, E., Dhanoa, M.S., and Theodorou, M.K., 1996. Prediction of in situ rumen dry matter disappearance of Ethiopian forages from an in vitro gas production technique using a pressure transducer, chemical analyses or in vitro digestibility. Animal Feed Science and Technology. 61: 73–87.

Singh, B., Sahoo, A., Sharma, R and Bhat, T.K. 2005. Effect of polyethylene glucol on gas production parameters and nitrogen disappearance of some tree forages. Animal Feed Science and Technology. 123-124: 351-364.

Theodorou, M.K., Williams, B.A., Dhanoa, M.S., McAllan, A.B. and France, J., 1994. A simple gas production method using a pressure transducer to determine the fermentation kinetics of ruminant feeds. Animal Feed Science and Technology. 48: 185-197.

Tilley, J.M.A. and Terry, R.A. 1963. A two stage technique for the in vitro digestion of forage crops. Jounal of British Grassland Society. 18: 104-111.

Van Milgen, J., Berger, L.L. and Murphy, J., 1993. An integrated, dynamic model of feed hydration and digestion, and subsequent bacterial mass accumulation in the rumen. British Journal of Nutrition. 70: 471-483.

Van Soest, P.J., 1994. Nutritional Ecology of the Ruminant, 2nd edn. OandB Books, Cotvallis, OR, p.476.

Wolin, M.J. 1960. A theoretical rumen fermentation balance. Journal of Dairy Science. 43: 1452-1459.

□□□

Chapter 17

Nutritional Management of Sheep under Thermal, Migratory and Transportation Stress

S.K. Sankhyan and O.H. Chaturvedi
Division of Animal Nutrition, Central Sheep and Wool Research Institute
Avikanagar- 304 501 (Rajasthan)

Stresses are part of life on the planet earth. Any factor affecting the normal life and life cycle of the living organisms is called stress. The frequency and severity of stress is gradually increasing with passage of time and in the future likely to increase further. On an average 28-30% of geographical area of India is vulnerable to drought and other climatic vagaries. Meteorologically 19% deviation in rainfall from the long term mean is considered normal in India. Deficiency in the range of 20 to 59% represents moderate and more than 60% severe drought (Samra, 2004). Since 1871, India has witnessed 22 major droughts and 5 of them were severe. Although, with time India has developed institutionalized system for monitoring, prevention, mitigation, preparedness, relief and impact analysis, as a result there were hardly any starvation or drought related human deaths after 1967. However, livestock causalities are immense, making livestock farming, vulnerable in event of continuous climatic and other stresses- either directly through the improper supply of feed and water, or indirectly by reduced income both during and after such environmental fluctuations. Deterioration of pasture and soil erosion are less obvious costs, but important, particularly in the long-term sustainability of production from ruminants.

Thermal stress

Although the sheep and goats are more tolerant to climatic extremes than other farm animals, still under acute climatic conditions they sustain themselves by compromising production. Alexander (1974) calculated from data of Bennett (1972) that adult sheep when dry, in a calm wind and with 10 cm of fleece could withstand -120°C ambient temperature. However, calculated cold tolerance for freshly shorn adult sheep (7 mm of fleece) would be only -15°C and when wet and exposed to a 7 m/s wind, similar sheep could withstand only 13°C. For lambs, Alexander (1968) suggested that heat loss would exceed summit metabolism at 23°C when a small lamb with a short fleece was wet and exposed to a 5.5 m/s wind. For a large lamb in the same condition, metabolism would match heat loss at approximately 4°C. Obviously, survival during cold is highly variable, depending on both the animal's ability to increase heat production and aspects of the environment affecting effective ambient temperature (EAT). Heat tolerance is even less defined than cold tolerance for sheep. Mount (1979) reports that sheep will survive acute periods of 40-60°C dry-bulb temperature, but successful growth and reproduction at that temperature has not been demonstrated and is unlikely. Since homeotherms must rely more on evaporative heat loss when exposed to EAT in the hot zone, factors affecting rate of evaporation (wind and humidity) are of major importance in determining survival during heat. Effect of thermal stress on nutrient intake and their requirement is described below:

Feed energy intake: Many factors affect the amount of metabolizable energy (ME) available to the animal. These include digestibility of the foodstuff, amount of the foodstuff consumed, and/or the ability of the animal to acquire food. In general, factors influencing amount of ME available for consequent use may be considered as feed intake. Exposure to heat reduces voluntary intake in sheep as it does in other species. Bhattacharya and Hussain (1974) reported that high ambient temperatures coupled with high humidity during the day, reaching a maximum of 32°C and 98%, respectively, reduced *ad libitum* intake in sheep, with depression most severe when the diets contained high levels of roughage. However, a later report from the same laboratory (Bhattacharya and Uwayjan, 1975) showed conflicting results when temperature was coupled with low humidity. The diversity of those findings supports the need to discuss results in terms of EAT rather than separating the effects of temperature and humidity during heat stress.

In general, voluntary intake increases during cold compared to Thermo neutral zone. Webster *et al.* (1969) reported increased food intake of sheep housed indoors as still air temperature fell. Soderquist and Knox (1967) reported higher dry matter intake at 0°C compared to 23°C in growing lambs. Ames and Brink (1977) reported increased dry matter consumption in lambs, whose critical temperature was 13°C, to be statistically higher at 10, 5, and 0°C, but no further increase was noted at -5°C. Those data clearly show that voluntary intake is increased above thermo-neutral values during mild cold, but that a limit in voluntary intake was reached before animals were severely cold stressed. For shorn lambs whose lower critical temperature was 13°C, Brink and Ames (1975) related dry matter consumption over a wide range of ambient temperatures (- 5 to 35°C) and found the following linear relationship:

$$DMI = 111.3 - 0.52T$$

(Where, DMI = daily intake ($g/W^{0.75}$), T = temperature in (°C)

The impact of fluctuating temperatures and the validity of mean daily temperature when the standard deviation of daily temperature is high has been studied by Giacomini (1979) where lambs exposed to a constant thermo-neutral temperature (15°C) were compared with lambs in fluctuating environments with a mean temperature of 15°C. When fluctuations were from 10 to 20°C, 5 to 25°C, or 0 to 30°C, feed intake was not different from constant 15°C temperature. Certainly the area of fluctuating temperature deserves more study. This is particularly important in the design of confinement systems where constant temperatures may result in patterns of feed intake different from those established during fluctuating temperatures.

Assuming some nutrient (e.g., vitamin and mineral) requirements are constant over wide ranges in temperature raises a concern that difference in intake can have a major effect on vitamin and mineral intake. When these nutrients represent a constant percentage of the diet, it is obvious that reduced intake may lead to deficiency. Care must be taken (and adjustments made when necessary) to meet the animal's requirement when intake varies. The same consideration must be made for various non-nutrient additives (antibiotic premixes, growth promoters etc.) when they are to be ingested at a constant rate daily. Obviously, diet adjustment for components that are not affected by the thermal environment should be altered in proportion to changes in rate of feed consumption. For this reason it is important that accurate estimates of voluntary intake during thermal stress be established.

Nutrient digestibility: Many authors have reported a positive relationship between ambient temperature and nutrient digestibility for ruminants. Although information relating diet digestibility to heat stress is not in total agreement, most data tend to support the hypothesis that digestibility is increased during heat stress. Some believe this results from decreased voluntary intake rather than from a direct effect of increased EAT. Ames and Brink (1977) used shorn lambs fed in controlled environmental chambers to determine the effect of ambient temperature on the digestibility of diet components. This study showed increased digestibility of dry matter, crude protein, and nitrogen- free extract as temperature rose from 15°C to 35°C. Crude fiber digestibility increased when temperature rose from 15 to 30°C, but was not increased at 35°C. No difference was found in ether extract digestibility during heat stress. Bhattacharya and Hussain (1974) reported that during heat stress sheep diets had lower digestibility except for crude fiber and nitrogen-free extract. They found that higher roughage (75%) diets were most affected. Perhaps variations in findings relating heat stress to diet digestibility are altered by roughage to concentrate ratio. Obviously, more knowledge is needed for different rations.

The dry matter digestibility lowered during cold (Blaxter and Wainman, 1961; Christopherson, 1976; Kennedy and Milligan, 1978; Young and Christopherson, 1974). Depressed digestibility with increased intake during cold is considered in combination, the advantages of the former would be partially offset by the latter. For example, increased consumption per unit of metabolic size from 10 to 0°C is 5.3%, but with decreased digestibility the net increase in digestible energy was only 2.7%. Christopherson (1976), who conducted extensive studies of digestibility during prolonged cold with both sheep and cattle, also found a temperature effect independent of level of intake. He reported that dry matter digestibility had a 0.31, 0.21, and 0.08 percent decline per °C cold stress for sheep, calves, and steers, respectively. Kennedy and Milligan (1978) suggest that cold effect on digestibility is greater with higher levels of food intake.

Energy requirement during cold stress: When exposed to EAT below the cool zone, energy expenditure must compensate for increased energy loss. Increased heat production during cold stress has been measured by several authors (Alexander, 1962; Bennett, 1972; Blaxter *et al.*, 1966; Graham *et al.*, 1959). Wind (Joyce and Blaxter, 1964), rain (Panaretto *et al.*, 1968) and wind and rain combinations (Blaxter *et al.*, 1966) have been shown to increase further the rate of heat loss of sheep exposed to cold. These findings suggest an apparent reduction in external insulation and result in increased rate of sensible heat loss when measured at a given thermal gradient. Use of effective ambient temperature measures such as wind-chill temperature (Ames and Insley, 1975) and insulatory value of the wetted fleece should provide similar estimates of heat loss When sheep are exposed to temperatures below the LCT, there are two factors that determine rate of heat loss: (1) thermal gradient between core temperature and ambient temperature, and (2) amount of insulation provided by tissue, fleece, and air. These factors can be used to estimate rate of heat loss, and therefore maintenance energy requirement for animals exposed to cold, by the following equation:

$$ME_m = {}_aW^{0.75} = b \times \Delta T/1,$$

Where, MEm = metabolizable energy for maintenance corrected for effective temperature (kcal ME/day), T = magnitude of cold (°C), i.e., difference between animal's lower critical temperatures and effective temperature, I = total insulation (°C/kcal/m^2/day), a = coefficient of maintenance requirement for animal in zone of thermoneutrality (kcal ME/day), b = surface area of animal (m^2) and Coefficient a is 127.8 kcal ME/day for sheep.

Table 1 shows the percentage increase in maintenance energy requirements at seven levels of insulation for five different weights. The system to estimate the listed values does have shortcomings and cannot be calculated without some error. First, the insulative value of the animal is not uniform over its entire surface. Indeed, small errors in estimating insulative value will lead to relatively large differences in energy required during cold. For example, Blaxter *et al.* (1959) reported conductive value of fleece (in similar sheep) ranges from 122 to 149 kcal/m2/24 h/°C/cm. That variation would result in a 111% error for a 50 kg lamb with 0.04°C/kcal/m2/day total insulation when estimating additional heat loss during cold. Second, the animal's ability to shunt blood to and from specific areas of the body reduces the accuracy of the estimates of insulation. Third, calculations assume that the animal is a sphere with no facing surfaces. When the system presented in above table is compared to observed increases in heat production for rather well defined sheep, the utility of the system can be assessed. Variations of up to 19.7% are noted; however, in each case insulative value was estimated, and increased metabolic heat production during cold exposure was measured for a relatively short period. While more work is obviously needed to improve estimates of insulation, in a general sense these data support increasing energy requirements of sheep based on estimated insulation and body weight.

Table 1 : Percent increase in maintenance energy cost per degree centigrade below lower critical temperature

Insulation (°C/kcal/m2/day)[a]	Sheep Weight (kg)				
	40	50	60	70	80
0.01	5.8	5.4	5.2	4.7	4.6
0.02	2.9	2.7	2.6	2.4	2.3
0.03	1.9	1.8	1.7	1.6	1.5
0.04	1.4	1.3	1.3	1.2	1.2
0.05	1.2	1.1	1.0	0.9	0.9
0.06	1.0	0.9	0.8	0.8	0.7
0.07	0.8	0.7	0.7	0.7	0.6

[a] Wool provides about 0.007°C/kcal/m2/day per cm depth (Blaxter *et al.*, 1959).

The options for increasing energy intake for animals fed *ad libitum* are more limiting than for those where adjustment can be accomplished by simply providing more feed. In this situation increasing caloric density by addition of fat or increasing relative amounts of feedstuffs with higher caloric densities (i.e., replacing roughages with concentrates) are possibilities. The former approach, however, is contrary to the notion of increasing heat increment during cold since fat is lower in heat increment compared with most feedstuffs. However, its high caloric density may still be used advantageously. The value of heat increment during cold has been mentioned previously, and, while this may prove valuable, it should be understood that heat increment for each unit of weight of roughages and concentrates is similar. However, heat increment is a higher percentage of digestible energy for roughages as compared with concentrates, so that calories supplied by the heat increment of roughage may be less expensive than those from a concentrate source. Consequently, from an economic standpoint energy costs may be reduced during cold by increasing roughages at the expense of concentrates. Moose *et al.* (1969) reported that feeds with high heat increments fed during cold have a sparing effect on net energy for production, thus allowing their use for gain. Brokken (1971) developed a model using the data of Lofgreen and Garrett (1968) to blend rations to improve performance during cold stress. This model is based on maximum use of heat increment and concludes that economic advantages do exist for altering rations during cold. The magnitude of this advantage is dependent upon relative ingredient prices, magnitude of cold, and the effect of cold on intake.

Energy requirement during heat stress: Expected increases in heat production during heat exposure of sheep have been reported, but little quantification of increased energy needs is available. During heat exposure, energy requirement increases because of energy expended during panting, sweat gland activity (Macfarlane, 1964) and the calorigenic effect of hormones. An additional factor when core temperature rises is the *Q*10 effect (Schmidt-Nielsen *et al.*, 1967). Whittow and Findlay (1968) calculated that the effect of increased rectal temperature accounted for as much as 62% of increased O_2 consumption in cattle and Ames *et al.* (1971) measured a 41% increase in O_2 consumption of sheep assuming *Q*10 = 2.0. It is apparent that increases during heat are nonlinear (Graham *et al.*, 1959) as opposed to linear increases during cold. Nonlinearity is to be expected because of the decreased efficiency of evaporative mechanisms and increased *Q*10 effect as heat stress becomes more severe (Ames *et al.*, 1971). More precise estimates of increased energy requirement during heat are further confounded by depressed appetite. The adjustment of diets during heat stress can be a practical approach toward minimizing the effect of heat even though increased maintenance requirement during heat is difficult to estimate accurately. McDowell (1972) and Brink and Ames (1978a) have reported nonlinear increases in maintenance energy during heat when maintenance is calculated as the difference between intake and gain.

Lofgreen (1974) confirmed the validity of formulating diets for relief of heat stress. His adjustment involved lowering heat increment of the diets while keeping net energy constant. These adjustments were accomplished by reducing the roughage content of the diets, adding dried beet pulp, and increasing fat content. Moose *et al.* (1969) found that low-concentrate diets (35%) had lowered heat increment than higher-concentrate diets (70%) when fed to lambs and reported that at temperatures above 25°C high heat increment can seriously impair the efficiency of diets containing higher percentages of roughage. Rea and Ross (1961), in a growing trial with lambs, concluded that lambs gain more rapidly in warm temperatures when given diets of 60% concentrate as compared to 40% concentrate.

Protein requirement of sheep: Protein requirement includes both that necessary to maintain nitrogen equilibrium (maintenance protein) and that needed for productive function. Ideally, dietary protein exceeding that needed for maintenance is used only for production (growth, wool, or milk); however, growth and other productive functions may be limited by available energy because of increased energy for maintenance during thermal stress. When energy is limiting, protein may then be catabolized and serve as an energy source (Crampton and Harris, 1969). Because of the relationship between energy and protein requirement, the direct effect of climate on energy requirement has a subsequent effect on protein required for growth or production. Data suggest no effect of thermal environment on protein required to maintain nitrogen equilibrium (Brink and Ames, 1978b). The frequently used protein-to-energy ratio for formulation of animal diets is not appropriate for describing diets during thermal stress when maintenance energy requirement and intake vary unless only protein and calorie values surplus to maintenance are used to calculate a ratio. Instead, when formulating diets with respect to the thermal environment, both energy and protein should be included to meet requirements for each nutrient separately, and the protein-to-energy ratio of the diet should be ignored. When energy requirement for maintenance increases (i.e., cold stress), Less energy is available for production, and consequently the protein-to-calorie ratio above maintenance levels increases. Ames and Brink (1977) have reported reduced protein efficiency ratio of lambs-during both cold and heat compared to thermo neutral zone (TNZ). Some workers have suggested a system for adjusting protein above maintenance to match expected growth rate of lambs exposed to thermal stress. When protein is adjusted, growth rate during thermal stress is not altered, but protein efficiency ratio is improved. When protein is a more expensive nutrient than energy, cost of gain is decreased. Table 2 indicates protein adjustments for a 27 kg lamb receiving a diet that is expected to result in 272 g average daily gain (ADG).

Table 2 : Protein adjustment for growing lambs

Deviation from Critical Temperature	Expected ADG (g)a	Maintenance Protein (g)b	Protein for Growth (g)	CP in Ration (%)c
20	54	33.2	17.0	2.4
15	132	33.2	41.0	5.8
10	195	33.2	60.8	8.6
5	236	33.2	73.6	10.4
Critical temperature	272	33.2	84.9	12.0
-5	222	33.2	69.3	9.8
-10	181	33.2	56.6	8.0
-15	136	33.2	42.5	6.0
-20	95	33.2	29.7	4.2

a- Ames *et al.*, 1971; b- Preston, 1966 ; c- Constant intake.

Thermal effects on lams performance

Exposure of sheep to thermal stress affects voluntary food intake and maintenance requirement as discussed previously. Obviously, average daily gain and feed required per unit of gain are also affected by thermal stress. Few studies have reported the effect of temperature on performance of growing lambs, but Ames and Brink (1977) conducted growth and efficiency studies for shorn lambs exposed to a wide range (- 5 to 35°C) of ambient temperatures. These lambs received a 50% concentrate (grain sorghum) and 50 roughage (alfalfa) diet.

Miscellaneous thermal factors affecting nutrition of sheep

The effects of high carbon dioxide levels on nutrition of sheep revealed reduced feed intake when exposed to 4% CO_2, but intake was inversely related to CO_2 concentration at exposure levels of 8, 12, 16, and 18%. Nutrient digestibility was not influenced by CO_2 levels up to 16%, but variable decreases were measured at 16 and 18% CO_2. Blaxter (1978) studied the effect of simulated altitude on sheep and found no difference in heat production or heat increment values when oxygen concentration in air was 150 ml/liter compared to 200 ml/liter. Confinement rearing of sheep has been estimated to reduce energy requirements by 30% (Parker, 1976). Direct measurement of heat production in commercial confinement management systems has not been done, but Young and Corbett (1972) reported that maintenance requirements were generally 60-70% greater for grazing sheep compared to housed animals. The need for a more precise estimate of effect of confinement on energy required for maintenance is needed. Harbers *et al.* (1975) reported that sheep acclimate to sound of 100 dB or less, however, intermittent noise was shown to increase nutrient digestibility during short-term exposure. Allden (1968) reported that feed consumption and utilization for weight gain were not affected in the long term by prolonged periods of under-nutrition. They reported that lambs subjected to restricted feed levels during the first 6 months of life failed to fully recover (in terms of weight) compared with lambs receiving adequate nutrition. However, when unlimited feed was available, when lambs were 6-12 months old, they completely recovered earlier weight loss. Graham and Searle (1975) held 4-month-old wethers at 20 kg live weight for 4 or 6 months then fed *ad libitum* to recover weight for age. They reported increased voluntary food intake during rehabilitation compared to controls. While heat production per unit metabolic size fell during weight stasis, it rose in the first month of recovery but remained less than controls. Gross efficiency was higher during the first week of recovery then returned to control values. Except for acute changes in intake and consequent efficiency during the first week of recovery following under nutrition, there appear to be no long-lasting nutritional differences in sheep receiving restricted levels of nutrition.

Migration stress

Migration of sheep takes place to overcome the stresses viz. feed and water scarcity, high environmental temperature or extreme cold. As soon as the sheep migrates from the stress is minimized to a negligible amount. Sheep migration is an ancient regular process in temperate and tropical regions of our country. The germination of vegetation in pastureland is either stopped or pasture is covered by snow due to extreme cold or heavy snow fall from December to March every year in temperate and hilly areas of the country. This results in feed scarcity due to in unavailability of pasture for suitable grazing of sheep. In this adverse condition of feed scarcity, sheep farmers along with their sheep migrate from temperate and hilly areas to plain areas during November-December every year. These migratory farmers graze their sheep on pastures available in plain area and subsequently return to their native areas during April. On the other hand sheep framers of tropical hot arid region in the condition of feed scarcity migrates along with their sheep to neighbouring states viz. Uttar Pradesh, Madhya

Pradesh, Haryana, Punjab etc. These migratory farmers graze their sheep on pastures available in the migratory area and subsequently return to their native areas during June. In general four types of migration Viz. short duration, long duration, long distance and short duration are prevalent in our country. Various types of migration are discussed below.

(i) *Short duration migration*: Under local adverse condition of occasional feed and water scarcity, sheep farmers along with their sheep migrate for a period of five to six months. These migratory farmers along with their sheep return to their native tract during favourable conditions. Short duration migration in arid regions has been in vogue since ages. The length of short duration migration depends on quantum of rainfall. The length of short duration migration increases during scarce rainfall, drought and famine while it decreases during good rainfall. Farmers along with their sheep leave their home tract in December and return to their home at the onset of monsoon.

(ii) *Long duration migration*: Some farmers along with their sheep migrate permanently for long duration due to locally deficit of fodder and pastureland. The local deficit of feed and pastureland persist for one or more years. As soon as the conditions happen congenial for sheep rearing, the farmers return to their native tract.

(iii) *Short distance migration*: Sheep farmers along with their sheep migrate to their neighbouring distracts or states due to local scarcity of feed and water. This type of migration takes place within a periphery of 200-300 km. For example, sheep of western Rajasthan migrate in the other districts of Rajasthan.

(iv) *Long distance migration*: This type of migration is of short as well as long duration. Possibility to occur long duration migration predominates during severe famine and drought conditions. Sheep farmers along with their sheep enter to their neighbouring states for distant places in search of feed and water. Farmers come back to their native tract as soon as the conditions return to normal for sheep rearing.

Nutrition management during migration

The study conducted in India established that the sheep fulfilled their requirements above maintenance from grazing during migration.

Thus, sheep are not under stress during migration as far as their maintenance requirement is concerned. However, nutrient requirements of ewes are higher during critical physiological stages viz. last quarter of lactation and early part of lactation. In view of poor pasture quality and high stocking density on grazing lands, such ewes remain underfed during gestation and lactation. Healthy lambs of optimum birth weight and their adequate nutrition through dam during pre-weaning phase is important for cost effective mutton production. Healthy lambs of comparatively higher birth weight suckling from optimum fed ewes grow faster and attain finishing weight at an early age. Therefore, the supplementation of ewes grazing on pasture is important for economic fat lamb production.

During gestation: The growth of fetus during first three and half months of pregnancy becomes slow and dam becomes able to maintain at normal level of feeding. In contrast, the growth of fetus becomes faster during later part of gestation (last six weeks of pregnancy). Therefore the nutrient requirement during later part of gestation with respect to DM, ME, DCP, Ca and P, respectively becomes 65, 90, 150, 160 and 165% higher than the maintenance. On the other hand, the biomass yield of community rangeland in most of the part of our country is low and insufficient to meet the nutrient requirement of ewes during later part of gestation. Besides the grazing on good pasture, concentrate supplementation @ 1% of body weight to ewes during last quarter of gestation enhanced their production performance, general condition as well as birth weight and growth rate of lambs. The birth weight of lambs born from concentrate supplemented ewes becomes higher from 800 to 850 g as compared to those not supplemented ewes (Chaturvedi *et al.*, 2001a; 2003). The subsequent daily gain of these lambs was also higher (15-45 g/day) during pre-weaning phase because the ewes reared on concentrate supplementation yielded higher milk (150-200 g/day) after parturition. Higher milk yield from concentrate supplemented ewes provided better nutrition to lambs during pre weaning phase.

During early part of lactation: The nutrient requirement of lactating ewes during first two months of lactation becomes twice of the maintenance requirement because mobilization nutrients towards milk production. In lactating ruminants, a complex interaction exists among the major substrates for milk synthesis i.e. acetate, glucose, amino acids and fatty acids and a multitude of regulatory hormones. The regulatory hormones those exert their influence on the galactopoietic process in epithelial cells of the mammary gland in maintaining milk secretion are insulin, prolactin, growth hormone (GH), thyroid hormone and glucocorticoides. Of these, insulin and GH are the key hormones in the homeorhetic control of lactation and are involved in the coordination of metabolism in body tissues. In fact, GH plays a significant role in the partitioning of nutrients away from tissue deposition and towards mammary gland for milk synthesis. Besides the grazing on good pasture, concentrate supplementation @ 1% of body weight to ewes during early part of lactation enhanced their production performance, general condition as well as growth rate of lambs. The daily gain of lambs nourished by supplemented ewes increased (25 g/day) due to higher daily milk yield by these ewes from 150-200 g (Chaturvedi *et al.*, 2003; 2007a). The lambs suckling from supplemented ewes got adequate nutrition during pre- weaning phase.

During gestation and early part of lactation: The nutrient requirements of ewes during last quarter of pregnancy and early quarter of lactation are higher due to the obvious reasons. Like the supplementation during late gestation or early lactation, concentrate supplementation @ 1% of body weight to ewes from last quarter of gestation to early part of lactation in addition to grazing also enhanced production performance and general condition of ewes as well as growth rate of lambs. The birth weight of lambs born from concentrate supplemented ewes was higher (1000 g) as compared to those not supplemented (Chaturvedi *et al.*, 2003). The growth rate of lambs nourished by supplemented ewes increased (55 g/day) due to higher daily milk yield by the ewes from 200-250 g (Chaturvedi *et al.*, 2003; 2007a). There exists a positive relationship between milk yield of the dams and pre weaning growth because the lambs meet their nutrient requirement from dam's milk (Singh *et al.*, 1973).

Feeding of lambs: Optimum feeding of lambs during pre and post weaning results in desired finishing weight at 5-6 months age for economic mutton production. The feeding methods of lambs during pre and post weaning are described below.

(i) *Pre-weaning phase*: It is established that nutrition of lactating ewes affects its milk yield which in turn influence the pre weaning growth. The efficiency of milk utilization for growth is during pre weaning phase ranges from 17 to over 30% in different studies (Sharma, 1998). Feeding management of lambs during pre weaning phase is a prerequisite for economic fat lamb production because it affects the finishing weight of fat lambs. Because of optimum biomass availability on the pastures, the desirable growth rate of pre weaner lambs is not achieved under field conditions. The lambs in the famers' flock achieve 68-78 g ADG. Under organized farm feeding management on *ad libitum* concentrate and free suckling, the pre weaning growth rate increased up to 172 g ADG in male Mutton synthetic lambs and 168 g ADG in female Malpura lambs (Arora *et al.*, 1986). ADG of Avivastra lambs maintained on free suckling and *ad libitum* creep mixtures varying in CP levels was 140 g with a feed conversion ratio of 1:3.4 during pre weaning phase (Santra and Karim, 1999). In another study, creep mixture containing 10% CP and 2.7 Mcal DE/kg feed was adequate to support 124 g ADG in pre weaner lambs (Karim *et al.*, 2001). An ADG of 156 g was achieved in pre weaning lambs maintained on free suckling to their dams and *ad libitum* feeding of creep mixture and *Zizyphus nummularia* (pala) leaves as source of roughage. Thus, besides the free suckling and good quality leguminous hay or dried tree leaves, creep mixture of 16% CP and 60% TDN should be offered *ad libitum* to lambs for their optimum growth during pre weaning phase. Creep mixture should be prepared by using ground maize, groundnut oil meal, sunflower oil meal, milk powder, wheat bran, mineral mixture and common salt 50, 15, 10, 5, 18, 1 and 1, respectively in parts. Besides, vitamin blend at the rate of 25 g per quintal and quality animal protein supplement should be included in creep mixture to balance the amino acids.

(ii) *Post-weaning phase*: During migration feeding of weaner lambs can be done under two feeding systems viz. extensive, semi intensive.

Extensive feeding system: Under field conditions, most of the farmers maintain their lambs under this system i.e. the lambs are maintained exclusively under grazing on degraded rangelands for 8-10 hrs. However due to inadequate nutrient supply through grazing alone, the lambs achieve 18-20 kg finishing weight at the age of 5-6 moths (Chaturvedi *et al.*, 2000; 2001b). Weaner lambs reared for mutton production should attain the finishing weight of 25-30 kg at 5-6 months of age otherwise it seems uneconomical in terms of benefit cost ratio. Therefore, economic fat lamb production does not permit to adopt the extensive feeding of lambs under field conditions.

Semi-intensive feeding system: Under this system of feeding management, fat lambs are grazed on rangelands for 8-10 hrs and thereafter, concentrate mixture @ 1.5 to 2.5% of the body weight is offered to fat lambs. This system of fat lamb feeding is followed by few farmers under field conditions wherein little of concentrates (barley, dal churi, bran) in the form of supplement is fed. However, the quantities of concentrates offered by the farmers remain low in terms of nutrient supply to exploit the production potential of lambs. Therefore, it is recommended that besides the free grazing of weaner lambs on rangeland, concentrate mixture @ 1.5 to 2.0% of their body weight would provide 25 to 30 kg finishing weight at 6 and 9 months of age, respectively (Karim *et al.*, 2004). Grazing with supplementation on established pasture has still higher production potential since established Cenchrus (*Cenchrus ciliaris*) pasture stocked as per carrying capacity with concentrate supplementation @ 1.5% of body weight provided 27.3 kg finishing body weight in fat lambs at 6 months age (Shinde *et al.*, 1995). In other studies, free grazing of weaner lambs on reseeded Cenchrus pasture with concentrate supplementation of 300 g/lamb/day provided 23.0-27.7 kg finishing weight and 80-106 g ADG with 9-12% feed conversion efficiency (Karim and Verma, 2000; Chaturvedi *et al.*, 2007b). The feed cost in terms of Rupee per kg gain ranged from 28 to 30 under semi-intensive feeding of lambs. Under field conditions, weaner fat lambs grazing on community rangeland with supplementation of concentrate mixture @ 1 to 1.5% of their body weight achieved 21.6 to 24.2 kg finishing weight with 54 to 127 g ADG (Chaturvedi *et al.*, 2000; 2005). The cost benefit ratio due to concentrate supplementation under farmers' field ranged from 1.45 to 1.75 indicating that farmers get additional profit of Rs. 1.45 to 1.75 on per Rupee spent. In general farmers spent Rupees 135 to 150 per fat lamb in terms of concentrate supplement and they get Rupees 300 to 400 more on a supplemented fat lamb. Thus, net profit per fat lamb ranges from Rupees 165 to 250 on selling of fat lambs. Concentrate mixture containing 10% DCP and 65% TDN should be used in supplementation of weaner fat lambs under semi-intensive feeding system. This concentrate mixture can be prepared by using maize, barley, groundnut oil meal, sunflower oil meal, wheat bran, mineral mixture, common salt and vitamin blend 25, 25, 15,15, 18,1 and 1, respectively in parts and vitamin blend (20 g/q). Further, the concentrate mixture can be made cost effective by using animal feed grade damaged wheat at the rate of 10 kg /q.

Transportation stress

It is important to look at the process of transporting animals, as many animals are injured or even die during transport. Also, many carcasses destined for slaughter are bruised, and this represents a huge loss to the livestock industries. In beef, losses from bruising and losses through death and serious injury of railed cattle are very costly.

Treatment of animals before transport: Animals are usually handled intensively before transport. They are grouped together, often in unfamiliar groups ready for loading onto a truck. Mixing of strange animals will cause restlessness and agonistic encounters leading to bruising. Mixing of unfamiliar animals at any stage results in increase in agonistic behaviour, poorer welfare and meat quality. Once the social organisation has been established, fighting diminishes. If sheep, cattle and pigs can be grouped together for two or three days before transporting so that they become familiar with each other, the stress of transporting will be much less. If young animals are familiarized with the yards and handling procedures, then the potential stress will be reduced. Groups of animals should be about the same size for transportation. One of the key factors is the handling by the stockman. If the animals are handled quietly and gently, the stress will be reduced. The design of yards to improve the flow of sheep is important. The use of dogs in herding sheep often causes the animals to stand alert as a primary response, often accompanied by a covert increase in heart rate (Baldock and Sibly, 1990). Drafting prior to transport is more stressful than dipping and drenching, and is represented by a significant increase in plasma cortisol levels. The use of a crush can often cause a greater stress response than drafting or penning.

Loading and unloading facilities: This is a critical area in the process of transport. Poorly designed loading ramps, over-use of force and lack of understanding of animal behaviour all contribute to both physical damage and stress. There is a difference in design for chutes used only for unloading trucks to those which are used for both loading and unloading. If at all possible, it is better to have a type of chute for loading and another for unloading. A chute used for unloading any type of livestock should be wide and straight to provide a clear, unimpeded path. This type of chute must never be used to load livestock. A chute used for loading only, should have high solid sides to prevent animals from seeing out, and a narrow curved single-file chute is the most efficient. If the chute is going to be used for loading and unloading, care must be taken not to curve it too sharply. If the chute has too sharp a curve the animals will often baulk and refuse to leave the truck because the chute appears to be a dead end. A common problem in poorly designed loading chutes is bunching and jamming of livestock at the junction between the single file ramp and the crowding pen. Bruises are prevented if this transition is smooth and gradual. Where a wide variety of trucks is going to be used, adjustable chutes are ideal, as they can be raised and lowered to load or unload the bottom or top deck. Straight raceways cause animals to baulk, because they perceive the truck as a dead end. There are conflicting data to suggest that loading animals from darkened to illuminated areas reduces stress or increases efficiency. Initially after loading, urination and defecation is very frequent but declines as transport begins. During rail transit, cattle rarely alter their position. They align their bodies at right angles to the direction of travel. In horses, transport by road over short and long distances is found to suppress feeding behaviour, elevate heart rate and lead to unnatural body postures causing weight loss and fatigue. Over-loading and under-loading of trucks increases bruising.

Transport and adjusting to a new environment: The actual transporting of an animal is probably one of the most traumatic periods of its life. It leaves the security of a known environment and is subjected to motion, changes in temperature, ventilation, noise levels, smells and changes in group size and density. Short transportation periods cause rises in sheep plasma cortisol of moderate to high levels (66 ng/ml) compared to minimal disturbance levels (36 ng/ml). Long transportation periods and a new environment cause complex changes in corticosteroid levels in both directions, which may extend over some months. Transport can cause physical bruising and damage. Besides, it also causes transit erythema (red skin due to urine soakage), transit tetany (metabolic upset caused by lack of food and water), transit or shipping fever (a bacterial infection (Pasteurellosis) in fatigued animals), and fatigue and exposure.

Behaviour of animals during transport and on arrival at new environment sheep: The effect of different modes of transport on the behaviours of sheep has been reviewed by Kilgour (1976).

(i) *Road transport:* Following completion of a road journey, lambs grazed briefly (2–3 hs) and spent the next 23 hrs resting, then returned to their field. Where animals have not been able to lie down, resting takes precedence over feeding or arrival (Ewbank, 1975).

(ii) *Air transport:* Little is known of the effects of flight on sheep or lambs, but one study suggests that unshorn sheep in two-tiered crates suffered some ventilation problems while the plane was not in flight.

(iii) *Sea transport:* The main problems seem to be in the handling of the sheep. Sheep must be conditioned to eat pellets before boarding the ship; hand-fed sheep that are used to this type of feed do not have this problem. Ship hygiene and Salmonella losses, poor ventilation with high temperatures and humidity, fluctuating and changing diets can all cause problems.

(iv) *Rail transport:* On a long rail trip, adult Merino sheep seldom lie down in railway trucks, even on a five-day journey. When rested after traveling for two to four days without water or food, no preference for either was shown, but after five days there was a preference for water. In the rest pens, only 0.4 kg of lucerne hay per sheep was eaten in 24 hrs. During long transportation where a lairage period is allowed, sheep require sufficient time to drink before a subsequent journey is undertaken (Jackson *et al.*, 1999).

If feed is provided during a break from transport, and sheep are not provided with sufficient drinking time, dehydration can result due to consumption of large amounts of dry feed (Jackson *et al.*, 1999). Sheep require a lairage of more than 8 hrs to gain any real benefit (Knowles, 1998). The behaviour of sheep generally is little changed under conditions of poor welfare, such as injury or overcrowding (Knowles, 1998). Thus sheep seem to be particularly tolerant of transportation compared with other farm animal species. During transportation of sheep by road, they ate less, ruminated less and lay down less (Ewbank and Kent, 1990). Sheep will ruminate while being transported and if they are transported at low enough densities, they will lie down and be able to rest to some extent. However, they do not lie down as much as they would in a static pen at a similar stocking density (Knowles, 1998). Driving conditions play a role in the behaviour of sheep during road transport. The rougher the journey, the more likely is bruising and the greater is the increase in cortisol levels (Ruiz-de-la-Torre, 2001). After a trip lasting 24 hrs, slaughter lambs did not return to normal drinking patterns until 14 hrs into recovery; normal eating patterns were not resumed until 16 hrs later and even after 24 hrs of recovery; the lambs were not standing as much as prior to transport (Knowles, 1998). Sheep that are to be transported by sea on journeys of less than 8 hrs should be fasted of water and food (18 hrs prior to departure) to reduce the incidence of death or sickness. On longer journeys, the sheep should be fed 2–3 hrs prior to the start of the journey (Shupe, 1985). Ewes introduced to a new flock show minimal grazing and increased vocalising and walking. The newly introduced sheep tend to remain at the edge of the flock (Baldock and Sibly *et al.*, 1990). Exposure to a familiar feed (e.g., hay) will increase the food and water consumption (up to 4.9 times) of sheep transported to a new environment (Hall *et al.*, 1993).

Nutrition management during transportation

Sheep are transported for the purpose of migration, sale and export. Sheep are either transported through walking or by a motor vehicle. In general sheep are transported on their feet for migration or short distance nearby animal fair for selling purpose. Sheep are transported from rural areas to mega cities for selling purpose. Most of these sold sheep are slaughtered for meeting the mutton requirement in these mega cities. It is established that sheep spend nearly 8 hrs in feeding or grazing, 8 hrs in rumination and 8 hrs in resting. A substantial reduction in rumination was observed during transportation. Hence, nutrient supply particularly energy and protein is also reduced at tissue level. This results in reduction of body weights and debility. Further, seller may get low price of their sheep to be sold. Sheep should be fed easily digestible diets containing higher density of nutrients prior to the overnight transportation. If sheep are transported for more than a overnight then there should be a facility of feeding above types of diets during day hours. Sheep should also be offered *ad libitum* clean and good quality drinking water. Feeding management helps in overcoming the transportation stress.

References

Alexander, G. 1962. Temperature regulation in the new-born lamb. V. Summit metabolism. Australian Journal of Agricultural Research 13:100.

Alexander, G. 1968. The environment and neonatal survival in sheep in Australia. In: Proc. Ecol. Soc. Australia 3:125.

Alexander, G. 1974. Heat loss from sheep. In: Heat Loss from Animals and Man (J.L. Monteith and L.E. Mount, Eds.), Butterworth, London.

Allden, W.G. 1968. Under nutrition of the Merino sheep and its sequelae. I. Growth and development of lambs following prolonged periods of nutritional stress. Australian Journal of Agricultural Research 19: 621.

Ames, D.R., and Insley, L.W. 1975. Wind-chill effect for cattle and sheep. Journal of Animal Science 40: 161.

Ames, D.R. and Brink, D.R. 1977. Effect of temperature on lamb performance and protein efficiency ratio. Journal Animal Science 44: 136.

Ames, D.R., Nellor, J.E. and Adams, T. 1971. Energy balance during heat stress in sheep. Journal of Animal Science 32: 784.

Ames, D.R., Brink, D.R. and Willms, C.L. 1980. Adjusting protein in feedlot rations during thermal stress. Journal of Animal Science 50: 1.

Arora, A.L., Prasad, V.S.S., Gupta, D.C., Maru, A., Gupta N. and Mahajan, J.M. 1986. All India coordinated research project on sheep breeding for mutton. Annual Report, Central Sheep and Wool Research Institute, Avikanagar Rajasthan, India.

Baldock, N.M., Sibly, R.M, 1990. Effects of handling and transportation on the heart rate and behaviour of sheep. Applied Animal Behaviour Science 28: 15-39.

Bennett, J.W. 1972. The maximum metabolic response of sheep to cold: Effects of rectal temperature, shearing, feed consumption, body posture and body weight. Australian Journal of Agricultural Research 23: 1045.

Bhattacharya, A.N., and Hussain, F. 1974. Intake and utilization of nutrients in sheep fed different levels of roughage under heat stress. Journal of Animal Science 38: 877.

Bhattacharya, A..N. and Uwayjan, M. 1975. Effect of high ambient temperature and low humidity on nutrient utilization and on some physiological responses in Awassi sheep fed different levels of roughage. Journal of Animal Science 40: 320.

Blaxter, K.L. 1978. The effect of simulated altitude on the heat increment of feed in sheep. British Journal of Nutrition 39: 659.

Blaxter, K.L. and Wainman, F.W. 1961. Environmental temperature and the energy metabolism and heat emission of steers. Journal of Agricultural Sciences (Cambridge) 56: 81.

Blaxter, K.L., Graham N. McC. and Wainman, F.W. 1959. Environmental temperature, energy metabolism and heat regulation in sheep. III. Metabolism and thermal exchanges of sheep with fleeces. Journal of Agricultural Sciences (Cambridge) 52: 41.

Blaxter, K.L., Clapperton, J.L. and Wainman, F.W. 1966. The extent of differences between six British breeds of sheep in their metabolism, feed intake and utilization, and resistance to climate stress. British Journal of Nutrition 20: 283.

Brink, D.R. and Ames, D.R. 1975. Effect of ambient temperature on lamb performance. Journal of Animal Science 41: 264.

Brink, D.R. and Ames, D.R. 1978a. Thermal stress and NEm, of lambs. In: 11th Annual Midwest ASAS.

Brink, D.R. and Ames, D.R. 1978b. Effect of thermal stress on protein for maintenance. In: 70th ASAS, p. 407.

Brokken, R.F. 1971. Formulating beef rations for improved performance under environmental stress. American Journal of Agricultural Economics 53: 79.

Chaturvedi, O.H., Mishra, A.S., Karim, S.A. and Jakhmola, R.C. 2000. Effect of supplementary feeding on growth performance of lambs under field condition. Indian Journal of Small Ruminants 6: 110-112.

Chaturvedi, O.H., Mishra, A.S., Santra, A., Karim, S.A. and Jakhmola, R.C. 2001a. Effect of supplementary feeding during late gestation on production performance of ewes grazing on community rangeland. Indian Journal of Animal Sciences 71: 714-717.

Chaturvedi, O.H., Bhatta, R., Verma, D.L. and Jakhmola, R.C. 2001b. Effect of supplementary feeding on growth performance of lambs grazing on community rangeland. In: Proc. IV National Seminar of Indian Society for Sheep and Goat production and Utilization (ISSGPU), November 9-11, Coimbatore, India. pp. 41.

Chaturvedi, O.H., Bhatta, R., Santra, A., Mishra, A.S. and Mann, J.S. 2003. Effect of supplementary feeding of concentrate on nutrient utilization and production performance of ewes grazing on community rangeland during late gestation and early lactation. Asian-Australasian Journal of Animal Sciences 16: 983-987.

Chaturvedi, O.H., Verma, D.L. and Mann, J.S. 2005. Benefit cost ratio and impact of concentrate supplementation to weaner lambs during active phase of growth. In: Proc. National Seminar on "Extension Methodological Issues in Impact Assessment of Agricultural and Rural Development Programmes", January 21-23, University of Agricultural Sciences, Bangalore, India. pp. 318-319.

Chaturvedi, O.H., Verma, D.L., Singh, N.P. and Mann, J.S. 2007a. Effect of concentrate supplementation on production performance of ewes grazing on community rangeland. Indian Journal of Animal Sciences 77: in press.

Chaturvedi, O.H., Kumar, S., Mishra, A.K., Arora, A.L. and Karim, S.A. 2007b. Effect of complete feed or grazing and supplementation of lambs on performance, nutrient utilization and feed cost of production. In: Proc. of International Tropical Animal Nutrition Conference Volume II, October 4-7, National Dairy Research Institute, Karnal (Haryana), India. p. 247.

Christopherson, R.J. 1976. Effects of prolonged cold and the outdoor winter environment on apparent digestibility in sheep and cattle. Canadian Journal of Animal Sciences 56: 201.

Crampton, E.W. and Harris, L.E.. 1969. Applied Animal Nutrition, 2nd ed. W.H. Freeman and Company, San Francisco.

Ewbank, R. 1975. The transport of animals by road. United States Animal Welfare. Symp. p. 3-9.

Ewbank, R. and Kent, J.E. 1990. The behaviour of road transported sheep. Journal of Applied Animal Behavioural Science 26: 294.

Giacomini, G. E. 1979. Effect of fluctuating temperature on lamb performance. Unpublished M.S. Thesis. Kansas State University, Manhattan.

Graham, N. McC. and Searle, T.W. 1975. Studies of weaner sheep during and after a period of weight stasis. I. Energy and nitrogen utilization. Australian Journal of Agricultural Research 26: 343.

Graham, N. McC., Wainman F.W., Blaxter, K.L. and Armstrong, D.G. 1959. Environmental temperature, energy metabolism, and heat regulation in sheep. I. Energy metabolism in closely clipped sheep. Journal of Agricultural Sciences (Cambridge) 52: 13.

Hall, S.G., Schmidt, B. and Broom, D.M. 1993. Feeding behaviour and the intake of food and water by sheep after a period of deprivation lasting 14 hours. Animal Science 64: 105-110.

Harbers, L.H., Ames, D.R., Davis, A.B. and Ahmed, M.B. 1975. Digestive responses of sheep to auditory stimuli. Journal of Animal Science 41: 654.

Jackson, R.E., Cockram, M.S., Goddard, P.J., Doherty, O.M., McGlip, I.M. and Warren, N.K. 1999. The effects of 24-hr water deprivation when associated with some aspects of transportation on the behaviour and blood chemistry of sheep. Journal of Animal Welfare 8: 229-241.

Joyce, J.P. and Blaxter, K.L. 1964. The effect of air movement, air temperature and infrared radiation on the energy requirements of sheep. British Journal of Nutrition 18: 5.

Karim, S.A. and Verma, D.L. 2000. Growth performance of weaner lambs under protocol of intensive feeding or grazing with supplementation. Indian Journal of Animal Sciences 71: 586-588.

Karim, S.A., Santra, A. and Singh, V.K. 2001. Preweaning growth response of lambs fed creep mixtures with varying levels of energy and protein. Small Ruminant Research 39: 137-144.

Karim, S.A., Santra, A. and Singh, V.K. 2004. Lamb feeding for mutton production. Central Sheep and Wool Research Institute, Avikanagar (Rajasthan), India.

Kennedy, P.M. and Milligan, L.P. 1978. Effect of cold exposure on digestion, microbial synthesis and nitrogen transformations in sheep. British Journal of Nutrition 35: 105.

Kilgour, R. 1976. Sheep behaviour: Its importance in farming systems, handling, transport and pre-slaughter treatment. In: Proc. Sheep Assembly and Transport Workshop. Western Australia, Department of Agriculture, Perth, October.

Knowles, T.G., 1998. A review of road transport of slaughter sheep. Veterinary Record 143: 212-19.

Knowltoh, P. H., W. H. Hoover, and B. R. Poulton. 1969. Effects of higher carbon dioxide levels on nutrition of sheep. J. Anim. Sci. 28:554.

Lofgreen, G.P. 1974. Ration formulation for relief from heat stress. In: 13th California Feeders Day, Imperial Valley. Experimental Station, El Centro, California. p. 81.

Lofgreen, G.P. and Garrett, W.W. 1968. A system for expressing net energy requirements and feed values for growing and finishing beef cattle. Journal of Animal Science 27: 793.

Macfarlane, W.V. 1964. Terrestrial animals in dry heat: Ungulates. In: Handbook of Physiology, Section 4, Adaptation to the Environment. American Physiology Society, Washington, D.C. p. 509

McDowell, R.E. 1972. Improvement of Livestock Production in Warm Climates. W.H. Freeman and Company, San Francisco.

Moose, M.G., Ross C.V. and Pfander, W.H. 1969. Nutritional and environmental relationships with lambs. Journal of Animal Science 29: 619.

Mount, L.E. 1979. Adaptation to Thermal Environment. University Park Press, Baltimore.

Panaretto, B.A., Hutchinson J.C.D. and Bennett, L.W. 1968. Protection afforded by plastic coats to shorn sheep. In: Proc. Australian Society of Animal Production 7: 264.

Parker, C.F. 1976. Feeding and breeding ewes in confinement housing. Ohio Sheep Day Report.

Preston, R.L. 1966. Protein requirements of growing-finishing cattle and lambs. Journal of Nutrition 90: 157.

Rea, J.C. and Ross, C.V. 1961. Effect of energy-protein relationship, physical form of feed and environmental temperature on lambs. Journal of Animal Science 20: 948.

Ruiz-de-la-Torre, J.L., Velarde, A., Diestre, A.., Gispert, M., Hall, S.J.G., Broom, D.M. and Manteca, X. 2001. Effects of vehicle movements during transport on the stress responses and meat quality of sheep. Veterinary Record 148: 227-29.

Samra, J.S. 2004. Review and analysis of drought monitoring, declaration and management in India. Working paper 84. International Water Management Institute. Colombo, Sri Lanka.

Santra, A. and Karim, S.A. 1999. Effect of protein levels in creep mixture on nutrient utilization and growth performance of pre weaner lambs. Small Ruminant Research 33: 131-136.

Schmidt-Nielsen, K., Crawford, E.C., Newsome Jr. A.E., Rawson, K.S. and Hammel, H.T. 1967. Metabolic rate of camels: Effect of body temperature and dehydration. American Journal of Physiology 212: 341.

Sharma, V.K. 1998. Influence of pre weaning nutrition on post weaning gain of lambs. Ph. D. Thesis. Chaudhary Charan Singh University, Meerut (U.P.), India.

Shinde, A.K., Karim, S.A., Singh, N.P. and Patnayak, B.C. 1995. Growth performance of weaner lambs and kids under intensive and semi-intensive feeding management. Indian Journal Animal Sciences 65: 830-833.

Shupe, W.L. 1985. Transporting sheep to pastures and markets. American Society of Agricultural Engineers. No. 85: 6008.

Singh, V.K., Tiwari, S.B., Singh, L.B. and Homode, J. 1973. Efficiency of milk production and its conversion into lamb weight in Malpura, Chokla and crossbred ewes. Indian Veterinary Journal 50: 1199-1204.

Soderquist, H.G. and Knox, K.L. 1967. Temperature-energy relationships in fattening lambs. Journal of Animal Science 26: 930.

Webster, A.J.F., Hicks, A.M. and Hays, F.L. 1969. Cold climate and cold temperature induced changes in the heat production and thermal insulation of sheep. Canadian Journal of Physiology and Pharmacology 47: 553.

Whittow, G. C., and J. D. Findlay. 1968. Oxygen cost of thermal panting. Am. J. Physiol. 214:94.

Young, B.A. and Christopherson. R. 1974. Effect of prolonged cold exposure on digestion and metabolism in ruminants. In: Proc. International Livestock Environment Symposium, Lincoln, Nebr p. 75

Young, B.A. and Corbett, J.L. 1972. Maintenance energy requirement of grazing sheep in relation to herbage availability. Australian Journal of Agricultural Research 23: 57.

□□□

Chapter 18

Stall Feeding System in Small Ruminants : Future Perspectives

U.B. Chaudhary*, T.K. Dutta, M.K. Tripathi, and P. Tripathi
Central Institute for Research on Goats, Makhdoom, Farah, Mathura, UP-281 122 (India)

Intensive feeding to small ruminants is a challenging job to the nutritionists, as this sector is coming up very fast as an entrepreneur to meet out the increasing demand of meat in Indian sub-continent. A marked imbalance between total ruminant livestock units and available permanent pastures exists in India. Attempts should be made to explore better utilization of small ruminant friendly feed resources. Conventional ingredients like grains and oilseed cakes are used mainly for milk production purposes from cows and buffaloes; therefore, small ruminants are forced to relish on traditional grazing and browsing materials. Hence, utilization of processed agricultural and agro-industrial by-products including enriched straws/hay for intensive small ruminant rearing system is the need of the hour. To increase the production potential of goats in terms of meat, milk and skin, it is necessary to incorporate proper feeding schedule under intensive or semi-intensive system of production. For proper growth of various breeds of small ruminants in India approximately 60-65 million tones of dry matter is required every year. If 40% concentrate is offered, the amount of concentrate will be around 24-26 million tones, whose availability is very scarce due to diversion of concentrate ingredients for milk production from cows and buffaloes. Indian farmers are reluctant to spend much on feeding practices; hence, research should focus on development of economic feeding schedule of small ruminants using cheaper and locally available feed resources for improved productivity under intensive system of production. Improvement of nutritional quality of existing feed and fodder through processing and conservation could be another option to increase the production potential. The small ruminant husbandry sector in India is not an organized sector like poultry; but, now-a-days many young entrepreneurs are coming up to set up goat/sheep units in India with scientific rearing practices; hence, development of suitable and economic feeding schedule for goats/sheep under different physiological stages is required.

Grazing land for small ruminants

Goat and sheep husbandry is an integral component of livelihood and life style of millions of small holder farmers in difficult areas of the country. Goats/sheep are reared on common property resources (CPR), rangelands, stubbles, wasteland and fallow land under extensive system. Moreover, sheep rearing in the country is not grain based and hence small ruminants do not compete with human and organized dairy sector for food and shelter rather live in absolute harmony with man and nature. Goat husbandry plays a significant role in supplementing family incomes and generating gainful employment in the rural unorganized sector particularly among the landless, small and marginal farmers and women besides providing cheaper and nutritious meat and milk to rural people. Total area available for grazing of sheep and goats in 1951 was 82.1 million ha, which included uncultivable land, fallow land and permanent pastures. The grazing land has now decreased to 43.3 million ha due to land reclamation for conventional agriculture and conversion of cultivable land to colonization. Total area under grazing has deceased by 47% during the last five decades while during the period the small ruminant population has increased by 105%. This has resulted in over stocking and over grazing of available land by the animals. Due to such problems, we must focus on development of economic feeding schedule for small ruminants in the country for greater sustainability of small ruminant husbandry sector and to meet out the demand of increasing human population by scientifically using locally available feed resources.

Intensive feeding to small ruminants

The intensive system of small ruminants feeding management includes grazing on developed pastures and/or feeding completely in stalls on cultivated fresh or conserved fodders, crop residues and concentrates. Although goats prefer to browse as compared to grazing, they are quite capable of making efficient use of cultivated pastures for meat and milk production. Stocking rates of 16 to 60 goats per hectare are feasible depending on the type of grass, rainfall pattern in the region, level of fertilization and the presence and absence of legumes and fodder trees. This system requires high labour and capital investment and is suitable for only intensive meat production from goats. In addition to providing better milk, growth and carcass quality it removes pressure from the grazing lands. Therefore, the present paper focuses on the nutritional requirements for small ruminants *vis-à-vis* production potential of goat/sheep under intensive system of management.

Pre-weaning growth

The colostrum has a greater role for proper growth and immunity of the newly born kids/lambs; which has a direct bearing on the immunity status during early stage of growth, as kids are very susceptible to *E. coli* and other enteric infection. It was observed that quality of goat colostrum may be improved when the pregnant does were fed with yeast culture (*Saccharomyces cerevisiae*), which may have direct bearing on the health of newly born kids (Table 1).

Table 1 : Effect of yeast culture (*Saccharomyces cerevisiae*) on chemical composition of colostrum in goat (Kumar and Dutta, CIRG, unpublished data)

Parameters	Control	Yeast culture
pH	6.54±0.04	6.39±0.04
Total solid	26.94±1.81	28.93±2.12
Fat	4.13±0.71	5.39±0.71
SNF	22.81±1.40	23.54±1.49
Protein	15.90±1.11	16.48±0.89
Lactose	6.0±0.73	6.18±1.08
Ash	0.91±0.04	0.88±0.03

The weight gain of suckling kids is closely associated with the level of milk intake during the early stages of the milk feeding period and declines with declining milk production. One unit of kid live weight gain results from 7 kg of goat's milk. Weaning of kids can take place at around 3 months of age, depending on the management system. With either artificial rearing or natural suckling the success of early weaning systems onto solid food depends on the state of rumen development at weaning which is governed by the ingestion of solid feed. Solid feed intake is negatively related to milk intake. Good quality creep feed and roughage should be available to kids from the age of three-four weeks onwards.

When the milk supply of goats is inadequate or absent or when it is necessary to remove the progeny as part of the management system artificial rearing is practiced with milk replacer. Milk substitute/ replacer can be given warm and should contain 16-24% fat and 20-28% protein for kids. The milk replacers (with 24% CP) developed at CIRG and simultaneously tested in other centers were found palatable and effective to maintain the normal growth of kids without any harmful effects (Dutta *et al.*, 2003a). However, growth performance with mothers's milk was found best in kids. When natural suckling is practiced the adoption of early weaning and partial suckling with the objective of increasing commercial milk yields is of great importance. However, the growth of the offspring should not be affected by the lower milk consumption. Milk replacer with added pre-biotic (Terre *et al.*, 2007) and pro-biotic (Fleige *et al.*, 2007) preparations improve pre-weaning performance, thus weaning weights. Addition of lectulose or mannan oligosaccharides (3%) in milk replacer and a probiotic at the rate of 10^9 CFU (colony forming unit)/kg after one week of birth increased intake, body weight and affect the morphology of the small and large intestine in pre-weaning stage. Experiments with varying plane of nutrition during pre-weaning phase, were conducted under feeding regimens of grazing (C0; Control), grazing and *ad libitum* creep mixture supplementation (C-AL; Concentrate) or grazing, *ad libitum* creep mixture and milk replacer supplementation (C-ALMR). Lamb during pre-weaning phage had a growth rate (ADG) of 90, 138 and 154 g/day, respectively in C0, C-AL and C-ALMR groups (Bhatt *et al.*, 2008). Lambs were allowed to suckle respective dam in morning and evening till 90 d of age, and fed *ad lib* green leaves of *Ailanthus excelsa* (AL) after grazing. The results revealed that milk replacer feeding did not have added advantage once lambs given free access to a creep mixture.

Birth weight of lambs is an indicator of pre-weaning performance but nutritional state of lamb during pre-weaning phase of growth influence the weaning weight. Weaning weight of the lambs has significant impact on post-weaning performance; thereby on finishing weight, carcass quality and quantity. Nutritional manipulation of pre-weaner lambs enhances performance (ADG up to 165 g) and weaning weight (17.4 kg) and varies with level of nutrition. The pre-weaner lambs maintained on free suckling and *ad libitum* creep mixture with varying levels of crude protein (CP) indicated that 18% CP in the creep mixture was adequate for the desired rate of gain of pre-weaner lambs. The lambs in pre-weaning phase, on an average consumed 83 g dry matter (DM), 12.0 g digestible crude protein (DCP) and 48 g total digestible nutrient (TDN)/kg $W^{0.75}$ amounting to 54 g DCP/Mcal digestible energy (DE) and had 140 g ADG. Early rumen development is also known to improve weaning weights. Live microbes feeding facilitate early establishment of rumen microflora and rumen development. Three yeast strains, *Kluyveromyces marximanus*, *Saccharomyces cerevisiae* and *S. uvarum*, and a mixed culture (1:1:1) were evaluated for their value as probiotics in lamb feeding. Lambs were offered *ad libitum* a creep mixture and *Zizyphus nummularia* leaves, and yeasts cultures (1.5-2×10^{10} live cells/ml) were dosed orally 1 ml/kg live weight. During 63 days of experiment, lambs gained at the rate of 165 g/day with mixed yeast culture feeding and lambs consumed 50 g DCP and 5.34 MJ ME (metabolizable energy) to harvest 165 g ADG. A diet containing 8.45 MJ ME and 80 g DCP in each kg of feed DM was found to be optimum for harvesting 165 g ADG and more than 16 kg weaning weights (Tripathi *et al.*, 2007a). Pre-weaner lambs consumed concentrate dry matter between 3.0 to 3.6% of live weight to have an ADG ranging from 137 to 163 g.

For rapid weight gains, creep diets must be palatable, contain high energy and adequate protein (14 to 18%), minerals (especially calcium, since grains are low in calcium, and ideal calcium to phosphorus ratio of the diet should be 2:1) and vitamin supplement. The relationship show that nitrogen intake between 13 to 17 g/day during pre-weaning phase of growth required for having a daily growth rate ranging from 120 to 160 g (Tripathi *et al.*, 2011b). Pre-weaner lambs require 7.5 to 9.5% DCP to achieve a daily growth rate of 120 to 175 g. Experiments conducted by Karim *et al.* (2001), Santra and Karim (1999), Bhatt *et al.* (2008) and Tripathi and Mishra (2008) revealed that the pre-weaning growth of lambs could be manipulated through optimized nutrition inputs. A daily gain of 137 to 163 g can be achieved with feed conversion (feed/gain) ratio (FCR) of 2.5 to 3.1 with dry matter intake of 3.6 to 4.0% of live weight and maintaining an intake of 42.2 to 59.9 g DCP and 4.19 to 5.91 MJ ME/day. The required dietary ME (MJ/kg) ranged between 8.0 to 8.9 and DCP between 7.5 to 8.5%. To harvest optimum growth rate of pre-weaner lambs, the fed ration must ensure nitrogen intake between 12 to 16 g/day. The N requirement was 109 mg (range 71 to 134 mg), while ME was 5.14 kJ (4.19 to 5.91) and DM 4.2 g (between 3.7 to 4.9 g) for each g of gain during pre-weaning phase of growth. An ADG of 150 g can be achieved in pre-weaner lamb with FCR of 2.66 from DMI (629 g/day or 3.6 % of BW) of a diet containing 8.22 MJ ME and 80 g DCP in each kg diet.

Nutrition for post-weaning/finisher small ruminants

Post-weaned kids: Energy plays a major role for post-weaned growth, however, balance of C:N should be maintained properly for optimum growth in kids. The dry matter requirements for one kg body weight gain were decreased in the groups of Beetal kids fed high-energy diets. The DCP and TDN intakes were lowered in the groups fed low protein-high energy diets. This suggested better FCE on low protein- high energy feeding regimes (Garg *et al.*, 1994). Saikia *et al.* (1995) observed ADG of 25, 48.61 and 68.33 gram on iso-nitrogenous diets fed to goats containing 15% CP and 60, 65 and 70% TDN. Saikia and Baruah (1997) also reported the daily gain in body weight lowest in low energy group and highest in high-energy group of crossbred goats. Goonewardene *et al.* (1998) and Shahjalal *et al.* (1992) also reported significantly higher ADG (27.5%) in goats fed high protein and high-energy diets than those fed low levels of protein and energy. The higher intake of energy and protein by goats resulted in higher FCE (Goonewardene *et al.*, 1998; Shahjalal *et al.*, 2000). Rekhate *et al.* (2004) found that daily live weight gain was considerably higher in Indian goats fed gram straw based pellets and fulfilled the requirement of goats growing at 108 g per day under stall fed condition. The complete feed pellet (CP% 12 and TDN 60%) containing *Cajanus Cajan* straw as basal roughage gave 51.11g ADG in weaned (5-10 months) Barbari kids (Dutta *et al.*, 2003b). Das and Ghosh (2007) observed that the ADG increased significantly ($P<0.01$) with increased level of concentrate supplementation and maximum ADG was observed when concentrate was supplemented @ 1.5% of body weight in Sikkim local male kids (3-6 months of age).

Several studies have been conducted on fattening of indigenous and crossbred kids under *ad libitum* feeding on concentrates including barley grain, maize grain, oil cakes, wheat and rice brans, molasses etc. and roughages including tree leaves, cultivated grasses and legumes in the ratio of 40:60, 50:50 and 60:40. The male kids weaned at 2-3 month age and fed under feedlot system achieved slaughter weights of 25 kg at 5 to 6 months age with a dressing % of 48 to 51 (Parathasarthy *et al.*,1984). Ration (60% roughage, Arhar straw based) with low protein-low energy (TDN 55%, CP 12%) was found economical to give more than 50g ADG with 10% FCE (gain/DMI) in post weaned Barbari kids (Prakash *et al.*, 2006). Supplementation of concentrate mixture containing CP19.51%, TDN 70.35% and blended with strategically added minerals increased nutrients intake, utilization of nutrients and growth performance in weaned kids with better quality carcass traits under semi-intensive system of management. Supplementation of such concentrate mixture tended to increase fat percentage in the carcass under intensive feeding (Dutta, *et al.* CIRG, unpublished data). Crop residues like cotton stalks can be incorporated in the rations of growing sheep and goats without any adverse effect and this type of feeding reduces the cost of feed for meat production (Reddy and Reddy *et al.*, 2003). Further, such feeding helps in rearing of sheep and goats under intensive system. Complete pelleted feed with 50% concentrate and 50 % roughage (*C. cajan*) may result into higher body weight gain by 25.34g/day with additional DM intake of 229 g/day/kid and 3.02 kg extra meat yield at 9 months of age over TMR fed Jamunapari kids (Singh *et al.*, 2010). Higher level of dietary energy (11.98 MJ ME/kg DM) was suggested for optimizing growth and reproductive performance of female goats under grazing condition (Hossain *et al.*, 2003). Rations prepared with agro-industrial by-products and new feed resources (siris pod-with seeds and cowpea pod-without seeds) were effective in Barbari kids with normal growth, although DCP intake was lower. However, Jamunapari and Marwari kids responded with lower TDN and DCP intakes coupled with lower weight gain considering the breed characteristics (Dutta and Singh, 2009).

The kids maintained under semi-intensive system reached the target live weight of 25 kg earlier than those under intensive system. The kids under semi-intensive required less feed for a kg of gain than those under intensive feeding. The dressing % was superior under intensive system. The bone and lean % was higher under semi-intensive and fat % under intensive system (Singh and Sahu, 1997). Average daily gains under intensive system were higher in lambs than kids while they were similar under semi-intensive system (Shinde *et al.*, 1995). The daily gains, milk intake, meat quantity and quality and feed efficiency were found superior in the Sirohi, Marwari and Kutchi kids maintained under semi-intensive as compared to those maintained under intensive or extensive system. The milk yield during 150 days of lactation was higher under intensive system than that under semi-intensive and extensive systems and in Sirohi does than that in Kutchi and Marwari does (Singh, 1993). Studies have shown that the low-grade roughages like straws and stovers added with little oil cakes, brans and mineral supplements may be very suitably compounded into complete feed blocks and pellets for goats. The technology of compounding complete feed blocks is advantageous in several ways. Feed blocks require less than one-third storage space as compared to the raw material and their transportation is easier and cheaper. Selectivity of ingredients by the animals from the feed blocks is avoided. Palatability and nutritive value of the ration is improved. Live weight gains and milk production are also improved under complete feeding technology. Some works under intensive feeding to post-weaned kids have been summarized in the table 2. Feeding of monensin to stall feeding goats was found detrimental to the rumen ciliate population (Chaudhary *et al.*, 2004). Daily ration consisting of barley straw 750 g crushed barley grain 160 g and cotton seed cake 150 g supplemented with common salt and mineral mixture may be used as maintenance ration for Barbari kids weighing about 28 kg (Upadhayay and Chaudhary, 2005). All roughage containing diet (cultivated green fodder and dry fodder) was found similar to the concentrate based diet, which may be economical also in goats (Chaudhary and Singh, 2004).

Silvipasture development initiatives on common lands/degraded lands can have significant impact on livestock feeding system and on the types and number of livestock that people keep. Three tier improved silvi-pasture system containing *Leucaena leucocephala, Dichrostachys nutan* and *Cenchrus ciliaris* increased dry matter intake, DCP, TDN and DE (Mcal/kg DM) by 7.6, 22.8, 14.17 and 13.04%, respectively over natural pasture in grazing Barbari goats (Sharma and Bhattacharya, 1993). At CIRG , Makhdoom a comparative study was carried out on natural pasture (ravine area grazing), *C. ciliaris* pasture and *Zyziphus* sp. + *C. cilaiaris* silvipasture under grazing condition; it was observed that goats grazed in silvi-pasture system had 6.7 times higher average daily body weight gain over natural system and 1.62 times over *C. ciliaris* pasture. However, dry matter intakes were 4.66,

4.46 and 3.46 kg per 100 kg body weight recorded in *Zizyphus sp.* + *C. ciliaris* silvi-pasture, *C. ciliaris* pasture and natural pasture, respectively.

Table 2 : Effect of feeding on growth, dressing percentage and meat composition in goats

Goat breed /region	Feeding system	ADG (g/d)	Dressing (%)	Meat protein (%)	Meat fat (%)	References
Barbari/UP	*Ad libitum* Complete pelleted feed (R:C=40:60)	88.53	45.61	20.18	2.56	Dutta and Das, 2008-09
Barbari/UP	*Ad libitum* Complete pelleted feed (R:C=60:40)	79.83	45.48	19.86	2.75	Dutta and Das, 2008-09
Barbari/UP	Concentrate mixture (CP 15%, TDN 65%) @ 2% of the BW + *ad libitum Cajanus* straw + 300-400 g green fodder	53.60	42.90	18.66	4.55	Dutta, *et al.*, 2003a
Barbari/UP	Grazing 5-6 h + Barley grain @ 2% of the body weight.	65.07	46.10	19.19	2.35	Dutta, *et al.*, 2008
Barbari/UP	Grazing 5-6 h + Concentrate mixture @ 2% of the body weight	75.65	49.12	18.84	2.97	Dutta, *et al.*, 2008
Barbari/UP	Concentrate mixture @2% of the body weight+ gram straw *ad libitum* + green fodder *ad libitum*	72.61	48.34	18.37	3.24	Dutta, *et al.*, 2008
Jamunapari/ UP	*Ad libitum* complete pelleted feed	90.23	47.56	-	-	Singh *et al.*, 2010
Jamunapari/ UP	*Ad libitum* TMR	64.89	44.71	-	-	Singh *et al.*, 2010
Bidari/ Karnataka	*Ad libitum* Complete pelleted feed (R:C=40:60) with CP 12% and TDN 55%	65.33	49.43	21.68	4.79	Dutta, *et al.*, 2003b
Non-descript (Mehboobnagri)/ AP	*Ad libitum* Complete pelleted feed (R:C=40:60) with CP 12% and TDN 55%	69.42	49.90	17.53	4.60	Reddy and Reddy, 2003 Dutta, *et al.*, 2003c
Non-descript/ Maharastra	*Ad libitum* Complete pelleted feed (R:C=40:60) with CP 12% and TDN 55%	70.27	51.18	19.57	5.67	Rekhate *et al.*, 2004 Dutta, *et al.*, 2003c

Dutta, *et al.*, 2003c

Intensive feeding to sheep

Sheep production around the world, including India is the grass/ range based production system. Stall-feeding to sheep for wool production is not an economical proposition hence neither practiced nor advocated. Stall-feeding for fat lamb production is the only system, which is in practice to have high quality and heavier carcass at an early age of animal that add health promoting bio-molecules to human food chain. The pre- and post-weaning growth of lambs manipulated under various nutrition and feeding protocols to optimize growth potential are discussed in the following section.

Nutrition and feeding of post-weaning lambs: Nutritional management during post weaning phase of growth decides the marketability of lambs for different purposes. Dry matter intake for feeder lambs varies between 3.5 to 4.0% of their body weight. Actual intake, however, depends on several factors, namely, age, size and condition, growth rate, amount of feed offered, competition for available feed, palatability, physical form of feed, energy and fibre content of feed, ambient temperature and humidity and availability of quality water. The post-weaning ration should be a high concentrate ration with a minimum of 16% crude protein, 0.6% calcium, and 0.30% phosphorus. The post-weaning diet should be high energy and should contain 18 to 20% protein (as-fed basis) for the first 3 weeks and 14 to 17% protein thereafter. It is doubtful whether higher levels of protein will result in sufficiently better lamb performance to justify the cost. Growth of post-weaning lambs can be manipulated by feeding of fermented feed, using mushroom by-product, rice bran and barley bran in the ratio of 50:20:25 fermented for 30 days at 60% moisture level. Feeding of dried fermented product up to 5% affected the growth performance, carcass traits, meat quality and altered fatty acid content favorably (Song *et al.*, 2007). Studies conducted at CSWRI, Avikanagar indicated that for harvesting desired finishing weight, khejri, ardu, pala leaves, conserved cultivated grasses and crop residues as roughage sources (Karim and Patnayak, 1991), maize, barley, jowar, bajra or its part replacement by livestock feed grade damaged wheat as energy (Karim and Patnayak, 1992; Tripathi *et al.*, 2007b) and groundnut cake, mustard cake (Tripathi *et al.*, 2001), til cake, cotton seed cake, gour korma or its part replacement by urea as protein (Karim and Patnayak, 1993) supplement in 50-60% concentrate based complete feed can be used in least cost ration formulation for intensive mutton production. Sole concentrate feeding is not recommended in intensive feeding because of higher incidence of enterotoxaemia. However, high concentrate feeding for enhanced growth of lamb, may induce rumen acidosis, which may impair growth performance of lambs. High concentrate diets supplemented with 1.5% sodium bicarbonates helps to maintain rumen pH near neutrality, which enhance growth by 35% (Tripathi *et al.*, 2004).

Crossbred lambs: Researchers (Karim and Santra, 2000; Santra and Karim, 2001; Tripathi *et al.*, 2001, 2007a; Santra *et al.*, 2002; Anil Kumar *et al.*, 2002 Singh *et al.*, 2006) conducted experiments on crossbred lambs to assess the growth performance and nutrient utilization to optimize growth of crossbred lambs. Crossbred lambs during post-weaning phase required dietary ME 10.4 MJ in each kg diet and DCP 10.44% to have average daily gain 112 g (46 to 162 g). Lambs consumed 74.68 g DCP and 886 g feed dry matter. N intake was 21.77 g/day accounting 0.194 g N intake for each g of gain, while ME and DCP intake was 84 kJ (range 78.8 to 95.9 KJ) and 0.51 g (range 0.35 to 0.60 g), respectively for each g of gain. Dry matter intake in crossbred lambs has poor relationship with average daily gain, Lambs consumed 7.26 g dry matter for each g of gain, with mean daily feed intake of 885.9 g for an average daily gain of 125.3 g, which ranged between 86 to 172 g/day. These lambs during post weaning phage of growth had dry matter intake 3.81, which ranged from 3.5 to 4.2% of live weight, while optimum DMI estimated to be 3.65% of live weight. With optimum dry matter intake lambs had ADG 136 g (108 to 162g/day) and feed conversion (kg feed/kg gain) 6.94 ranging from 5.7 to 8.17 under optimum nutrition.

Native lambs: Native lambs during post weaning phase of growth attained an average daily gain of 123g, which ranged from 74 to 186g under optimum nutritional manipulations. Under various experimental protocols, lambs consumed daily 21.2g of N (12.7 to 28.0g), 783g of feed DM (528 to 1040 g), 7.3 MJ of ME and 65.3 g of DCP, which accounted respectively to 0.177 g of N (range 0.166 to 0.307 g), 6.6 g of feed DM (4.97 to 9.78 g), 59.6 kJ of ME and 0.62 g of DCP intake for each g of gain. The mean DCP level among various diet fed to weaner lambs ranged between 7.3 to 9.9% with mean DCP of 9.04%, however 7.3% dietary DCP seems optimum for having better rate of growth. In comparison to cross bred lambs, the native lambs have better opportunity to improve live weight gain beyond 180 g/day by manipulating dry matter intake, which has linear relationship with average daily gain. The DMI in terms of per cent of live weight ranged from 2.9 to 5.0% with mean value of 3.68%. However, optimum DMI for better growth was worked out to be 2.9 to 3.5% of BW. Maintaining a DM intake between 2.4 to 5.0 with mean of 3.52 %, the native lambs had an ADG of 142 g (97.6 to 196 g). The feed conversion ration of lambs can also be predicted using developed mathematical equation for native lambs. The Dietary requirement for native lambs for higher growth rate was worked out in each kg diet is 9.5 MJ ME and 9.04 % DCP to harvest an ADG of 124 g with feed conversion ratio of 6.92 (Bhatt *et al.,* 2011; Dutta *et al.,* 2008; Tripathi *et al.,* 2004, 2006, 2007a; Tripathi and Karim, 2011; Raghuvansi *et al.,* 2007; Karim and Santra, 2000; Santra and Karim, 2000, 2002; Santra *et al.,* 2002).

Nutritional manipulation experiments carried out under stall-feeding during pre- and post-weaner phase of lambs growth to optimize mutton production show that the pre- and post weaning growth of lambs can be manipulated through optimized nutrition inputs (Tripathi *et al.,* 2011a,b). During pre-weaning growth, a daily gain of 137 to 163 g can be achieved with feed conversion (feed/gain) ratio of 2.5 to 3.1, dry matter intake of 3.6 to 4.0% of live weight and maintaining an intake of 42.2 to 59.9 g DCP and 4.19 to 5.91 MJ ME/ day. The required dietary ME (MJ/kg) ranged between 8.0 to 8.9 and DCP 7.5 to 8.5%. To harvest optimum growth rate of pre-weaned lambs the fed ration must insure nitrogen intake between 12 to 16 g/ day. The lambs during post-weaning phage of growth had dry matter intake 3.81, which ranged from 3.5 to 4.2% of live weight, while optimum DMI estimated to be 3.65% of live weight. With optimum dry matter intake, lambs had ADG 136 g (108 to 162g/day) and feed conversion (kg feed/kg gain) 6.94 ranging from 5.7 to 8.17 under optimum nutrition. Native lambs during post-weaning phase of growth attained an average daily gain of 123 g, which ranged from 74 to 186 g under optimum nutritional manipulations. The dietary requirement of native lambs for higher growth rate in each kg diet was 9.5 MJ ME and 9.04% DCP to harvest an ADG of 124 g with feed conversion ratio of 6.92. With the available research, it was evident that, in comparison to cross bred lambs, the native lambs had better opportunity to improve live weight gain beyond 180 g/ day by manipulating dry matter intake, which had linear relationship with average daily gain. The dietary N intake supported live weight gain at higher levels of intake. Therefore, genetic potential of native lambs for mutton production was found to be similar and on some occasions better than the crossbred lambs if exploited under optimum nutrition and management.

Nutrition for reproduction: Inadequate nutrition, particularly of energy, depressed the reproductive performance of extensively or intensively managed sheep and of Indian breeds of goats. Sexual maturity of sheep and goats is advanced by good feeding and the energy stimulates oestrus activity within the normal breeding season, ovulation rate, fertilization and survival of ova and the maintenance of the resultant embryos to term as viable lambs. Body condition at mating, achieved over a longer period i.e. the period between one reproductive cycle and the next, has a greater effect on ovulation rate and barrenness than flushing (i.e. increasing the level of nutrition in the immediate pre-mating and mating period). High producing dairy ewes or goats, require a dry period to achieve maximum prolificacy.

The level of feeding after weaning of female lambs or kids intended for replacements depends on the age at mating. Usually lambs or kids are mated for the first time when they reach 60–80% of their mature weight. This weight is accomplished with proper feeding and management at the age of 8–10 months in France, Norway, India and Cyprus. There is a very slow growth of foetus during the first 100 days of gestation with more than 80% taking place during the last 8 weeks of gestation. Stress in pregnant goats during late pregnancy increased with increasing kidding percentage as indicated from the total birth weight of kids as a percentage of the dam's weight which was 8, 13.5 and 18.5 for goats giving birth to singles, twins or triplets, respectively. Foetal energy requirements in the final stage of pregnancy are 1.5MJME/kg foetus/day. This means that a 50 kg ewe carrying twins would have an energy requirement of about 2.5 to 3 times that of a non-pregnant ewe. However, these full requirements are not recommended and 25% lower requirement would reduce birth weight of lambs by only 10% which is acceptable on both biological and economic considerations. Low levels of energy during late pregnancy lead to pregnancy toxaemia particularly in goats. However, high levels of feeding during pregnancy can lead to pregnancy toxaemia in sheep and kidding difficulties. The performance of Damascus goats in the last stages of pregnancy was similar with either medium (15.7MJME/day) or high (20.1 MJME/day) levels of energy, but a low level of energy (11.3MJME/ day) resulted in pregnancy toxaemia.

Reducing methane production for higher goat productivity: Ruminal methane production is a nutritionally wasteful process that represents a significant energy loss to the host animal. Usually 6-15% of the gross energy in the feed is lost through methane production depending on the level of feeding, composition of the diet and digestibility. Therefore, researches on rumen methanogenesis and its inhibition were conducted with the aim of increasing feed efficiency; more energy and carbon would become available for volatile fatty acids (VFA) production in rumen, by shifting electron flow from methane to propionate production. Recently, it has become clear that methane has an important role in global warming and destruction of the ozone layer. Methane is more efficient in absorbing infrared energy than carbon dioxide, therefore, despite its very low concentration; the contribution of methane to global warming is not negligible.

The effect of starch based and fiber based concentrates on enteric CH_4 production (Lovettet *et al.*, 2005) demonstrated that increased fiber based concentrate use at pasture reduced enteric methane per kilogram of animal product. An increased proportion of starch in the diet changes ruminal volatile fatty acid concentration in such a way that less acetate and more propionate is formed and the supply of hydrogen for methanogenesis is limited the pH decreases as the proportion of propionate increases which reduces methanogenic activity (Walichnowski and Lawrence, 1982) Concentrate feeding has shown to reduce methane output by reducing the protozoa population (Van Soest, 1982). However increased levels of concentrates may result in health problems. Ruminants offered *ad libitum* diets rich in starch, or infused with a single dose of a soluble carbohydrate (such as glucose) tends to exhibit increased propionate production, lower methane production and a decreased acetate/propionate ratio. This shift in rumen fermentation pattern has been attributed to an increase in the rate ruminal fermentation, which favors the production of propionate over methane.

The proportion of concentrate within the diet has been reported to be negatively correlated with methane emissions. Lovettet *et al.* (2005) demonstrated that increased fiber-based concentrate use at pasture reduced enteric methane per kilogram of animal product (19-26 and 16.02g of CH_4 1 kg of fat-corrected milk). A positive response to high levels of starch-based concentrate (grains) on methane reduction has also been reported by others (Beauchmin and MC Jin, 2005). An increased proportion of starch in the diet changes ruminal volatile fatty acid concentrations in such a way that less acetate and more propionate is formed and the supply of hydrogen for methanogensis is limited. Also, the pH decreases as the proportion of propionate inverse, which reduces methanogenic activity (Walichnowski and Lawrence, 1982). However, increased levels of concentrates may result in health problems e.g. acidosis. The cost of production in the case of concentrate feeding limits their use in low cost systems.

Benchaar *et al.* (2001) used a modeling approach to assess the effectiveness of different existing nutritional strategies to reduce methane production from ruminants simulated statelier included dry matter intake. Forage to concentrate ratio, nature of concentrate (fibrous versus starchy concentrate) type of starch (slowly versus rapidly degraded) forage species (legume versus grass) forage maturity, forage processing, and upgrading and supplementation of poor quality pages (straw) methane production was reduced (-7% and 40%) by increasing dry matter intake and the proportion of concentrate in the diet. The use of more digestible forage (less mature and processed forage) resulted in a reduction of methane production, methane production was lower with legume than with grass forage (-28%). legumes feeding generally have higher dry matter intake and produce more milk solids, this reduces methane emissions per unit of milk or meat production, Hegarty (1999) fund that methane production per gram of live weight gain was reduced significantly when animals were shifted from low digestible pasture to high digestible pasture. Methane emissions per unit of fed intake can be reduced by use of grass cultivars selected for improved animals performance.

Conclusion

Landless, small and marginal farmers rear goats/sheep in the Indian subcontinent. Therefore, considering the economic condition of the farmers we have to develop feeding schedule which should fit the economic viability of these farmers. Since, the grazing area/ rangeland in the country is gradually reducing and at the same time human demand for meat is increasing; therefore, to match this gap we have to develop suitable economic feeding schedule for small ruminants under stall feeding/intensive system. However, following approaches should be taken for stall feeding to small ruminants:

- Locally available and non-competitive (with large ruminants) feed ingredients should be selected for economic ration computation for small ruminants under stall-feeding.

- Community land should be enriched with seeding/reseeding of legume and non-legume grasses on regular interval for greater sustainability of the pasture. Panchayeti Raj (system) should take the key role for such enrichment of community grazing land in the villages for higher and quality fodder yield.
- For commercial goat/sheep farms scientific feeding schedule should be developed for pre and post weaning kids; pregnant and lactating animals for ensuring higher growth and milk production.
- Breed specific packages for feeding should be developed for meeting out the nutritional requirements of goats/sheep under different agro-climatic conditions of the Indian sub-continent.

References

Anil Kumar, G.K., Panwan, V.S., Yadav, R.R. and Sihag, S. 2002. Mustard cake as a source of protein for growing lambs. Small Ruminant Research 44: 47-51.

Benchaar, C., Pomar, C. and Chiquette, J. 2001. Evaluation of diet strategies to reduce methane production in ruminants: a modeling approach. Canadian Journal of Animal Science 81: 563-574.

Beauchemin, K.E. and Mc Jin, S.M. 2005. Methane emissions from feedlot cattle fed barley or com diets. Journal of Animal Science 83: 656-661.

Bhatt, R.S., Tripathi, M.K., Verma, D.L. and Karim, S.A. 2008. Effect of different feeding regimes on pre-weaning growth rumen fermentation and its influence on post-weaning performance of lambs. Journal of Animal Physiology and Animal Nutrition 93: 568-573.

Bhatt, R.S., Soren, N.M., Tripathi, M.K. and Karim, S.A. 2011. Effect of different levels of coconut oil supplementation on performance, digestibility, rumen fermentation and carcass traits of Malpura lambs. Animal Feed Science and Technology 164: 29-31.

Chaudhary, U.B. and Singh, Nawab. 2004. Rumen protozoal population and fermentation pattern as affected by all roughage diet in goats. Indian Journal of Animal Sciences 74: 292-295.

Chaudhary, U.B., Upadhayay, R.S. and Singh, Nawab. 2004. Effect of feeding monensin and vitamin E on rumen fermentation in goats. Indian Journal of Animal Sciences 74: 980-982.

Das, A. and Ghosh, S.K. 2007. Effect of partial replacement of concentrates with jackfruit (*Artocarpus heterophyllus*) leaves on growth performance of kids grazing on native pasture of Tripura, Indian. Small Ruminant Research 67: 36-44.

Dutta, T.K. and Das, A.K. 2008-09. Project report of XI/NFRPT/-2 entitled "Development of feeding strategies for goats under intensive and semi-intensive systems. In: Annual Report 2008-09, Central Institute for Research on Goats, Makhdoom, Farah, Mathura, UP, pp 58-62.

Dutta, T.K. and Singh, N.P. 2009. Voluntary feed intake, growth, rumen fermentation and nutrient utilization in different breeds of Indian goats reared under intensive system. Indian Journal of Animal Sciences 79: 311-315.

Dutta, T.K., Rao, S.B.N. and Singh, Nawab. 2003a (Eds.). Technical Report on "Development and evaluation of milk replacers in kids under different geo-climatic regions of India". Central Institute for Research on goats, Makhdoom, Farah, Mathura, UP.

Dutta, T.K., Agnihotri, M.K. and Singh, Nawab. 2003b. (Eds.). Technical Report on "Response of feeding complete broiler rations in different Indian kids for optimum growth and quality chevon production". Central Institute for Research on goats, Makhdoom, Farah, Mathura, UP.

Dutta, T.K., Tripathi, P. and Singh, N. 2008. Final Report of AP-Cess funded project on "Development of supplementation strategies for goats under field condition" Central Institute for Research on Goats, Makhdoom, Farah, Mathura, UP.

Fleige, S., PreBinger, W., Meyer, H.H.D. and Pfaff, M.W. 2007. Effect of lectulose on growth performance and intestinal morphology of pre-ruminant claves using milk replacer containing *Enterococcus faecium*. Animal 1: 367-373.

Garg, M.C., Narang, M.P. and Chauhan, J.S. 1994. Effect of plane of nutrition on growth and nutrient utilization in Beetal kids. Indian Journal of Animal Production and Management 10: 147-151.

Goonewardene, L.A., Okine, E., Patrick, N., Patrick, D., and Day, P.A. 1998. Effects of feeding high protein and high energy diets to six breeds of goats. In: Proc. 8th World Conference on Animal Production, Seoul National University, Seoul, 1: 204-205.

Hegarty R.S. 1999. Mechanisms for competitively reducing ruminal methanogenesis. Australian Journal of Agricultural Research 50: 1299–1306.

Hossain, M.E., Shahjalal, M., Khan, M.J. and Hasanat, M.S. 2003. Effect of dietary energy supplementation on feed intake, growth and reproductive performance of goats under grazing condition. Pakistan Journal of Nutrition 2: 159-163.

Karim, S.A. and Patnayak, B.C. 1991. Feeding different roughage sources in complete feed of lambs. Annual Report, CSWRI, Avikanagar, Rajasthan, India, p. 38.

Karim, S.A. and Patnayak, B.C. 1992. Growth performance of weaner lambs on rations with different energy sources. Annual Report, CSWRI, Avikanagar, Rajasthan, India, p. 25.

Karim, S.A. and Patnayak, B.C. 1993. Performance of weaner lambs on rations with different protein sources. Annual Report, CSWRI, Avikanagar, Rajasthan, India, p. 20.

Karim, S.A. and Santra, A. 2000. Growth performance of Malpura and cross bred lambs under intensive feeding. Small Ruminant Research 37: 287-291.

Karim, S.A., Santra, A. and Sharma, V.K. 2001. Pre-weaning growth response of lambs fed creep mixture with varying levels of energy and protein. Small Ruminant Research 41: 137-144.

Lovette, D.K., Stack, L.J., Lovell, S., Callan, J., Flynn, B. and Hawkins, M. 2005. Manipulating enteric methane emissions and animal performance of late-lactation dairy cows through concentrate supplementation at pasture. Journal of Dairy Sciences 88: 2836-2842.

Parthasarthy, M., Singh, D. and Rawat, P.S. 1984. Performance of feedlot kids on different dietary regimen. Indian Journal of Animal Sciences 54: 130-131.

Prakash, B., Dutta, T.K. and Siddiqui, I.A. 2006. Effect of plane of nutrition on nutrient utilization and performance of Barbari kids. Indian Journal of Animal Nutrition 23: 29-33.

Raghuvansi, S.K.S., Prasad, R., Tripathi, M.K. Mishra, A.S., Chaturvedi, O.H., Misra, A.K., Saraswat, B.L. and Jakhmola, R.C. 2007. Intake, performance, nutrient utilisation, rumen fermentation and rumen microbial enzymes of lambs maintained on complete feed blocks or grazing and supplementation. Animal (Cambridge) 1: 221-226.

Reddy, G.V.N. and Reddy, J. Linga. 2003. Effect of cotton stalks based complete diet on growth and carcass characteristics in sheep and goat in field condition. Indian Journal of Animal Nutrition 20: 97-100.

Rekhate, D.H., Madavi, V.B., Dhok, A.P. and Patil. 2004. Evaluation of arhar and gram straw based pelleted complete feed in goat. Indian Journal of Animal Nutrition 21: 257-260.

Saikia, G. and Baruah, K.K. 1997. Feed conversion efficiency and relative cost of growth production of crossbreed (Beetal x Assam local) goats fed three levels of energy. Small Ruminant Research 17: 279-282.

Saikia, G., Baruah, K.K., Buragohain, S.C., Saikia, B.N. and Pathak, N.N. 1995. Feed intake, utilization of nutrients and growth of Assamese x Beetal fed three levels of energy. Small Ruminant Research 15: 279-282.

Santra, A. and Karim, S.A. 1999. Effect of protein levels in creep mixture on nutrient utlisation and growth performance of pre-weaner lambs. Small Ruminant Research 33: 131-136.

Santra, A. and Karim, S.A. 2000. Growth performance of faunated and defaunated Malpura weaner lambs. Animal Feed Science and Technology 86: 251-260.

Santra, A. and Karim, S.A. 2001. Nutrient utilization and growth performance of cross bred lambs under intensive feeding. Small Ruminant Research 41: 277-282.

Santra, A. and Karim, S.A. 2002. Nutrient utilization and growth performance of defaunated and faunated lambs maintained on complete diets containing varying proportion of roughage and concentrate. Animal Feed Science and Technology 101: 87-99.

Santra, A., Karim, S.A. and Chaturvedi, O.H. 2002. Effect of concentrate supplementation on nutrient intake and performance of lambs of two genotype grazing a semi arid rangeland. Small Ruminant Research 44: 37-45.

Shahjalal, M., Galbraith, H. and Topps, J.H. 1992. The effect of changes in dietary protein and energy on growth, body composition and mohair fiber characteristics of British Angora goats. Animal Production 54: 405-412.

Shahjalal, M., Bishwas, M.A.A., Tareque, A.M.M. and Dohi, H. 2000. Growth and carcass characteristics of goats given diets varying protein concentration and feeding level. Asian-Australasian Journal of Animal Science 13: 613-618.

Sharma, K. and Bhattacharya N.K. 1993. Silvipastoral system in relation to goat farming, Asian livestock XVIII 10: 111-114.

Shinde, A.K., Karim, S.A., Singh, N.P. and Patnayak, B.C. 1995. Growth performance of weaner lambs and kids on intensive and semi-intensive feeding management. Indian Journal of Animal Sciences 65: 830-833.

Singh, N.P. 1993. Milk yield and composition in three goat breeds under three systems of feeding management. In: VI Animal Nutrition Research Workers Conference, OUAT, Bhubaneshwar, September13-16.

Singh, N.P. and Sahu, B.B. 1997. Chevon production in three goat breeds under two feeding systems. Indian Journal of Animal Sciences 67: 87-89.

Singh, S., Kundu, S.S., Negi, A.S. and Singh P.N. 2006. Cow pea (*Vigna unguiculta*) legume grain as protein source in the ration of growing sheep. Small Ruminant Research 64: 247-254.

Song, Y.M., Lee, S.D., Chowdappa, R., Kim, H.Y., Jin, S.K. and Kim, I.S. 2007. Effect of fermented Oyster mushroom (*Pleurotus ostreats*) by-product supplementation on growth performance, blood composition and meat quality. Animal 1: 301-307.

Terre, M., Calvo, M.A., Adelantado, C., Kocher, A. and Bach, A. 2007. Effects of mannan oligosaccharides on performance and microorganism feacal counts of calves following an enhanced growth feeding program. Animal Feed Science and Technology 137: 115-125.

Tripathi, M.K. and Karim, S.A. 2011. Effect of individual and mixed yeast culture feeding on growth performance, nutrient utilisation and microbial protein synthesis in lambs. Animal Feed Science and Technology 155: 163-178.

Tripathi, M.K. and Mishra, A.S. 2008. Glucosinolate in animal nutrition: A Review. Animal Feed Science and Technology 132: 1-27.

Tripathi, M.K., Mishra, A.S., Misra, A.K., Mondal, D. and Karim, S.A. 2001. Effect of substitution of groundnut with high glucosinolate mustard (*Brassica juncea)* meal on nutrient utilization, growth, vital organ weight and blood composition of lambs. Small Ruminant Research 39: 261-267.

Tripathi, M.K., Santra, A., Chaturvedi, O.H. and Karim, S.A. 2004. Effect of graded levels of $NaHCO_3$ supplementation on ruminal fluid pH, feed intake, nutrient utilization, growth performance and blood biochemical constituents of lamb on high concentrate diets. Animal Feed Science and Technology 111: 27-39.

Tripathi, M.K., Karim, S.A., Chaturvedi, O.H. and Singh, V.K. 2006. Effect of *ad libitum* tree leaves feeding with varying levels of concentrate on intake, microbial protein yield and growth of lambs. Livestock Research for Rural Development 18: 1-6.

Tripathi, M.K., Karim, S.A., Chaturvedi, O.H. and Verma, D.L. 2007a. Effect of different liquid cultures of live yeast strains on performance, ruminal fermentation and microbial protein synthesis in lambs. Journal of Animal Physiology and Animal Nutrition 92: 631-639.

Tripathi, M.K., Chaturvedi, O.H., Karim, S.A., Singh, V.K. and Sisodiya, S.L. 2007b. Effect of different levels of concentrate allowances on rumen fluid pH, nutrient digestion, nitrogen retention and growth performance of weaner lambs. Small Ruminant Research 72: 178-186.

Tripathi, M.K., Mondal, D., Somvanshi, R. and Karim, S.A. 2011a. Haematology, blood biochemistry and tissue histopathology of lambs maintained on diets containing an insect controlling protein (Cry1Ac) in Bt-cotton seed. Journal of Animal Physiology and Animal Nutrition (In press).

Tripathi, M.K., Tripathi, Prabhat and Karim, S.A. 2011b. Nutrient requirement and feeding of lambs for mutton production under tropical climates: a review. Indian Journal of Small Ruminants 17: 1-17.

Upadhayay, R.S. and Chaudhary, U.B. 2005. Intake and utilization of nutrients by goats fed barley grain and cotton seed cake. Indian Journal of Animal Sciences 74: 330-332.

Van Soest, P.J. 1982. Nutritional ecology of the ruminant. O and B Books Inc, Corvall.

Walichnowski, Z. and Lawrence, S.G. 1982. Studies into the effects of cadmium and low pH upon methane production. Hydrobiologia 91–92: 1573–5117.

□□□

Chapter 19

Epidemiology and Management of Gastrointestinal Helminths in Small Ruminants - An Update

D. Singh and C.P. Swarnkar
Division of Animal Health, Central Sheep and Wool Research Institute, Avikanagar – 304 501 (Rajasthan)

India is characterized by high ecological diversity as evident by variable climatic conditions from hot-humid to hot-dry, arid to semi-arid and plain to hills. Animal rearing in India has so far been subsidiary to the agriculture. However, small ruminants has provided sustenance to rural economy, particularly in areas where crop and dairy farming are not economical and play an important role in the livelihood of a large proportion of small and marginal farmers and landless labourers. Livestock are tangible assets for nearly 65% of the rural population and provide them nutrition and regular income. Though, India is having 61.47 millions sheep and 124.36 million Goats (Census, 2003), their productivity is not up to the mark. India cannot afford to be a poor performer in livestock production considering the vast genetic diversity of our livestock and qualified human resources at our command. Despite the existence of rich animal genetic resources in the country, the per capita availability and consumption of livestock products is lower as compared to developed countries. The reason behind this are many, like large animal population with rapidly diminishing grazing lands and consequent overstocking, poor nutrition, traditional husbandry practices accompanied by clinical or sub-clinical mixed infections and poor exploitation of genetic potential. Investment for improved feeding, genetic and productivity improvements are all constrained severely by the negative impact of diseases on the animal system, rendering such investments largely unfruitful. In recent years, in addition to increase in productivity, ensuring safety of animal products from pathogens including parasites has received greater attention particularly because of the need for meeting the requirement for trade and also due to the implication of liberalized trade regulations of WTO.

Parasitism in grazing animals is a major problem severely limiting their productivity throughout the World, but the effect of parasitism may be more severe in tropical countries like India. An exhaustive review commissioned to prioritize animal health research for poverty reduction in the developing World, by an international donor consortium consisting of the WHO, OIE and FAO concluded that gastrointestinal (GI) parasitism had the highest global index as an animal health constraint to the poor. Across host species, helminthosis was top ranked followed by neonatal mortality, FMD and ectoparasitism (Davis *et al.*, 2009). Detailed economic evaluations repeatedly show that the major losses due to parasites are on animal production, rather than on mortality (McLeod, 1995). In many instances, these costs exceed the costs of losses due to the major "killer" diseases due to viruses and bacteria (Anon, 1991). The total annual cost of parasitism was estimated to $ 222.0 million in the Australian sheep industry (McLeod, 1995), while in USA, the economic losses in ruminants due to parasites are estimated at more than $ 3.0 billion per year (Smith, 2002). Nari *et al.* 1997 estimated annual costs of parasites to the sheep industry in Uruguay to the tune of US$ 41.8 million. Within sub-Saharan Africa, de Haan and Bekure (1991) estimated that endoparasites cause mortality and production losses to the order of $ 2.0 billion per annum. McLeod (2004) estimated annual costs of roundworm parasites in selected Asian countries and found that roundworm-inflicted production losses to sheep production were at the maximum of $ 5.6 million / year in Indonesia followed by Nepal and Philippines. Substantial annual economic losses to the tune of $ 103.0 million and $ 111.0 million were estimated to be inflicted by roundworm infection in small ruminants of India and Australia, respectively (McLeod, 2004). Gazehegan (1992) estimated a loss of US$ 400 million due to helminthosis in Ethiopian meat industry. With the approach of partial farm budgeting Singh *et al.* (2011) estimated that under natural challenge of infection, the overall annual loss per adult and yearling sheep was Rs. 125.78 and Rs. 94.29, respectively in sheep flocks of Rajasthan. Based on sheep population (Census, 2003) the total annual loss in Rajasthan was estimated to be Rs. 1191.71 million. The contribution to loss was comprised of losses in mutton production (59.56%), increased susceptibility for mortality (16.57%), premature culling (11.25%), reduced fertility (7.97%) and decreased wool yield (4.65%).

Often parasite causes diseases but several factors such as type of parasites, disease resistance in host and environmental conditions influences the importance and severity of parasitic diseases. The presence of gastrointestinal (GI) helminths in an animal however, does not mean that they are necessarily the cause of any overt disease in that animal, thus it become essential to assess the type and level of parasitism in a flock to determine the significance of parasitic infection and to recommend the most cost-effective feasible control / management programme. Modern anthelmintics, together with an understanding of epidemiology, immune responses and nutritional requirements of sheep, currently enable to manage the problem satisfactorily. However, the rising emergence of anthelmintics resistance strains of parasites is challenging the ability of the animals to produce and maintain high level of productivity. On a "worm-for-worm" basis, *H. contortus* is generally considered the most pathogenic parasite of small ruminants (Soulsby, 1986). Although it occurs in mixed infections with other nematode parasites, it invariably dominates the faecal egg counts (FEC) and often approaches 90% of egg contamination on pastures under prevailing conditions of high temperature and humidity, which are the norm in the humid tropics / sub tropics. However it is now apparent that *H. contortus* is becoming more important in the temperate regions of the world, with the apparent change in weather conditions that favour this parasite (Waller *et al.* 2004). Thus much of the problems associated with parasite infections in small ruminants, problems in their control and problems of anthelmintic resistance, relate specifically to this single species of nematode parasite. Keeping in mind above scenario, the present communiqué highlights the pattern of epidemiology of GINs and feasible options for their managements.

Issues in epidemiology and management of parasites

The epidemiological studies demonstrated considerable variation between and within flocks in FEC and indicate regional differences in nematode parasite epidemiology and host exposure to nematodes, worthy to note when devising control programme. Since long in worm control practice it has been recommended that all animals in a flock should be drenched with an anthelmintic at the same time. However, this strategy has turned out to be unsustainable and researchers now favour a selective approach where only those animals in need of anthelmintic intervention actually receive medication. This selective approach is highly compatible with host-parasite-environment interaction. Worm burdens are highly aggregated in hosts with about 20-30% of animals harbouring about 80% of all the worms. Majority of parasitologists now considered levels of *refugia* as the single most important factor contributing to selection for anthelmintic resistance in parasites (van Wyk, 2001). Treating animals with low worm burdens does little to control parasites, but removes an important source of *refugia,* thereby accelerating the evaluation of resistance (Singh and Swarnkar, 2008). There is a paradigm shift in the way to deal with parasites - away from flock control and the chemical 'big hit' approach to something more akin to parasite management i.e. "living with worms". Following three strong reasons for looking at reducing the use of anthelmintics for adult sheep are:

- In the adult sheep, the level of immunity to most worms is high, apart from during the peri-parturient period. This means the ewes maintains a relatively low population of parasites so that any anthelmintic treatment will exert a very high selection pressure. On this basis, we should be advising against unnecessary treatment of ewes.
- There is a need to maintain a population of parasites within the overall population in *refugia*. Adult sheep are the obvious candidates for the maintenance of a population of parasites in *refugia,* because their immune system controls the number of worms.
- Nutrition both in terms of current levels of nutrient intake and past nutritional level, was seen as a vital component in the need to treat ewes. An assessment of the adequacy of nutrition (body condition scores) could, therefore be used as a guide to the need for anthelmintic treatment.

The insight into extent and severity of worms, rampant emergence of anthelmintic resistance in them and un-sustainability of chemotherapeutic based worm control programme, rose following issues before us:

i. Reset / set objective for epidemiology of parasites
ii. Need to consider double-edged problem in worms and their management
iii. Identify and harvest benefits of soft targets available in epidemiology

Epidemiology of gastrointestinal nematodes (GINs)

It is governed by weather conditions and management systems that regulate the development and survival of exogenous stages of parasites. In India, though several studies were performed on epidemiology of GINs but on reviewing the information it was realized that comprehensive studies on different aspects of epidemiology are limited. Further, in majority of studies there were a number of lacunae like lack of objective of study (whether for academic purpose or for formulation of control strategies), reporting of point prevalence only, small sample size, limited to incidence only, failure to quantify the magnitude of intensity, poor correlation with climatic observations, failure to correlate finding with management and rearing practices of livestock, status of pasture infectivity, drug-use pattern etc.

Incidence means the study of the dynamic changes which occurs both with in host and environment. Only incidence has little significance in the epidemiology of GINs as it may remain continuously higher throughout the year without noticeable ill-effect on host or in flock. The study only on incidence pattern of GINs fails to differentiate the animals harbouring varying degree of infection i.e. an animal having a single parasite in body is also considered at par with the animals possessing thousands of parasites. The magnitude of intensity of infection indicates the pathological level of GI parasitism in a flock situated in locality under consideration. It is directly related with the animal factors (age, nutrition, immunity etc), management practices (reproductive, grazing, rearing etc), herbage larval burden, climatic variations and agro climatic conditions. Analysis and correlation of intensity of GIN infection with managemental practices provide base for formulating the efficient worm management programme.

In temperate and sub-temperate Himalayan region, the common GI parasites encountered were *Haemonchus contortus, Trichpstrongylus axei, T. colulobriformis, Bunostomum trigonocephalum, Skrjebima ovis, Cooperia punctata, Oesophagostomum, Chabertia, Trichuris, Nematodirus, Marshallagia* and *Strongyloides.* (Dhar and Das, 1982; Jithendran, 1994, 1998; Mittra *et al.*, 1998; Katoch *et al.*, 1998; Bhat *et al.*, 2007). The coprological studies revealed an annual prevalence of GI helminths ranging from 59.83 to 94.30% depending upon the year and location of the study area (Khajuria *et al.*, 2005, 2006, 2010; Nasreen *et al.*, 2005; Yadav *et al.*, 2006; Sharma *et al.*, 2007; Wani *et al.*, 2011). The overall frequency distribution of infected animals exhibited that majority of small ruminants (68.22%) harboured low level of intensity followed by 29.82% with moderate intensity of infection. Only 1.96% of the animals found to posses high intensity of infection. Young animals were found to have lower incidence compared to adult in J&K (Yadav *et al.*, 2006; Wani *et al.*, 2011). Pandit *et al.* (2003) reported 75.92 and 88.39% incidence of GINs in farm and field flocks of sheep in Kashmir valley. The seasonal incidence ranged from 70.87% in autumn to 83.82% in summer under farm conditions and from 84.36% (summer) to 92.24% (autumn) under field conditions. The results of majority of studies in Jammu region exhibited maximum incidence during monsoon (88.54%) followed by summer (83.15%) and minimum (76.01%) in winter (Yadav *et al.*, 2006; Khajuria *et al.*, 2010). However, in Kashmir region, Nasreen *et al.* (2005), Tariq *et al.* (2008) and Wani *et al.* (2011) observed higher incidence (84.60%) during summer followed by spring (80.00%), winter (72.00%) and autumn (60.00%). Yadav *et al.* (2006) observed that intensity of infection ranged from 1418.18 epg (winter) to 2302.33 epg (monsoon). The increase in strongyle egg count during spring coinciding with lambing season suggested occurrence of PPR in the region and this is responsible for contamination of pasture during spring which intern contribute to the build up of infection in lambs (Dhar *et al.*, 1982). This is further supported by findings of retrospective study by Darzi *et al.* (2004) who reported that among the adult sheep, deaths due to haemonchosis were mostly in females particularly during post-partum period. Khajuria *et al.* (2006), observed significant influence of altitude on incidence of strongyle worms with maximum (74.88%) in plain belt (1000-1500′ above MSL) followed by 70.84% in middle zone (1500-4000′ above MSL) and minimum (20.51%) in high altitude (4000-6000′ above MSL). Agnihotri *et al.* (2010) observed only 17.85% incidence of GIN in Chegu goats at higher altitude (Lahaul and Spiti). In migratory flocks of Himachal Pradesh, the incidence of

GINs was 94% with peak intensity of infection during July-September (Jithendran, 1998). In adult animals, rise in FECs was occurred during March-April while in lambs from June to September. From Himachal Pradesh, Sharma *et al.* (2007) reported maximum incidence in the rainy and summer season and lowest in the winter season in Gaddi sheep. The intensity of infection was maximum (1323.75 epg) during rainy season followed by 865 epg in summer and minimum of 722.50 epg in winter. Based on a retrospective study in Corriedale sheep at Kashmir, Darzi *et al.* (2004) noticed higher death rate in lambs due to haemonchosis compared to adult sheep. The outbreak of parasites induced mortality and morbidity occurred mostly in rainy and winter season in migratory flocks of Himachal Pradesh (Katoch *et al.*, 1998; Mittra *et al.*, 1998). Khajuria *et al.* (2009) reported an outbreak of parasitic gastroenteritis in small ruminants in Jammu with 80% morbidity and 8% mortality during the month of March, 2007.

From Uttarakhand, on faecal examination, Yadav *et al.* (2004) reported 60.7 and 63.4% incidence in sheep and goats, respectively. However, in another study, Banerjee *et al.* (2004) reported higher prevalence (84.63%) in goats. Yadav *et al.* (2007) studied comparative epidemiology of GINs in goats reared in Tarai and Hill region of Uttarakhand and found higher incidence (66.89%) in Tarai compared to Hill region (33.31%). The maximum incidence was during September in Tarai and during June in Hills. The intensity of infection was significantly higher (8023 epg) in goats of Tarai than that of Hills (1047 epg). From organized goat farm situated at high altitude of Uttarakhand, Ram *et al.* (2007) found 87.0% incidkgce for GINs. The seasonal intensity was maximum (1717 epg) during monsoon followed by summer (838 epg) and minimum in winter (775 epg). Like-wise, Pant *et al.* (2009) reported an overall prevalence of helminths to the tune of 96.00% in Tarai region. The prevalence of *Haemonchus* spp was more (95.00%) in flocks at organized farms than flocks of villages (76.92%). The analysis of data generated in All India Network Programme on GI Parasitism showed that in sheep annual incidence was maximum in Tarai region (70.7%) followed by 60.0% in Plains and minimum (47.8%) in Hills. Similar pattern was observed in goats (75.4% in Tarai, 52.1% in Plains and 42.1% in Hills). Based on over the years, the trends of monthly incidence in sheep flocks exhibited higher incidence during July to October and January to March in Plains, during April to November in Tarai and during June to December in hills (Fig.1). On the other hand the variation in monthly was non-significant in goats of Plains and Tarai, however in Hill region showed two peaks during June to September and in March (Fig.2). The magnitude of intensity of strongyle infection in sheep flock revealed higher FECs in August, August to September and July to September in Plains, Tarai and Hills, respectively (Fig.3). In goat flocks, higher FECs were observed during May, September-October and August in Plains, Tarai and Hills, respectively (Fig. 4).

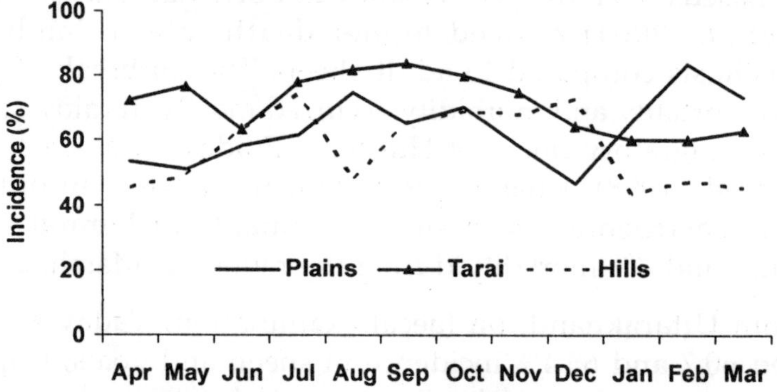

Fig. 1 : Incidence of strongyle infection in sheep of Uttarakhand (on faecal examination)

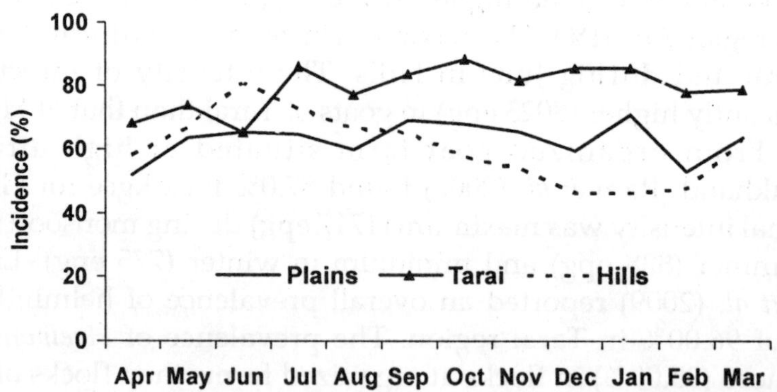

Fig. 2 : Incidence of strongyle infection in goats of Uttarakhand (on faecal examination)

North-Eastern Himalayan region has high rainfall with super humid climate and ideal optimum temperature for faster propagation of the parasites and is known endemic zone for the metazoan parasites (Sharma and Godara, 2010). In a survey in Assam, Talukdar (1996) recorded 17 species of nematodes in goats. The nematode recorded on autopsy from goats were identified as *H. contortus* (90.1%), *Trichuris*

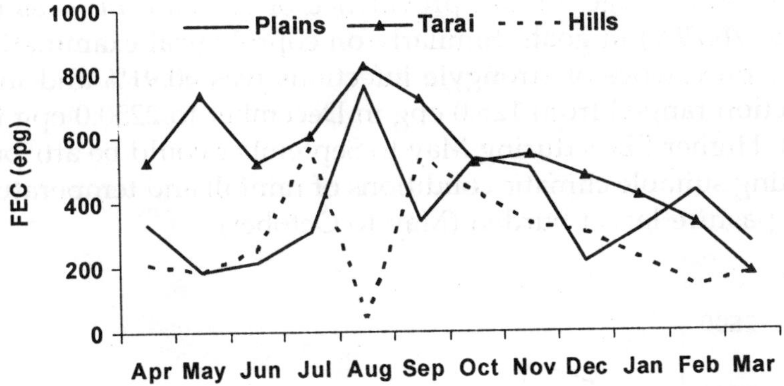

Fig. 3 : Intensity of strongyle infection in sheep of Uttarakhand

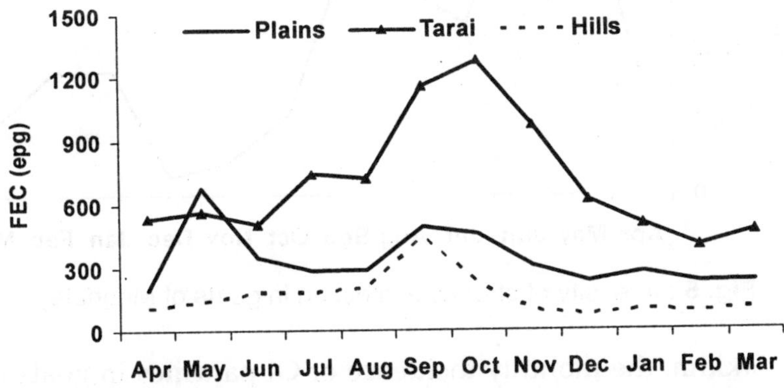

Fig. 4 : Intensity of strongyle infection in goats of Uttarakhand

ovis (88.0%), *B. trigonocephalum* (78.3%), *T. colubriformis* (55.4%), *T. axei* (46.5%), *O. columbianum* (43.2%), *Ostertagia circumcincta* (42.5%), *O. venulosum* (33.5%), *Gongylonema pulchurum* (29.5%), *Trichuris globulosa* (27.5%), *Gaigeria pachyscelis* (19.7%), *S. papillosus* (13.5%) and *Skerjabinema ovis* (3.4%). Pal and Bandyopadhyay (2004) observed 77.13% incidence in goats in Sikkim with mean FEC of 1166.7 epg. Though, prevalence was higher during summer and autumn compared to winter and spring, the intensity of infection was at the maximum during autumn (September-November). In organized sheep farm of Arunachal Pradesh, Sarvananan *et al.* (2006) observed 43.66% incidence of GIN. The incidence was 52.00% in goats at farms in Meghalaya with the seasonal variation ranging from 34.48% in winter to 57.14% in summer (Laha *et al.*, 2010). The findings of All India Network Programme on GI Parasitism exhibited that on abattoir surveys, an average annual prevalence of *H. contortus* was 67.37% (56.52 to 76.79%) in goats. Similarly on coprological examination, the average prevalence of strongyle infections was 60.91% and intensity of infection ranged from 125.0 epg in December to 2250.0 epg in June (Fig. 5). Higher FECs during May to September could be attributed to prevailing suitable climatic conditions of rainfall and temperature and higher pasture larval burden (May to October).

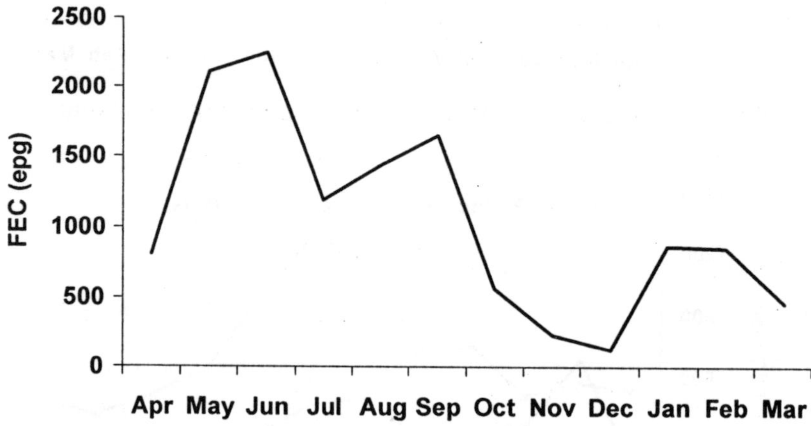

Fig. 5 : Intensity of strongyle infection in goats of Meghalaya

In Sikkim, the monthly incidence of GI parasites in goats ranged from 27.0% in January to 81.3% in August (Fig. 6). There was distinct seasonal variation with maximum incidence (79.4%) in summer followed by 73.2% (autumn), 64.6% (spring) and minimum (30.8%) in winter. Similarly intensity of strongyle infection remained drastically low from December to February and start rising from March to reached peak (2320.4 epg) in September (Fig. 7). The pattern suggested occurrence of hypobiosis as well as spring-rise phenomenon. Further an inverse relationship was noticed between incidence and altitude with maximum of 70.54% (sub tropical high humid zone) followed by 58.52% (temperate humid zone), 27.27% (sub-alpine low humid zone) and minimum of 18.36% (alpine dry zone). From Orissa, Subudhi *et al.* (2006) observed 83.98 to 87.00% incidence of GI parasites. Higher incidence of GINs was reported during monsoon season (Mishra *et al.*, 1974). In Bihar, Kumari *et al.* (2010) found 89.00 and 79.33% incidence of GI helminths (predominantly *H. contortus* and *T. colubriformis*) in sheep and goats, respectively.

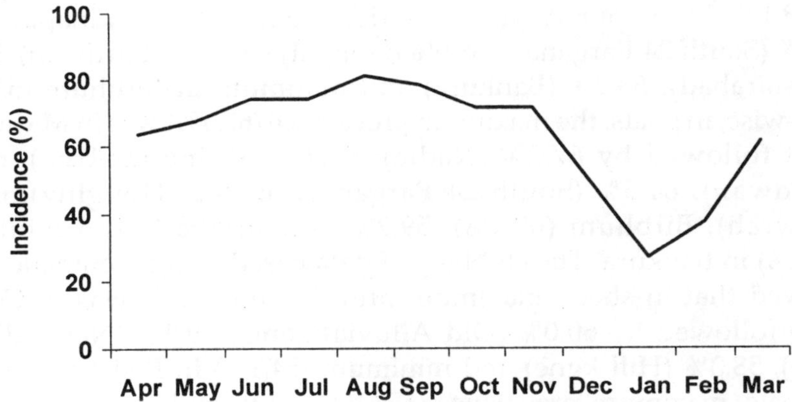

Fig. 6 : Incidence of GI parasites in goats of Sikkim (on faecal examination)

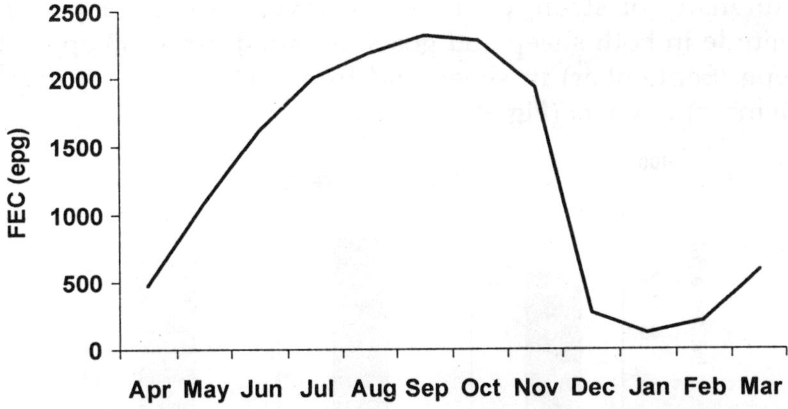

Fig. 7 : Intensity of strongyle infection in goats of Sikkim

Bandyopadhya (1999) reported the overall prevalence of *Haemonchus* spp to the tune of 45-60% in sheep and 40% in goats from West Bengal. The other GI nematodes recorded were *Bunostomum, Trichuris* and *Strongyloides* spp. The data collected from 2001-11 in West Bengal, revealed that average annual prevalence of GI helminths was 66.85 and 65.21% in sheep and goats, respectively with minor variation between years (55.63 to 81.21% in sheep and 50.46 to 77.89% in goats). Almost similar incidence was observed on abattoir survey (69.73% in sheep and 73.49% in goats). The seasonal profile exhibited relatively higher incidence (73.47 and 74.99%) during monsoon in both the species followed by during winter and summer (Fig. 8). The region-wise maximum prevalence in sheep (68.5%) was in Nadia followed by 68.1% (Midnapur-West), 68.0% (Howrah), 67.8% (Midnapur-East), 67.7% (South 24 Parganas), 66.9% (Houghly), 64.4% (Burdwan), 56.1% (Mushirabad), 53.2% (Bankura) and minimum in Birbhum (53.2%). Like-wise, in goats, the maximum prevalence (67.4%) was in Midnapur-West followed by 67.2% (Nadia), 66.2% (Midnapur-East), 64.6% (Burdwan), 64.5% (South 24 Parganas), 64.0% (Houghly), 63.7% (Howrah), Birbhum (60.1%), 59.2% (Mushirabad) and minimum (53.2%) in Bankura. The clubbing of data based on agro climatic zones showed that in sheep maximum prevalence (66.5%) was in Coastal zone followed by 60.0% (Old Alluvial zone), 59.3% (New Alluvial zone), 58.3% (Hill kgne) and minimum (54.1%) in Red letarite zone. In goats, maximum prevalence (65.6%) was in Hill zone followed by 64.9% (Tarai zone), 64.0% (Coastal zone), 60.6% (New Alluvial zone), 57.5% (Red letarite zone) and minimum (53.7%) in Old Alluvial zone. The intensity of strongyle infection revealed similar pattern and magnitude in both sheep and goats. It varied from 453 epg (May) to 944 epg (September) in sheep and from 453 epg (May) to 937 epg (September) in goats (Fig. 9).

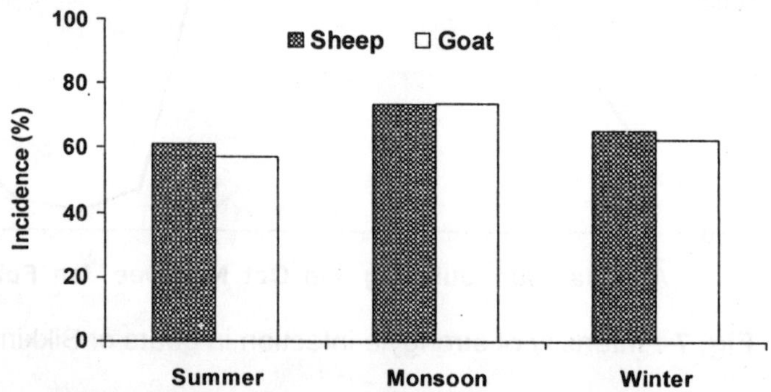

Fig. 8 : Incidence of strongyle infection in small ruminants of West Bengal

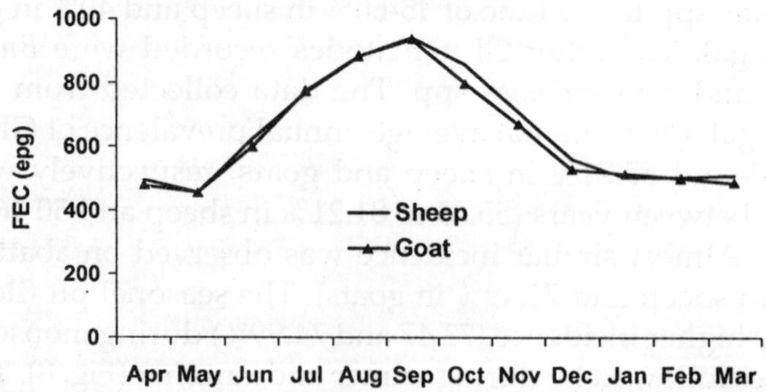

Fig. 9 : Intensity of strongyle infection in small ruminants of West Bengal

In Northern plains, the predominant nematode was *Haemonchus contortus* followed by *Trichostrongylus, Osophagostomum* and *Bunostomum* spp. (Thaper, 1956; Nadakal, 1961; Patnaik *et al.*, 1973; Bali and Singh, 1977). An outbreak of parasitic gastroenteritis was encountered in small ruminants from Punjab with 43.1 and 11.2% morbidity and mortality, respectively (Bal *et al.*, 2007). The incidence of *H. contortus* was maximum during July-October and minimum during March-June (Gupta *et al.*, 1987). In UP, Shankar *et al.* (2010) observed 60.70 and 68.89% incidence of GIN in goats and sheep, respectively. The seasonal analysis exhibited maximum incidence during monsoon followed by winter and minimum in summer. However, from farm flocks in the similar region (CIRG, Makhdoom), Arora *et al.* (2006) observed an overall prevalence of 44.32% in goats with monthly variation ranging from < 20.00% (January, May and October) to 72.56% (September). The seasonal incidence at farm was high during monsoon (42.95%) followed by summer (34.67%) and winter (16.22%). In the same fashion, intensity of infection was minimum (595.66 epg) during winter followed by 623.73 epg in summer and 1049.73 epg during monsoon. In a survey of different sheep and goat farms in UP during 2001-02, the incidence of GI parasites was 53.11 and 64.08%, respectively. Among sheep farms maximum prevalence (86.32%) was recorded at Pashulok followed by at CIRG (82.85%), IVRI (75.00%) and Navagarh, Varanasi (23.64%). Similarly among goat farms, it was maximum (77.77%) at IVRI followed by CIRG (71.85%) and Kushi Nagar, Gorakhpur (27.77%). Among field flocks, during 2010-11 in Rohilkhand region (UP), the incidence of GIN ranged from 67.65% in sheep to 68.08% in goats. The incidence was higher during March and August in sheep and during December to March in goats. Two peaks (July-October and December-January) were observed for intensity of infection in sheep compared to single peak during October in goats. On abattoir survey, higher recovery of *H. contortus* and *Trichostrongylus* spp was during October to March while of *Oesophagostomum* spp during February-March.

In semi-arid Western region, rainy season happened to be from July to September and peak GIN infection reported was during monsoon and post-monsoon period (Singh *et al.*, 1997a). In a retrospective study on necropsied sheep at CSWRI, Avikanagar (semi-arid Rajasthan), Swarnkar *et al.* (1996) reported an overall incidence of abomasal worms to the tune of 56.39% followed by *O. columbianum*

(7.89%), *Trichuris* spp. (1.13%). The common nematode species were *H. contortus, T. axei, T. columbriformis, O. columbianum, S. papillosus* and *Trichuris* spp. Like wise on routine screening of sheep flocks from semi-arid Rajasthan during 2004-10, an annual prevalence of 69.7% was observed by Swarnkar *et al.* (2010). Higher prevalence was encountered during monsoon and post-monsoon (hot and humid climate) than summer (hot and dry) and winter (cold and humid) season. The monthly prevalence remained at the lowest (47.0%) in March and in subsequent months rose gradually to reach at peak (84.3%) in October and then declined thereafter. From other localities in similar agro climatic conditions, Godara and Sharma (2010) reported an overall prevalence of 35.71% for GIN in sheep and goats. On long-term monitoring of sheep flocks in Rajasthan, Swarnkar *et al.* (2008) observed that annual incidence of strongyle worms remained around 55.0% and 65.0% in field and farm flocks, respectively. A marginally higher incidence was noticed in semi-arid conditions under both the management systems. Among farm flocks the incidence was higher (>65.0%) from May to November in semi-arid region and from July to November and April in arid region. Similarly in field flocks >65% incidence was observed from June to October in both the agro climatic regions (Fig. 10). In all types of management and agro climatic conditions, the seasonal incidence was highest (70-80%) during monsoon followed by summer and lowest during winter.

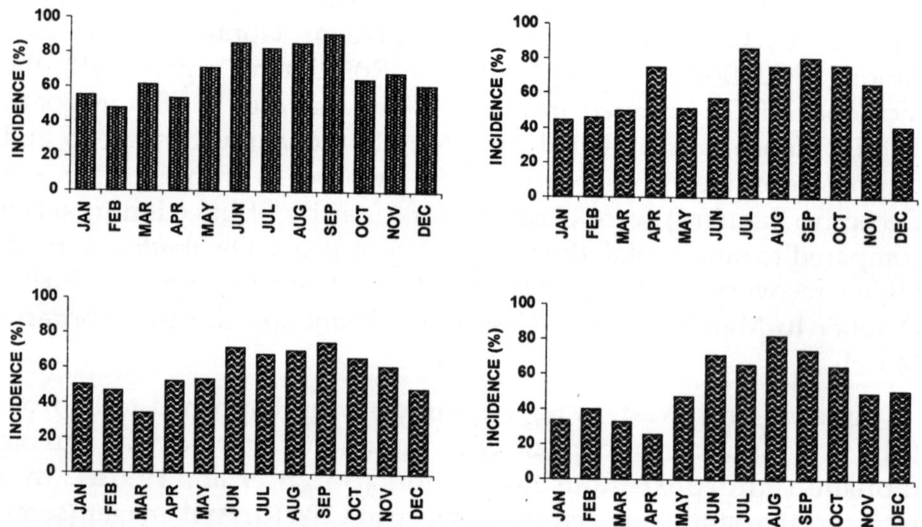

Fig. 10 : Incidence of strongyle infection in sheep flocks of Rajasthan (on faecal examination)

In farm flocks of semi-arid region, high FECs occurred from late May to early September in adult sheep and from August to early November in young sheep (Singh *et al.*, 1997a). Almost similar trend was noticed in field flocks (Khan *et al.*, 1999). The long-term average revealed that in semi-arid Rajasthan, the monthly FEC varied from 128.37 epg (February) to 1753.10 epg (July) in farm flocks and from 87.65 epg (March) to 1012.50 epg (September) in field flocks. In arid Rajasthan, the monthly FEC ranged from 194.39 epg (March) to 2314.64 epg (October) in farm flocks and from 59.20 epg (April) to 1429.22 epg (August) in field flocks (Fig. 11). The intensity of strongyle infection remained higher during July to September only. In general the initial rising trends in FEC occurred in June is probably due to resumption of development of hypobiotic worms with in the host, giving peak of infection in July and provide the source of pasture contamination during monsoon. The decline in FEC in the following months may be due spontaneous occurrence of self-cure phenomenon following acquisition of fresh wave of infection from pasture and expulsion of old worms. The magnitude of FEC during the period from November to May revealed that there is occurrence of hypobiosis and absence of periparturient rise in FECs (Swarnkar *et al.*, 2008).

The work conducted under All India Network programme on GI parasitism in Madhya Pradesh showed annual incidence of 78.6 and 65.0% in adult goats and kids, respectively. The monthly incidence remained higher during the period from July to December (Fig. 12). The zone-wise analysis for incidence in adult goats exhibited maximum (75%) in Vindhya plateau followed by 68% in Satpura area, 63% in Grid area and Malva plateau, 60% in Narmada valley, 50% in Chhattisgarh plain and Northern Chhattisgarh, 49% in Satpura hills and minimum of 43% in Bundelkhand area. These findings were further strengthened by magnitude of intensity of infection which remained higher during July to December (Fig. 13). From Chhattishgarh, Pathak and Pal (2008) observed overall prevalence of GI helminthes to the tune of 85.22% in goats and seasonal prevalence to the level of 94.60% in monsoon, 85.50% in summer and 63.15% in winter.

From Maharashtra, Deshpande and Deshpande (2005) reported 33.59 and 29.66 % incidence of GINs in sheep and goats, respectively. The annual prevalence of GI parasites in different region ranged from 45.69% to 65.85% in goats (Chavan *et al.*, 2008; Palampalle *et al.*, 2009). Based on slaughter house study, Sutar *et al.* (2010) reported an annual incidence of 62.75% in goats.) In general, majorities of the studies

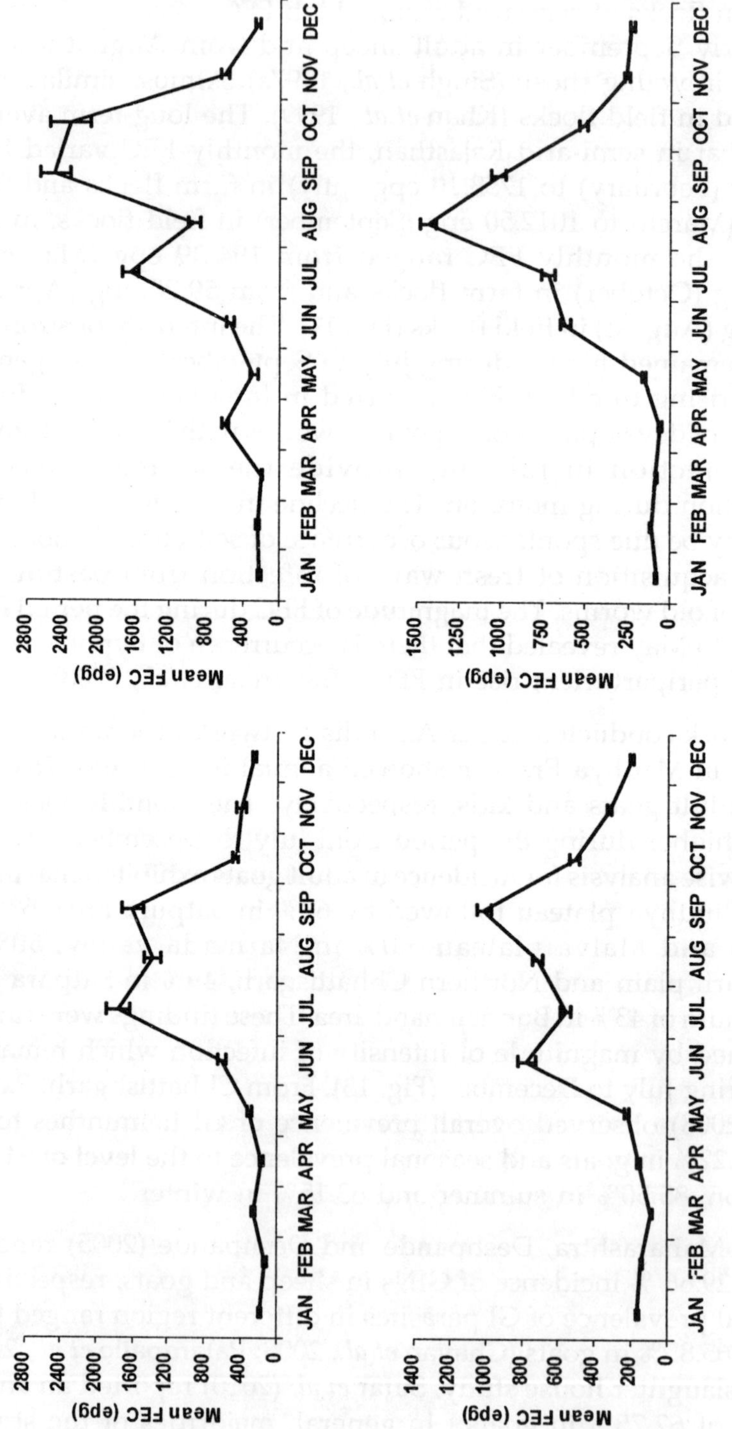

Fig. 11 : Intensity of strongyle infection in sheep flocks of Rajasthan

revealed maximum incidence and intensity during monsoon followed by winter and minimum in summer (Kalwaghe *et al.*, 2009; Sutar and Khan, 2011). Higher incidence was noticed in male and young goats. Further, goats were reported to have higher intensity of infection compared to sheep.

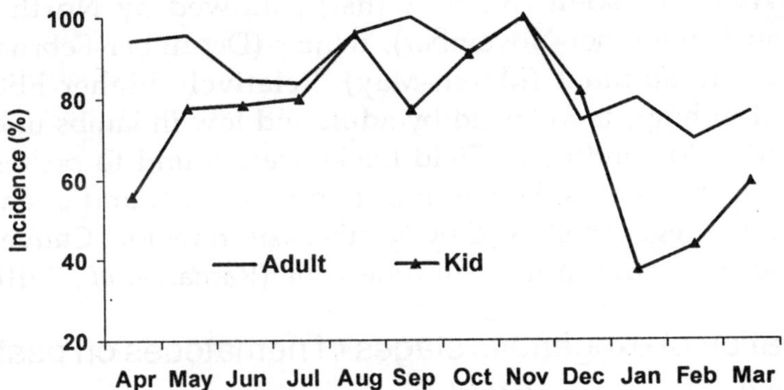

Fig. 12 : Incidence of GI parasites in goats of Madhya Pradesh (on faecal examination)

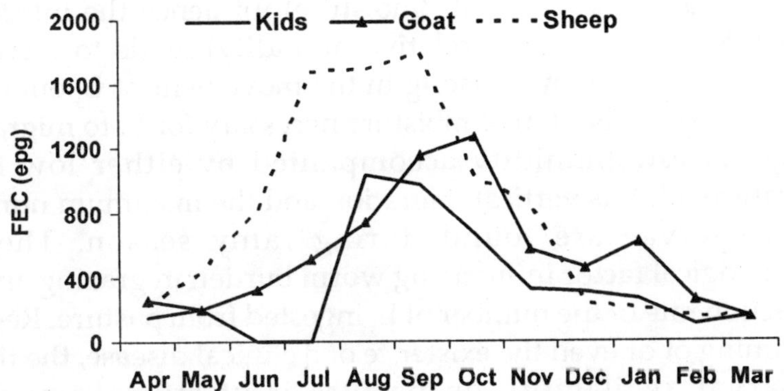

Fig. 13 : Intensity of strongyle infection in small ruminants of Madhya Pradesh

Peak parasitism was recorded in the month of November to January in Southern Humid region. The prevalent parasites were *H. contortus, T. colubriformis, O. venulosum* and *Strongyloides* spp. In Nigiri hills (Tamil Nadu), Soundarajan and Iyne (2003) observed 26.43% prevalence of helmintic infection on necropsy of sheep. The seasonal analysis exhibited maximum prevalence (44.33%) during south-west monsoon followed by 24.74% during north-east monsoon, 23.00%

during summer and minimum of 7.22% during winter. From Puducherry, on faecal examination, Das *et al.* (2006) reported 56.0% incidence of GIN in goats. Based on long term observations (2001-11) from different agro climatic regions of Tamil Nadu, the average annual incidence was 72.6 and 64.6% in sheep and goats, respectively. The seasonal analysis exhibited maximum incidence and intensity during South-West monsoon (June-August) followed by North-Eastern monsoon (September-November), winter (December-February) and minimum in summer (March-May). Relatively higher FECs were observed in hoggets followed by adult and low in lambs under both form and field conditions. Field flocks were found to posses higher FECs than farm flocks. Higher infection rate was found in animals of high rainfall region followed by North-Eastern region, Cauvery Delta zone and minimum in high altitude zone (Raman *et al.*, 2010).

Translation of exogenous stages of nematodes on pasture

The incidence of nematode parasites in an area is directly related to the ability of pre-parasitic stages to withstand the environmental conditions. Translation of exogenous stages of parasites comprised of development, survival and dissemination of infective larvae on pasture. Both temperature and rainfall (moisture) influence the infectivity of pastures. Rain (moisture / relative humidity) tends to increase the infectivity of pasture by assisting in the movement of L_3 out of faeces and by providing the film of moisture necessary for L_3 to migrate on to herbage. A low humidity accompanied by either low or high temperature inhibits vertical migration and the maximum numbers of infective larvae are found during rainy season. The major epidemiological factor influencing worm burden in grazing animals is the infection rate or the number of L_3 ingested from pasture. Regardless of the timing of or even the existence of a clinical disease, the timing of peak larval availability on pasture is of crucial importance. Development of L_3 and their availability for ingestion by host was optimum at about 25°C when adequate moisture is present. The optimum conditions for translation of *H. contortus* includes total monthly rainfall of more than 50 mm and a mean monthly maximum temperature over 18.3°C. *Trichostrongylus* spp. requires a total monthly rainfall of over 50 mm and mean monthly temperature of 12.8 to 18.3°C for their translation on pasture (Gordon, 1953). The bioclimatographs for *H. contortus* showed suitable climatic conditions for translation of exogenous stages of parasites were from June to September and July to August in semi-arid and arid Rajasthan, respectively (Swarnkar and Singh, 2011). The favourable conditions prevail during May to October in Madhya Pradesh and from February to November in Sikkim. From southern region, there was bi-modal parasitic activity on pasture in western (April-May, August-September), high rainfall, Cauvery delta and southern zones (April-June, August-December) while in northern zone favourable conditions prevails from March to November.

In temperate and sub-temperate climate eggs deposited over prolong period in winter, spring or early summer may result in large number of larvae being available to grazing animals in spring, summer, autumn, respectively depending on their temperature-rainfall relationship. Typical seasonal rise in nematode worm burden in host and on pasture was observed following monsoon accompanied with moderate temperature during July makes the environment favourable for the development, survival and dissemination of exogenous stages leading to high rise of GINs in host and infective larvae on pasture during the period from July to September. In Himachal Pradesh, monsoon rains triggers by mid-June with moderate temperature and makes the environment favourable for development and survival of free-living stages on pasture (Jithendran, 1998). In Uttarakhand pasture larval burden (PLB) was higher during September-October. Higher PLB was observed during May to October in Meghalaya and from July to October in Sikkim. In Northern plains the climatic conditions suitable for development, survival and dissemination of infective stages are during monsoon (June-October) causing high incidence of GIN with peak intensity during monsoon and post-monsoon period (Bali and Singh, 1977; Ahmed and Ansari, 1987). In Rohilkhand region of UP, the pasture infectivity was higher during the period from September to January. In Madhya Pradesh, PLB was higher from August to December. Dey *et al.* (2008) from organized goat farm in Chhattishgarh exhibited that period from June to August were most favourable for translation of nematodes and FECs reached to maximum during July.

In Rajasthan, rains occur during July-August but the mean maximum temperature was more than 20°C throughout the year in semi-arid region. The coproculture and PM worm count revealed low level of *T. axei* during March-June and August-October, respectively (Singh *et al.*, 1997a). However, due to favourable climatic conditions in arid Rajasthan the *Trichostrongylus* spp ova develop easily to L_3 during winter (Singh and Swarnkar, 2003; Swarnkar and Singh, 2011).

In semi-arid Rajasthan, it was observed that infective larvae of *H. contortus* remained for maximum period of time (9 weeks) on pasture during September (Swarnkar *et al.*, 1997). High temperature during summer was found unsuitable for development of nematode ova. Like wise winter climate was also unsuitable and restricted their development. Sanyal and Gaur (1984) observed lowest pasture contamination in the month of December and attributed it to harsh climatic as a result of low temperature and sparse rainfall. The pasture contamination by grazing ewes from January to March took 4 months to become parasitologically barren following preventing the grazing in April.

Hypobiosis (arrested / inhibited larval development)

It means temporary cessation in development of a nematode parasite at a precise point in its parasitic phase of development. The abomasal nematodes like *H. contortus* and *T. axei* and small intestinal worms such as *T. colubrifirmis, Cooperia and Nematodirus* spp are capable of interrupting or arresting their development at the L_4 stage and persisting for long period in a state of dormancy. On return of favourable conditions they resume their development and become normal egg laying adults. Though occurrence of this phenomenon in nematode parasites in Rajasthan has not been established but the epidemiological profile so far available (very low FECs and adult worm count from November to May followed by sudden increase in FECs in June in spite unfavourable climatic conditions on pasture for larval survival) is suggestive of occurrence of hypobiosis in nematode parasites (Singh *et al.*, 1997a; Swarnkar *et al.*, 2008). From Haryana, Gupta *et al.* (1986, 1987) reported absence of hypobiosis. In Madhya Pradesh, a decline in intensity from November to June indicates possible occurrence of hypobiosis. At Kodai hills in Tamil Nadu, Sanyal (1988, 1989) observed that in spite of low herbage larval burden and low FEC in February the sudden rise in eggs and worm count in March were attributed to occurrence of hypobiosis in of *H. contortus*, which may become the potential source of pasture contamination in spring coinciding with the lambing.

Periparturient Rise in Faecal Egg Count

The periparturient rise of worm egg count in faeces of lactating ewes is a well recognised phenomenon and usually observed within a period extending from 2 weeks prior to lambing to 8 weeks post-lambing (Michel, 1976). This phenomenon is postulated to be associated with temporarily impairment of acquired immune-responsiveness in lactating ewes (O'Sullivan and Donald, 1970). Isolated reports on spontaneous elimination of worms and peri-parturient rise (PPR) of GIN in certain geographical areas in India are available. Increase in strongyle egg count occurred in March-April coinciding with lambing season in Kashmir Valley suggested occurrence of PPR phenomenon. The PPR was found responsible for contamination of pasture during the spring season which inturn contribute to the built up of infection in lambs (Dhar *et al.*, 1982). The exact cause of PPR is not known, if this is due to resumption of development of arrested worms or due to an increase in number of newly acquired infection by the host consequent to loss of resistance. Similarly hypobiotic behaviour of *H. contortus* at Kodai Hills in Tamil Nadu (Sanyal, 1988) resulted in sudden increase in eggs and worm counts in March in spite of fact that the larval burden on pasture and egg counts in animals remained lower in February. Brunsdon and Vlassoff (1982) postulated that freshly acquired infection from contaminated pasture / corral was the major source of infection in lactating ewes, resulting in PPR in spring season. Gupta *et al.* (1986) reported that agro-climatic conditions of Haryana were favourable for development of trichostrongylid larvae on pasture leading to occurrence of PPR in sheep (Gupta *et al.*, 1987) during February-April. In Rajasthan, the agro-climatic conditions does not favour the development of strongyle larvae during December-June (Swarnkar *et al.*, 1997) resulting in non-availability of source of infection for ewes and absence of typical PPR (Singh *et al.*, 1997a). Further, Swarnkar *et al.* (1998) observed non-significant difference in FEC in different breeds of sheep over the 12 weeks post-lambing and ruled out presence of PPR phenomenon in this region. Like-wise, the studies on lambing pattern in field flocks of Rajasthan revealed that majority of ewes in flocks are in lambing / lactation during October to February and agro climatic conditions of the state does not favour the development and dissemination of worms from December to June resulting in non-availability of source of infection for lactating ewes (Swarnkar and Singh, 2010). Thus, the strategic anthelmintic drench as practiced by farmers in the month of February-March could be withdrawn without hampering the flock productivity. Further, avoidance of deworming during this period enables survival of susceptible parasites with in the host (as hypobiotic) which in turn leads to help in reducing selection pressure for anthelmintic resistance and maintaining the efficacy of anthelmintics by increasing the size of *refugia* (Singh and Swarnkar, 2008).

Over-dispersion phenomenon in faecal egg counts

GI parasite populations in small ruminants are highly aggregated and over-dispersed within the host, with around 80% of the worms found in only 20-30% of the host, whilst the vast majority of host posses low worm burden (Hoste *et al.*, 2002). In sheep flocks of Rajasthan it was observed that even during favourable monsoon season (July-September) around 20-30% and 50% of animals in field and farm conditions, respectively had FECs to the tune of >1000 epg. Other wise in rest of seasons, majority of animals had either < 200 epg or free of infection (Swarnkar *et al.*, 2008). In recent times, it has been recognized that the phenomenon of parasite over-dispersion could be put to good use if those animals suffering from level of infection sufficient to cause considerable production loss or health effects, can be identified and treated individually (Singh and Swarnkar, 2010). Keeping in mind the issues arising in epidemiology and management (as described above) it become essential for researcher to develop some mechanism in order to harvest the benefits of over-dispersion in FECs in a flock. The available information on different alternate approaches of worm management (Singh and Swarnkar, 2007) revealed that existence of this phenomenon can be used in form of targeted selective treatment and for breeding for resistance / resilience to parasites ultimately with the aim to increase the size of *refugia,* maintain anthelmintic efficacy and cost-effective worm management (Singh and Swarnkar, 2008).

Paramphistomosis

It is caused by immature stages of various species of paramphistomes and responsible for massive losses due to reduced weight gain and productivity in endemic areas. The aquatic snail intermediate host species in India identified are *Indoplanorbis exustus, Lymnaea luteola, Gyranulus convexiusculus, Digoniostoma pulchella* (Dutt, 1980; Gupta *et al.*, 1985; Jitendran and Krishna, 1999). The cercariae are predominantly released from snail during July/August to December/January. Immature paramphistomosis has been characterized by dueodenal inflammation and high mortality and recorded for the first time in small ruminants from Punjab (Baldrey, 1906; Walker, 1906). The majority of species were recorded from sheep in many states like Haryana (Gupta *et al.* 1985), Himachal Pradesh (Jitendran and Katoch, 2003), Gujarat (Hafeez and Avsathi, 1987), Uttar Pradesh (Prasad and Verma, 1999), Punjab (Dutt, 1980; Hassan *et al.*, 2005), Bihar (Varma, 1957). It was observed that *Paramphistomum epiclitum* and *Gatrothylax crumenifer* are the predominant species with 50-70% prevalence in different agro climatic regions of India (Chaudhri, 2006). Gupta *et al.* (1985) reported incidence of immature paramphistomosis to the tune of 31.1% in small ruminants from Eastern Haryana with 25-60% mortality. Based on faecal examination, the results of an epidemiological study during 1977-1982 in Haryana revealed 9.5% incidence in sheep and goats (Guptal *et al.*, 1985) while it was 1.79% (sheep) and 0.85% (goats) from Punjab (Hassan *et al.*, 2005). However, incidence was three times higher (28.4%) on examination of slaughtered sheep and goats (Gupta *et al.* 1985). Recently, Yadav *et al.* (2010) reported an overall prevalence of 6.86 and 3.69% in sheep and goats, respectively from NCR, Delhi. The peak prevalence was during May (29.0%) in sheep and during February (8.24%) in goats. Prasad and Verma (1999) observed incidence of adult paramphistomes to the tune of 8.06% in sheep and 7.97% in goats slaughtered at abattoir of Bareilly (UP). From Madhya Pradesh, Agrawal *et al.* (2004) reported an annual prevalence of adult paramphistomes to the extent of 13.07% in goats. In West Bengal, the incidence of adult paramphistomes ranged from 51.8% in goats to 55.9% in sheep (Manna *et al.*, 1994). In southern region, Hafeez and Rao (1978) from Andhra Pradesh reported incidence rate of 15.08% in sheep. On abattoir survey, Das *et al.* (2006) recorded 28.73 and 20.73% incidence in sheep and goats, respectively.

The overall annual incidence of paramphistomes in sheep ranged from 1.6% in arid Rajasthan to 7.5% in semi-arid Rajasthan. The monthly rate of prevalence also exhibited significant variability with two peaks in a year (June and August) in semi-arid compared to a single peak during August in arid Rajasthan. The occurrence of higher incidence from June to September in semi-arid region is suggestive of facts that animal pick up infection in the month of February-March and the clinical manifestation due to immature amphistomes expected to occur in the month of April-May (Swarnkar *et al.*, 2008). The incidence of adult flukes was higher during May to September in Haryana, Uttar Pradesh and Jammu region and from July to October in Punjab. Like-wise higher incidence was observed during summer in north-western temperate Himalayan region (Tariq *et al.*, 2008). In J

& K, the epidemiological pictures revealed that infection manifest a definite seasonal pattern with 2 peaks, first during February-March and second during July-September. The mature flukes were seen at high rate from May-September whereas immature flukes were seen from October-April with the peak from November-February. Similarly, in West Bengal, it was higher during November to February (Ghosh and Datta, 2005). Immature paramphistomosis occurred from October to April with the peak from November to February in Punjab and Haryana (Chhabra *et al.*, 1978).

Clinical outbreaks of paramphistomosis are usually confined to the drier months. During this period, the snail population become concentrated around natural sources of water and as these areas may provide the only dry season grazing, animal may become heavily infected. Most of the cercariae were released from snail in the autumn / spring period. Circumstantial evidence indicates that clinical cases are often preceded by flooding of grazing area which carries released cercariae over the paddocks so that metacercariae are distributed over the grazing area. In dry weather snail habitats can shrink leaving metacercariae available to grazing animals along with their margin and clinical outbreaks are usually confined to the drier season. The continuous high rise in the incidence during monsoon is indicative of regular intake of infection during drier months through grazing, stocking and watering the flocks in the vicinity of snail habitats. In contrast to semi-arid region, the infection of paramphistomes seems to be sporadic in nature in arid region due to limited existence of snail habitats, practice to feed the flock on top feed or crop stubbles during drier months and having provision of water from tube wells (Swarnkar *et al.*, 2008). The metacercariae are resistant to desiccation and transportation of contaminated fodder for animals of hilly areas found as possible mode for spread of infection (Jithendran and Krishna, 1999).

Fasciolosis

It is caused by *Fasciola gigantica* (plain areas) and *F. hepatica* (hilly areas) and is characterized by anaemia, hypoproteinaemia, submandibular oedema, reduced body weight and digestive disturbances. *Lymnaea auricularia* is main snail intermediate host and shedding of cercariae were observed from August to January in Haryana and from September to February in UP. Outbreaks of fasciolosis have been reported in sheep in Uttranchal (Katiyar and

Tewari, 1962), Jammu and Kashmir (Pandit *et al.*, 1991), Haryana (Chaudhri *et al.*, 1991), Andhra Pradesh (Rao and Madhubala, 1998) and in Tamil Nadu (Soundarajan and Iyue, 2005). The outbreaks in Punjab and Haryana were occurred during the month of March and April (Chaudhri *et al.*, 1991; Dhand *et al.*, 2004). In Kashmir, it was observed that majority of slaughtered sheep had mixed infection (58.8%) of both the *F. gigantica* and *F. hepatica* with the prevalence varying from 25 to 100% in sheep and 0.66% in goats (Sharma, 2003). The magnitude of infection in sheep and goat was higher (51.3% and 14.3%) in Kashmir valley compared to 12.48% and 5.83% in Jammu region (Sharma *et al.*, 1989; Khajuria and Kapoor, 2003). Further, Yadav *et al.* (2006) observed very low level (3.08%) incidence in sheep from plan and irrigated areas of Jammu region. In Himachal Pradesh, region-wise incidence ranged from 7.4% in Kangra valley (Jithendran, 1996) to 65.8% in Rewalsar area (Mathur, 1986). In a survey under NATP in different regions of India, the prevalence of *Fasciola* eggs ranged from 0.57% to 20.41% in sheep (3.88%) and from 0.31% to 18.44% in goats (2.87%). The incidence was higher in winter in sub-temperate Himalayan region (Bhatia *et al.*, 1989; Jithendran and Katoch, 2003). From Uttaranchal, Kumar *et al.* (2007) reported 3.87 and 2.62% prevalence of *F. gigantica* infection in sheep and goat, respectively. In hill region peak prevalence was notice during winter while in tarai region it was during monsoon in sheep and during winter in goats. Higher prevalence in tarai region may be due to the availability of well irrigated low-lying marshy lands and green pasture alongside rivers and water bodies. The lower prevalence in hill region might be due to migration of animals to alpine pasture during summer. In J & K, the seasonal prevalence of fasciolosis was studied by dividing the whole state in to 3 agro-climatic zones. The animals of sub-hilly and orchards zone, picked up infection during autumn while grazing in paddy fields after return from alpine pasture and incidence increased to 48.95% in winter. In irrigated, low lying marshy and inundated zone, the rate of infection in summer was low because of the fact that sheep migrate to up hills where chances of re-infection remain less. Low prevalence in hilly and migratory zone is due to fact that sheep are reared mainly on non-paddy hay. Another study revealed that in hilly tract of state acute outbreaks of fasciolosis occurred in winter month (January-February), whereas in plains though it occurs between October-March but higher incidence was noticed during March-May. Relatively low incidence of flukes in Jammu region than Kashmir region was attributed to dry arid conditions of the region which were not suitable for breeding of snail intermediate host.

From arid and semi-arid region of Rajasthan, Swarnkar *et al.* (2008) observed an overall incidence of *F. gigantica* in sheep flocks to the tune of 0.2 and 0.1%, respectively on faecal examination. The relatively marginal higher incidence in arid region is due to higher migration rate of sheep flocks to the adjoining fluke prone states like UP, MP, Haryana etc. The monthly egg shedding pattern exhibited higher incidence in June (semi-arid region) and February (arid region) indicating possible period of ingestion of metacercariae during March in the vicinity of snail habitats in semi-arid Rajasthan. In arid region, migratory sheep found to pick up infection during November-early December and in May-June during their grazing around water reservoirs. Feeding of moist hay, green fodder from low lying areas, drinking of water possibly passing through the channels flooded with infected snails are major contributor to transmission of infection.

Schistosomosis

Blood flukes, (predominantly, *Schistosoma indicum*) are responsible for causing hepatointestinal schistosomosis and recorded from Madhya Pradesh, Haryana, Punjab, Rajasthan, Uttar Pradesh and Himachal Pradesh (Sharma and Dwivedi, 1976; Lodha *et al.*, 1981; Agrawal, 1986; Chaudhri *et al.*, 2006). In addition, *S. spindale* from Himachal Pradesh (Jithendran and Krishna, 1999) and *Orientobilharzia turkestanicum* from Kashmir (Bali *et al.*, 1976) were also reported. The intermediate host is *I. exustus* snails. Mishra and Agrawal (1998) reported high infectivity of snails during August to December in Madhya Pradesh. The higher incidence in rainy season may be due to re-exposure of the old cases to the cercariae, which might have triggered the immunological reactions in already infected animals (Chaudhry, 2006). The incidence of *Schistosoma* infection is found to increase with increasing avenues of water conservations, irrigation and with increase in the population density of animals. Among sheep flocks of Rajasthan, Swarnkar *et al.* (2008) observed an overall annual incidence of *S. indicum* (on the basis of faecal examination) to the tune of 0.3 and 0.5%, respectively in arid and semi-arid conditions. The higher incidence during May to September in semi-arid region is suggestive of that flocks pick up infection during February-March when the environmental and managemental conditions favours cercarial shedding from snails and proximity of host to the water reservoirs.

On the other hand a single distinct peak during August in arid region indicates that cercarial shedding and infection to final host occurs during the period from April to June. Variation in managemental practices and water reservoirs are main reason behind very low incidence during summer in arid region compared to semi-arid region. On faecal examination, Cherian and D'Souza (2009) observed 6.76% incidence of schistosomosis in sheep in Karnataka.

Dicrocoeliosis

It is caused by *Dicrocoelium dendriticum* and widely prevalent in hilly regions of India only. In spite of probably being more common than *Fasciola,* it is considered a little known disease that is often underestimated by researchers and veterinarians, mainly due to fact that it produces mild clinical symptoms and is often masked by the pathological effects of mixed parasitism in grazing livestock. It's incidence in small ruminants ranged from 1.92 to 4.18% in Jammu region (Khajuria and Kapoor, 2003; Yadav *et al.,* 2006) while in Kashmir, it was 1.06% in sheep (Makhdoomi *et al.,* 1995). In Himachal Pradesh, Jithendran and Bhat (1996) observed 4.1% (in goats) to 8.1% (in sheep) incidence on faecal examination while Kaur *et al.* (2009) recorded 2.0% prevalence of *D. dendtricum* in sheep. Similarly on necropsy examination, incidence rate is higher in sheep (24%) compared to goat (12%). Seasonal pattern exhibited higher incidence during rainy season in Jammu (Yadav *et al.,* 2006) and during autumn and winter in Himachal Pradesh (Jithendran and Bhat, 1996). The eggs are highly resistant to the action of low or high temperature and drying, thus capable of surviving on the pasture, soil and in faeces for 1-2 years. The terrestrial snails are found in dry low land / mountain pasture, hence restricting its occurrence in hilly region. Further the infection is often maintained in wild life, which may serve as a source of infection to livestock. The egg elimination in faeces peaked during winter whereas peak infection in snails was noticed during spring. Jithendran and Katoch (2003) observed that migratory flocks acquired infection from infected ants on pasture during migration to high altitude in summer and thus brought infection to the non-endemic areas of the Kangra valley in winter season.

Worm management

In attempting to consider the future of worm management in small ruminants, we inevitably need to consider both our past and our current situation. Two of the most relevant thoughts on the matter come from Sigmund Freud who considered "Only a good-for-nothing is not interested in his past" and Friedrich Nietzsche who stated that "Every past is worth condemning". Given the wide regional variation that exists between sheep management systems and the different parasites that inhabit them, it is hardly surprising that there are no universally applicable "blueprint" approaches to the control of nematode infestations. This in turn, means that farmers, their veterinarians and/ or specialist advisors have to choose worm control strategies that suit the unique situation that each farm presents in terms of its prevalent parasites, their epidemiology and the structure and management of the farm. The management of GI parasites is based on three approaches as described below.

a. Kill the parasites in the host: In order to restore production in flock and to break the dynamics of infections, this approach involve use of chemical means. At present, these diseases are largely controlled by using anthelmintics and the world-wide annual expenditure on anthelmintics is over USD 3 biilion (Jackson *et al.*, 2009). However, a high frequency of treatments, discriminate use, en-mass treatment in small ruminants, the exclusive reliance on one family of anthelmintics, under-dosing etc have been identified as main factors contributing to increase the pressure of selection on nematode populations and hence, favouring the development of anthelmintic resistances (Singh *et al.*, 2002; Swarnkar and Singh, 2010). Nowadays, the farmers have to face a double challenge, (i) to control the parasites and (ii) to avoid the diffusion and the development of anthelmintic resistance within the worm populations.

   Strategic treatments: It is most commonly practiced and consists of en-mass treatment of flock on the basis of historical knowledge of parasite epidemiology (eg. drenching at pre-monsoon, monsoon, post-monsoon, around lambing etc). This practice found to be costly and labour intensive along with responsible for causing severe increase in selection pressure for anthelmintic resistance, gradual decline in efficacy of anthelmintics and reduction in quantum of refugia.

   Targeted treatments: It involves treatment to whole flock at the most appropriate times bearing in mind the need to maintain refugia. The targeted treatment approach serves to reduce the numbers of treatments given to a flock and thus minimise pasture contamination with resistant genotype. Further, it lead to an increased interval between treatments, allowing susceptible genotypes a better opportunity to establish on pasture and so reduce the risk of heterozygous mating and producing homozygous resistant offspring (Cringoli *et al.*, 2008). In Rajasthan, the experience gained after over the years by application of anthelmintic drench during mid to late monsoon suggested rise in refugia and better efficacy of anthelmintics for prolonged period.

The days of being able to control GIN in small ruminants by treating with anthelmintics at frequent intervals are nearing an end. Unless we dramatically change the ways we use anthelmintics, there may be no effective anthelmintics remaining when that time comes. Thus, if anthelmintics are to remain a viable component of GIN control, a fresh approach will be needed. Ultimately, GIN parasite control in small ruminants must be practiced with an eye to the future and in this direction the another approach is implementation of targeted selective treatments in flock.

Targeted selective treatments (TST): It exploit both epidemiologically appropriate treatment times and involves selective treatment of only those animals that will most benefit from treatment, leaving rest of the flock untreated. TST is directed towards those animals that are susceptible or that most contaminate pasture and this requires the ability to identify these individuals within a flock (Jackson and Coop, 2000). Particularly, in the population of *H. contortus* in order to maintain the susceptibility of anthelmintics by reducing the selection pressure and allowing the maintenance of susceptible worms in *refugia*, the FAMACHA method has been developed (van Wyk and Bath, 2002). This method consists of an animal's conjunctiva, which may vary by five categories of colour that correlate with micro-haematocrit measurements.

In India, a color chart based on ocular mucous membrane, microhaematocrit and intensity of infection in sheep was developed at CSWRI, Avikanagar. The implementation of TST approach in farm flocks exhibited that only an average of 22.93% animals were drenched / annum compared to 100% drenching in targeted treatment approach. The application of TST is feasible and effective not only in managing the haemonchosis but also help in increasing the size of *refugia* which may ultimately resulted into both maintenance of drug efficacy against parasites and sizeable reduction in the cost of worm management in sheep flocks (Swarnkar *et al.*, 2010). TST particularly aims at treating only those animals unable to withstand current worm challenges, is not only exceptionally affordable in relation to other conventional control programmes, but will also help to delay selection for anthelmintic resistance (Sanyal, 2009), reduced selection pressure, lower drug residues in animal products and lower costs of worm management. The main disadvantages are the difficulty and time spent on selecting animals in need of treatment and the possibility of lower production (Cabaret, 2008). Although the system is labour intensive and is suitable for the identification of infection by haematophagous parasites only, the benefits include the ability to make the decision to treat 'sheep-side', it is low cost and require low levels of expertise and training for implementation.

b. *Improve the host response against nematodes*: Two main components composed the host response to the trichostrongyles, i.e. the resistance and the resilience. Resistance is defined as the ability of the host to regulate the nematode populations. On the other hand, resilience refers to the aptitude of a host to withstand the negative effects of nematode infections and to maintain productions under parasitic challenge. The major options to improve these 2 facets of the host responses are either genetically or nutritionally based.

   Genetics of resistance and resilience to nematode infection: Differences in the level of GI infections between breeds have been documented both in sheep (Gray, 1997) and in goats (Jackson, 2000). In most studies, the main phenotypic measurement used for selection of the responding animals has been the level of nematode egg excretion i.e. FEC. This was usually found to be moderately repeatable and heritable (Hunt *et al.*, 2008). Worm resistant animals can be found in any flock, whether they are in a wormy, high rainfall environment or a dry area as demonstrated in sheep breeds like East Africa Masai, Florida Native, Barbados Blackbelly, St. Croix and others (Baker, 1996). The largest source of genetic variation in resistance is between sheep within a flock, rather than between different flocks (Kumar *et al.*, 2006). The heritability of resistance to GIN infection in sheep, as measured by FEC varied from 0.01 to 0.50. Using FEC as phenotypic marker for within breed selection of resistant and / or susceptible animals at CSWRI, Avikanagar it was observed that this trait is low to moderately heritable (Singh *et al.*, 1999, 2009; Swarnkar *et al.*, 2008; Prince *et al.*, 2010). Creation of divergent lines either resistant (R-line) or susceptible (S-line) could be possible through regular screening for FEC at naïve and exposed stage of infection and selection of progenies. The analysis of data for intensity of strongyle infection in divergent lines over the years exhibited that in both the breeds animals of R-line had lower monthly FECs compared to their counterparts in S-line. The animals of S-line required strategic as well as tactical anthelmintic intervention while animals of R-line were maintained without any anthelmintic intervention.

The relevant investigation to identify QTLs for resistance to GIN was arranged in 1979 in New Zealand (Diez-Tascon *et al.* 2002). Different studies showed that the QTLs for resistance are localized on chromosome 3, 6, 8 (Beh *et al.*, 2002; Crawford *et al.*, 2006). In Germany the study on QTL for resistance to parasites in Rhönschaf sheep showed significant association between parameters of resistance (FEC) and the markers *OarCp73, DYMS1* and *BM1815*. The *DYA* gene (belonging to the class IIb subregion of the MHC) closely linked to the microsatellite *DYMS1*, is a possible candidate gene for resistance to *H. contortus* in sheep (Janssen *et al.*, 2002). Three loci appear to be associated with parasite resistance, INFG on chromosome 3 (Coltman *et al.*, 2001), MHC on chromosome 20 (Paterson *et al.*, 1998) and the adenosine deaminase gene on chromosome 13 (Gulland *et al.*, 1993). Special attention is paid to the MHC class II molecules that induce the immune response in case of extracellular infection. The widest polymorphism among the MHC genes is found in *locus DRB*. This gene encodes the beta chain of the DR molecule, protein found in high concentrations on the surface of antigen-presenting cells. The first commercial genetic marker (WormSTAR™) for worm resistance was recently released and marketed by Catapult Genetics of Pfizer Animal Health in New Zealand (www.catapultsystems.co.nz). The WormSTAR™ marker explains approximately 2.3-3.6% of the genetic variation for the

FEC traits, 4.8-5.5% of the live weight traits, 3.7% for the wool traits and 6.2% for lean weight (McEwan *et al.*, 2008).

Interactions between nematode infections and host nutrition: The presence of the different nematode species in the various parts of the digestive tract is usually associated with: (i) a decrease in food consumption; (ii) a malabsorption/maldigestion syndrome; and (iii) changes in the host metabolism (Hoste *et al.*, 1997; Swarnkar and Singh, 2005). Recent studies have brought evidence showing that manipulation of the host nutrition could represent an option to improve the host resistance and or resilience to parasites. Several studies, performed in small ruminants, have underlined the possible antiparasitic effects of plant secondary compounds on nematodes. Amongst these secondary metabolites, tannins, present in some legume forages or in woody plants composing the vegetation of rangelands have been investigated. Results from both *in vivo* and *in vitro* studies suggest an action of tannins on the biology of the most prevalent worm species in small ruminants (Athanasiadou *et al.*, 2003; Paolini and Hoste, 2003; Swarnkar *et al.*, 2009).

c. *Limit the contamination of host by decreasing contact with the infective larvae*: The last option to control nematode infections in small ruminant aims at avoiding contact between susceptible host and a large number of infective larvae.

Types of pasture: Depending upon the level of worm larvae, pastures can be classified in following three categories (Michel, 1982):

i. *Clean pasture*: It is the pasture free from infection in the sense that susceptible animals grazing on it will not become a source of contamination. If worm free animals are put on such pasture it will remain safe for the rest of the season. Sanyal (1986) observed that clean pasture provided after winter drenching could be grazed for more than 3 months, however clean pasture after rainy season in June showed high infectivity in the second month of grazing and concluded that rotation of grazing on pasture should be made at the point so that pasture larval burden should not exceed 40 per kg of forage.

ii. *Safe pasture*: It is not sufficiently heavily infested to affect the production of susceptible animals grazing on it but such animals will become a source of contamination. The safe pastures are those which grazed only by young animals during summer.

iii. *Potentially dangerous pastures*: These are liable to carry an infestation sufficient to impair the production of susceptible animals.

Grazing management systems: The different practices of pasture management are based on one of the three strategies of management i.e. preventive, evasive or diluting strategy.

i. *Pasture rotation system*: To optimize the pasture growth and productivity, use of pasture for grazing in form of rotation is rapidly increasing. It involves subdivision of pasture in which each paddock is grazed for a short time and then rested for as relatively much longer time. The resting time should be framed in such a way that most of the infective larvae originating from the previous grazing to have died off. It is achievable in tropical climate where larval survival times are short compared to temperate environment where 3-9 months resting period is required to reduce the pasture infectivity. In Rajasthan, the grazing system of farmers is automatically of rotational in nature depending upon the availability of fodder (although not perfectly systematized). It has been observed that farmers put their animals on community grazing land / forest with the onset of monsoon where animals are drenched during mid-monsoon and continued on the same up to October. After harvesting of kharif crop the flocks are moved on such field to utilize crop stubbles for a period of one month. From November onward the flocks were again moved to community grazing land, forest or maintained on top feed with intermittent grazing on crop stubbles after rabi harvesting (Swarnkar *et al.*, 2008).

ii. *Safe pasture system*: The numbers of larvae on pasture are reduced over the time by resting the pasture during the period when they are normally being re-contaminated or through the growing and harvesting of a crop of hay or silage followed by a period of regrowth. This approach is only suitable in combined crop and livestock production system but if combined with the use of anthelmintics (dose and move system) it may increase the selection pressure for anthelmintic resistance.

iii. *Alternate grazing system*: To the extent that two or more host species in any given environment do not share common parasite species, alteration between the species can be a successful tool of improving worm control. Using alternate grazing for parasite control is based on different age groups of the same species (taking advantage of higher resistance in older animals) or different species (little cross infectivity between species and reduced susceptibility of different host species) grazing the pasture in sequence. It cannot be recommended as a standalone strategy (Barger *et al.*, 1994). In area where *T. axei* is not a major concern, alteration between small ruminants and cattle would be successful. In *H. contortus* predominant area, though the parasite infects cattle but fail to cause any disease, thus small ruminants and cattle alteration works. However in environment where *H. placei* infect cattle great caution should be exercised if their pastures are used for grazing by small ruminants, as this species is pathogenic in all hosts (Barger, 1999). This approach is less efficient in controlling parasitism in temperate climate compared to tropical and subtropical regions because cool and moist weather prolongs the larval survival. It has been observed that intensity of GIN in farmer's flock was low compared to farm flocks. One of the reasons behind this finding is that in rural area farmers graze all types of animals on same community grazing land in contrast to mono-specific grazing in organized farms.

iv. *Pasture resting*: It consists of preventing the animals from grazing in the same field or paddock. Since too low or too high temperature kill the infective larvae, cold and dry (hot dry) period can be relied upon to reduce or extend rest periods. In semi-arid conditions at least 2 month resting is essential compared to 6 month in cool, moist environment. In semi-arid Rajasthan, study with tracer lambs exhibited that sheep grazed during monsoon on spring contaminated-summer un-grazed pasture had very low FEC and worm count compared to those placed on continuously grazed contaminated pasture. The pasture larval burden was higher in general pasture than summer un-grazed pasture. Thus, resting the contaminated pasture during summer found to effectively control the pasture larval burden (Singh *et al.*, 1997b).

v. *Dose and move*: During 1970's, this strategy was central to the maintenance of clean grazing. Sheep were treated as they were moved on to clean pasture to prevent contamination.

Unfortunately this practice is highly selective for anthelmintic resistance (Abbott *et al.*, 2004).

Which solutions for which systems?

The choice of the various solutions to combine is also dependent on the system and on the objectives of production. Clearly, the criteria used to characterise a production system, both those related to the flock (size, stocking rate, breed) or to the environment (physical, pedo climatic, technical) are also main factors known to influence parasitism with nematodes. On the other hand, the environmental factors, associated with the different types of production system, also condition the applicability of various methods of parasite control. For example, regulation on the use of drugs and on the choice of anthelmintics is usually more drastic in ruminants producing milk than in those bred for meat or fibre. In addition, the threshold of acceptable parasitism is generally lower in intensive systems where the objectives of production have to be achieved in order to ensure the economy of the farm than in more extensive systems. Consequently, the need for measures to control nematode infections will differ between the farming systems. In extensive systems, the low stocking rates associated with the dilution of parasites, the incorporation of rangelands, the use of indigenous breed more adapted to the local environment and the flexibility obtained through the flock management, should allow to mainly rely on pertinent application of plan of surveillance. In more intensive systems, methods of control are more likely to be needed. Nowadays, it should be based on selective use of anthelmintic associated with management of pastures but it is reasonable to assume that some of the currently explored alternative approaches would lead to field application and will be incorporated in parasitism management. Unless veterinarians take an active and leading role in the education of small ruminant owners and help to implement these new approaches to parasite control, there may be no effective anthelmintics remaining when that time comes.

SWOT analysis on epidemiology and management of GI parasites

Efficient and effective management of GI parasites is only possible after surveillance has provided sufficient information to understand the prevailing epidemiological factors influencing transmission. Knowledge of the seasonal population trends and availability of infective larvae of nematode parasites is crucial for developing control programs that are appropriate for livestock owners.

Strength: Collection of data since long, observations in different livestock species and investigations in varied agro-climatic conditions of India.

Weakness: Lack of sound objective in most of the studies, application of erratic and haphazard methodology, no synchronization in methodology used by researchers in different states, short-term duration of studies, lack of observations on simultaneous studies on regulation of exogenous stages in given environment, lack of formulation of worm management programme and its validation, lack of integration between parasitologists, epidemiologist and statistician, lack of effective monitoring mechanism for standard anthelmintics (type of salt, formulation, sale, efficacy etc) and use of anthelmintics as a ready-made recipe in health camps and other programme organized by different institutions under various developmental activities.

Opportunities: Extensive infrastructural, financial and man-power facility under Network programme, region based collaborating centers and availability of variety of software / modules for analysis and interpretation.

Threats: Require long time to formulate management programme and its validation, role/interest of pharmaceutical companies in implementation of such programme, poor linkage between research organizations and state AH department, changing scenario of climate and management practices led to frequent reformulation and uncontrolled migration of livestock across the states.

Conclusion

"WORMS" - **W**isely thinking on **O**pportunities and **R**esources available with us and their integration into formulation of programme for parasite **M**anagement with the aim of **S**ustainability in production. Internal parasites continue to be a threat to health and productivity of small ruminants. The parasites of major concern were *Haemonchus*, *Trichostrongylus* and *Oesophagostomum* throughout the country. As the number of worm genera and species with anthelmintic resistance are growing it warrants systematic study of the reasons associated with failure of worm control measures. Control of GI helminths presents a difficult challenge following wide-spread emergence of anthelmintic resistance and is further complicated by recent and radical changes in approach to worm management (Sanyal, 2009). There must be regional worm control programmes based on detailed epidemiological and ecological studies of nematode infections of livestock in a variety of locations / agro-climatic conditions. These programmes should include: time and type of anthelmintic to be used, rotation of anthelmintic, if required, monitoring the efficacy of anthelmintic used and economic assessment of a control programme. As a new concept, the proposal to limit anthelmintic treatments to only part of a group will require some communication effort to achieve adoption. Although at present most animal managers take pains to ensure that every animal receives a treatment, experience with refugia-based strategies shows that new approaches can be palatable if new recommendations involve little additional work and there is minimal risk of disease or significant production loss. An advantage of targeted treatment systems may be that they are easier to comprehend and implement than other sustainable approaches. The benefit of avoiding expensive whole-flock treatment is likely to have additional appeal, especially to resource-poor farmers.

The veterinary advisors and parasitologists are the groups that have to take on the primary role. The advisors in particular, with their regular contact with farmers and the position of trust they have earned, have to make a sustained effort to make farmers aware of the need for change by giving frequent warnings of the dangers inherent in a drug-dominated worm control strategy and by encouraging them to adopt an incremental approach of holistic internal parasite management. An appropriate and sustained continuing education is essential. Parasitologists need to establish and then emphasize the relative economic importance of different worm species in each area. They should certainly continue to research practical alternatives to chemical control as experience has shown that nothing is static and the worms too will adapt to changed circumstances. The advice that is given must be simplified and practical, and should be fully integrated with other priorities and realities and not stand-alone or contradict economic imperatives. The predominance of *H. contortus* and use of all types of anthelmintic revealed that there is a great need to educate farmers and extension workers on appropriate anthelmintics to be used in their localities; moreover, there should be regular camps, ghosti / meetings, seminars and visits in rural areas by qualified veterinarians.

References

Abbott, K.A., Taylor, M. and Stubbings, L.A. 2004. Sustainable worm control strategies for sheep: A technical manual for Veterinary Surgeons and Advisors. SCOP, Context Publication, UK, p 43.

Agnihotri, R.K., Sharma, D., Dogra, P.K., Moudgil, A.K. and Sen, D. 2010. Incidence of gastrointestinal parasites in Chegu goats in tribal area of Lahual and Spiti of Himachal Pradesh. In: XX National Congress of Veterinary Parasitology, CCS HAU, Hisar, 18-20 February, p. 7.

Agrawal, M.C. 1986. Nasal schistosomiasis - A review. Helminthological Abstracts 61: 373-381.

Agrawal, M.C., Vohra, S., Gupta, S. and Singh, K.P. 2004. Prevalence of helminthic infection in domestic animals in Madhya Pradesh. Journal of Veterinary Parasitology 18: 147-149.

Ahmad, M. and Ansari, J.A. 1987. Prevalence of gastrointestinal nematodes of sheep in Aligarh. Indian Veterinary Medical Journal 11: 165-170.

Anon. 1991. Report of the FAO Expert Consultation of the Helminth Infections of Livestock in Developing Countries. Rome Italy 23-27 September, Food and Agriculture Organisation of the United Nations, Rome. AGA 815. p 32.

Arora, N., Sharma, S.D., Vihan, V.S. and Kumar, A. 2006. Seasonal changes in gastrointestinal parasitic infection of goat reared at an organized farm in semi-arid zone. Indian Journal of Small Ruminants 12: 37-41.

Athanasiadou, S.A., Kyriazakis, I., and Jackson, F. 2003. Can plant secondary metabolites have a role in controlling gastro intestinal nematode parasitism in small ruminants? In: 6th International Symposium on the Nutrition of Herbivores, Mérida, Mexico, 18-24 October.

Baker, R.L. 1996. Characterization and utilization of sheep and goat breeds that are resistant to helminths. In: Sustainable Parasite Control in Ruminants (Eds. L.F. Le Jambre and M.R. Knox), ACIAR Proceeding No. 74: 172-177.

Bal, M.S., Mahajan, V., Verma, S, Alka and Sharma, S. 2007. Outbreaks of parasitic gastroenteritis in sheep and goats. Journal of Veterinary Parasitology 21: 93-95.

Baldrey, F.S.H. 1906. Some problems on sheep diseases. Journal of Tropical Veterinary Science 1: 387.

Bali, H.S., Kwatra, M.S. and Fotedar, D.N. 1976. Studies on pathology of some helminth borne diseases in sheep of Kashmir. Journal of Animal Health and Production 4: 1-2.

Bali, M.K. and Singh, R.P. 1977. Studies on the prevalence of *Haemonchus contortus* in sheep and goat in Hissar. Haryana Agricultural University Journal of Research 7: 143-148.

Bandyopadhya, B. 1999. Gastrointestinal parasitic infections of sheep and goat at Salboni, West Bengal. Journal of Veterinary Parasitology 13: 79-80.

Banerjee, P.S., Godara, R., Kumar, R.R. Yadav, C.L., Garg, R., Kumar, S. and Vatsya, S. 2004. Seasonal incidence of gastrointestinal nematodosis in goats at Pantnagar. In: XV National Congress of Veterinary Parasitology GBPUAT, Pantnagar, 25-27 October, p 33.

Barger, I.A. 1999. The role of epizootiological knowledge and grazing management for helminth control in small ruminants. International Journal for Parasitology 29: 41-47.

Barger, I.A., Siale, K., Bank, D.J.D. and Le Jambre, L.F. 1994. Rotational grazing for control of gastrointestinal nematodes of goats in a wet tropical environment. Veterinary Parasitology 53: 109-116.

Beh, K.J., Hulme, D.J., Callaghan, M.J., Leish, Z., Lenane, I., Windon, R.G. and Maddox, J.F. 2002. A genome scan for quantitative trait loci affecting resistance to *Trichostrongylus colubriformis* in sheep. Animal Genetics 33: 97-106.

Bhat, M.S., Sudhan, N.A., Shahardar, R.A. and Mir, A.Q. 2007. Prevalence of gastrointestinal nematodosis in Kashmir valley. Journal of Veterinary Parasitology 21: 89-91.

Bhatia, B.B., Upadhaya, D.S. and Juyal, P.D. 1989. Epidemiology of *Fasciola gigantica* in buffaloes, goats and sheep in Tarai region of Uttar Pradesh. Journal of Veterinary Parasitology 3: 25-29.

Brunsdon, R.V. and Vlassoff, A. 1982. Parasite control – a rensed approach. In: Internal Parasites of Sheep (A.D. Ross, Ed.), Animal Industries workshop, Lincoln College, pp 53-64.

Cabaret J. 2008. Pro and cons of targeted selective treatment against digestive-tract strongyle of ruminants. Parasite 15: 506-509.

Census. 2003. Livestock Census. Department of Animal Husbandry, Dairying and Fisheries, Ministry of Agriculture, New Delhi.

Chaudhri, S.S. 2006. Epideiological trends of snail borne infections in small and large ruminants. In: XVII National Congress of Veterinary Parasitology, Puducherry, 15-17 November, pp 27-42.

Chaudhri, S.S., Gupta, R.P. Kumar, S. and Singh, J. 1991. A note on outbreak of fasciolosis in sheep in Eastern Haryana. Haryana Veterinarian 30: 148-150.

Chaudhri, S.S., Singh, S. and Singh, A. 2007. Epidemiology of hepatointestinal schistosomiosis in ruminants of some Northern states of India. Indian Journal of Animal Sciences 77: 288-292.

Chavan, P.B., Damle, P.S., Waghode, H.J., Bendre, M.U., Kurve, V.P. and Maske, D.K. 2008. Seasonal prevalence of gastrointestinal parasitism in goats at Nagpur. Veterinary World 1: 360.

Cherian, S. and D'Souza P.E. 2009. Prevalence of schistosomosis in sheep in Karnataka. Journal of Veterinary Parasitology 23: 93-94.

Chhabra, R.C., Gill, B.S. and Dutt, S.C.1978. Paramphistomiasis of sheep and goats in Punjab and its treatment. Indian Journal of Parasitology 2: 43-45.

Coltman, D.W. 2001. What microsatellites can tell us about disease resistance in free-living sheep populations: the genetics of resistance to nematodes in naturally parasitised Soay sheep from St. Kilda, Scotland. Biennial Symposium Northern Wild Sheep and Goat Council 12: 85.

Crawford, A.M., Paterson, K.A., Dodds, K.G., Diez Tascon, C., Williamson, P.A., Roberts Thomson, M., Bisset, S.A., Beattie, A.E., Greer, G.J., Green, R.S., Wheeler, R., Shaw, R.J., Knowler, K. and McEwan, J.C. 2006. Discovery of quantitative trait loci for resistance to parasitic nematode infection in sheep: I. Analysis of outcross pedigrees. BMC Genomics 7:178.

Cringoli, G., Veneziano, V., Jackson, F., Vercruysse, J., Greer, A.W., Fedele, V., Mezzino, L. and Rinaldi, L. 2008. Effect of targeted anthelmintic treatments on milk production of dairy sheep naturally sheep infected by gastrointestinal strongyles. Veterinary Parasitology 156: 340-345.

Darzi, M.M., Mir, M.S., Pandit, B.A., Nashiruddullaj, N. and Bhat, A.S. 2004. A retrospective study of naturally acquired haemonchosis in sheep. Journal of Veterinary Parasitology 18: 143-145.

Das, S.S., Kumar, D. and Sreekrishnan, R. 2006. prevalence of helminths parasites in ruminants in and around Puducherry. In: XVII National Congress of Veterinary Parasitology, Puducherry, 15-17 November, p. 67.

Davis, G., Genini, S. Bishop, S.C. and Giuffra, E. 2009. An assessment of the opportunities to dissect host genetic variation in resistance to infectious diseases in livestock. Animal 3: 415-436.

de Haan, C. and Bekure, S. 1991. Animal health services in sub-Saharan Africa: initial experience with alternative approaches. World Bank Technical Paper No. 134, Washington DC, World Bank, pp 49.

Deshpande, A.V. and Deshpande, P.D. 2005. Gastrointestinal nematodiosis in sheep and goats of Marathwada region. In: XVI National Congress of Veterinary Parasitology, Anjora, Durg, 6-8 December, p. 17.

Dey, S., Sanyal, P.K., Mukherjee, K., Sarkar, A.K., Patel, N.K., Mandal, S.C. and Pal, S. 2008. Caprine parasitic gastroenteritis in semi-organized farming conditions. Journal of Veterinary Parasitology 22: 77-78.

Dhand, N.K. singh, J., Aradhana and Sandhu, K.S. 2004. Fasciolosis in sheep and goats: an outbreak and treatment. Journal of Veterinary Parasitology 18: 77-78.

Dhar, D.N. and Dash, P.K. 1982. Lung worm and strongylate nematode infections in sheep in the Kullu Valley (Himachal Pradesh). Indian Journal of Parasitology 6: 53-55.

Dhar, D.N., Sharma, R.L. and Bansal, G.C. 1982. Gastrointestinal nematode infections in sheep in Kashmir. Veterinary Parasitology 11: 271-277.

Diez-Tascon, C., Macdonald, P.A., Dodds, K.G., McEwan, J.C. and Crawford, A.M. 2002. A screen of chromosome 1 for QTL affecting nematode resistance in ovine outcross population. In: Proc. 7th World Congress on Genetics Applied to Livestock Production, Montpellier, France, pp. 13-37.

Dutt, S.C. 1980. Paramphistomes and paramphistomiasis of domestic ruminants in India. A. Singh (Ed.) Punjab Agricultural University Press, Ludhiana, Punjab, p 162.

Gezahegn, L. 1992. Report to the Ministry of Agriculture, Addis Ababa, Ethiopia, p 28.

Ghosh, J. D. and Datta, S. 2005. Prevalence of gastrointestinal trematodes of ruminants in West Bengal. In: XVI National Congress of Veterinary Parasitology, Durg, 6-8 December, p 30.

Godara, R. and Sharma, R.L. 2010. Parasitic infections in livestock at Jaipur. Journal of Veterinary Parasitology 24: 192-193.

Gordon, H. McL. 1953. The epidemiology of helminthosis in sheep in winter rainfall regions of Australia I. Preliminary observations. Australian Veterinary Journal 29: 337-348.

Gray, G.D. 1987. Genetic resistance to haemonchosis in sheep. Parasitology Today 8: 253-255.

Gulland, F.M., Albon, S.D., Pemberton, J.M., Moorcroft, P.R. and Clutton-Brock, T.H. 1993. Parasite-associated polymorphism in a cyclic ungulate population. Proceeding of Royal Society of London B Biological Sciences 254: 7-13.

Gupta, R.P., Chaudhri, S.S., Ruprah, N.S. and Yadav, C.L. 1985. Epizootiology of paramphistomiasis in sheep and goats. Indian Journal of Animal Sciences 55: 14-19.

Gupta, R.P., Ruprah, N.S. and Yadav, C.L. 1986. Some observations on the spring-rise phenomenon in sheep of Haryana (India). Indian Veterinary Journal 63: 449-453.

Gupta, R.P., Yadav, C.L. and Choudhary, S.S. 1987. Epidemiology of gastrointestinal nematodes of sheep and goats in Haryana, India. Veterinary Parasitology 24: 117-127.

Hafeez, M. and Avsathi, B.L.1987. Incidence of ruminal amphistomes of certain domestic ruminants in and around Gujarat. Gujarat Veterinarian 15: 18-20.

Hafeez, M. and Rao, B.V. 1978. Studies on amphistomes and amphistomoasis in sheep and goats. Journal of Research, APAU, 5: 1-5.

Hassan, S.S., Kaur, A., Joshi, K. and Juyal, P.D. 2005. Epidemiology of paramphistomosis in domestic ruminants in different districts of Punjab and adjoining areas. Journal of Veterinary Parasitology 19: 43-46.

Hoste, H., Huby, F. and Mallet, S. 1997. Strongyloses gastro intestinales des ruminants : conséquences physiopathologiques et mécanismes pathogéniques. Le Point Vétérinaire 28: 53-59.

Hoste, H., Chartier, C. and Le Frileux, Y. 2002. Control of gastrointestinal parasitism with nematodes in dairy goats by treating the host category at risk. Veterinary Research 33: 531-545.

Hunt, P.W., McEwan, J.C. and Miller, J.E. 2008. Future perspectives for the implementation of genetic markers for parasite resistance in sheep. Tropical Biomed 25: 18-33.

Jackson, F. 2000. Options for the sustainable control of gastrointestinal nematode infections in goat production systems in Europe. In: Proc. 7th International Conference on Goats, Tours, France, 15-21 May, pp 789-792.

Jackson, F. and Coop, R.L. 2000. The development of anthelmintic resistance in sheep nematodes. Parasitology 120: S95-S107.

Jackson, F., Bartley, D., Bartley, Y. and Kenyon, F. 2009. Worm control in sheep in the future. Small Ruminant Research 86: 40-45.

Janssen, M., Weimann, C., Gauly, M. and Erhardt, G. 2002. Association between infections with *Haemonchus contortus* and genetic markers on ovine chromosome 20. In: Proc. 7th World Congress on Genetics Applied to Livestock Production, Montpellier, France, pp. 13-11.

Jithendran, K.P. 1994. Gastrointestinal parasitism in Gaddi sheep and goats in Kangra Valley, Himachal Pradesh. Journal of Hill Research 7: 9-12.

Jithendran, K.P. 1996. Occurrence of hydatidosis and various liver fluke infections in sheep and goats in Kangra valley: An abattoir survey. Journal of Veterinary Parasitology 10: 63-67.

Jithendran, K.P. 1998. Epidemiology of gastrointestinal nematodes in migratory sheep and goats in North-West humid Himalayan region. Indian Journal of Animal Sciences 68: 894-896.

Jithendran, K.P. and Bhat, T.K. 1996. Prevalence of dicrocoeliosis in sheep and goats in Himachal Pradesh, India. Veterinary Parasitology 61: 265-271.

Jithendran, K.P. and Katoch, R. 2003. Helminthic infections of livestock and wild animals in Himachal Pradesh. In: Helminthology in India (M.L. Sood, Ed.), International Book Distributors, Dehradun (Uttranchal), India, pp 341-362.

Jithendran, K.P. and Krishna, L. 1999. Fresh water snails with larval trematodes in Kangra Valley, Himachal Pradesh. Journal of Veterinary Parasitology 4: 51-53.

Kalwaghe, S.T., Khandare, L.M., Deshpande, P.D. and Narladkar, B.W. 2009. Study of round worm infection of ruminants, faecal culture and faecal egg count of Marathwada region. In: XIX National Congress of Veterinary Parasitology, Ludhiana, 3-5 February, p 44.

Katiyar, R.D. and Tewari, H.C. 1962. Acute fasciolosis amongst sheep in Kummaon hills. Indian Veterinary Journal 39: 382-386.

Katoch, R., Mittra, S., Agnihotri, R.K. and Sharma, A.K. 1998. Winter strongylosis in sheep and goats at high altitude: A sporadic occurrence. Indian Veterinary Journal 75: 362-363.

Kaur, A., Chhabra, S., Ashuma, Singh, N.K. and Juyal, P.D. 2009. Occurrence of *Dicrocoelium dendriticum* in sheep in an outbreak in Himacjal Pradesh. Journal of Veterinary Parasitology 23: 89-90.

Khajuria, J.K. and Kapoor, P.R. 2003. Prevalence of parasites in sheep and goats at Katua-Jammu. Journal of Veterinary Parasitology 17: 121-126.

Khajuria, J.K., Katoch, R., Yadav, A., Borkataki, S. and Singh, A. 2010. Prevalence of gastrointestinal helminths of sheep and goats of low-altitude sub tropical zone. In: XX National Congress of Veterinary Parasitology, 18-20 February, Hisar, p 15.

Khajuria, J.K., Sabberwal, C.S., Kappor, P.R., Gupta, S., Katoch, R., Yadav, A. and Vohra, S. 2005. epidemiological studies of helminths parasites in sheep of Katua district (Jammu). In: XVI National Congress of Veterinary Parasitology, 6-8 December, Anjora, Durg, p 32.

Khajuria, J.K., Sabberwal, C.S., Kappor, P.R., Katoch, R., Yadav, A., Vohra, S. and Soodan, J.S. 2006. Prevalence of helminths parasites in goats of Katua district (Jammu). In: XVII National Congress of Veterinary Parasitology, 15-17 November, Puducherry, p 78.

Khajuria, J.K., Yadav, A., Vohra, S., Katoch, R. and Sood, S. 2009. An outbreak of parasitic gastroenteritis in sheep and goats at RS Pura Jammu. In: XIX National Congress of Veterinary Parasitology, 3-5 February, Ludhiana, p 33.

Khan. F.A., Swarnkar, C.P., Singh, D., Jayasankar, J. and Bhagwan, P.S.K. 1999. Ovine gastrointestinal parasitism in farmers flock under semi-arid conditions of Rajasthan. Indian Journal of Small Ruminants 5: 65-70.

Kumar, S., Swarnkar, C.P., Singh, D., Kolte, A.P. and Singh, V.K. 2006. Genetic resistance to parasitic nematodes – A review. Indian Journal of Small Ruminants 12: 131-145.

Kumar, R.R., Garg, R., Yadav, C.L., Banerjee, P.S., Godara, R. and Kumar, S. 2007. Prevalence of fasciolosis in sheep and goats in Uttaranchal. Journal of Veterinary Parasitology 21: 15-16.

Kumari, S., Sinha, S.R.P., Sinha, S., Hoda, M.Z., Mandal, K.G. and Sharma, S.K. 2010. Incidence of gastrointestinal helminthoses in sheep and goat in Patna (Bihar). Journal of Veterinary Parasitology 24: 97-99.

Laha, R., Das, M., Goswami, A., Bardoloi, R.K. and Kharguria, G. 2010. Prevalence of gastrointestinal parasitism in Assam hill goats of Meghalaya. In: XX National Congress of Veterinary Parasitology, Hisar, 18-20 February p 10.

Lodha, K.R., Raisinghani, P.M., Sharma, G.D., Pant, U.V., Arya, P.L. and Vyas, U.K. 1981. Note on an outbreak of ovine pulmonary schistosomiasis in the arids of Rajasthan. Indian Journal of Animal Sciences 51: 382-385.

Makhdoomi, D.M., Shugufta, N., Mandey, S.D. and Molve, B. 1995. Incidence of different ovine gastrointestinal parasites in Kashmir. Indian Veterinary Journal 72: 898-900.

Manna, A.K., Pramanik, S. and Mukherjee, G.S. 1994. Incidence of paramphistomosis in West Bengal. Indian Journal of Animal Health 33: 87-89.

Mathur, P.B. 1986. A note on Fasciolosis in sheep in Himachal Pradesh. Indian Journal of Veterinary Medicine 6: 120-121.

McEwan, J.C., Weston, N.K., Payne, G.M., O'Sullivan, N.H., Auvray, B.N.E.E. and Dodds, K.G. 2008. Patent: Ovine identification method number 556506, http://www.iponz.govt.nz

McLeod, R.S. 1995. Costs of major parasites to the Australian livestock industries. International Journal of Parasitology 25: 1363-1367.

McLeod, R.S. 2004. The economic impact of worm infections in small ruminants of Southeast Asia, India and ustralia. In: Worm Control for Small Ruminants in Tropical Asia (R.A. Sani, G.D. Gray and R.L. Baker, Eds.), ACIAR Monograph 113, Australia, pp. 23-33.

Michel, J.F. 1976. The epidemiology and control of some nematode infections in grazing animals. Advances in Parasitology 14: 355-397.

Michel, J.F. 1982. Some thoughts on control of parasitic gastroenteritis. In: Biology and Control of Endoparasites (Eds, L.E.A. Symons, A.D. Donald and J.K. Dinnen), Academic Press, New Yark, pp. 113-131.

Mishra, A. and Agrawal, M.C. 1998. Role of *Indoplanorbis exustusi* snails in spreading schistosomiasis in endemic area. Indian Journal of Animal Sciences 68: 107-110.

Mishra, S.C., Das, D.N. and Mohapatra, G.S. 1974. Seasonal distribution of gastrointestinal helminths in sheep of Orisa. Indian Journal of Animal Health 13: 25-28.

Mittra, S., Agnihotri, A.R. and Nagpal, K.B. 1998. Sporadic deaths in migratory flocks of sheep due to strongyle nematodes. Himachal Veterinary Journal 1: 32-34.

Nadakal, A.M. 1961. Pregnancy and seasonal fluctuation of infection of sheep with certain helminth parasites in Northern India. Journal of Parasitology 47 (suppl): 87.

Nari, A., Salles, J., Castell, D. and Hansen J.W. 1997. Control of gastro-intestinal nematodes in farming systems of Uruguay. In: Proc. Biological Control Workshop (J.W. Hansen, and P.J. Waller, Eds.), FAO Technical Series Report No. 141. pp. 89-94.

Nasreen Shugufta, Jeelani Syed Gh. And Hakeem, Munir. 2005. Incidence of gastrointestinal nematodes in sheep in Kashmir valley. Journal of Veterinary Parasitology 19: 27-29.

O' Sullivan, B.M. and Donald, A.D. 1970. A field study of nematode parasite populations in the lactating ewes. Parasitology 61: 301-315.

Pal, P. and Bandyopadhya, S. 2004. Prevalence of gastrointestinal nematodosis in goats in Sikkim. Journal of Veterinary Parasitology 21: 93-95.

Palampalle, H.Y., Katamwad, S.S., Narladkar, B.W., Patil, P.S. and Kadam, D.P. 2009. Prevalence of nematohelminthiosis in Osmanbadi breed. XVII National Congress of Veterinary Parasitology, Ludhiana, 3-5 February, p 62.

Pandit, B.A., Mir, A.S. and Banday, M.A.A. 1991. An unusual recovery of *Fasiola gigantica* in the lungs and duodenum of sheep. Indian Veterinary Journal 68: 192.

Pandit, B.A., Shahardar, R.A., Darzi, M.M., Banday, M.A.A. and Bhat, A.S. 2003. Survey of gastrointestinal nematodes in sheep of Kashmir valley. Indian Journal of Small Ruminants 9: 39-42.

Pant, K., Rajput, M.K.S., Kumar, J., Sahu, S. Rajkumari, V and Gangwar, P. 2009. Prevalence of helminthes in small ruminants in Tarai region of Uttarakhand. Veterinary World 2: 265-266.

Paolini, V. and Hoste, H. 2003. How secondary compounds can have a role as an alternative way to control gastro intestinal nematodes in ruminants? In: Proc. 6th International Symposium on the Nutrition of Herbivores, Mérida, Mexico, 18-24 October.

Paterson, S., Wilson, K. and Petmberton, J.M. 1998. Major histocompatibility complex variation associated with juvenile survival and parasite resistance in a large ungulate population (*Ovis aries* L.). In: Proc. National Academy of Science, USA 95: 3714-3719.

Pathak, A.K. and Pal, S. 2008. Seasonal prevalence of gastrointestinal parasites in goats from Durg district of Chhattisgarh. Veterinary World 5: 136-137.

Patnaik, B., Mathur, P.B. and Pachlag, S.V. 1973. Helminths in sheep in semi-arid zones with particular reference to Rambouillet breed. Gujarat Veterinary Journal 7: 38-43.

Prasad, A. and Verma, T.K. 1999. On the prevalence and community dominance among paramphistomes infecting domestic ruminants. Journal of Veterinary Parasitology 13: 129-133.

Prince, L.L.L., Gowane, G.R., Swarnkar, C.P., Singh, D. and Arora, A.L. 2010. Estimates of genetic parameters for faecal egg count of *Haemonchus contortus* infection and relationship with growth traits in Avikalin sheep. Tropical Animal Health and Production 42: 785-791

Ram Hira, Sharma, A.K., Singh, S.K., Meena, H.R. and Rasool, T.J. 2007. Seasonal nematode egg out put in goat at high altitude of Uttaranchal. Journal of Veterinary Parasitology 21: 73-74.

Raman, M., Bharathi, R. Silva, Basith, S. Abdul and John Lalitha. 2010. Epizootiology of gastrointestinal helminths in sheep and goats of Tamil Nadu. Indian Journal of Small Ruminants 16: 74-78.

Rao, P.B. and Madhubala, K. 1998. Outbreak of fasciolosis in sheep with pulmonary involvement. Indian Veterinary Journal 75: 183-184.

Sanyal, P.K. 1986. Annual Report (1986). Central Sheep and Wool Research Institute, Avikanagar, Rajasthan.

Sanyal, P.K. 1988. Preliminary studies on hypobiosis - a diapause phenomenon of *Haemonchus contortus*. Indian Veterinary Medical Journal 12: 111-114.

Sanyal, P.K. 1989. Hypobiosis in *Haemonchus contortus* in South Indian sub temperate climate. Indian Journal of Animal Sciences 59: 1224-1227.

Sanyal, P.K. 2009. Automated technology transfer for sustainable control of parasitic gastroenteritis in small ruminants: A review. Indian Journal of Small Ruminants 15: 134-155.

Sanyal, P.K. and Gour, D. 1984. Studies on pasture sampling on the availability of ovine strongyle larvae in sub temperate Tamil Nadu. International Journal of Animal Science 4: 167-170.

Sarvananan, B.C., Pandey, B., Kotaktalware, M.A., Bandyopadhya, S., Pourouchottamane, R. and Bora, M. 2006. Study on prevalence of parasitic infection in organized sheep farm in Arunachal Pradesh. In: XVII National Congress of Veterinary Parasitology, Puducherry, 15-17 November p 55.

Shankar, D., Tiwari, J. and Sachan , B. 2010. Study of gastrointestinal helminthoses in different ruminant animals of Mathura district of UP. In: XX National Congress of Veterinary Parasitology, Hisar, 18-20 February, p 10.

Sharma D., Katoch, R. and Agnohotri, R.K. 2007. Gastrointestinal helminths in Gaddi sheep. Journal of Veterinary Parasitology 21: 141-143.

Sharma, D.N. and Dwivedi, J.N. 1976. Pulmonary schistosomiasis in sheep and goats due to *Schistosoma indicum* in India. Journal of Comparative Pathology and Therapeutics 81: 449-454.

Sharma, R.L. 2003. Helminthic diseases of livestock in Jammu and Kashmir. In: Helmintic Diseases in India. (M.L. Sood, ed.) International Book Distributors, Dehradun pp 231-245.

Sharma, R.L. and Godara, R. 2010. Metazoan diseases of livestock in the Greater Himalayan region of India and their diagnosis – An overview. Journal of Veterinary Parasitology 24: 1-16.

Sharma, R.L., Dhar, D.N. and Raina, O.K. 1989. Studies on prevalence and laboratory transmission of Fasciolosis in animals in the Kashmir valley. Veterinary Journal 145: 57-61.

Singh, D. and Swarnkar, C.P. 2003. Gastrointestinal nematodiasis in grazing ruminants. In: Sustainable Animal Production, (R.C. Jakhmola and R.K. Jain, Eds.), Pointer Publishers, Jaipur (Rajasthan), pp 264-297.

Singh, D. and Swarnkar, C.P. 2007. Alternative methods of control of gastrointestinal nematodes in small ruminants. In: Small Ruminant Emerging Diseases, Containment under WTO regime, (V.S. Vihan, Ashok Kumar, V.K. Gupta and N.P. Singh, Eds.), Satish Serial Publishing House, Delhi, pp. 269-304.

Singh, D. and Swarnkar, C.P. 2008. Role of refugia in management of anthelmintic resistance in nematodes of small ruminants - A review. Indian Journal of Small Ruminants 14: 141-180.

Singh, D. and Swarnkar, C.P. 2010. Harnessing the advantages of over-dispersion in faecal egg counts through targeted selective treatment and breeding for diseases resistance. In: XX National Congress of Veterinary Parasitology, Hisar, 18-20 February.

Singh, D., Swarnkar, C.P., Khan, F.A., Srivastava, C.P. and Bhagwan, P.S.K. 1997a. Epidemiology of ovine gastrointestinal nematodes at an organised farm in Rajasthan, India. Small Ruminant Research 26: 31-37.

Singh, D., Swarnkar, C.P., Khan, F.A. and Bhagwan, P.S.K. 1997b. Infectivity of spring contaminated – summer ungrazed pasture for gastrointestinal nematodes in sheep. In: IX National Congress of Veterinary Parasitology, Ludhiana, p 64.

Singh, D., Swarnkar, C.P., Khan, F.A., Jayasankar, J. and Bhagwan, P.S.K. 1999. Heritability of faecal egg counts in Avikalin sheep. Indian Journal of Animal Sciences 69: 983-985.

Singh, D., Swarnkar, C.P. and Khan, F.A. 2002. Anthelmintic resistance to gastrointestinal nematodes of livestock in India. Journal of Veterinary Parasitology 16: 115-130.

Singh, D., Swarnkar, C.P., Kumar Sushil, Prince, L.L.L. and Arora, A.L. 2009. Performance of Avikalin sheep selected for resistance to *Haemonchus contortus*. Journal of Veterinary Parasitology, 23: 23-27.

Singh, D., Swarnkar, C.P. Prince, L.L.L. and Pathak, K.M.L. 2011.Economic analysis and impact of gastrointestinal nematodes on sheep production in Rajasthan. Directorate of Knowledge Management in Agriculture, ICAR, New Delhi, pp 1-84.

Smith, S.M. 2002. AGRI-FOCUS July. http://grant-adams.wsu.edu.

Soulsby, E.J.L. 1986. Helminths, Arthropods and Protozoa of Domesticated Animals. 7th Edn., Baillìere Tindall, London.

Soundarajan, C. and Iyue, M. 2003. Seasonal prevalence of helminthic infection of sheep in Nilgiri hills. Indian Journal of Small Ruminants 9: 144-145.

Soundarajan, C. and Iyue, M. 2005. Pulmonary fasciolosis in sheep due to *Fasciola gigantica*. Journal of Veterinary Parasitology 19: 65-66.

Subudhi, M.S., Panda, D.N., Panda, M.R. and Mohanty, B.N. 2006. Incidence of gastrointestinal helminths in sheep and goats in the costal belt of Orissa. In: XVII National Congress of Veterinary Parasitology, Puducherry, 15-17 November, p. 76.

Sutar, A.U. and Khan, M.R. 2011. Seasonal prevalence of gastrointestinal parasites in sheep of rural areas of Ahmednagar district of Maharashtra. Asian Journal of Animal Sciences 6: 21-22.

Sutar, A.U., Kengar, S.B., Patil, S.S. and Khan, M.R. 2010. Prevalence of gastrointestinal parasites in goats of Ahmednagar district of Maharashtra. Veterinary World: 3: 456-457.

Swarnkar, C.P. and Singh, D. 2005. Nutritional interventions in management of gastrointestinal nematodes in small ruminants. In: Proc. FAO Symposium on "Integrated Animal Parasite Management : From Academic Interest to Reality" Durg, December 6-8, pp 41-54.

Swarnkar, C.P. and Singh, D. 2010. Worm control practices, anthelmintic use and its implication on anthelmintic resistance in gastrointestinal nematodes of sheep in Rajasthan. Indian Journal of Animal Sciences 80: 593-600.

Swarnkar, C.P. and Singh, D. 2011. Role of bioclimatographs in forecasting of strongyle infection in Rajasthan. Indian Journal of Animal Sciences 81: 216-223.

Swarnkar, C.P., Khan, F.A., Singh, D., Sharma, S.R. and Bhagwan, P.S.K. 1998. Some observations on periparturient rise in ewes at an organised farm. Indian Veterinary Journal 75: 781-784.

Swarnkar, C.P., Singh, D., Khan, F.A., Srivastava, C.P. and Bhagwan, P.S.K. 1997. Development and survival of *Haemonchus contortus* larvae on pasture under semi-arid conditions of Rajasthan. Journal of Veterinary Parasitology 11: 37-41.

Swarnkar, C.P., Singh, D., Lal Krishna and Khan, F.A. 2008. Epidemiology and Management of Gastrointestinal Parasites of Sheep in Rajasthan. CSWRI, Avikanagar pp 1-145.

Swarnkar, C.P., Singh, D. and Solanki, V. 2010. Prevalence of gastrointestinal parasites of sheep in semiarid Rajasthan: a field study. Indian Journal of Small Ruminants 16: 221-227.

Swarnkar, C.P., Singh, D., Srivastava, C.P., Bhagwan, P.S.K. and Dimri, U. 1996. A retrospective study on ovine gastrointestinal helminthoses under semi-arid condition. Journal of Veterinary Parasitology 10: 15-21.

Swarnkar, C.P., Singh, D., Kumar Sushil, Mishra, A.K. and Arora, A.L. 2009. Study on Malpura sheep selected for resistance to *Haemonchus contortus*. Indian Journal of Animal Sciences 79: 577-581.

Swarnkar, C.P., Singh D. and Solanki, V. 2010. Prevalence of gastrointestinal parasites of sheep in semiarid Rajasthan: a field study. Indian Journal of Small Ruminants 16: 221-227.

Talukdar, S.K. 1996. Prevalence of anthelmintic infection of goat in Assam. Journal of Veterinary Parasitology 10: 83-86.

Tariq, K., Chisti, M.Z., Ahmed, F and Shawl, A.S. 2008. The epidemiology of paramphistomes in sheep (*Ovis aries L.*) in the north west temperate Himalayan region of India. Veterinary Research Communication 32: 383-391.

Thaper, G.S. 1956. Systematic survey of helminth parasites of domestic animals in India. Indian Journal of Veterinary and Animal Husbandry 26: 211-271.

Van Wyk, J.A. 2001. Refugia - overlooked as perhaps the most potent factor concerning the development of anthelmintic resistance. Onderstepoort Journal of Veterinary Research 68: 55-67.

Van Wyk, J.A. and Bath, G.F. 2002. Practical methods of identifying individual animals for anthelmintic treatment within a group. Veterinary Research 33: 509-529.

Varma, A.K. 1957. On a collection of paramphistomes from domestic animals in Bihar. Indian Journal of Veterinary Science 59: 231-234.

Walker, G.K. 1906. A preliminary note on a gillar- a disease affecting sheep and goats. Journal of Tropical Veterinary Science 1: 410.

Waller, P.J., Rudby-Martin, L., Ljungström, B.L. and Rydzik, A. 2004. The epidemiology of abomasal nematodes of sheep in Sweden, with special reference to overwinter survival strategies. Veterinary Parasitology 122: 207-222.

Wani, Z.A., Shahardar, R.A. and Shahnawaz, M. 2011. Prevalence of nemathelminth parasites in sheep of Ganderbal district of Kashmir valley. Journal of Veterinary Parasitology, 25: 26-29.

Yadav, A., Khajuria, J.K. and Raina, A.K. 2006. Seasonal prevalence of gastrointestinal parasites in sheep and goats of Jammu. Journal of Veterinary Parasitology 20: 65-68.

Yadav, C.L., Banerjee, P.S., Godara, R., Kumar, R.R. and Kumar, S. 2004. Incidence of gastrointestinal nematodosis in Uttaranchal. In: XV National Congress of Veterinary Parasitology Pantnagar, 25-27 October, p 33.

Yadav, C.L., Kumar, R.R., Vatsya, S. Garg, R. and Banerjee, P.S. 2007. Epidemiology of gastrointestinal nematodosis in goats of Uttarakhand, India. In: XVIII National Congress of Veterinary Parasitology Jammu, 7-9 September, p 85.

Yadav, C.L., Kumar, R.R., Vatsya, S. and Garg, R. 2010. prevalence of amphistomosis in ruminants in national capital region, India. Journal of Veterinary Parasitology 24: 125-127.

□□□

Chapter 20

Genetics of Disease Resistance in Small Ruminants : Scope and Future Application

P.K. Rout
Central Institute for Research on Goats, Makhdoom
Farah- 281 122, Mathura (UP)

Disease biology and disease genetics

Disease is the economically important issue and is the major reason for genotype and phenotype gap. Infectious disease has major adverse effects on livestock production and animal welfare, worldwide. Despite the traditional disease control measures, losses attributable due diseases contribute to impede the livestock industries. The costs of disease are estimated as 10-20% of turnover within the livestock sector in the developed world and 35-50% in the developing world (more than Rs. 14,000 crores in India). All animal production systems are subjected to challenges by infectious disease and all animal production systems are liable to large production losses from disease. Disease also poses threats across species barriers as diseases in one species may act as reservoirs for infections in other species. In particular, animal infections pose zoonotic threats to human health. The control or management of infectious disease is currently achieved by several mechanisms, including (i) chemical intervention, notable examples being anthelmintics for nematode parasite control, acaricides for tick control and antibiotics for the control of many bacterial diseases, (ii) vaccination, (iii) sanitation and disinfection and (iv) culling, isolation and control of the movements of animal and/or animal products. Disease control or management using genetics, i.e. exploiting genetic variation amongst hosts in disease resistance (in the most general sense) is increasingly looked upon as an additional way of controlling many diseases, complementing or sometimes replacing existing strategies.

Disease is one of the most important biological constraints to livestock production in all over the world. Loss of production performance, mortality and the cost of drugs are the major concerns for farmers and Industries. Moreover, the foremost pressure to breed for disease resistance is the evolution of resistance in parasites to chemical or vaccine control measures. Important examples include:

- The evolution of resistance to anthelmintics by nematodes in all major sheep producing countries. This threatens sustainable sheep production throughout the world. Resistance has developed to all classes of anthelmintics and no new classes are being produced by pharmaceutical companies.
- The evolution of resistance to antibiotics by bacteria. This threatens the efficacy of antibiotics in many production systems. This is especially problematic in intensive production systems where antibiotics are used to control unknown and sometimes sub-clinical disease problems.
- The evolution of resistance to anti-protozoal compounds. For example, there is widespread resistance to drugs used to control animal trypanosomosis.
- The evolution of acaricide resistance by populations of ticks, leading to greater problems of tick infestation and tick-borne diseases.
- The evolution of vaccine resistance. For example, each new generation of vaccines against Marek's disease has apparently been followed by strains of ever more virulent viruses.

Predicting the consequences of breeding animals for disease resistance is qualitatively different from predicting the consequences of breeding animals for a production trait. A safe assumption with most production traits is that animals express their trait independently of other animals in the herd or flock. This is not always the case with resistance to infectious diseases, where animals may infect each other either directly or indirectly. Hence, the expression of infection or disease status between individual animals within the same population is not independent of each other, depending upon the dynamics or epidemiology of the disease. Therefore, the consequences of genetic improvement will depend upon both the genetic makeup of the host population and the epidemiology of the disease. The diseases of livestock were ranked according to their importance (Table 1).

Table 1 : Top-ranked diseases according to their impact on the poor, by species (from Perry *et al.*, 2002)

Rank	Cattle	Sheep/Goats	Poultry	Pigs
1.	Foot and mouth disease	Helminthosis	Newcastle disease	Ecto-parasites
2.	Nutritional deficiency	PPR[2]	Helminthosis	Helminthosis
3.	Reproductive disorders	Haemonchosis	Coccidiosis	Swine fever
4.	Haemorrhagic septicemia	Neonatal mortality	Ecto-parasites	Neonatal mortality
5.	*Brucella abortus*	Respiratory complexes	Neonatal mortality	Foot and mouth disease
6.	Trypanosomosis	Sheep and goat pox	Fowl cholera	African swine fever
7.	Liver fluke	Ecto-parasites	Infectious coryza	Cystcercosis
8.	Anthrax	Anthrax	Fowl pox	*Brucella suis*
9.	CBPP[1]	Liver fluke	DVE[3]	Trypanosomosis
10.	*Toxocara vitulorum*	Heartwater	Nutritional deficiency	Japanese B encepthalitis

1. Contagious bovine pleural pneumonia. 2. Peste-des-petits ruminants. 3. Duck virus enteritis

Mechanisms of disease resistance

The onset of disease is often the result of complex interaction between the genotype, pathogen and its environment. Generally two types of resistance have been described in all the infectious diseases. (1) Resistance to infection means that the mechanism that prevent the organism to penetrate into living host cell i.e first line of defense or cellular resistance. Examples of such resistance are absence of receptor in the cell membranes for retroviruses of subgroup A, B, C, D, E and absence of cell receptor for K88 antigen in pig. (2) Second type resistance / second line of defense is the resistance to the disease process or effects of infestation in host in response to pathogen infection.

Exploiting genetic variation in disease resistance

Genetic resistance may be found with discrete or continuous phenotypic variation and inherited by simple Mendelian mechanism or polygenic inheritance. Genetic resistance to infection or tolerance of infection may, in some cases, be due predominantly to a single gene. Examples include resistance to *Escherichia coli* diarrhoea in pigs and the PrP gene, which is associated with resistance to scrapie in sheep. In other cases, resistance or tolerance is due to the combined effects of several or many genes. Examples of this include nematode resistance in ruminants, mastitis resistance in dairy cattle and sheep, and trypanotolerance in locally adapted breeds of cattle. Although resistance and tolerance are sometimes qualitative phenomena, as in the case of *E. coli* diarrhoea in pigs, more often they are quantitative phenomena. That is, they show continuous variation from one extreme to the other. Continuous variation is seen when resistance or tolerance is due to the combined effects of several genes. Disease resistance tends to be specific to particular diseases rather than general to all diseases. This is because genetic resistance to different diseases is controlled at least to a major degree by different mechanisms. Thus, different genes will generally influence resistance to unrelated diseases. However, similar genes may influence resistance to closely related infections. An example is the often-observed strong genetic correlation between resistance to different species of gastrointestinal nematode parasites.

Exploiting genetic differences in resistance, i.e. using host genetic variation to reduce the transmission of infection has the benefit of reducing the incidence of infection in the target population. This reduces the effects of disease and may also reduce transmission of infection to other populations. Using genetics to assist in the management of the clinical signs of disease, i.e. genetically increasing the tolerance of a population to infection will be effective in reducing the incidence or the effect of disease in the target population. However, it may not decrease the prevalence of the parasite. Hence, the disease incidence or prevalence in other populations in the same environment will not be affected. In worst-case scenarios, the presence of infection in the environment may be masked. For example, in the case of zoonoses, using genetics to manage tolerance of infection would be unwise as it may lead to human disease threats being unrecognized.

A critical issue is the need for disease resistance genes (more correctly, gene variants) or QTL to assist in selection for disease resistance. Clearly, actual disease resistance gene variants or QTL (or even genomic predictors) have the benefit of enabling the selection of animals without exposing them to infection. For many diseases molecular techniques may be the only way of enabling effective selection for disease resistance. For others, such as mastitis or nematode parasites, a combination of phenotypic measurement and genetic markers may be the optimal approach.

Genetic epidemiological modeling

Impacts of infectious diseases in livestock species present a considerable challenge for profitability in a production system. Complex interactions occur between the host animal population and the pathogen, and these interactions will vary temporally, spatially and with the host genotype. Moreover, the infection and subsequent host immune-response processes are multi-factorial. In order to predict the effect of any factor, including treatment strategies or genetic selection of resistant hosts, on an infectious disease at the population level, an epidemiological model is required. This model should capture and quantify the dynamics of the disease and allow the impact of various factors affecting the disease severity and epidemiology to be predicted. Major uses of epidemiological models have traditionally included (i) evaluating the effects of various control strategies, e.g. vaccination or management options, on the disease severity, (ii) evaluating the impact of local weather conditions on the disease severity and (iii) evaluating the impact of various chemotherapy strategies on likely evolution of drug resistance in the pathogen.

The application of mathematics to the study of infectious diseases was pioneered by David Bernoulli in 1760. Hamer (1906) postulated that the course of epidemics depends on the contact rate between susceptible and infected individuals, one of the most important concepts in epidemiology. Ronald Ross (1908) translated the problem from a discrete-time model to a continuous-time framework in his work on the dynamics of malaria. Subsequently much of the theory used to develop epidemic models has been based on differential calculus used to describe rates of transmission or processes, or on stochastic approximations to such equations.

Modelling approaches: General principles

Epidemic models must define the pathways of transmission shown in figure below.

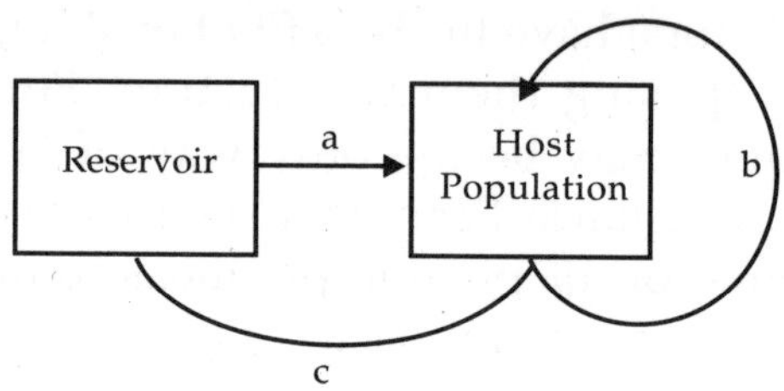

Not all pathways are relevant to all diseases, and some of the pathways ways may be considerably more complex than shown here. For example, pathway **c** may involve intermediate hosts. All infections must initially arise from some reservoir of infection. The transmission of infection from the reservoir may be 'continuous' or sporadic. Once infection is in the host population it may follow several transmission pathways. Typically, but not exclusively, microparasitic infections will be transmitted by direct animal-to-animal contact along pathway **b,** whereas macroparasitic infections will be transmitted via some external host, vector or reservoir. There are many diseases where pathway **a** is important and continual, and pathways **b** and **c** are non-existent or trivial.

Examples include trypanosomiasis and mastitis caused by environmental contamination. Sub clinical disease challenges in intensive production systems, addressed using the concept of generalised immunity, may also fit into this framework. Diseases where pathway **b** is critical, with sporadic infection from the reservoir (pathway **a**) include viral diseases. Diseases where pathways **a** and **c** are critical, i.e. a continuous flow of infection between the host population and the reservoir, include nematode infections in ruminants, where the reservoir is the pasture, and some bacterial diseases.

Approaches to epidemic modelling vary dramatically according to the disease scenario. Models take many forms, with the main aim being to describe the disease patterns in relation to events that may change either deterministically or stochastically. Inputs into the models may be explanatory variables describing the infection process or simply empirical relationships between observed phenomena - sometimes with no strong theoretical justification. Classic applications of models using empirical relationships are the weather based models describing helminth infection in cattle, sheep and goat. In these models, the parasite epidemiology is calculated as a function of the prevailing weather conditions in any particular season, and inputs to the model include a database of meteorological records over many years.

A critical issue when considering epidemic modelling is whether to take a deterministic or stochastic approach. Within animal breeding contexts both approaches generally yield the same expected outcome, although the stochastic approach can yield a greater richness of output - sometimes for less stringent understanding of the underlying processes. In epidemiological modelling, outputs from stochastic and deterministic models can differ dramatically quantitatively and qualitatively. For example, minor epidemics that arise and die out without intervention are predicted by stochastic models but not deterministic models. Both approaches have a role to play: deterministic models may give initial insight into a problem, however stochastic models are required to represent the diversity of outcomes possible from epidemics, and quantify epidemic risks under different circumstances.

Status of disease resistance genetic improvement programs

The best-known examples are for scrapie and nematode resistance in sheep, tick resistance, mastitis resistance in cattle. For nematode resistance there are breeding programs underway in New Zealand, Australia and the UK; tick resistance is an integral part of cattle breeding programs in subtropical Australia; mastitis resistance, either in terms of clinical cases of mastitis or reduced somatic counts, is incorporated into many dairy cow and sheep breeding programs. Breeding for resistance to post-weaning *E. coli* diarrhoea in pigs, where the causal mutation or closely linked markers are known, has been undertaken in some selection programs. Perhaps the most far-reaching example of breeding for disease resistance has been selection for scrapie resistance, based on PrP genotype, which has been practised in several countries in Western Europe.

The first indication of genetic variation for disease resistance often comes from the observation that some breeds or populations have the ability to tolerate endemic diseases or to survive an epidemic disease that more susceptible breeds cannot. The possible source of genetic variation between breed, strains, families and individuals should be analyzed. The source of genetic variation in important diseases in farm animals will give an idea about the nature of variation and inheritance of the trait in the population. The application of breeding for resistance to diseases should consider all the factors in relation to impact on production, control strategy and zoonotic potential.

The susceptibility of sheep to ovine lentivirus infection such as Maedi/visna has long been known to be subject to distinct genetic variation. Scrapie is associated with major gene in sheep. British goats were more susceptible to capripox challenge than north Yemen Black goat. The susceptibility of British sheep breed to Bluetongue virus infection revealed that Soya sheep were most susceptible and died before showing any clinical symptoms, whereas Dorset horn and Merino developed several clinical signs before death. The indigenous sheep and cattle breeds of Kenya were relatively resistant to rift valley fever as compared to exotic animals imported for breed improvement programme.

Bacterial diseases that has been analyzed for disease resistance include anthrax, brucellosis, caseous lymphadenitis, enterotoxaemia, pasterulosis, salmonellosis and dermatophilosis in sheep and mycoplasmosis in goat. Genetic variation to many bacterial diseases has been described in studies between small ruminant breeds and within breeds and flocks. Genetic resistance to foot rot in sheep has been well recognised and the heritability of resistance to foot rot has been reported in specifically designed experiment in Merino sheep. Breed differences in susceptibility to Jhone's disease in goat have been reported in different countries. Genetic variation to parasites has been found both within and between host populations and for a number of important parasite species including nematode worm, coccidian, flies and ticks. Variation in resistance to gastrointestinal nematodes (GIN) between breeds and within breeds have been reported and reviewed by Kassai and Streter and by Gray and colleague. In goats, the resistance to *H. contortus* has been reported by different researchers. In the case of small ruminants in the tropics this is well illustrated by the resistance and/or tolerance of a number of sheep breeds to GIN infections including the Red Maasai in East Africa, the Djallonke in West Africa, the St. Croix and Barbados Blackbelly in the Caribbean, the Javanese Thin Tail in Indonesia and the Garole in India. The heritability estimates for resistance to GIN (assessed by faecal egg counts) estimated from the relatively susceptible Romney and Merino breeds in New Zealand and Australia. The potential impact of quantitative trait loci (QTL) associated with resistance to helminthes (*Trichostrongylus colubriformis*) infection has been carried out in Merino sheep, Thin tail sheep of indonesia and Black face sheep of Scotland.

National scenario

In small ruminants, some reports of breed differences to disease susceptibility from herds maintained by research institute and universities have been reported, however most of the studies are not aimed to assess genetic variation in breeds. Comparative disease susceptibility to Sheep pox, Blue tongue, Ovine adenovirus, FMD and haemonchosis has been reported. Malpura and Chokla breeds were less susceptible to sheep pox in comparison to Sonadi and Nali. Malpura, Marwari, Sonadi and Nali breeds were less susceptible to Blue tongue in comparison to exotic breeds. Nellore, Mutton synthetic breeds of sheep were highly susceptible to FMD, whereas Malpura and Mandya were lowly susceptible to FMD. Similarly in goats, breed differences in resistance to Goat pox, FMD, Johne's disease, colibacilosis have been reported. Results of analysis of data in natural infection revealed that Sirohi was less susceptible to Goat pox in comparison to Kutchi and Marwari. Barbari was less susceptible to FMD than Jamunapari and Jakhrana. Jamunapari goats are less susceptible to JD than Barbari goats. Jamunapari kids were less susceptible to colibacilosis than Barbari kids. Barbari goats were more susceptible to pneumonia than Jamunapari goats under similar system of management.

Genetic resistance to GIN (*H. contortus*) in goats has been initiated at CIRG, Makhdoom. Indicator traits for resistance to GIN have been established in Indian goats. The study showed the variability in resistance pattern in response to natural *H. contortus* infection in selected flocks of Barbari and Jamunapari goats and established genetic correlation with indicator traits and growth parameter. Age related Immunity to nematodes (*H. contortus*) does not exist in Indian goats as observed in sheep. Genetic modelling including FEC, PCV and bodyweight at 9 months of age was proposed for getting optimum productivity as well as reduced pasture contamination, thereby fulfilling all the indicators of sustainable livestock production. Increase in parasite infection (particularly *H.contortus*) occurs during pregnant and lactating stages of goat and susceptibility to infection during pregnant and lactating stages varies with respect to breed. Therefore the management decisions should be taken to get better kid weights and milk yield while the goats are under parasite challenge. Moreover highly susceptible breeds should not be introduced in humid zones for breed improvement purpose.

Breeding for disease resistance experiment has been mainly conducted in temperate regions. The breeding objective for small ruminants in tropical production systems will be different from those in temperate production systems. The genetic variation among indigenous sheep or goat breeds in the tropics is likely to be larger than that found among breeds of small ruminant in temperate regions. We must utilize the breed variation most efficiently to improve the performance of our stock and to check mortality as well as sub clinical infection. We have not yet evaluated our genetic resources for genetically based resistance in different agro-climatic zones and production system.

Future scope and application

We need to analyze the patterns of host resistance to infection in relation to genetic and epidemiological factors, using different modelling approaches according to the available data. Therefore, it is essential to establish the base line data in relation to the environmental conditions and analyze the resistance patterns. The statistical and mathematical models will enable the host genetic factors and environmental factors to be disentangled, and this will assist in the control of nematode infection in livestock. To enable finer scale dissection of genetic resistance and potentially allow more precise genetic selection, we can analyse the association of various molecular markers (microsatellite and SNP) with indicator traits of nematode infection, and analyse their contribution to controlling GI parasite infections under Indian conditions.

Small ruminant productivity in India varies greatly in all respects in different agro-climatic zones. For enhancing productivity, it is equally important to give greater attention to the biological attributes of indigenous breeds and need to be exploited for local advantage. The productivity of different goat and sheep breeds in different production systems gives a close look to their importance for conservation. So it is necessary to characterize and evaluate the performance of the different breeds in different production systems. We also have to develop strategy to maintain productivity of goats and sheep with reference to geographic shift of production system from temperate and dry areas to warmer, more humid and disease prone environment. Our indigenous goat and sheep population has not been characterized and evaluated for genetic-based disease resistance in natural population. Therefore, we must evaluate our stocks for the disease resistance parameter with respect to geographic, climatic and production system. Parasitic characterization of field condition as well as host response in kids up to 1 year of age and in different physiological condition should be carried out.

References

Baker, R.L. 1998. A review of genetic resistance to gastrointestinal nematode parasites in sheep and goats in the tropics and evidence for resistance in some sheep and goat breeds in sub humid coastal Kenya. Animal Genetics Resources Information Bulletin 24: 13-30.

Baker, R.L., Mwamachi, D.M., Audho, J.O., Aduda, E.O. and Thorpe, W. 1998. Resistance of Galla and Small East African goats in the sub humid tropics to gastrointestinal nematode infections and the periparturient rise in faecal egg counts. Veterinary Parasitology 79: 53-64.

Bishop, S.C. and Wolliams, J.A. 2010. On the genetic interpretation of disease data. PLoS ONE 5: e8940.

Bishop, S.C., Jackson, F., Coop, R.L. and Stear, M.J. 2004. Genetic parameters for resistance to nematode infections in Texel lambs and their utility in breeding programmes. Animal Science 78: 185-194.

Bishop, S.C. and Morris C.A. 2007. Genetics of disease resistance in sheep and goats. Small Ruminant Research 70: 48-59.

Bishop, S.C. and Stear, M.J. 1999. Genetic and epidemiological relationship between productivity and disease resistance: gastro-intestinal parasite infection in growing lambs. Animal Science 69: 515-524.

Bishop, S.C. and Stear, M.J. 2003. Modelling of host genetics and resistance to infectious diseases: understanding and controlling nematode infections. Veterinary Parasitology 115: 147-166.

Chauhan, K.K., Rout, P.K., Singh, P.K., Mandal, A., Singh, S.K. and Roy, R. 2003. Genetic resistance of Barbari and Jamunapari kids to natural infection with gastrointestinal nematodes. Tropical Animal Health and Production 35: 397-408.

Over, H.J., Jansen, J. and Von Olm, P.W. 1992. Distribution and impact of helminth diseases of livestock in developing countries. Food and Agriculture Organization of the United Nations Animal Production and Health paper 96.

Perry, B.D., Randolph, T.F., McDermott, J.J., Sones, K.R. and Thornton, P.K. 2002. Investing in animal health research to alleviate poverty. ILRI, Nairobi, Kenya, p 148.

Rout, P.K., Sharma, D.K., Saxena, V.K., Singh, S.K. and Roy, R. 2002. Resistance of Jamunapari and Barbari goat breeds to natural infection with gastro-intestinal nematodes. Indian Journal of Animal Sciences 72: 770-773.

Vagenas, D., Bishop, S.C. and Kyriazakis, I. 2007. A model to account for the consequences of host nutrition on the outcome of gastrointestinal parasitism in sheep: logic and concepts. Parasitology 134: 1263-1277.

Vagenas, D., Bishop, S.C. and Kyriazakis, I. 2007. A model to account for the consequences of host nutrition on the outcome of gastrointestinal parasitism in sheep: model evaluation. Parasitology 134: 1279-1289.

Vagenas, D., Doeschl-Wilson, A., Bishop, S.C. and Kyriazakis, I. 2007. Exploration of the effects of host genotype and nutrition on the genetic parameters of lambs challenged with gastrointestinal parasites. International Journal for Parasitology 37: 1617-1630.

□□□

Chapter 21

Neonatal Mortality in Small Ruminants : Issues and Management

V.K. Gupta[1] and Ashok Kumar[2]

[1]Senior Scientist (Immunology), [2]Principal Scientist (Veterinary Medicine), Division of Goat Health, Central Institute for Research on Goats, Makhdoom- 281 122, PO Farah, Mathura (U.P.)

Expulsion from the uterus at birth arguably exposes lambs/kids to the greatest physiological challenges they will face in their lives. Nevertheless, when pregnancy, birth and/or the newborn are managed scientifically, the majority of newborns are healthy and vigorous and show few if any signs of debility. In some cases, however, survival of the foetus during birth and of the newborn afterwards depends upon the individual operating at the limits of its physiological capacity. Some of these newborns survive, but with chronic functional impairment, some are forced beyond their physiological limits and die (Smith and Sherman, 1994).

During the past 50 years, fundamental and applied research, driven primarily by economic considerations, has clarified much about the causes and prevention of neonatal mortality in small ruminants and has provided practical means for minimising neonatal losses. Accordingly, with human intervention, neonatal mortality rates can usually be kept below 15%, but without it, rates of 30–50% or more commonly occur. To date, however, there has been no systematic or comprehensive analysis of the welfare compromise the newborns of small ruminant species may experience before death or during sickness due to different causes. One of the key indicators of the efficiency of a small ruminant production system is the degree to which lambs and kids survive to a marketable age and/or to a sustainable reproductive life. Low survival rates may be signs of serious problems in such a system; they may be indications of a very low standard of husbandry. They may also be among the major causes of a reduced rate of multiplication of animals and poor return to capital invested. Thus, knowledge of postnatal losses is a prerequisite for a good understanding of the production system of interest and to the adequate diagnosis of the related constraints. In any livestock production system, certain diseases and production constraints can be anticipated on the basis of accumulated experiences. An understanding of some of these management practices and common disease problems is helpful to accomplish good neonatal health. In general, great emphasis would have to be placed on kid/lamb rearing techniques to reduce neonatal mortality and diseases that inhibit the rapid, efficient growth of young kids/lambs such as pneumonia, coccidiosis and gastrointestinal parasites (Donkin and Boyazoglu, 2004; Sharif *et al.*, 2005).

Management issues

A major obstacle to newborn's survival is hypothermia/ hypoglycaemia and infectious diseases due to delayed or an inadequate intake of colostrum. Failure of passive transfer of maternal antibodies to newborns leads to an increased disease incidence and death throughout the postnatal period. The does/ewes in late pregnancy should receive their vaccination for enterotoxemia, pox and tetanus. The vaccine will both protect the doe/ewes and ensure high levels of antibodies in the colostrum, which will subsequently protect the newborn kid/lambs. Therefore, kidding/lambing should be a well-anticipated event, not an unexpected surprise. Being prepared for routine processing of kids/lambs at birth, such as dipping navels, colostrum feeding and being ready to respond to emergencies will reduce neonatal mortality. In goats surviving the neonatal period, diseases that inhibit rapid, efficient growth are pneumonia, coccidiosis and gastrointestinal parasites.

Neonatal mortality rates

Neonatal mortality is defined as death of young during the first 3-7 days after birth, however, the majority of deaths occur within the first 1-2 days. The overall mortality rates reported are variable and in some cases include much wider variability. For instance, although the range for overall kids/lamb mortality in India is 10–25%, between different farms in a particular region the range can be as wide as 5-70%. Kid mortality rates from birth to weaning can be as high as 85%. Litter size can have major effects on mortality rate, as single and twin lambs/kids are much less likely to die than triplets. Monotocous and ditocous animals such as sheep and goats have fewer offspring with each pregnancy, which allows a greater maternal investment to maximise survival rates (Sreedhar, 2009; Turkson *et al.*, 2004).

Major causes of neonatal mortality

The major factors that predispose newborn farm animals to death are similar in the different species, but the prevalence of each cause and its precise manifestation may differ between species. Here we describe the major causes which affect neonates of small ruminant species most.

Hypothermia: It commonly precedes neonatal death in most small ruminants, but the reduced body temperature itself is not necessarily the primary cause of death. Indeed, hypothermia, which occurs when body heat loss exceeds heat production, has several causes in the newborn.

a. Cold exposure – excessive heat loss: Healthy newborns which increase their heat production to maximum levels in response to cold exposure nevertheless become hypothermic when the ambient conditions are so cold that heat loss from their bodies exceeds heat production. In such cases, cold exposure is the primary cause which leads to death from hypothermia. Healthy newborn lambs are more resistant to body cooling than are kids because of a higher heat production capacity per unit body weight and a lower surface area to body weight ratio, as well as generally better skin insulation in lambs (wool) than in kids (hair). The maximum rate of heat production per unit body weight is greater in newborn lambs than in other newborn species.

b. *Placental insufficiency – impaired heat production*: A small placenta in sheep impedes oxygen supply to the foetus and causes chronic foetal hypoxaemia which, in its turn, chronically elevates plasma lactate concentrations and the haematocrit. A small placenta also restricts nutrient supply, leading to low foetal plasma glucose and fructose concentrations and reduced foetal growth rates. These well-established effects of placental insufficiency in foetal lambs are also likely to occur in foetal kids. Postnatally, heat production is inhibited for at least 6-8 hr in low-weight newborn lambs which have markedly elevated plasma lactate concentrations and haematocrits and such lambs are susceptible to hypothermia (Hossain *et al.*, 2004).

c. *Acute intrapartum hypoxaemia / dystocia – impaired heat production*: Hypoxic inhibition of heat production can also occur in newborn lambs in which placental size has not been restricted, but in such cases it is due to umbilical cord compression and/or protracted labour. This form of fetal hypoxaemia occurs acutely during birth and elevates plasma lactate concentrations. Thus, the primary cause of hypothermia in these cases is umbilical cord compression and/or protracted labour.

d. *Inhibited heat production and immaturity at birth*: Some hypothermic lambs have impaired heat production which is not due primarily to chronic or acute hypoxaemia. Their impaired heat production, which distinguishes these lambs from fully competent lambs that have experienced excessive heat loss, may be due to immaturity of their thermogenic mechanisms through premature birth and/or through reduced thyroidal and adrenocortical support for postnatal metabolic activity, indicated by their low plasma thyroid hormone and cortisol concentrations, respectively.

e. *Starvation of the newborn – impaired heat production*: Starvation means a total lack or insufficient intake of colostrum/milk. It occurs in newborn lambs and kids when they fail to suck adequately due to weakness, competition with litter mates or inadequate mothering, or when colostrum/milk production is deficient. First, newborn and young animals become hypoglycaemic as their body energy reserves are depleted. This causes cerebral compromise in warm conditions and inhibits heat production, which leads to hypothermia in cold conditions. Second, the gut of the starved newborn does not exhibit the accelerated cellular maturation, enhanced functional capacity and increased growth normally seen in the gut of fed animals during the first 1-3 days after birth. Accordingly, colostrum composition and accelerated postnatal gut development are likely to be similar in all the species considered here. However, it is not known whether starvation for a few hours followed by colostrum or milk feeding causes persistent deleterious effects on gut function. Third, starvation deprives newborns of their only significant source of immunoglobulins, which are present in colostrum in high concentrations. Epithelial cell renewal on the villi of the small intestines is largely completed during the first 48-72 hr after birth and is considered to be largely responsible for "gut closure" (the loss of the immunoglobulin-absorbing capacity of the small intestine), which is usually complete by 24-48 hr after birth in lambs. Thus, when colostrum intake is delayed significantly or the immunoglobulin content of ingested colostrum is low, newborns lose opportunities for optimal absorption of protective immunoglobulins, and when they are starved they receive none (Srivastava *et al.*, 2009).

Maternal underfeeding: Underfeeding pregnant goat/sheep can have deleterious effects on foetal and/or newborn lambs by adversely affecting placental size, foetal growth, deposition of foetal fat reserves for use after birth, maternal udder development and colostrum/milk production. A delay in the onset of sucking by such lambs, which have low birth weights, is therefore more likely to lead to starvation-induced hypothermia than in normal-weight lambs. This is also the case in goats (Soares *et al.*, 2010).

Mis-mothering: It leads to starvation of the newborn. It occurs in sheep and goats due to a range of reasons. These include failure to establish an effective mother–young bond through inexperience (primiparas), debilitating maternal under nutrition during late pregnancy or dystocia-induced maternal exhaustion (Mathews, 1999).

Infections: Various infections affect neonates of small ruminants at various stages. These are:

a. *Prenatal disease*

Foetal diseases: Diseases of the foetus during intrauterine life, e.g. prolonged gestation, congenital defects, abortion, foetal deaths with resorption or mummification.

Parturient diseases: Diseases associated with dystocia causing cerebral anoxia, injuries of skeleton and soft tissues.

b. *Postnatal diseases*

Early postnatal diseases: Occurs within 48 hr after birth e.g. malnutrition due to poor mothering, hypothermia due to exposure to cold, low vigour in neonates due to malnutrition, specific disease (Naval ill and collibacillosis).

Delayed postnatal diseases: Occurs within 2-7 days after parturition e.g. mammary incompetence resulting in starvation, increased susceptibility to infections (lamb dysentery, colibacillosis and septicaemia) due to hypoglobulinaemia.

Late postnatal disease: Occurs within 1-4 week of life e.g. White muscle disease, enterotoxaemia.

Newborn lambs and kids absorb protective immunoglobulins from ingested colostrum during the first 24-48 hr after birth before "gut closure" occurs; they do not acquire immunoglobulins prenatally across the placenta. At birth the newborn is thrust from a sterile into an infective environment. Consequently, any factors that impede colostrum intake and hinder the acquisition of immunoglobulins increase the newborn's susceptibility to gut, respiratory, systemic and other infections in lambs and kids. Such infections may lead to diarrhoea, "watery mouth", pneumonia, pleurisy, septicaemia, peritonitis, septic arthritis and other conditions which are usually debilitating and are often fatal. Some economically important neonatal infections of kids/lambs are described.

Entropion: It (turned under eyelids) occurs most frequently and is most damaging to lambs. It is an inherited condition and appears in most breeds. One treatment is to remove a small section of the skin about 3/8 inches below the bottom eyelid, which will draw down the eyelid when the skin heals. The eyelid also can be clipped or drawn down with thread. Failure to correct the condition will lead to an unthrifty lamb that may remain blind.

Polyarthritis: It is arthritis involving one or more leg joints. It may or may not produce pus about the joint. Bacteria causing it are *Corynebacterium pseudotuberculosis* (the same bacteria that cause caseous lymphadenitis in ewes). The organism enters the body through the umbilicus or through docking or castrating wounds. To prevent polyarthritis, disinfect the navel cord and proper care should be taken during docking and castration. Treatment with antibiotics is only moderately successful.

Urinary calculi: It occurs in feedlot lambs and rams on high grain rations and in creep-fed lambs. Mortality is 80–90% of those affected. The usual cause is improper calcium: phosphorus ratio. High grain rations result in a Ca: P ratio of 1:2 or 1:3. To avoid incidence of urinary calculi, the ratio of Ca: P in lamb rations should be 1.5:1 cr 2:1. The addition of 0.5% ammonium chloride to the grain ration is an effective preventive measure.

Sore mouth: It (contagious ecthyma) is caused by a virus. Herpes ulcers develop on the lip and tongue of the lamb and on the udder of the ewe. An abrasion on the lips seems to contribute to its incidence. It is more prevalent in lambs raised on rubber nipples. Vaccinate (autogenous vaccine) if infected sheep running with susceptible sheep (young lambs). For most sheep it is of little concern. Other than with lambs, let it run its course. The use of antibiotics is ineffective (Kumar *et al.*, 2004).

Pneumonia: Pneumonia, the number one kid/lamb disease, occurs because of a lack of colostrum, ingestion of "mastitis milk," or because ewes are heavily infected with pasteurella (99% are infected, so the organism is always present). A lamb contracts pneumonia because it can't stand such stresses as too little milk, draft, dampness, and ammonia off a manure pack. Diagnosis of sick, unthrifty young kid/ lambs is relatively simple, because 90% of the time they are either starving or have pneumonia. Strive for early detection and start antibiotic treatment before the lungs have been permanently damaged. Treatment for pneumonia is to inject the animal with antibiotics (tetracycline, penicillin, or streptomycin) plus sulfamethazine. Adequate selenium and vitamin E help the kid/lamb withstand pneumonia.

Baby lamb scours: Scours are due to one of many bacteria (*Clostridium perfringens* type C, *Escherichia coli, Salmonella* spp). To minimize the problem, an adequate intake of colostrum (~ 250 to 350 ml) is absolutely essential. Scours may hit the lamb the first day of life. The lamb succumbs due to added stress (draft, ammonia, poor ventilation). Vaccinate the ewe four weeks before lambing to prevent the scour due to clostridium organisms. Treatment of affected cases with a tetracycline orally, injection of penicillin or tetracycline (IM) is successful (Kumar *et al.*, 2002; Kritas *et al.*, 2003).

White muscle disease: The cause of white muscle disease (muscular dystrophy) is a lack of selenium or vitamin E or both. Lack of vitamin

E is more likely to be the cause. Signs are lambs born dead or weak, or lambs that are unable to rise or walk or that do so stiffly. It may affect six- to eight-week-old lambs. Very often the fastest gaining lambs are affected. To prevent white muscle disease, feed salt containing 90 ppm selenium, feed salt fortified with 100000 IU vitamin E per 45 kg salt, or inject young lambs with selenium and vitamin E on day 1 and day 10.

Coccidiosis: It usually occurs in kids/lambs four weeks or older. It is caused by protozoa. Kids/Lambs usually show blackish, blood-tinged diarrhoea and are reluctant to eat. Treat it with amprolium or sulfamethazine. Monensin (15 g/ton) in feed prevents its occurrence. Bovatec, 40 g/ton of feed is also effective. Electrolyte-baking soda is supportive treatments (Kanyari, 1988).

Enterotoxaemia: It can kill goat/sheep of all ages but usually kills only those that consume high levels of carbohydrates. Feedlot mortality for vaccinated kids/lambs is 0.5% compared to 5-10% in unvaccinated kids/lambs. *Cl. perfringens* type D, one type of bacteria that causes enterotoxaemia, is most prevalent in feedlot or in creep-fed lambs. Symptoms are sudden death, occasional pushing and staggering and apparent blindness. For an outbreak, vaccinate with type D toxoid on day 1 and again 12-14 days later, and reduce grain until the vaccine takes effect. *C. perfringens* type C causes a type of enterotoxaemia that usually is accompanied by bloody scours. Mortality may be high. It usually occurs among fast gaining lambs during the first three weeks. Ewes vaccinated three-four weeks before lambing provide antibody protection in their milk. Acidosis caused by high grain intake which lowers the rumen pH from about 7.2 to 5.2–5.8 causing kids/lambs to discontinue eating, pain and if sufficiently severe, death. Purging with mineral oil or a bicarbonate drench is effective.

Floppy kid syndrome: The affected kid is normal at birth and develops a sudden onset of muscular weakness (flaccid paresis or paralysis) or ataxia at 3 to 10 days of age. Cases tend to occur most commonly late in kidding seasons. Affected kids are depressed, cannot use their tongues to suckle but can swallow and have marked paradoxial metabolic acidosis. There are no signs of diarrhoea and respiratory disease. The clinical signs of paresis/paralysis/ataxia in 3 to 10-day old kids and supporting blood chemistry value are diagnostic features. The causative agents have not been identified. However, infection and endotoxaemia could likely be the cause. Differential diagnoses include white muscle disease, abomasal bloat, colibacillosis, septicaemia, or enterotoxaemia. Early detection and correction of a base deficit as well as good supportive care are critical. Since the etiologic agent is not known, no preventive or treatments, aside from correction of electrolyte imbalance and supportive care, is recommended. Less severe cases are most commonly treated by owners with oral bicarbonate at the onset of signs. Kids may need to be fed milk by stomach tube. More severe cases may require blood chemistry and intravenous fluid. A mixture of 2 teaspoons of baking soda, ½ teaspoon salt in a quart of water has been used successfully.

Neurological diseases

a. *Bacterial meningitis*: The kids/lamb can't stand and its rear quarter is weak. The brain is infected. Antibiotics may help but the prognosis is guarded.

b. *Polioencephalomalacia:* The disease occurs in feedlot animals on high grain rations and is caused by bacteria in the rumen that deprives the animals of thiamine. In contrast to enterotoxaemia, the lamb lives one–three days. Infected lambs flex back their heads and peddle their legs. Thiamine injection may produce a dramatic response if lambs are treated early (Mahmoud *et al.*, 2004).

c. *Listeriosis:* An aerobic bacteria, *Listeria spp*, which frequently occurs in silage, causes this disease. The animal move in circle. Antibiotic treatment may save a small percentage of infected goat/sheep. Feeding high quality, mold-free silage will not cause the disease.

d. *Rabies:* Rabies (Rhabdo virus) spread by bite of infected animals. In this species, furious form is less common in comparison to dogs. Dumb form is clinically characterized by ataxia, swaying of hindquarter, tenesmus, paralysis of anus, loss of voice, paralysis and death. This disease must be differentiated with listeriosis.

e. *Tetanus:* It is caused by *Clostridium tetani*, which persists in the soil of most farms. Next to horses, sheep are the most susceptible farm animal. The bacteria are anaerobic, so wounds in which air contact is limited are most susceptible to tetanus. Docking and castrating with rubber rings increase the incidence of infection. Disinfecting docking and castrating wounds will minimize it. Infected animal become stiff, move with a straddled gait, and usually die. Vaccinating with tetanus toxoid and anti-toxin prior to docking is effective.

Principles of control and prevention of infectious diseases of newborn kids/lambs

(a) Removal of the cause of diseases from the environment

- The newborn should be born in an environment which is clean, dry and conducive for the animal to get up after birth and such the dam.
- Swabbing of the navel with tincture iodine to prevent the entry of infection.
- Disinfection of the uterus before conception is also necessary. Examination of swabs from the uterine contents before and after treatment in suspected animals.

(b) Removal of the newborn from the infected environment

- Transfer the newborn to a non-infected environment either temporary or permanently in cases of overcrowding of coral.
- Removal of the newborn away from the main kidding/lambing ground.
- Diseased newborn should be transferred with his dam to another shed during the period of treatment and convalescence.

(c) Increasing and maintaining the non – specific resistance of the newborn

- Ingestion of colostrums from dam is as important as it is the only one source of immunoglobulin to newborn.
- Intake of colostrum in neonate should be about 80 ml / kg body weight at 6 hr of age.
- Special nutritional and housing requirements.
- Isolation of newborn animals in rearing unit within few days after birth.
- Provision of suitable environment.

(d) Increasing the specific resistance of the newborn

- Vaccinate dam before parturition to stimulate the production of specific antibodies for subsequent transfer to the newborn via the colostrum. This includes the principles of diseases which occur during the first month of life in animals born alive at term.

Injuries

Traumatic injuries can be sustained during birth, especially when foeto-pelvic disproportion and/or mal-presentation occur and reduce the viability of the newborn. Human intervention during dystocia may increase the incidence of such injuries, which include brain damage (cerebral haemorrhage due to compression of the skull in the birth canal), liver damage, fractures (jaw, spinal column, ribs and limbs), dislocations (limbs) and abrasions.

Animal welfare implications of neonatal problems

Despite the substantial amount of research into the causes and prevention of neonatal mortality and morbidity in small ruminants, some of which has been mentioned above, attention to date has been focused almost entirely on seeking and assessing solutions, not on the welfare impact of the nature of neonatal death and/or morbidity. This is not surprising as most of such work was done before the mid-1980s, and only after that animal welfare begin to assume the significance in our thinking today. Those involved were not indifferent to suffering in the newborn; with their primary focus on taking practical steps to minimise the problems, when successful, they also minimised any associated welfare compromise.

References

Donkin, E.F. and Boyazoglu, P.A 2004. Diseases and mortality of goat kids in a South African milk goat herd. South African Journal of Animal Science 34: 258.

Hossain, S.M.J., Sultana, N., Alam, M.R. and Hasnath, M.R. 2004. Reproductive and productive performance of Black Bengal goat under semi-intensive management. Journal of Biological Sciences 4: 537-541.

Kanyari, P.W.N. 1988. Coccidiosis in goats and aspects of epidemiology. Australian Veterinary Journal 65: 257-258.

Kritas, S.K., Burriel, A.R., Tzivara, A.H., Govaris, A., Kyriakis, Karatzias, H. and Vlemmas, J. 2003. Prevention of scours in neonatal kids after modification of management and experimental vaccination against *Escherichia coli*. Small Ruminant Research 50: 51-56.

Kumar, A., Rana, R., Vihan, V.S., Barua, S., Gupta, Vinod and Tewari, H.A. 2004. Epidemiological features observed in contagious pustular dermatitis in kids. Indian Journal of Animal Sciences 74: 1113-1115.

Kumar, A., Vaid, R.K., Rana, R., Vihan, V.S. and Gupta, Vinod K. 2002. Descriptive epidemiology of colibacillosis in Barbari kids under semi intensive system. Indian Journal of Animal Sciences 72: 237-236.

Mahmoud, O.M., Haroun, E.M. and Omer, O.H. 2004. An outbreak of neurofilariosis in young goats. Veterinary Parasitology 120: 151-156.

Matthews, J. 1999. Diseases of Goats. Blackwell Science, Japan.

Sharif, L., Obeidat, J. and Al-Ani, F. 2005. Risk factors for lamb and Kid mortality in sheep and goat farms in Jordan. Bulgarian Journal of Veterinary Medicine 8: 99-108.

Smith, M.C. and Sherman, D.M. 1994. Goat Medicine. Lippincott William and Wilkins London.

Soares, C.M., Simões, S.V.D., Medeiros, J.M.A., Riet-Correa, F. and Pereira Filho, J.M. 2010. Passive immunity, colostrum Ingestion and mortality of Moxotó kids raised under extensive and intensive breeding systems. Arquivo Brasileiro de Medicina Veterinária e Zootecnia 62: 544-548.

Sreedhar, S. 2009. Factors affecting mortality of kids in Andhra Pradesh. Indian Journal of Small Ruminants 15: 253-256.

Srivastava, A.K., Singh, Charan and Kumar, Praveen. 2009. Influence of breed, sex, season, age, type of birth and birth weight on mortality rate in crossbred kids under stall fed conditions. Indian Journal of Small Ruminants 15: 156-162.

Turkson, P.K., Antiri, Y.K. and Baffuor-Awuah, O. 2004. Risk factors for kid mortality in West African Dwarf goats under an intensive management system in Ghana. Tropical Animal Health and Production 36: 353-364.

□□□

Chapter 22

Meat Production and Value Addition - Where We Stand ?

S. Sureshkumar, D. Santhi and A. Kalaikannan
Veterinary College and Research Institute, Namakkal,
Tamil Nadu Veterinary and Animal Sciences University
Tamil Nadu-637 002

Livestock sector plays a critical role in the livelihood of India's rural population and is one of the most important components of agriculture which serves as an exclusive source of animal protein in human diets. It provides employment to over 300 million of rural population and contributing enormous amount of draught power and biomass production. This sector thus plays a crucial role in national economy and contributes 7.35% of National GDP, with major share of global livestock population comprising of 172.45 million cattle, 106.63 million buffaloes, 65.71 million sheep, 126 million goats, 13.8 million pigs and 0.65 million poultry (FAOSTAT, 2009). In recent years, livestock output has grown at a rate of about 5% a year, higher than the growth in agricultural sector and acting as an important growth leverage. Despite great potential and large livestock population, Indian meat industry has not yet taken its due share. Because, it is highly in the unorganized sector and most of the productions takes place in the local slaughter-houses which are unhygienic, poor in infrastructure, and lacking basic facilities thus not meeting the export standards. Hence, it is necessary to either improve/modernize the existing slaughter houses or establish new ones to provide safe and wholesome meat, while gainfully utilizing animal by-products, and alleviating environmental concerns.

Since 1995, production of meat and meat products showed a steady growth of 4% / annum. Currently, the processing level of buffalo meat is estimated at 21%, poultry at 6% and marine products at 8% levels. According to the Ministry of Food Processing Industries (MoFPI), about 3% of meat is processed out of which only 1% is converted into value added products like sausages, ham, bacon, luncheon meat, kababs, meat balls etc. However, this could be an under-estimate, since a very large proportion of meat processing takes place in unregistered cottage meat processing units and small establishments, which cater solely for local needs.

Meat production and processing – India's prospects and retrospect

Animals, which are generally used for production of meat, are cattle, buffaloes, sheep and goat, pigs and poultry. Out of 5.8 million tonnes in India, buffalo contributes about 30% of total meat production followed by poultry (11.5%), goat (10.2%), sheep (10%) and cattle (5%). The livestock presently slaughtered in India include 45.5 million goats, 19.8 million sheep, 3.6 million buffaloes, 2.6 million cattle and 6.1 million pigs per annum (AHS Series-12, 2010). Rabbit meat is used as a specialty meat in Kerala and some other states. In India, cattle meat production is largely a by-product system of livestock production utilizing spent animals at the end of their productive life. Poultry meat is the fastest growing animal protein in India.

There are around 4000 municipal slaughter houses in the country and 30 abattoirs/meat processing plants. These 30 abattoirs/meat processing plants are exclusively export oriented units and are registered with the Agricultural and Processed Food Export Development Authority (APEDA). Additionally, 74 meat processing and packaging units are also registered with APEDA. These meat processing and packaging units receive dressed carcasses from approved municipal slaughter houses for the export of meat. According to industry sources, approximately 7 slaughter houses are expected to be added by the end of 2012. In addition, a large proportion of meat production is slaughtered in houses or small-unlicensed establishments.

Meat production is constrained by lack of productivity augmenting technologies and socio-religious taboos. Breeding efforts are yet to capitalize on the genetic stock of the indigenous breeds. The yawning gap between the existing slaughter rates and potential off-take for certain species merits urgent attention. There are many other reasons for the slow growth of the meat industry, including the negative attitude of public towards meat on account of misinformation campaign, and socio-political considerations. Most of the meat is sold in the domestic market without proper sanitary inspection by the veterinarians. Mostly small animals, sheep, goat and pigs are slaughtered in unregistered slaughter houses in small numbers ranging from 2-10 by the individual butchers and meat is sold as fresh on the same day. However, large numbers are slaughtered in the modern state-of-the-art abattoirs following world class sanitary and phytosanitary measures. Meat production is intimately linked to leather production, in which India has acquired second position in the world after Italy and fifth largest exporter of bovine meat in the world.

Beef and carabeef: According to Livestock Census (2007), buffalo constitute approximately one third of India's total bovine population. Buffalo are preferred for their high milk fat content and their adaptability to Indian agricultural conditions. Indian dairy farmers typically earn a bonus for producing buffalo milk as well as increased market rate for animals due to the availability of export oriented modern slaughter facilities. As the world's largest dairy consumer, India's bovine herd continues to be fuelled by domestic dairy demand and generates additional bovine meat production as an increasing herd raises the pool of animals available for slaughter. In addition, a strong global demand for price-competitive bovine meat generates new incentives for slaughter facilities to salvage previously under-utilized animals, which in turn increased future production forecast to 7% higher than present 3.3 million tonnes (Ritambhara Singh, 2011). The production has been growing at the rate of 6% in last five years (Table 1). There is a spectacular demand of Indian buffalo meat in the international market, because of its leanness thus exports more than 500,000 tones. The export of buffalo meat has been growing at a compound annual growth rate (CAGR) of about 8% (MoFPI). Indian buffalo meat is exported to more than 60 countries. Prominent among those are Africa (Angola, Congo, Cote D. Ivories, Gabon, Ghana etc.), CIS (Azerbaijan, Georgia, and Uzbekistan) Vietnam, Malaysia, Philippines and the Middle East (Ritambhara Singh, 2011). Exporters are also working to gain market access in countries like Russia and Indonesia. Over 90% of buffalo meat exports are boneless and the rest as carcasses or portion. India's total export earnings during 2007-08 were around two billion dollars from livestock and poultry products and 1.8 billion dollars from marine products in which buffalo alone contributes 90%.

Even though, buffalo has not been exploited fully as a meat animal in India, about 86% of the world buffalo meat production is in Asia and mostly from old and culled animals (Singh and Barwal, 2010). Buffalo meat is surplus in India and there is a vast scope to set up modern slaughter facilities and cold store chains in meat. According to the Ministry of Food Processing Industries, the state of Uttar Pradesh in India is the largest producer and exporter of buffalo meat, accounting for roughly 70% of the production while South India produces around 17% of the total buffalo meat with the largest share from Andhra Pradesh.

India's cattle and buffalo population is made up of small holdings distributed among millions of farmers and is characterized by a "low-input/low-output model," which emphasizes low-cost or no-cost feed rations. Industry sources indicate that buffalo meat production will likely peak within the next two to three years, as Indian buffalo meat prices achieve parity with competing producers. Buffalo meat is mostly processed and exported in large scale abattoirs due to the lack of high demand in domestic markets. According to the Ministry of Food Processing Industries, processing levels in buffalo meat (20%) and poultry (6%) are quite low as compared to most developed countries.

Mutton and Chevon: Small ruminants (sheep and goat) are numerically important domesticated animals in arid and semi-arid regions of Asia. Goats / sheep constitute a very important species of livestock in India, mainly on account of their short generation intervals, higher rates of prolificacy and improved marketability and their contribution to the development of rural folks (APEDA, 2010). However, the future of the goat and sheep industry as a significant economic activity will also be very dependent on the standards of living in the countries, where there is a market for the goat products. In recent years, it received substantial improvement due to the local initiatives of quality labels and production of innovative products. Goat and sheep meat forms about 4.9% in quantity and about 9.7% in value terms of the total meat exports (Global Agrisystem, 2011).

Table 1 : India: beef exports (Source: Global Trade Atlas; Courtesy: Ritambhara Singh, 2011)

Partner Country	Quantity (Metric tons)				
	2006	2007	2008	2009	2010
Vietnam	18,163	39,151	92,258	111,166	90,773
Malaysia	75,376	52,325	50,553	48,214	79,865
Egypt	5,911	26,560	43,567	28,590	69,779
Saudi Arabia	27,102	35,310	25,599	24,274	47,634
Philippines	46,407	51,365	53,036	41,479	43,828
Jordan	36,125	20,835	15,465	12,503	41,742
Kuwait	41,746	40,315	31,203	28,363	36,234
United Arab Emirates	30,543	26,887	18,416	16,594	31,757
Angola	42,571	47,863	29,870	17,082	19,916
Myanmar	37	12	0	286	19,800
Algeria	0	30	0	0	18,158
Iran	21,719	12,238	12,112	5,391	18,023
Iraq	1,610	5,370	2,982	7,436	17,652
Syria	168	0	1,702	6,496	13,929
Congo	13,785	10,576	13,997	12,148	12,377
Oman	11,487	11,962	11,501	8,027	11,351
Georgia	10,981	11,214	8,189	6,563	9,427
Lebanon	1,689	5,068	6,448	6,830	8,823
Gabon	7,198	7,653	6,234	5,837	7,913
Senegal	7,617	7,825	5,119	4,814	5,054
Qatar	4,253	2,904	4,076	4,116	4,624
Ghana	5,712	9,489	6,425	3,674	4,492
Thailand	109	99	77	0	3,855
Azerbaijan	7,283	3,271	4,241	2,823	3,819
Mauritius	3,700	3,361	4,001	2,974	3,189
Pakistan	23,055	13,049	3,701	2,939	2,967
Bahrain	3,071	2,692	2,322	1,932	2,849
Armenia	1,500	4,346	5,570	3,717	2,793
Yemen	3,243	3,163	1,368	1,314	2,450
Cote d Ivoire	7,403	5,025	4,176	3,783	2,430
Equatorial Guinea	1,262	1,366	1,266	1,098	2,056
Comoros	1,486	1,702	2,007	1,786	1,945

Tajikistan	781	2,790	1,762	2,196	1,681
Brunei Darussalam	915	1,641	1,972	954	1,231
Turkey	1,512	943	306	158	836
Namibia	168	393	1,181	281	813
Indonesia	0	0	0	0	683
Liberia	674	449	452	254	655
South Africa	28	1	0	1	598
Uzbekistan	976	897	624	196	577
Maldives	531	548	311	186	530
Singapore	1547	0	0	0	525
Germany	144	37	12	7	450
United Kingdom	7	1	0	0	433
Afghanistan	3,655	3,390	1,745	464	405
Hong Kong	645	572	83	4,063	360
Seychelles	71	53	333	219	336
Benin	0	0	58	29	316
Canada	0	0	0	0	280
Sierra Leone	893	838	503	255	263
Mozambique	784	1,237	57	0	252
United States	7	0	121	67	193
Albania	58	1,110	1,425	726	141
China	4,186	948	630	363	27
Greece	3,258	1,560	512	0	0
Others	3,004	4,065	771	2,036	1,952
World Total	**486,157**	**484,499**	**480,339**	**434,704**	**655,041**

The poor man's cow goat has tremendous potential to be projected as the 'Future Animal' for rural prosperity under the changing agro-geo climatic conditions and depleting resources. There are over 880 million goats around the world, out of which India has over 126 million goats (14.31%) of 23 defined and non-descript breeds that are adapted efficiently in different agr-climatic conditions spread all over the country (CIRG, 2011). In the last few years, commercial goat rearing under intensive and semi-intensive system of production is attaining significance due to its economic potential and the assured revenue had attracted many farmers, self-help group women, educated youths, etc. to take up the goat enterprise on a commercial scale. Due to this a number of commercial goat farms have been established in different regions of the country. Goats are hardy, disease resistant and widely adapted. They thrive well and reproduce well in tropical, cold, humid as well as dry regions. Their small size compared to cattle and buffaloes permit them to be maintained on a limited area. The breeding animals are inexpensive. Goats consume a wide variety of grasses, weeds, forbs, bushes, shrubs, tree leaves and crop residues that would otherwise go waste and cause pollution. Goat is an efficient converter of the sparse vegetation available in wastelands, community grazing lands of arid, semi-arid and mountainous regions into milk, meat, skin, fibre and manure while utilizing traditional and under employed manpower. They are gentle and easy to control.

The goat meat production has doubled (9.3% to 18.3%) during the last decade. The country is the second largest meat producer in the world sharing 10.41% goat meat production. The goat sector contributes 14,453 crores to the agricultural economy of the country through meat (6851 crores), milk (4588 crores), skin (648 crores), etc. which accounts for around 8% of the GDP from livestock sector (CIRG, 2011). In addition, the goat sector generates about 4% rural employment and about 20 million small and marginal farmers' and landless labourers' families depend on goats for their livelihood partially or completely. The numbers of goats in the top ten countries, the ratio of goats to sheep and their percentages from the total number in the world is given below:

Continent	Number (million)		Ratio		Percentage of world total	
	Goat	Sheep	Goat	Sheep	Goat	Sheep
China	149.4	136.4	1	0.91	17.3	12.7
India	125.7	65.0	1	0.51	14.6	6.0
Pakistan	56.7	27.1	1	0.48	6.6	2.5
Bangladesh	56.4	1.6	1	0.02	6.5	0.2
Nigeria	53.8	33.9	1	0.63	6.2	3.1
Sudan	43.1	51.1	1	1.19	5.0	4.7
Iran	25.3	53.8	1	2.13	2.9	5.0
Ethiopia	21.8	25.0	1	1.15	2.5	2.3
Mongolia	20.0	18.4	1	0.92	2.3	1.7
Indonesia	15.8	8.4	1	0.53	1.8	0.8
World	861.9	1078.2	1	1.25		

(Source: FAOSTAT, 2008; Courtesy: Mahmoud Abdel Aziz, 2010)

The current status and future needs of sheep production had been clearly depicted by CSWRI (2011) which states that mutton production is not increasing with the rising global demand for meat, which is expected to be doubled by 2030. Universally, little attention has been given to sheep husbandry that has led to sharp rise in mutton price. Indian sheep produces average 10 kg carcass as against world's average of 17 kg. Further, climate change in the recent past has influenced sheep production resulting in reduction of flock size and early age disposal of surplus male lambs. Mutton production was 125 million kg in 1980-81, 230 million kg in 2001-02, 263 million kg currently, which will be around 316 million kg by 2020 and 356 million kg in 2030. During the period mutton requirement in the country would be 533.5 million kg by 2020 and 579.5 million kg in 2030 indicating deficits of 31.2 and 37.2% by 2020 and 2030, respectively. The problem will further aggravate if present trend of early slaughter of lambs will continue. The export of mutton from India is primarily done in three forms:

- Chilled / frozen carcasses
- Frozen boneless(pieces/cubes)
- Frozen with bone (pieces/ cubes)

The major export from India is primarily in the lamb and sheep meat category and the percentage shared out of total export, by various forms is as follows (Courtesy: Global Agrisystem, 2011):

Category	Export Qty(MT)	Share %
Carcasses of lamb (chilled fresh)	669.90	13.47
Meat of sheep with bone(chilled fresh)	591.24	11.89
Boneless meat of sheep (chilled fresh)	674.60	13.56
Carcasses of lamb (frozen)	2.25	0.05
Carcasses of sheep (frozen)	717.63	14.43
Meat of sheep with bone (frozen)	529.57	10.65
Boneless meat of sheep (frozen)	333.186	6.70
Meat of goats (chilled fresh)	130.22	2.62
Carcasses of sheep (chilled fresh)	1324.97	26.64
Total	**4973.60**	**100.00**

Pork: Pork production in India is limited, representing only 7% of the country's animal protein sources. Production is concentrated mainly in the north-eastern corner of the country and consists primarily of backyard and informal sector producers (Thom Wright, 2011). The market for imported pork products in India is limited to the Hotel, Restaurant and Institutional sector (HRI), as well as other niche and specialty markets. Industry sources have indicated that Indian pork imports consist almost entirely of processed product and estimate that annual imports on a calendar year basis are approximately 150 tons annually. When compared to 17th census, the pig population decreased from 14 million in 2003 to 12 million heads.

Large White Yorkshire (LWY) is most extensively used exotic breed in India which is a prolific breeder and suitable for the purpose of cross breeding. Prasad *et al.* (2011) had reported that LWY took 28.7% less time and gained 50% higher body weight during sexual maturity as compared to the local breed. Number of piglet produced per farrowing was 41.9% higher in LWY than local. The net profit per pig was also 79.0% higher in LWY than local. Even though pig farming is still less constrained with social taboos, costly ration, high piglet mortality and lack of good marketing facilities, numbers of entrepreneurs are coming forward to venture into this sector in the recent years.

Poultry: The poultry industry is among the faster growing sectors rising at a rate of 8% per year. India is the fifth largest producer of egg and ninth largest producer of poultry meat. India was positioned 17th in the world poultry production. The Indian poultry production is considered to be the cheapest in the world. The industry is moving from largely unorganized to a few large organized sector players. The organised sector of poultry industry is contributing nearly 70% of the total output and the rest 30% in the unorganized sector (MoFPI). The broiler industry is well dominated in southern states in our country with nearly 60-70% total output coming from these states (MoFPI). Vertical integration of poultry production and marketing has lowered costs of production, marketing margins and consumer prices of poultry meat. Broiler production grew at an annual percentage growth rate of 8.35% from 2001 (1.25 million metric tons) to 2010 (2.65 million metric tons). Production is projected to grow 2% in 2011 compared to the previous year (Table 2). Per capita consumption has grown from 1.22 kg in 2001 to 2.26 kg in 2010, an increase of 185%. (USDA, 2011).

Table 2 : India: broiler production and consumption (1000 MT)

	2001	2003	2005	2007	2008	2009	2010	2011*
Production	1,250	1,500	1,900	2,240	2,490	2,550	2,650	2,700
Domestic	1,252	1,498	1,899	2,239	2,489	2,549	2,649	2,699
Per Cap (kg)	1.22	1.42	1.74	1.99	2.18	2.20	2.26	2.30

*Forecast; Source: Foreign Agricultural Service, Official USDA Estimates

The Indian broiler sector operates almost completely as a live-bird market. Manual poultry processing accounts for more than 90% of consumption. Traditional poultry dressing facilities at the wholesale or retail level are completely manual, with no sanitary measures taken for the dressing floor or the workers. There is some demand for frozen or chilled poultry products from hotels, fast food restaurant chains and some urban consumers. About 6% of poultry meat is sold in processed form, of which only about 1% undergoes processing into value-added products (ready-to-eat/ready-to-cook).The modern poultry processing sector in India consists of more than 12 firms, which are mostly operated by poultry integrators located in or near major urban areas. These firms use imported equipment and follow hygienic procedures, including monitoring employee health, water supplies, sanitary conditions and refrigeration facilities. Leading broiler integrators in India are as follows:

- Venkateswara Group, Pune
- Suguna Poultry Farms Ltd, Coimbatore
- Pioneer Poultry Group, Coimbatore
- Godrej Agrovet Ltd, Mumbai
- Shanthi Processing Plant, Tamil Nadu

These companies account for nearly 40% of broiler industry integrators and contracts. Transition from a live-bird market to a chilled/frozen poultry product market is an important factor in the future expansion of broiler production. Expansion of the poultry industry could create potential trade and investment opportunities.

Rabbit: Rabbit as a small animal has been ascribed as "micro livestock". Rabbit husbandry has vast potential to improve the socio-economic status of the rural poor and to provide fond security in terms of low cost animal protein. A female rabbit, through its progenies can produce up to 80 kg of meat per year i.e. 2900 to 3000% of her live weight (Risam *et al.,* 2005). Rabbit husbandry was introduced in the sub-temperate Himalayan region of the country way back in seventies whereas now the demands has picked up in broiler rabbits for meat in Southern region. Rabbit production though a recent venture in the country, it has promising scope for meat production. Broiler rabbit can play a major role as an alternative source of white meat under scenario of growing demand of meat in the country. We have already achieved 2 kg target finishing weight at 12 weeks of age with 30 g ADG and 30% feed conversion efficiency. Therefore, rabbit production deserves better attention in future policy for meat production (CSWRI, 2011). Preparation of rabbit meat products is not commercialized though a very few research had been carried out. Non conventional meats such as rabbits have therefore, drawn attention as promising alternative sources of meat. There is a need for the research and development has to be undertaken to strengthen and popularize rabbit as backyard farming and for large scale commercial production and processing under provision of contract farming.

Value addition

Sustained livestock production to provide livelihood and ensure food and nutrition security to a large population is dependent on efficient utilization of livestock products. Processing meat to value added products contribute to sustained demand for meat and efficient marketing of meat to earn reasonable returns from meat animals by the farmers. In India processed meat is sold as frozen and chilled while frozen meat is mainly meant for export and chilled meat is consumed in the domestic market. The domestic market is mostly catered by municipal slaughter houses and unauthorized slaughter facility and the export-oriented facilities, registered with the APEDA, are eligible to process meat for export purposes. Export oriented processed meat is transported in refrigerated vans/ containers from processing units to port locations and is stored in cold storage near port locations, from where the product is shipped to destination markets. There are about 170 processed meat units, producing a number of meat products mostly as small scale units and licensed under Meat Food Products Order, 1973.

Value addition is a vital avenue for effective utilization of livestock resources with increased demand and higher returns. There would be increased trade opportunities for India due to increasing demand for processed/value added meat products globally, because of its convenience and variety as well as change in life style of the consumers, which in turn assures the farmers a regular off take of their produce at reasonable prices. Even though it involves a larger component of labour, India has the advantage of availability of low cost laborers (Anjaneyulu *et al.*, 2004). Processing and value addition of meat leads to improved and efficient utilization of low value meat such as trimmings, edible by products spent animals' meat, etc. The subsequent handling and transportation is comparatively better with processed meat products. Fuelled by a booming retail sector, the market for processed meat is growing at an estimated 15-20% per annum.

The mutton processing industry is still in a nascent stage of growth. Presently 96% of the production is sold as fresh mutton. Only 3% is processed and sold as frozen or other value added products. Two types of processing techniques are adopted for export purpose i.e. fresh/chilled and frozen. The Indian market for processed pork products is small, and the majority of this market is supplied through imports. Although there are some local companies which manufacture processed products such as sausages and bacon, quantities are limited. Poultry Industry in India is constantly on the rise given the use of modern techniques and changing from live bird to fresh chilled and frozen product market. Poultry products account for more than 75% of the non-vegetarian items consumed in India. The introduction of new poultry products and perceptible shift in eating habits are moving people to branded foods such as cold cuts, breaded and coated snacks, marinated snacks, chicken nuggets, canned chicken curry, freeze dried chicken pulao, meat soup, powder omlette and scrambled egg mixtures, sandwich, pizza, burger and dial-a-chicken and fast food joints.

The processed and semi-cooked meat products include corn beef, meat loaf, sausages, curries, bacon, ham, cutlet-mix, chicken-n-ham and salami. Sausages, one of the most popular products range come in varieties such as cocktail sausage, pork sausage, chicken pepperoni sausage and masala sausage. Some of the initiatives have also been taken to produce organic rabbit, duck and turkey meat. The processed meat sector, formerly regulated by the MoFPI, is now regulated by the Food Safety and Standards Authority of India (FSSAI) through the Food Safety and Standards Rules and Regulation, 2011. These regulations were enforced nationwide with effect from August 5, 2011, repealing the Meat and Meat Products Order (MFPO), 1973. The Food Safety and Standards Regulations (FSSR), 2011 contain standards and regulations for meat and meat products. The FSSR 2011 requires registration and licensing of meat processors and other food operators in the meat value chain. It also enforces sanitary maintenance and controls stages of meat (including fish and poultry) products production. These standards equally apply to domestic and imported meat and meat products.

Value added traditional meat products: Traditional meat products are highly popular and play a pivotal role in human nutrition. Meat consumers relish them by virtue of their appealing physical, textural and sensory attributes. Traditional meat and chicken based fast foods like meat balls (koftas), kababs, tikka, chicken tandoori (roast), biryani, curries, pickles, enrobed and battered products are attracting greater consumer response. Gushtaba and Rista popular traditional Kashmiri products are also being well received in other major cities. A variety of value added convenience traditional meat products are being processed at fast food corners, restaurants, star hotel etc. and are liked by many for their freshness. Many entrepreneurs have priority programmes on meat based fast foods to cater the ever growing needs of present youth.

Indigenous meat products are poised for continuous growth in the country. In big cities, there is an ever increasing demand for, warm and serve and ready to eat convenience fast foods as evident from the growth of fast food parlours and restaurants. These foods occupy considerably less space at retail outlets and can be served within a matter of few minutes. Estimate suggest that the sales turnover of these products is 30-50 times that of all the Western type foods marketed in India through various modes of marketing outlets.

Meat consumption

Despite a strong culture of vegetarianism, India sees a sharp rise in consumption of meat in recent years. Indians are shunning their religious taboo about consuming different types of meat, as their diets change and hygiene improvement in the processing industry. As per the FAO, Indians' per capita consumption of meat is running at 5.0 to 5.5 kg a year, reflecting a wider taste for protein-rich diets from animal proteins.

Beef: In spite of its big potential for meat productions owing to its huge livestock population, the Indian meat industry has not grown in the early years due to socio-religious concerns. Indian consumption of buffalo meat averages approximately two kilograms per person per year and consumption in India forecasted around 2 million tons which is 2.5% more than 2011. For non-vegetarian Indians, poultry meat, fish, and mutton are the most preferred meats. Despite an increase in overall consumption, per capita consumption has not changed much due to increasing human population (Ritambhara Singh, 2011). The reported compounded average growth rate during the last two decades was only about 4.6% as against 21.0% during the last few years (Ranjhan, 2004). This growth was fuelled by the increase in buffalo meat exports of about 159,703 MT in 1995-96 to as much as 456,907 MT in 2008-2009 (APEDA, 2010).

Chevon and mutton: Goat meat (chevon) is preferred over other meats because it is leaner and there are no religious taboos against its consumption. Because of leanness, Indian chevon is preferred meat in the world market. Despite the limitations of availability for export, the quantity of chevon being exported has increased recently to around 12% of total chevon production. Besides these, global consumption of sheep meat (mutton) is forecasted to grow at 1.5-2.0% per annum over the next ten years (OECD, 2010). This growth is expected to be driven by developing regions increased per capita consumption levels from 1.6 kg to 1.8 kg due to income level shift and population growth. In contrast to the same, in the developed world consumption is expected to remain flat in volume terms as per capita consumption of mutton has declined over the past 30 years.

Pork: The pork consumption pattern in India is explained by Thom Wright (2011). Indian pork consumption can be divided into two segments *viz.* fresh pork and imported pork products. The major proportion of pork consumption is the locally raised fresh pork meat, which is limited to unorganized sector. Consumption of fresh local meat is limited to north eastern India and low income group of other regions due to cultural perception. The next segment of the pork market deals with high-value imported products. These products include sausages, ham, bacon and canned meat products, as well as small quantities of frozen meat which is limited to Indian hotels and speciality shops catering to international business travellers, tourists and high income group. The popularity of processed pork products amongst wealthier Indian consumers may be related to the popularity of Italian cuisine in India. The pork consumption regions of India are Assam, Meghalaya, Nagaland of North-East, Goa, Karnataka, Andhra Pradesh, Tamilnadu, Kerala, Bangalore of Southern India and Tangra

Chinatown of West Bengal. North East India has much higher pork consumption that the rest of the country.

Poultry meat: The poultry meat production and consumption in the domestic market is slated to grow and contribute and much to the meat processing sector in the country. From backyard activity to the current factory production, the poultry sector has undergone a paradigm shift. Poultry meat consumption is showing the fastest growth due to low cost relative to mutton and fish. The rise of quick service restaurants in India which delivers variety meat products especially from chicken is also a driver of non-vegetarian consumption of poultry products. Inspite of 5.3% increase in meat production during the last decade the per capita consumption does not changed much which gives a tremendous opportunity for India to promote meat consumption in domestic market.

Rabbit meat: Rabbit meat is popularly termed as game and favorably relished with other meats. Though there is no religious taboo with respect to rabbit meat, it could not attract consumers in India due to its high price and it could not compete with broiler chicken. India has, enormous unconventional meat resources including rabbits and harvesting of these can provide a far greater volume of cheaper sources of protein of higher biological value to the people.

Constraints

In India, both demand and production of goat meat have shown steady increase during the last decade and despite the rising production trend, country would need to double the number of goats to meet the projected requirement of goat meat for growing human population in the coming decades. However, the increase in livestock number would definitely put more stress over limited natural resources. Management of feed and fodder resources is crucial for the future development of goat production in the country. There is very little scope for increasing the area under fodder production, keeping in view the priority for food grains, pulses and oil seeds. Therefore, concerted efforts are required to develop technology for enhancing per animal productivity, besides increasing the productivity of fodder per unit area and utilization of the waste lands and newer non-conventional feed ingredients for goat production. Innovative research strategies need to be formulated to ameliorate impact of climate changes on health and productivity of animals. Research programmes for conservation and genetic improvement of indigenous goat resources and use of molecular genetics in understanding gene expression and gene variability and causes of genetic diversity need to be strengthen. Food management, food safety and value addition studies and green house gas mitigation technologies are important to address issues pertaining to eco-friendly sustainable goat production system. The unorganized market system is a major hurdle for goat farmers to fetch remunerative price. There is an absolute necessity for market oriented livestock production system and *vice versa*.

Constraints to livestock husbandry include the scarcity of good breeding stock, inadequate veterinary and extension services, lack of credit and access to markets. Focusing more assistance on small holder farmers would improve impact on the poor. Value-based holistic community development with self-help groups may create a foundation for increasing farmer incomes by providing a forum for education, mutual support and developing markets (CIRG, 2011). The Central Institute for Research on Goats, Makhdoom has detailed the constraints to livestock industry. Improved technologies are not adopted by sheep and goat owners due to lack of awareness to due to poverty, illiteracy and little or lack of decision making process. Lesser availability of elite breeding males, effective vaccines, grazing lands and feed resources are the other weaknesses. The sheep and goat farmers are exploited by the middlemen in marketing of surplus animals for meat markets. Slaughter of large number of animals is carried out in mostly in unauthorized places due to unavailability of sufficient modern abattoirs for hygienic slaughter. There is great scope for rearing sheep and goat for meat production under semi-intensive and intensive systems of management. The reproduction rate, multiple births, growth, slaughter weight, dressing percentage, bone: meat ratio and survivability can be significantly improved which in turn will provide higher returns to the goat owners. Majority of the goat population is nondescript that is capable of producing very less meat and milk. With shrinking resources and increasing demand of meat and milk, there is urgent need to genetically improve and manage these animals through modern scientific. Although, there is a need to utilize between breeds genetic differences for higher yields, greater emphasis is required on improvement of adapted indigenous breeds/types because of valuable adaptive traits they have developed over long periods of time through natural selection. Breeding strategies for enhancing goat meat and milk production in the country is needed. Food processing industry has been facing constraints like non-availability of adequate critical infrastructural facilities like cold chain, packaging and grading centres, adequate quality control and inefficient supply chain, shortage of processable varieties of farm produce, seasonality of raw material, high inventory carrying cost, high taxation, high packaging cost, affordability and cultural preference for fresh food.

There is a need to integrate meat quality component in to breeding and genetic selection as well as nutrition and management studies. Developing a method to select animals for increased muscle mass is necessary for faster genetic progress on muscling attributes. It is necessary to analyze the effect of breed, diet, geographical region on palatability, flavor, tenderness attribute of meat and cheese quality and fatty acid composition of milk to understand better quality goat for meat and milk type. In pork industry, Due to constraints in marketing channels and the absence of a comprehensive cold chain system, stocks of fresh and frozen pork meat for export are very meager. Pork importer restricts their supply to formal sector buyers on a consignment basis and do not maintain stocks of imported pork products because of uncertainty in supply and demand chain.

Promotional programmes

Government of India (GOI): The Government of India initiated a major program with a focus on genetic improvement entitled "National Project on Cattle and Buffalo Breeding (NPCBB)" in October 2000 for a period of 10 years. Given the success of this project, the GOI has decided to continue this program through the 11th Five Year Plan period (2007-2012). Based on the assessments and recommendations made by the GOI Standing Committee of Parliament and the Planning Commission, Department of Animal Husbandry and Dairying launched two major schemes under the 11th Five Year Plan. These schemes are "The Salvaging and Rearing of Male Buffalo Calves Scheme" and "The Utilization of Fallen Animals Scheme". These schemes are funded by the National Bank for Agricultural and Rural Development (NABARD) and are being launched in a bid to achieve a growth rate of 10% for the meat sector in the 11th Five Year Plan period. The Salvaging and Rearing of Male Buffalo Calves scheme promotes the rearing of male buffalo calves for meat production and to develop linkages with export oriented slaughterhouses. The states of Andhra Pradesh, Bihar, Chhattisgarh, Jharkhand, Kerala, Madhya Pradesh, Maharashtra, Orissa, Rajasthan, Uttar Pradesh, Punjab and

West Bengal are targeted as priorities. The salvaging scheme is expected to generate a substantial quantity of meat hides and by-products and also provide employment in feed, fodder, meat, leather and various input services. The utilization of fallen Animals scheme proposes to establish carcass utilization centers in animal density matrix areas and is expected to provide employment to the rural poor.

The GOI has launched the National Mission for Protein Supplements in the 2011-12, with an allocation of more than $65 million. This mission will take up activities to promote animal based protein production through livestock development, dairy farming, pig farming, goat rearing and fisheries in selected blocks of the country. The Ministry of Agriculture, GOI had implemented the Central Sector Scheme "Integrated Development of Small Ruminants and Rabbits" during 2010-11 and rest of XI Plan period for the creation of small ruminant development fund to foster area / cluster-based integrated development as viable commercial activity, for strengthening of infrastructure, human resources, institutions and rearers' organizations for rapid improvement of small ruminants and rabbits, for Developing skill-pool of NGOs for taking up development projects on PPP mode and for resource mapping in 126 identified districts for sheep, goat and rabbits rearing and in terms of raw material source as well as meat consumption pattern and development of 108 clusters for intensive development of sheep, goat and rabbit during XI Plan.

Schemes of the ministry of food processing industries: In order to improve abattoir conditions, the National Meat and Poultry Processing Board, under the MoFPI, has taken up an initiative to provide consultancy to build around 160 modern abattoirs across the country. The first abattoir under the initiative has already started working in the Dholpur district of Rajasthan. MoFPI schemes under 11th Plan schemes are as follows:

(a) *Scheme for infrastructural development*: It has got 3 components, namely Mega food parks, Integrated cold chain and Setting up/ Modernization of abattoirs. Mega food park component aims to provide a mechanism to bring together farmers, processors and retailers and link agricultural production to the market so as to ensure maximization of value addition, minimization of wastages and improving farmers' income. The primary objective of the scheme is to facilitate establishment of an integrated value chain, with processing at the core and supported by forward and backward linkages. The scheme envisages financial assistance in the form of grant-in-aid @ 50% of the project cost excluding land component in general areas and 75% in North Eastern Region and difficult areas subject to a maximum of Rs.50.00 Cr. per project.

(b) *Scheme for cold chain, value addition and preservation infrastructure*: To encourage setting up of cold chain facilities and backward linkages in the country and to provide integrated and complete cold chain and preservation infrastructure facilities without any break, from the farm gate to the consumer, MoFPI has launched a plan Scheme during 11th Plan to provide financial assistance to project proposals received from public/private organizations for integrated cold chain infrastructure development. The initiatives are aimed at filling the gaps in the supply chain, strengthening of cold chain infrastructure, establishing value addition with infrastructural facilities like sorting, grading, packaging and processing for horticulture including organic produce, marine, dairy, poultry, etc. The scheme envisages financial assistance in the form of grant-in-aid @ 50% of the total cost of plant and machinery and technical civil works in general areas and 75% for North Eastern Region and difficult areas subject to a maximum of Rs.10.00 Cr.

Flow diagram for setting up of cold chain facilities / supply chain

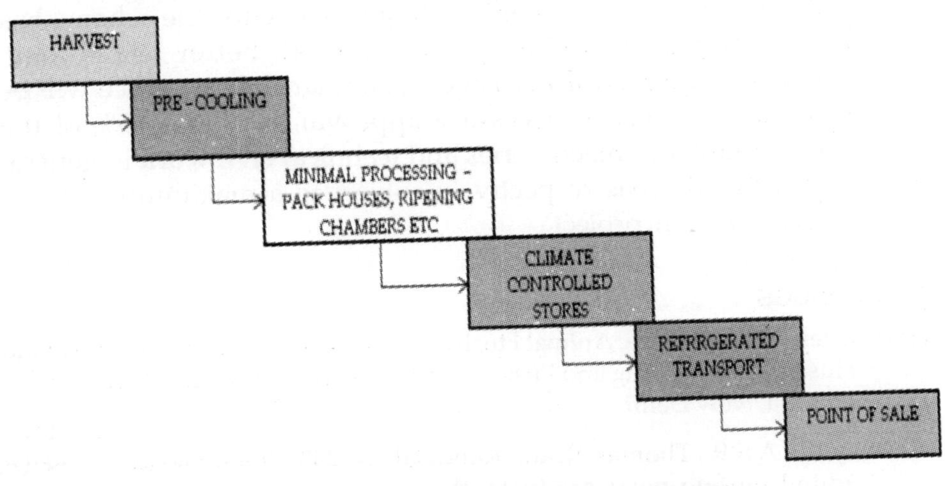

Courtesy: Annual Report, 2010-11, MOFPI.

Cold Supply Chain

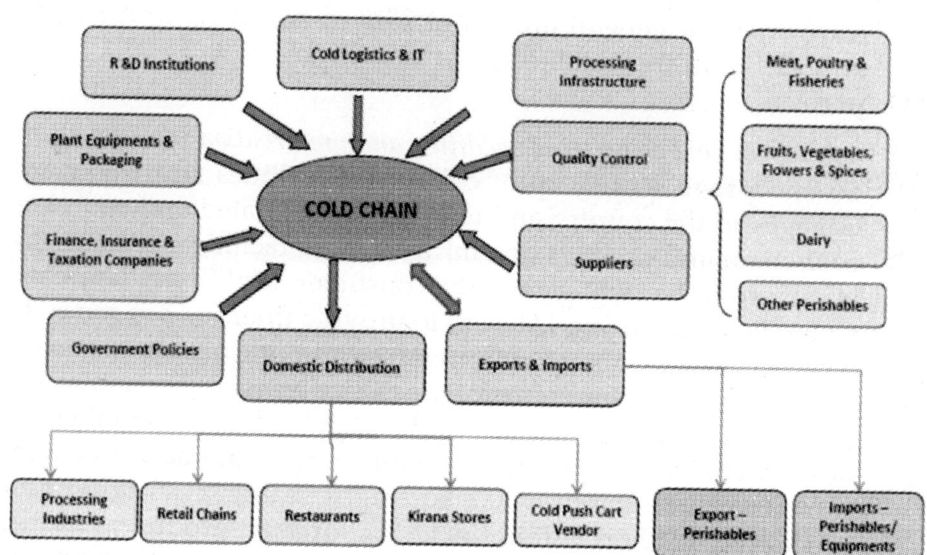

(c) *Scheme for setting up/ Modernization of abattoir*: MoFPI had launched the modernization of existing abattoirs/establishment of modern abattoirs, under the 11th Five Year Plan (2007-2012) which is expected to continue in the 12th Five Year Plan Period (2012-2017). MoFPI is also administering another scheme for technology upgrading, establishment and modernization of processing plants. Based on the detailed discussion with stakeholders, industries and state governments, the scheme has been modified to induct private capital, better technology, backward and forward linkages. The financial assistance will be provided, subject to necessary approval, 50% and 75% of the cost of plant and machineries and technical civil work in general and difficult areas respectively subject to a maximum of Rs.15 crores for each project.

References

AHS Series -12, 2010. Basic Animal Husbandry Statistics, Department of Animal Husbandry Dairying and Fisheries, Ministry of Agriculture, Government of India, New Delhi.

Anjaneyulu, A.S.R., Thomas, R. and Kondaiah, N. 2007. Technologies for value added buffalo meat products- A review. American Journal of Food Technology 2: 104-114.

APEDA, 2010. India Export Statistics. Agricultural and Processed Food Products Export Development Authority, Ministry of Commerce and Industry, Government of India, New Delhi.

CIRG, 2011. Vision 2030, Central Institute for Research on Goats, Makhdoom, UP, India.

CSWRI, 2011. Vision 2030, Central Sheep and Wool Research Institute, Avikanagar, Rajasthan, India.

FAOSTAT 2008. Summary of world food and agriculture statistics. http://faostat.fao.org/

FAOSTAT 2009. Summary of world food and agriculture statistics. http://faostat.fao.org/

Global Agrisystem, 2011. Madhya Pradesh State Agro Industries Development Corporation Ltd.

Mahmoud Abdel Aziz, 2010. Present status of the world goat populations and their productivity, Lohmann Information 45: 42.

OECD-FAO. 2010. Agricultural outlook 2010-2019. Organisation for Economic Co-Operation and Development, FAO, UN.

Prasad, R., Singh, A.K. and Singh Lakhan, 2011. Higher adaptability and economic return from pigs overshadows social taboos. Indian Research Journal of Extension Education 11: 103.

Ranjhan, S.K. 2004. Commercial production of buffalo meat with social agenda. In: Proc. 7th World Buffalo Congress, Manila, Philippines, 1 : 1-7.

Risam, K.S., Das, G.K. and Bhasin, V. 2005. Rabbit for meat and wool production in India: A review. Indian Journal of Animal Sciences 75: 365-382.

Ritambhara Singh, 2010. Livestock and Products Annual, New Delhi, India. GAIN Report Number: IN1082, USDA Foreign Agricultural Service, Global Agricultural Information Network.

Ritambhara Singh, 2011. Livestock and Products Annual, New Delhi, India. GAIN Report Number: IN1184, USDA Foreign Agricultural Service, Global Agricultural Information Network.

Singh, C.V and Barwal, R.S. 2010. Buffalo breeding research and improvement strategies in India. In: Proc. 9th World Buffalo Congress, Argentina

Thom Wright, 2011. Pork – Annual, New Delhi, India, GAIN Report Number: IN1128, USDA Foreign Agricultural Service, Global Agricultural Information Network.

USDA, 2011. International Egg and Poultry Review 14: 34.

□□□

Chapter 23

Small Ruminant Meat in India : Production and Export Prospects

Suresh A.
National Centre for Agricultural Economics and Policy Research,
Pusa, New Delhi- 110 012

India is blessed with a large livestock population, contributing substantially towards the food, nutrition and livelihood security of millions of rural poor. The demand for the livestock products is fast increasing, irrespective of the income group, both in rural and urban areas. Further, the export demand for Indian livestock products is also on rise. Given the high income elasticity of demand for livestock products like milk, egg and meat, much of the incremental production diverts towards domestic consumption driven by factors like high per capita income growth, change in taste and preference of the consumers and increasing urbanization (Birthal and Taneja, 2006). Because of the insufficiency of the production to meet the domestic demand and policy rigidities against export, the export of livestock products including meat remained quite insignificant even during early 1980s. The opening up of the economy and subsequent policy support to boost livestock products export boosted the export prospects. Given the vast population of livestock in the country, India stands to gain from the export of meat and meat products, with advanced processing technology, institutional innovation in marketing and favourable export policy. In this context, Government and private sector took active interest in investment in livestock sector and the livestock production has undergone considerable change to be qualified to term as "revolution", particularly in case of milk and to an extent in case of meat (more so in case of poultry meat). However, even after these revolutions, the domestic production could not catch with the ever increasing demand, resulting in high inflation of proteins of animal origin. This would have serious implications on the food and nutritional security of the country. In this context, the production of the small ruminants needs to be augmented to cater to the domestic as well as export demand, besides supporting the livelihood security of the marginalized sections.

Small ruminant meat has always been highly valued by consumers, in India and abroad as well, and priced higher compared to meats of poultry and buffalo. As on 2010, international prices of lamb meat was 380 cents per kg, which was comparable with that of chicken and beef at about 141 and 250 cents per kg, respectively (World Bank, 2010). Indian small ruminant meat is highly preferred in major export destinations mainly on account of its leanness and organic nature of production (Suresh *et al.*, 2008). One of the strategies to meet the surging internal and external demand for small ruminant meat is through their population expansion (Ranjhan, 2010). Though India is home to vast small ruminant population, its expansion is fraught with constraints arising from institutional, technological and social fronts (Ray, 1999; Kumar and Pant, 2003; Bhatia, 2005). In this context the present chapter delves upon three issues, viz. (1) The production and export of meat in India and role of small ruminant meat in it (2) The prospects of increasing its production and export.

Growth in meat production in India

The domestic meat production increased from 2.6 million tonnes in 1980 to 4.4 million tonnes in 2009 registering an absolute increase of about 1.8 million tonnes (Table 1). Compared to 1980, the production of all the meat items increased, with the largest absolute increase in case of buffalo meat (0.61 million tonnes) followed by poultry meat (0.59 million tonnes). As on 2009, buffalo meat accounted for about one third of the total meat production in India, followed by poultry meat (17%), small ruminants (sheep and goat together for about 16-17%) and pigs for about 11%. Compared to 1980s, major changes in the composition occurred in case of poultry meat and cattle meat.

While the share of poultry meat increased by about 12%, that of cattle meat declined by the same extent. The growth in the poultry meat production was triggered mainly by the private initiatives (Ramaswami *et al.*, 2006), while decline of cattle meat has to do much with the legal ban on its slaughter and social taboo against its consumption. The growth in the meat production has close correspondence with the growth of the livestock population as can be observed in the following session.

Livestock population in India

Over a quarter century (1982-2007), the population of all the livestock increased, albeit with wide variations among species and inter-census periods (Table 2). The highest increase in population occurred in poultry, from 208 million heads to 649 million heads registering growth over 212%. The annual growth rates always remained closer to 4% during all the inter-census periods under consideration. The high growth rate was mainly due to technological breakthrough in breeding, feeding and health, institutional innovations in the form of contract farming in the case of broilers and layers, vertical integration, high credit facility and increased demand for white meat (Ramaswami *et al.*, 2006).

Table 1 : Trend in meat production in India ('000 Tonnes), 1980-2009

Year	Buffalo	Cattle	Goat	Pig	Sheep	Poultry	Total Meat
1980	820. 5	853.4	302.4	261.5	153.8	132.2	2626.8
	(31.2)	(32.5)	(11.5)	(10.0)	(5.9)	(5.0)	(100.0)
1990	1078.5	1035.9	430.0	413.0	181.2	325.0	3590.5
	(30.0)	(28.9)	(12.0)	(11.5)	(5.5)	(9.1)	(100.0)
2000	1255.8	981.4	469.0	465.9	220.8	454.9	3994.8
	(31.4)	(24.6)	(11.7)	(11.7)	(5.5)	(11.4)	(100.0)
2009	1427.5	885.8	478.8	481.1	239.8	726.6	4400.5
	(32.4)	(20.1)	(10.9)	(10.9)	(5.4)	(16.5)	(100.0)

Basic data source: FAOSTAT accessed on 11 Nov 2010. Note: Figures in parenthesis indicates percentage to the total

The population increase of the small ruminants during the periods was also commendable- from 49 to 72 million in case of sheep and 72 to 141 million in case of goat. Major impediment in increasing the small ruminants' population is the dwindling area and productivity of pastures (Ray, 1999; Pasha, 1991). There were many initiatives to conserve the pastures and to increase their productivity through various central and state Government programmes (GOI, 2007), albeit with limited success. The population surge in case of buffaloes - closer to 50% over a quarter century- is also worth mentioning. With mechanization of agricultural operations, buffaloes were being displaced from draft use. Unlike cattle, the social prohibition towards buffalo slaughter is not intense. These factors, combined with increased abattoir facilities for handling buffalo slaughter and meat processing has contributed to increased buffalo meat production (Ranjhan, 2010).

Table 2 : Population and growth of livestock in India, 1982-2007

Year / time period	Cattle	Buffalo	Sheep	Goat	Pig	Poultry
	Population (million heads)					
1982	192.5	69.8	48.8	95.3	10.0	207.7
1992	204.6	84.2	50.8	115.3	13.0	307.1
2003	185.2	97.9	61.5	124.4	13.6	489.0
2007	199.1	105.3	71.6	140.5	11.1	648.8
	Increase in population in 2007 over 1982 (per cent)					
	3.4	50.9	46.7	47.4	11.0	212.4
	Growth rate (per cent per year)					
1982-1992	0.6	1.9	0.4	1.9	2.7	4.0
1992-2003	-0.9	1.4	1.8	0.7	0.4	4.3
2003-2007	0.6	1.9	0.4	1.9	2.7	4.0

Basic Data Source: Livestock Census, Various Issues

Contribution of small ruminant meat in the total livestock production

During the five year period of 2004-05 to 2008-09, the total value of output from livestock sector measured in 2004-05 constant prices increased from Rs 1747 billion to Rs 2075 billion at an annual growth rate of 4.4% (Table 3). The contribution of mutton increased from Rs 98 billion to Rs 119 billion at the rate of about 4.7%, well above the overall livestock sector growth rate. The share of mutton in the total value amounted to 5.6% and has remained almost same during the four year period. However, the growth performance of mutton in comparison with other meat items shows that there is much to improve in the performance of small ruminants. For example, during the four year period, the total meat sector grew at the rate of 6.8% and much of the growth has been contributed by poultry, beef and processed products.

Table 3 : Value of output from livestock sector, at 2004-05 prices (Rs Crores)

Item	Value of output		Share to total (%)		Compound annual growth rate (%)
	2004-05	2008-09	2004-05	2008-09	
Milk Group	122983	142447	70.4	68.6	3.7
Meat Group	30030	38477	17.2	18.5	6.5
Meat	25920	33561	14.8	16.2	6.8
Beef	2910	3603	1.7	1.7	5.8
Mutton	9814	11904	5.6	5.7	4.7
Pork	1755	2162	1.0	1.0	4.9
Poultry	11441	15892	6.5	7.7	9.0
Meat Products	933	1169	0.5	0.6	5.6
By- Products	3177	3571	1.8	1.7	3.1
Eggs	5858	7365	3.4	3.5	6.5
Wool and Hair	333	352	0.2	0.2	1.4
Dung	11296	12024	6.5	5.8	1.5
Cocoons and honey	1749	1967	1.0	0.9	3.2
Increment in stock	2455	4902	1.4	2.4	18.9
Total value	174704	207534	100.0	100.0	4.4

Basic Data Source: Basic Animal Husbandry Statistics, 2010, Government of India

Small ruminant meat production

With a production of 0.72 million tonnes, India accounted for only 5.45% of world small ruminant meat production (Table 4). It can be observed that at global level, small ruminant meat production registered an increase of about 5.50 million tonnes between 1981 and 2008, contributed mainly by sharp increase in Asian countries. One noteworthy development is the production increase in China by about

3.33 million tonnes in a span of just over a quarter century, thereby contributing to the extent of 29% of the global production. The deliberate effort of that country to increase small ruminant meat production through increase in the population and intensive production practices helped achieve this. The simple factor of high meat production at comparable prices helped China gaining edge on export front also.

Table 4 : Production of small ruminant meat across major countries in the world

Country/year	Meat Production (in 000 Tones)				Share in world meat production (%)			
	1981	1991	2001	2008	1981	1991	2001	2008
Australia	579	678	726	710	7.59	6.87	6.35	5.41
Bangladesh	25	80	132	214	0.33	0.81	1.15	1.63
China	476	1181	2721	3806	6.24	11.97	23.81	29.01
India	471	619	693	715	6.18	6.27	6.06	5.45
Iran	232	344	444	496	3.04	3.49	3.88	3.78
New Zealand	627	560	564	599	8.23	5.67	4.93	4.57
Nigeria	95	171	366	416	1.25	1.73	3.21	3.17
Pakistan	289	519	480	415	3.79	5.26	4.20	3.16
South Africa	162	168	140	131	2.12	1.70	1.23	1.00
Spain	181	244	251	166	2.37	2.47	2.20	1.27
Sudan	121	124	272	341	1.59	1.26	2.38	2.60
Turkey	349	367	351	320	4.58	3.72	3.07	2.44
UK	259	385	267	326	3.40	3.91	2.34	2.48
USA	153	165	101	105	2.01	1.67	0.89	0.79
World	7622	9867	11430	13120	100.00	100.00	100.00	100.00

Basic Data Source: FAOSTAT

The supply of small ruminant meat is closely dependent on their population. The population growth of small ruminants is largely a function of current stocking rate, carrying capacity of grazing lands and the demand for livestock products (Ray, 1999), besides supportive institutional mechanisms. A broad picture regarding small ruminant population and their growth in India is provided in Table 5. As per 2007 livestock census, India possesses 212 millions of small ruminants constituted by 140 million goats and 72 million sheep. With 35 million population (25 million sheep and 10 million goats) Andhra Pradesh leads the total small ruminants accounting for 16.6% of total population in India, closely followed by Rajasthan with 33 million, accounting for 15.4% (constituted by 22 million goats and 11.2 million sheep). Between these two censuses the small ruminant population in India increased by 26 million - from 186 to 212 million- contributed by 16 million goats and 10 million sheep. The highest increment of small ruminant population was witnessed in case of Andhra Pradesh (7.5 million), Rajasthan (5.8 million) and Karnataka (4.0 million), in that order. On the other hand, population decline was observed in case of Uttar Pradesh and West Bengal, among the major states. These developments have resulted in an aggregate growth rate of 2.68-2.48% for goats and 3.09% for sheep. Among the major small ruminant breeding states, above 4% growth has been registered by Andhra Pradesh, Karnataka, Rajasthan and Tamil Nadu; besides less populated states like Assam and Jharkhand. It can be observed that between the last two livestock censuses, goat population increased in all the states, but for Maharashtra and West Bengal; whereas, sheep posted negative growths in seven states. The Table also provides some indicators of prospects of increasing their population- the ratio of small ruminants to number of human beings and small ruminants to land available for grazing and cultivation (no./ha), the former proxies the localized demand and the latter for the stocking rate. It may be noted that in case of the small ruminants to man ratio, six out of 15 states posted less than national average values, whereas it was seven in case of small ruminants to land values. These figures indicate that there exists considerable scope for increasing the small ruminant population in many states. By organized efforts it might be possible to enhance the carrying capacity and optimize the stocking rate, and thereby enhancing the small ruminant meat supply.

India's meat and meat products' export

The export of livestock products from India has gained considerable attention of researchers during recent years, both at global and at national level. Globally the demand for livestock products, particularly for meat is on rise, owing to the rise of per capital income in many developing countries (Delgado *et al.*, 1999). Kumar *et al.* (2007) reported that as on 2006, the share of export revenue of livestock products was 0.8% of the total exports, 7.4% of total agricultural exports and 2.4% of the GDP of livestock origin. They exhibited an increasing trend since 1982. During 2002-04, out of exports of livestock and livestock products worth US$ 472 million, the share of milk (equivalent) was about 14%, whereas that of meat and meat preparations was about 72% (Bardhan, 2007). Major commodities of economic significance other than milk and meat were eggs, "hair and wool", and "hides and skin". Of these, the share of eggs in total livestock products exports was about 10% as on 2002-04, where as that of "hair and wool" and "hides and skin" was less than one per cent.

Table 5 : Population and growth of small ruminants in major states in India

States	Population ('000) (2007 Census)			Share (%)	Growth rates between 2003 and 2007			SRs to man ratio*	SRs to land (No/ha)**
	Goat	Sheep	SRs		Goat	Sheep	SRs		
Andhra Pradesh	9626	25539	35165	16.58	8.93	3.62	4.92	0.36	1.89
Assam	4320	354	4674	2.20	7.66	15.79	8.16	0.12	0.97
Bihar	10167	218	10385	4.90	1.39	-10.59	1.02	0.12	1.46
Gujarat	4640	2002	6642	3.13	0.43	-0.59	0.12	0.13	0.42
Himachal Pradesh	1241	901	2142	1.01	1.98	-0.54	0.87	0.34	0.72
Jammu & Kashmir	2068	4127	6195	2.92	0.13	3.89	2.54	0.54	4.23
Jharkhand	6592	483	7075	3.34	5.55	-6.60	4.38	0.21	1.42
Karnataka	6153	9558	15711	7.41	6.53	5.67	6.00	0.22	1.08
Madhya Pradesh	9014	390	9404	4.43	2.05	-6.51	1.60	0.14	0.47
Maharashtra	10391	2909	13301	6.27	-0.55	-1.22	-0.70	0.14	0.55
Orissa	7127	1818	8945	4.22	4.20	2.34	3.80	0.20	1.06
Rajasthan	21503	11190	32693	15.41	5.05	2.16	4.01	0.48	1.10
Tamil Nadu	9275	7991	17265	8.14	2.55	7.40	4.63	0.22	1.97
Uttar Pradesh	14793	1188	15980	7.53	2.71	-3.74	2.14	0.09	0.81
West Bengal	15069	1577	16646	7.85	-4.30	0.68	-3.89	0.25	2.88
All India	140537	71558	212096	100.00	2.48	3.09	2.68	0.18	1.01

Basic data source: Livestock Census, GoI (2003 and 2007); Agricultural Statistics at a Glance, various issues, Ministry of Agriculture, GOI; * indicates ratio calculated as per 2003 livestock population and 2001 human population, ** indicates the number of small ruminants per ha of land available for grazing and cultivation.

Compared to many other livestock products, meat exports enjoy high prospects due to competitiveness. Kumar (2009) indicated that under exportable hypothesis all the meat products from India except poultry meat were competitive in the world market and the competitiveness was the highest in case of bovine meat. This compares well with exported milk products like butter, whole milk powder and skimmed milk powder which were far from being competitive. Another major concern that has attracted the attention of the researchers is the increasing focus towards food safety measures imposed by the importing countries. This issue has become pertinent since the inception of WTO wherein SPS measures were given increased thrust. India has been facing impact of increasing non- tariff measures manifested in the form of refusals of its consignments on account of contamination, filthiness, unsanitary conditions, inadequate labeling, and use of unsafe additives (Kumar *et al.,* 2007).

India's share in world export of meat is very low (Table 6). As on 2008, the world meat export accounted for about US$ 107 billion, of which the highest individual contribution was by Brazil (13%), followed by USA (11%) and Germany (9%). With an export value of about US $1.2 billion, India's share was only one per cent. India mainly exports meat of bovines, sheep, goat, poultry and swine in various forms like fresh, chilled, frozen, salted, smoked etc. During 2009-10, India exported meat items worth Rs 6325 Crores (Rs 2606 Crores at 1993 prices) (Table 6). Since 1981, India made impressive strides in export of meat items, both in quantity and value terms. It was to the tune of 0.53 lakh tonnes in 1980-81, and increased to the level of 5.5 lakh tonnes by 2009-10 accounting for about 12% of total meat production in India. The corresponding values were Rs 64 Crores in 1980-81 and Rs 6525 Crores in 2009-10. As on 2009-10, about 86% of Indian meat export (in value terms) was contributed by bovine meat either in fresh, chilled or frozen form. Since meat items are liable to quick spoilage during long distance transport, lion's share of the lots are exported in frozen form, accounting for almost 95% of total bovine meat export. During early 1980s, the export was mainly in the form of fresh/ chilled meat. The export of frozen bovine meat was near absent during 1980-81, but it increased to 4.7 lakh tonnes by 2009-10. Availability of frozen technology offered significant boost to India's meat export. Mutton/ chevon constituted about 12% of total meat export. The case of poultry meat is quite interesting - despite contributing to 17% to the total meat production, its contribution in meat export is meager. As on 2009-10, the export was only about 13 lakh kg worth Rs 60 Crores. The major factor that might have contributed to the lower export is the poor competitiveness of Indian poultry sector as we could see later in this paper. Though pigs contributed about 10 % of the total meat production in India, its export is conspicuous by its near absence. The share of other processed meat items like fresh, chilled or frozen edible offal and salted and/or smoked meat is also very less compared to other meat items.

Table 6 : Export value of meat of major countries, 1981- 2008 (Values in million US $, share in per cent)

Country/year	1981		1991		2001		2008	
	Value	Share	Value	Share	Value	Share	Value	Share
Argentina	888.4	4.2	864.3	2.4	347.6	0.8	2060.9	1.9
Australia	1768.6	8.5	2433.7	6.8	3113.6	7.1	5701.1	5.3
Brazil	852.2	4.1	877.7	2.5	2848.7	6.5	14089.5	13.2
Canada	478.0	2.3	786.2	2.2	2841.9	6.5	3878.4	3.6
Denmark	2263.1	10.8	3403.5	9.5	3619.2	8.3	5605.0	5.2
France	1527.7	7.3	3205.1	9.0	2835.7	6.5	5128.6	4.8
Germany	1348.4	6.4	3008.6	8.4	2414.4	5.5	9714.5	9.1
India	74.7	0.4	92.6	0.3	262.6	0.6	1239.5	1.2
Ireland	764.9	3.7	1374.2	3.9	1376.3	3.2	3316.8	3.1
Netherlands	2634.8	12.6	5003.0	14.0	3352.7	7.7	9169.9	8.6
New Zealand	1383.3	6.6	1510.3	4.2	1792.1	4.1	3323.9	3.1
Poland	208.6	1.0	188.5	0.5	329.7	0.8	2888.9	2.7
USA	1174.8	5.6	3171.4	8.9	6713.2	15.4	11783.5	11.0
Others	5561.8	26.6	9747.9	27.3	11844.9	27.1	29235.1	27.3
World	20929.3	100.0	35666.9	100.0	43692.6	100.0	107135.6	100.0

Basic Data Source: FAOSTAT accessed on 13th January 2011

Small ruminant meat export

The small ruminant meats are exported in the form of fresh and chilled lambs and sheep, boneless mutton, frozen lamb and sheep and chevon (Table 8). The Table depicts the quantity and value of export of the small ruminant meat items from India during the time period spanning from 1990-91 to 2009-10. The export of the small ruminant meat from India increased manifolds during the last two decades. During 1990-91, India exported meat amounting for below 0.01 million tonnes and it surged to 0.08 million tonnes by 2009-10. The

Table 7 : Structure of meat and meat products export from India, 1980-81 to 2009-10

Meat products	Quantity (in lakh Kg)				Value (Rs. Crores)			
	1980-81	1990-91	2000-01	2009-10	1980-81	1990-91	2000-01	2009-10
Total live animals *	8.8	520.0	50.6	7.6	8.5	0.6	6.5	79.9
					(13.3)	(0.4)	(0.4)	(1.3)
Fresh and/or	35.7	84.4	574.4	116.3	3.3	14.1	278.9	108.9
chilled bovine meat	(6.7)	(11.48)	(18.5)	(2.1)	(5.1)	(10.0)	(19.1)	(1.7)
Frozen bovine meat	0	549.2	2305.9	4730.5	0	92.6	1096.1	5328.2
	(0.0)	(74.69)	(74.36)	(86.4)	(0.0)	(65.6)	(75.0)	(84.2)
Fresh, chilled	2	0	0	5.1	0	0	0	2.8
and/or frozen swine meat	(0.0)	(0.0)	(0.0)	(0.1)	(0.0)	(0.0)	(0.0)	(0.0)
Mutton/chevon	13.8	83.3	119.0	522.5	1.91	31.3	78.2	737.3
	(2.6)	(11.3)	(3.8)	(9.6)	(3.0)	(22.2)	(5.3)	(11.7)
Fresh,	0	6.2	0.1	62.8	0	0.98	2.0	53.6
chilled/frozen edible offal	(0.0)	(0.8)	(0.0)	(1.2)	(0.0)	(0.7)	(0.0)	(0.9)
Poultry meat	9	0	0	12.6	1.0	0	42.0	6.0
	(0.0)	(0.0)	(0.0)	(0.2)	(0.0)	(0.0)	(0.1)	(0.1)
Salted and or	26.3	1.3	0.6	7.1	4.2	1.5	2.4	8.5
smoked meat	(5.0)	(0.2)	(0.0)	(0.1)	(6.5)	(1.1)	(0.2)	(0.1)
Other meats	454.8	0.5	0	0.4	46.1	0.1	0	0.2
	(85.7)	(0.1)	(0.0)	(0.0)	(72.1)	(0.1)	(0.0)	(0.0)
Total meat items	530.6	735.3	3101.1	5472.6	64.0	141.0	1462.5	6325.2
(excluding live animals)	(100.0)	(100.0)	(100.0)	(100.0)	(100.0)	(100.0)	(100.0)	(100.00)

*In case of live animals the quantity is in '000 nos.; Figures in parenthesis indicates percentages to the total; Basic data source: Monthly Statistics of Foreign Trade, Directorate General of Commerce, Intelligence and Statistics, Ministry of Commerce.

corresponding increase value increase has been from Rs 31 Crores to 718 Crores. After adjusting for inflation it converts to Rs 318 Crores as per 1993-94 prices. The table clearly indicates that the export of the small ruminant meat is dominated by boneless mutton (36 % in quantity terms and 40% in value terms), followed by fresh/ chilled sheep (about 17% in quantity terms and 19% in value terms). At this juncture it is worthwhile to mention that we are retaining the classification adopted by Directorate General of Commerce, Intelligence and Statistics to study the commodity groupings, rather than modifying with some other criteria. Over years, Indian small ruminant meat export composition underwent gradual structural changes. The share of sheep/ lamb exported in frozen/ fresh/ chilled form in total export quantity declined from 77% in 1990-91 to 80% 2000-01, and further to 34% in 2009-10. The corresponding change in value share was from

83 to 78% and further to 37%. During this period, the share of boneless mutton increased from 10 to 40%. The export of chevon was quite low and it contributes to only about 14% of total export value as on 2009-10, but its share in overall export is on increase.

Table 8 : Quantity and value of export of small ruminant meat from India, 1990-91 to 2009-10

Article	Quantity (tonnes)			Value (Rs Lakhs)		
	1990-91	2000-01	2009-10	1990-91	2000-01	2009-10
Fresh and/or chilled lamb*	2125	1232	2784	705	944	2784
Fresh or chilled sheep*	353	2044	13787	125	1558	13787
Fresh /chilled sheep with bone+	1916	460	5166	548	3132	5166
Boneless mutton	1700	1223	28990	307	1089	28990
Frozen lamb*	106	2379	126	31	260	126
Frozen sheep*	540	623	1093	91	432	1093
Frozen sheep with bone+	2280	2775	4750	1095	2302	4751
Frozen sheep without bone	432	766	5100	182	893	5110
Chevon	12	420	9965	4	361	9965
Total	9463	11922	79337	3126	10972	71772

*These are concise nomenclature derived from classification provided by DGCIS, Basic Data Source: As Table 3

A vivid picture of the transition can be obtained from the growth and instability depicted in Table 9. In order to avoid the effect of price rise on the growth rate, nominal values of export were converted into real values by using whole sale price index with base year of 1993-94. The growth estimates were arrived at by using triennial ending averages to smoothen the fluctuations. The analysis has been carried out for a time span of about two decades; from 1990-91 to 2009-10. Further, the entire time period has been divided into two reflecting two distinct decades- 1990s and 2000s. The overall average annual growth rate was 3.71% during 1990-91 to 2009-10, with growth rates of 5.35% during 1990s and 12.41% during 2000s. During the overall period, all commodity groupings with the exception of fresh/ chilled sheep, boneless mutton and chevon experienced negative growth. The highest growth during this period was observed for fresh/ chilled sheep (16%), followed by boneless mutton (10.33%). Positive and statistically significant growth rate has been recorded during 1990s and 2000s only by fresh/ chilled sheep. During 2000s fresh/ chilled sheep and boneless mutton posted high growth- more than 19%. The case of boneless mutton is noteworthy. It posted moderate growth of 6.71% during 1990s, followed by a whopping 19.54% during 2000s. The growth in the latter period was statistically insignificant as it was associated with high standard error. This was reflected in the instability estimates also. The overall export instability in values terms was 55%; it was closer to 20% in 1990s and 58% in 2000s. As noted earlier, boneless mutton, the major export item during the recent period, exhibited high instability of 136% during the entire period and 107% during 2000s. Chevon registered a growth rate of 10% during the entire period, but with high instabilities.

Table 9 : Growth and instability of export of small ruminant meat from India (TE ending, constant prices, 1993-94 = 100) (%)

Name of Article	Growth			Instability		
	1990-91 to 1999-00	2000-01 to 2009-10	1990-91 to 2009-10	1990-91 to 1999-00	2000-01 to 2009-10	1990-91 to 2009-10
Fresh and/or chilled lamb	-3.86 NS	1.76 NS	-5.97***	24.19	51.13	36.29
Fresh or chilled sheep	17.42***	19.30***	16.04***	10.32	33.91	55.36
Fresh /chilled sheep with bone+	-5.58 NS	-11.94*	-3.99*	36.04	56.25	50.00
Boneless mutton	6.71**	19.54 NS	10.33***	21.69	106.55	136.36
Frozen lamb*	8.97 NS	-16.43**	-2.40 NS	121.73	32.87	110.11
Frozen sheep*	2.84 NS	-20.60**	-9.60***	47.32	49.22	52.27
Frozen sheep with bone+	11.76***	-0.21 NS	-2.68 NS	14.74	51.30	43.68
Frozen sheep without bone	12.25**	-4.14 NS	-2.81 NS	32.30	82.77	58.47
Chevon	33.46***	16.04 NS	10.09***	38.05	163.75	169.21
Total	5.35**	12.41**	3.71**	19.60	58.13	55.49

* CRCS and half CRCS +other cuts· ***, ** and * indicates P<0.01, 0.05 and 0.10, respectively; Basic Data Source: As Table 3

The above analysis brings forth an alarming situation of incremental exports being met out from the domestically available meat net of export. Though the small ruminant meat registered production increase, it is not sufficient enough to cater to the surging domestic and external demand. It can be noted that between 1990-91 and 2009-10, small ruminant meat production increased only by 0.11 million tonnes, compared to 0.35 in case of buffalo meat and 0.40 in case of poultry meat. The export demand for small ruminant meat was ruling high to the extent that the incremental export was more than the incremental small ruminant meat production. This can be ascertained by a simple analysis of the data already used. As on 1990-91 about 1.55% of the domestic small ruminant meat production was exported. This increased marginally to 1.73% by 2000-01 and further to 11.04% by 2009-10. The average increase of small ruminant meat production between 1990-91 and 2000-01 was about 78600 tonnes; the incremental export during this period was closer to 2458 tonnes constituting for 3.13% of incremental production. On the other hand, the incremental production during 2001-09 was about 29000 tonnes; the incremental export was about 60000 tonnes, accounting for 209% of incremental production. This clearly indicated the incremental export was met largely from the meat which was already available for domestic consumption net of export. This in turn has contributed to price rise of small ruminant meat in the domestic market this has contributed to high price rice also. This has been the major reason for lower export of Indian small ruminant meat. An analysis of the wholesale price index of mutton over a decade of time period (1997-98 to 2007-08) indicated that it has risen by about 45%. The year on year inflation calculated with this data indicated positive values during all the time period except for the year 2001-02. This compares well with poultry meat, where 7 out of 11 years reported negative price growth (Table 10).

Table 10 : Annual change in wholesale price index of meat/ fish products in India (per cent)

Commodity	1997 -98	1998 -99	1999 -00	2000 -01	2001- 02	2002 -03	2003 -04	2004 -05	2005 -06	2006 -07	2007 -08
Eggs	9.9	-4.3	4.8	2.2	1.1	-3.0	-1.8	1.4	1.8	8.8	14.8
Poultry	-3.6	6.3	-6.5	-2.4	-1.6	-12.2	-10.6	-7.8	-4.3	4.2	3.4
Mutton	6.1	5.6	0.5	5.0	-3.9	2.2	3.9	6.6	3.9	8.6	6.5
Pork	2.2	-0.6	0.8	3.0	0.7	-6.7	0.1	0.5	8.0	13.6	26.8
Marine fish	23.2	7.5	-9.7	5.6	-3.8	0.9	5.1	1.5	6.3	11.6	17.3
Inland fish	23.1	4.0	22.1	15.3	11.3	10.4	-11.5	6.1	25.2	-4.7	-8.3

Basic Data Source: Economic Advisor, Ministry of Commerce, Government of India.

Competitiveness of Indian small ruminant production

The differential between international price *vis a vis* the domestic price is the most important factor that affects the competitiveness of trade (Chand, 2002). Figure 1 illustrates the trend in the producer price of goats and sheep in major producing countries. Though the comparison of the producer prices is a crude method of ascertaining the competitiveness compared to other measures like nominal protection coefficient, it helps in ascertaining the trend, that are not complicated with the nuances of variables like tariffs and transportation costs. It can be observed that the producer prices of goat and sheep in India is competitive compared to most of the countries. Among major goat producing countries, only Australia and Thailand (along with Brazil and Germany) are more competitive than India in terms of producer prices. In case of sheep India is more competitive than most countries- the notable exception being Australia, the major sheep producer. China is equally competitive with India in case of both goat and sheep. This trend clearly indicates that Indian small ruminant meat production is competitive at producer level. Similar results were reported in earlier studies also (Kumar, 2009).

As has been mentioned earlier, the demand for the small ruminant meat in India is bound to rise. By 2020, the demand for total meat would be around 8-9 million tonnes (Table 11). The situation would exert pressure on the small ruminant sector to respond to the situation.

Table 11: Demand for livestock products (million tonnes)

Commodity	1983	1999-2000	2020
Milk	34.6	73.4	132.0-140.0
Total meat	1.7	3.1	8.0-9.0
Beef and buffalo meat	0.5	0.8	
Mutton and goat meat	0.8	1.0	
Pig meat	0.1	0.2	
Poultry meat	0.2	0.7	
Eggs (million numbers)	6.6	19.3	49.7

(Data Source: Birthal and Taneja, 2006)

The aforesaid discussion clearly brings out the urgency to improve domestic small ruminant meat production. Increasing the sheep population and its average body weight at slaughter age are important strategies in this regard. However, expansion of small ruminant population is severely constrained due to many structural reasons, the major one being scarcity of grazing lands. Small ruminants depend heavily on the availability of pastures for grazing resources (Pasha, 1991). The area and productivity of pastures is dwindling; it warrants concerted efforts to conserve the pasture resources and improve its productivity (Singh *et al.*, 2005; Suresh *et al.*, 2010). In a study conducted in Rajasthan, it was observed that majority of the animals are disposed before attaining 6 months of age. This is a major coping mechanism to overcome fodder scarcity. Interventions from institutional side in conserving the feed / fodder resources and timely availability of it to the needy at affordable rate are the need of the hour. The technological progress in the sphere of animal nutrition and feed technology has to be harnessed to make this a reality.

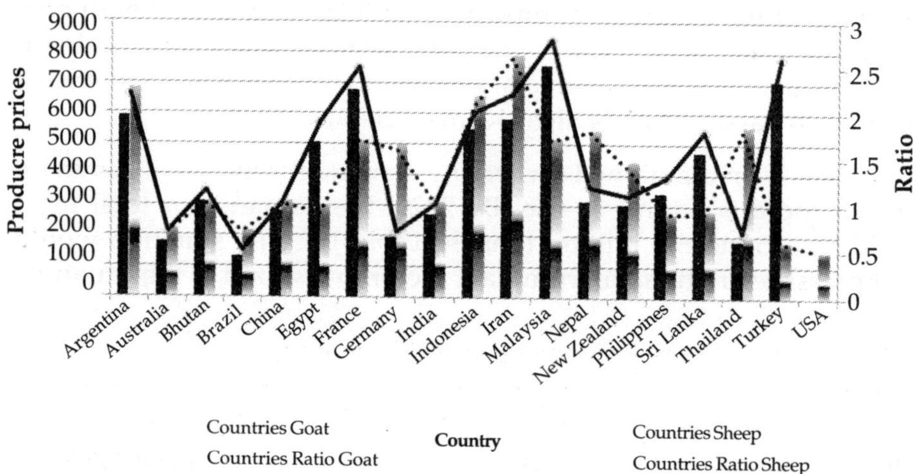

Fig. 1 : Producer prices of small ruminant meat in major producing countries (Source: Own estimation)

Status of animal feed in India

The major hindrance in the prospects of the small ruminant production is the scarcity of the fodder and feed resources. For the livestock sector as a whole the supply- demand gap of dry fodder, green fodder and concentrate as on 2007 was estimated at 40, 36 and 57%, respectively (GOI, 2008). This gap is bound to rise in the coming years, unless corrective measures are undertaken. It is reported that the by 2020, the demand for the green fodder would rise to 855 million tonnes whereas that of the dry fodder and concentrate would touch 526 and 55.7 million tones, respectively. Of this the demand by the small ruminants would be around 128 million tonnes of green fodder, 12 million tonnes of dry fodder and 4.5 million tonnes of concentrate mixture (Table 12). However, the prospects of small ruminants getting better feed than the current availability is dismal. This situation needs immediate attention of the policy makers and concerned official, as the body weight growth of the Indian small ruminants are quite low, compared to the world average (Table 13).

Table 12 : India's livestock demand to 2020

Animal category	Population (million)	Green fodder (Mt)	Dry fodder (Mt)	Concentrate (Mt)
Cattle	185.6	369.0	291.0	24.7
Buffalo	113.5	348.2	214.8	26.2
Sheep	73.8	43.1	5.1	1.1
Goat	156.6	85.7	11.4	3.4
Others	1.6	9.1	3.9	0.3
Total	513.2	855.1	526.3	55.7

(Source: Dikshit and Birthal, 2010)

Table 13 : Trend in body weight of small ruminants across world

Country	Sheep			Country	Goat		
	1961	2008	% increase over 1960		1961	2008	% increase over 1961
Argentina	171	111	-37	Bangladesh	70	70	0
Australia	178	212	19	Brazil	111	114	3
Brazil	157	160	2	China	99	137	38
China	100	150	50	India	100	100	0
India	120	120	0	Indonesia	100	100	0
Iran	159	180	13	Iran	140	140	0
New Zealand	167	177	6	Mexico	107	169	58
Nigeria	110	110	0	Mongolia	140	139	-1
Pakistan	121	150	24	Nigeria	127	127	0
South Africa	120	188	57	Pakistan	109	170	56
Sudan	174	160	-8	Somalia	130	130	0
Turkey	127	159	25	Sudan	130	130	0
UK	202	195	-3	Turkey	137	154	12
USA	177	111	-37	Tanzania	120	120	0
World	149	157	5	World	107	124	16

Source: FAOSTAT

Much of the fodder for the small ruminants is originating from common grazing land. However, the areas under the grazing lands are on steady decline over years. Table 14 provides the area under total grazing lands in India. The overall availability of the total grazing lands declined from 35 million ha in 1970-71 to 26 million ha in 2008-09. Sharp decline in the area was observed in many states including many small ruminant producer states like Andhra Pradesh, Maharashtra, Rajasthan, Uttar Pradesh and West Bengal. It needs constant attention to conserve the remaining grazing lands and to improve the productivity. This would contribute a long way in increasing the nutritional status of the small ruminants.

Table 14 : Area under grazing lands in India (000 ha)

States	1970-71	1980-81	1990-91	2000-01	2008-09
Andhra Pradesh	2492	2107	1885	1673	1518
Bihar	890	823	789	770	842
Gujarat	2929	2838	2773	2840	2833
Haryana	98	60	54	60	71
Himachal Pradesh	1397	1186	1309	1711	1699
Kerala	240	196	131	75	102
Madhya Pradesh	5460	4929	4413	3995	3719
Maharashtra	3363	2761	2727	2454	2411
Orissa	1927	1244	2182	1317	1211
Punjab	93	52	57	22	15
Rajasthan	7928	8256	7501	6629	6053
Tamil Nadu	964	693	648	730	702
Uttar Pradesh	2682	2149	1882	1811	1765
West Bengal	607	574	159	98	94
Jammu & Kashmir	388	374	338	338	345
India	35128	32311	30217	27737	26507

The areas coming under permanent pastures and other grazing lands, land under miscellaneous tree crops and groves not included in the net area sown and cultivable waste land as per the land use classification. Data Source: Centre for Monitoring Indian Economy, Various publications.

Small ruminant diseases

Growth in the small ruminant production cannot be sustained unless animals are protected against diseases. Over years India could make considerable progress to keep diseases under control. The devastating diseases that affect the ruminants like Rinder Pest was eradicated. But a number of other diseases like foot and mouth diseases, Peste des petits ruminants, Bluetongue, sheep and goat pox, enterotoxaemia etc affects the small ruminants and make considerable economic loss to the farmers. Table 15 depicts the reported incidence of various small ruminant diseases in 2008. Given the weak institutional mechanism to report the disease emergence correctly, the figures might be under estimates. The sudden emergence of the disease needs its management strategy at community level, as the small ruminants are raised on common grazing lands. The veterinary facility at the grass root level needs to be strengthened to meet the emerging situations.

Table 15 : Disease wise incidence of livestock diseases in India during the year 2008

Disease	No. of Outbreak	No. of Attack	No. of Death
Foot and mouth disease	–	425	5
Peste des petits ruminants (PPR)	165	4496	1092
Bluetongue	132	2903	342
Sheep pox and goat pox	63	2279	689
Anthrax	–	516	471
Contagious caprine pleuropneumonia	3	405	40
Blackleg/Black quarter	–	0	0
Distomatosis (liver fluke)/ Fascioliasis	–	53	0
Enterotoxaemia	281	2673	888
Mange	–	14	0

Source: Animal health division, Department of Animal Husbandry and Dairying and Fisheries

Conclusion

The livestock sector contributes to the food, nutritional and livelihood security of millions, besides the foreign exchange reserved in terms of export of various livestock products including meat. The growth in Indian meat sector is driven largely by buffalo and poultry meats. The role of small ruminant sector needs particular attention as it is closely linked with marginalized sections of the society and the high value attached to the small ruminant meat. The domestic and external demand for Indian small ruminant meat is high, and is posed to register further growth. Indian small ruminant meat is highly preferred in export markets due to lean meat and organic nature of production, and India has achieved impressive strides in export front. It is observed that the population of the small ruminants has increased considerably between 2003 and 2007 census - with mixed results across states and marked increase in southern part of the country. However, the export of the small ruminant meat has grown faster than the population growth to the extent that the incremental export was over and above the incremental production. This situation warrants the small ruminant sector to make use of the positive signals and augment its production. Indian small ruminant meat production is competitive at breeder level compared to other major producers. However, to bridge the supply-demand gap of the small ruminant meat, the sector needs special attention, particularly in terms of nutrition and veterinary care, notably disease management. This requires the attention of both public and private sectors, in terms of investment in development activities and identifying the potential areas of research and extension so as to explore the synergies.

References

Bardhan, D. 2007. India's trade performance in livestock and livestock products. Indian Journal of Agricultural Economics 62: 411-425.

Bhatia, J., Pandey, U.K. and Suhaga, K.S. 2005. Small ruminant economy of semi-arid region in Haryana. Indian Journal of Agricultural Economics 60: 163-183.

Birthal, P.S. and Taneja, V.K. 2006. Livestock sector in India: Opportunities and challenges for small holders. In: Proc. ICAR-ILRI International Workshop, NCAP, New Delhi and ILRI, Nairobi.

Chand, R. 2002. Trade Liberalisation, WTO and Indian Agriculture, Mittal Publication, New Delhi.

Delgado, C., Rosaegrant, M., Steinfeld, H., Ehui, S. and Courbois, C. 1999. Livestock 2020: The New food revolution: International Food Policy Research Discussion Paper EPTD 28, Washington DC.

Dixit, A.K. and Birthal, P.S. 2010. India's livestock feed demand: Estimates and projections. Agricultural Economics Research Review 23:15-28

Food and Agricultural Organization. 2010. FAOSTAT website.

Government of India. 2003. Livestock Census. Department of Animal Husbandry, Dairying and Fisheries, Ministry of Agriculture.

Government of India. 2007. Report of Working Group on Livestock and Animal Husbandry, 11th Five Year Plan, Planning Commission.

Government of India. 2008. Annual Report. Department of Animal Husbandry, Dairying and Fisheries, Ministry of Agriculture.

Kumar, A. 2009. India's livestock sector trade: Opportunities and Challenges. Policy Brief 24. National Centre for Agricultural Economics and Policy Research, New Delhi.

Kumar, A., Staal, S.J., Singh, N.P. and Singh, D.K. 2007. Livestock sector trade of India: Surging momentum in the new liberalized regime. Indian Journal of Agricultural Economics 62: 396-410.

Kumar, S. and Pant, K.P. 2003. Development perspectives of goat rearing in India-Status, Issues and Strategies. Indian Journal of agricultural economics 47: 754-757.

Pasha, S.A. 1991. Sustainability and viability of small and large farmers: Animal husbandry and common property resources. Economic and Political Weekly 26: A27-A30.

Ramaswami, B., Birthal, P.S. and Joshi, P.K. 2006. Efficiency and distribution in contract farming: The case of Indian poultry growers. Markets, Trade and Institutions Discussion Paper No. 91, International food Policy Research Institute, Washington DC.

Ranjhan, S.K. 2010. India's Meat Industry: Perspectives. Food and Agricultural Organization.

Ray, S. 1999. Declining production conditions of raw wool: Analysis of emerging conflicts in sheep husbandry in Rajasthan. Economic and Political Weekly 34: 1209-1214.

Singh, V.K., Suresh, A., Gupta, D.C. and Jakhmola, R.C. 2005. Common property resources, rural livelihood and small ruminants in India: A review. Indian Journal of Animal Sciences 75: 1027-1036.

Suresh, A., Gupta, D.C. and Mann, J.S. 2008. Returns and economic efficiency of sheep farming in semi-arid region of Rajasthan. Agricultural Economics Research Review 21: 227-234.

Suresh, A., Gupta, D.C. and Mann, J.S. 2010. Degradation of common pastures: An economics perspective of its Impact on livestock farming and coping strategies. Agricultural Economics Research Review 23: 47-56.

World Bank. 2010. Pink Sheet. Commodity Outlook.

□□□

and ca
Sheep
sheep
wool
second
count
world
when
million
million
produ
and la
major
produ
tradit
parts
breitsc

Chapter 24

Pelt Production Counts and Discounts

A.K. Shinde
Meat Science Section, Central Sheep and Wool Research Institute
Avikanagar-304 501 (Rajasthan)

Sheep husbandry plays an important role in livelihood security and economic sustenance of poor farmers in dry region of the country. Sheep provides meat, wool, milk, and/or pelts. Pelts from some of the sheep breeds are by-products of lamb production. In India, meat and wool are primary produce of sheep and milk, skin and pelt are secondary produce. Pelt producing sheep breeds are not found in the country. A total almost 540 millions sheep skins were produced in the world in 2008 (FAOSTAT, 2011). Half of these were produced in Asia, where China is the most important manufacturer. In Africa about 90 millions, in Europe 80 millions, in Australia and New Zealand 66 millions, in America 26 millions and in India 57 millions skins were produced. These figures are closely related to the number of sheep and lambs slaughtered in the different parts of the world. The great majority of all sheep skins in the world are processed into leather products by the tanning industry but special pelt products have a long tradition with Karakul, Icelandic and Gotland sheep breeds in certain parts of the world. Fur from fetal Karakul lambs is called: broadtail, breitschwanz (German) and karakulcha, or simply cha (Russian,

Uzbek). The fur from newborn karakul sheep is called: Karakul (also spelled caracul), Swakara (coined from South West Africa Karakul), Namikara or Nakara (from Namibian Karakul), Astrakhan (Russian), Persian lamb, Agnello di persia, (Italian) and Krimmer (Russian).

Pelt producing breeds

Karakul is one of the most important sheep breed raised for production of high quality pelts and is widely spread in Russia, Afghanistan, Namibia, South Africa, Iran and Rumania (Nel, 1991). Karakul sheep breed originates from the Middle East and is a fat-tailed desert sheep breed kept for production of Persian lamb pelts. Other sheep breeds used for pelt production are the Gotland in Sweden (Näsholm, 2005, 2008), the Icelandic sheep (Eythorsdottir, 1999), the Grey Shiraz and Zandi in Iran (Nanekarani *et al*.., 2010), the Romanov in former USSR, and the Wrzosowska in Poland (Flamant *et al*.., 1982).

Pelt production trend

In South West Africa, the interest for pelt production with Karakul increased during the period from 1930 to 1980 and in 1979 about 5 million pelts were exported to Europe. However, due to lifestyle changed, the pelt industry almost collapsed during the 1980's (Schoeman, 1998). In 1997 again the pelt prices increased and pelt garments became more popular. There are approximately 4.4 million Karakul sheep in Turkmenistan, mainly reared by the shepherds and about 1.5 million in southern Kazakstan. Karakul sheep are well adapted to arid desert conditions, mainly maintained on degraded pastures of Kyrgyzstan. Uzbekistan has a large population of Karakul sheep. Karakul sheep is kept primarily for meat and pelts (Astrakhan) from lambs is produced by slaughter at birth or in some cases, deliberately aborted before birth. The wool produced from pelt producing sheep is mostly coarse and has little utility in textile and mostly used for making felt. The trade was declined in Kazakstan as a consequence of the demise of the former USSR. Final processing and manufacture of pelts into garments was carried out in Russia in the Soviet period and Russian buyers are still the main purchasers of raw pelts from Central Asia. Since independence, Turkmenistan was producing about 750-770 thousand Karakul adult pelts annually until 2000. A small number of pelts were used by private small industries for lining coats and the majority of them were exported. Turkmenistan has a state-owned pelt processing plant, which processed 15% of annual pelt production, while quality of products is poor. The small numbers of pelts produced were exported mainly to Russia in the raw state. The depressed state of the Karakul industry in Turkmenistan was exacerbated by the presidential decree in 2000 due to banning of slaughter of Karakul lambs until such time as the size of the breeding flock was significantly increased. Only pelts from still born lambs and lambs dying within a few days of birth are currently traded. In Kazakstan herders are trying to increase Karakul sheep in the desert regions, as these are well adapted to the environment and their meat has a market premium. Nationally they have considerable knowledge and expertise in the breeding of Karakul sheep. Moreover slaughter of lambs at an early age reduced the burden on ewes nursing the lambs. Martins and Peters (1992a) found that early pelting of the lambs increased ewe weight and shortened the lambing interval.

Breeding strategies for pelt production

Pelt quality can be evaluated at an early age of new-born Karakul lamb and selection of breeding animals is possible before the animals are sexual mature (Greeff *et al..*, 1993a). Pelt traits for the Karakul are described by many authors (Nel, 1991; Schoeman, 1998). Individual Karakul breeders are specialized and focusing on a particular curl type and certain colours. Karakul pelts are black, grey, white or brown with black as the dominant colour. According to genetic studies, five loci (A, B, E, S and W-locus) are involved in the expression of these coat colours (Schoeman, 1998). Besides the colour and curl type, pattern, hair quality and hair length are the most important Karakul pelt traits as described by Nel (1991) and Schoeman (1998) as:

(i) Curl indicates the amount of curl in new-born lamb and varies from almost smooth to completely curly covering. Water-silk, shallow curl, shallow and pipe curl are desirable type.

(ii) Pattern of curl is an important trait and expresses the attractiveness of the curl. It is determined by the arrangement of the hair follicles and skin wrinkles.

(iii) Hair quality is of importance for the durability of the pelt garment and is affected by texture, lustre, and thickness of the fibre. A shiny, silky fibre with some degree of elasticity is preferred in pelt.

(iv) Relatively short hair is desired.

Curl size, lustre, texture, pelt or skin thickness and hair thickness are important traits in Karakul pelts (Albertyn and Schoeman, 1993; Schoeman, 1998). Greeff *et al.*. (1993b) studied correlated responses in selection for pelt traits in Karakul sheep. They concluded that unfavourable genetic relationships between the pelt traits are not significant and breeding should focus on improvement of pattern and eliminate unwanted hair quality.

Birth weight, pelt weight, reproductive performance, and length of the breeding season are some of other traits of importance in Karakul breeding. Schoeman (1998) studied estimates of heritability and genetic correlations for important Karakul pelt traits. The study indicated an unfavourable genetic relationship between hair quality score and pattern score. For hair quality therefore the breeding aims at intermediate values and both silkiness and some degree of elasticity is desired. Schoeman (1998) argued that disassortative mating are important in Karakul pelt breeding. It was also mentioned that constructed flock-specific selection indices were not used to a great extent by the breeders.

Besides for pelt production the lambs also can be raised for meat production. From a study with Karakul in the Kalahari deserts in Botswana (Martins and Peters, 1992c) meat production with purebred Karakul was as good as with local meat breeds or crosses between Karakul and the local breeds. The pelts from purebreds were better than those from the crosses and it was concluded that pelt production with purebred Karakul sheep can be a flexible, ecological, and economic alternative to use pasture in semi-arid regions.

Pelt production with sheep breeds in Australia and New Zealand are major contributors to sheep production worldwide and export most of their sheep products. Pelts are treated as by-products from the main production of meat and wool in both countries and the great majority of sheep and lamb skins are exported either raw or processed (Bray and Gonzalez-Macuer, 2010; Cottle, 2010). The Australian sheep population is characterized by large numbers of Merino and Merino-derived breeds that have mainly been selected for wool production, although meat production has gained increased emphasis in recent years (Cottle, 2010). Gordon (1995) described the majority of Australian skins as not suited for high quality leather production due to the high density of wool follicles which results in reduced strength of tanned leather. Further the skins of Merinos and Merino-crosses are often characterized by ribby patterns which increase the risk of shearing scars. The ribs cannot be flattened after tanning and may severely affect leather quality (Gordon, 1995; Scobie *et al..,* 2005). Pelts from fine wool Merinos are fell mongered mainly for the wool and pelts are of low value (Cottle, 2010).

The breeds used for specialized pelt production are hardy and adapted to certain environments, the Karakul to dry conditions and the Gotland to the marginal grass-land resources in Sweden. The nature of Karakul sheep being non-selective grazers (Nel, 1991) makes them robust under poor conditions. For the Gotland breed the hardiness is an important part of the breeding goal. Both breeds are characterized by a good fertility, although achieved in different ways. Gotland sheep are seasonal breeders and the ewes give birth to two or three lambs in one litter per year, whereas Karakul ewes can breed out of season with three lambing within two years. The Karakul ewes usually get only one lamb per lambing. The practice to remove the lambs from their mothers contributes to the hardiness of the Karakul ewes (Nel, 1991; Martins and Peters, 1992a). Karakul sheep are assumed to be resistant to internal parasites and foot-rot (Ibragimov *et al..,* 2007), although under cold rainy and windy weather they are susceptible to several diseases (Nel, 1991).

For Karakul pelt quality, on average medium high heritability have been found (Schoeman, 1998). For this breed there was a huge variation in the estimates from different studies and suggested that genetic differences due to fixation of pleiotropic genes existed between the flocks. Hair quality is a very important trait and a shiny, silky and coarse hair is desired together with uniform hair quality. Curl size is another trait and curls of intermediate size are preferred. Under the current breeding plan with Gotland sheep, size of curl may increase more than desired (Näsholm, 2005) and the author discussed possible ways to improve hair quality while keeping size of curl as well as thickness and shade of fleece at optimum levels. Restricted selection indexes and disassortative mating were suggested. Thickness or weight of the pelt is of importance in Karakul, Gotland, and Icelandic sheep and a light weight pelts are preferred. Breeding for thickness of fleece in Got-land sheep may increase the weight of the pelts. Low to moderate heritabilites for weight per unit area have been presented for Icelandic sheep (Adalsteinsson *et al..,* 1982; Adalsteinsson, 1983; Eythorsdottir, 1999) indicating a possible inclusion of this trait in the breeding programs. However, measuring of this trait that is only possible after slaughter, is labour- and time consuming, and has so far not been introduced in Gotland breeding. Genetic correlations between pelt quality traits other important production traits are generally low and breeding for pelt quality will not cause unfavourable effects on other traits.

Pelt production and utility

The lamb pelts are produced either through slaughter of lambs of pelt sheep within 24 to 48 hrs of birth or from unborn lambs removed through slaughter or through caesarian operation at about 130 to 140 days of pregnancy. The pelts produced from unborn lamb known as broad (fat) tailed Persian are thin and lustrous and valuable than the best type pelt produced through slaughter after birth. The lamb pelts fetch $25-50 per pelt in the international market depending upon size, ornament and colour. Good quality pelts of sur and grey colour sell at the rate of $40-50 per pelt, its lightness, large size, lustre and colour provide better price in the international market. Silky feel and lustre characteristics of pelt provide better option for many kinds of high priced garments such as overcoats, jackets and suits. The trimmings of pelts are used for making collars for gowns and dresses etc. Karakul pelts are used for making caps worn by Muslims as a symbol of religious sentiments. Pelts caps sell for Rs. 5-10 thousand in the international market. In the world of fur fashion, garments made of the pelts of fetal and newborn lambs are gaining popularity in recent years. In India, lamb pelts are in good demand in Jammu and Kashmir for conversion into various products like caps, collars, ladies and children coats and other garments, not for the tourist and elite societies but also for export.

The majority of Karakul skin are produced in Bokhara (erstwhile USSR), Afghanistan, South West Africa, Bessarabia, Shiraz (Iran), Baghdad and Salzfelle (Iraq). Swakara is a trade name for pelts of South West African Karakul. Swakara pelts are produced in Namibia, Republic of South Africa, and to a small extent in Botswana (Martins and Peters, 1992b). Fur from newborn karakul lambs is frequently referred to as Persian lamb, the first karakul pelts was exported from Central Asia to Europe via Persia, and this is how they named Persian lamb. The most basic distinction of Karakul lamb pelt lies in their textures which are determined by the age of slaughter. The look, feel and texture of the pelt provide price in the market. Fetal lamb fur is lightweight and flat, with a wavy texture and luminous sheen, rather like crushed velvet. Fur from newborn lambs is thicker, with a tight-patterned, curly texture. There are many gradations of pelt characteristics between fetal and newborn lamb, depending on the stage of development. The fur taken from a fetus 15 days before the natural birth is smoother than that of a fetus taken 5 days before birth. Similarly, the curled texture of a newborn lamb is tighter and glossier 3 hrs after birth than it is 3 days later. The texture, pattern, and lustre are the most important qualities for the fur trading. The smoothness and lustre of the fur from fetal karakul sheep provides higher price than that of newborn lambs. The price of the pelt is determined by its quality as reflected by colour, ornament (curl type, size, tightness etc) lustre and weight. The size of the curl is completed during pregnancy. The pelts are classified into various types such as jacket, ribbed and cacucasion on the basis of curl pattern. The present demand in the market is for light colour pelts.

The pelts with medium fibre diameter (Merino and cross-breeds) are often processed as wool skins for use as rugs, car seat covers, shoe lining, etc., where the main quality criterion is a dense and bulky wool cover (Gordon, 1995). Medical sheepskins are specialty woolskins that are treated to withstand repeated washing at high temperatures and intended for hospital use (Jolley *et al..*, 2004). The New Zealand sheep flock is comprised of many breeds that are mostly raised for meat production and the majority of pelts end up in various leather products, depending on quality and price fluctuations (Scobie, 2010). Passman and Sumner (1987) studied the suitability of pelts from different sheep breeds for processing into woolskins vs. leather. They suggested that pelts with high loose wool bulk were best suited for shearling (double-face) skin production. These pelts were not as well suited to leather tanning as other pelts in the study. Genetic parameters on pelt traits relevant to woolskin or shearling skin production were not found in the literature on sheep breeds in New Zealand and Australia.

Indian experience

Experimental work on lamb pelt production was taken up at the Carpet wool and Karakul Pelt Production Division of CSWRI at ARC, Bikaner (Rajasthan) with the importation of Karakul sheep from Uzbekistan (erstwhile USSR). A Karakul pelt production experts were invited to stay at Bikaner for one year to help in evaluation and processing of pelts. Indian coarse carpet wool breeds like Malpura and Sonadi were evaluated for lamb pelts but the curls were found to be more open and mostly white in colour. The crosses of Karakul with Indian coarse carpet wool breeds were initiated at Bikaner in hot arid climate. One flock of Karakul sheep was also maintained in cold arid climate of Jammu and Kashmir at Sheep Breeding Farm, Kargil.

At Bikaner, crossbreeding of Marwari, Sonadi and Malpura ewes with Karakul ram was undertaken and half bred as well as $3/4^{th}$ crossbreds were produced. Crossbreeds ($3/4^{th}$) produced satisfactory quality pelts with different colours comparable with those of purebred Karakul. The population was stabilized through *inter-se* mating and selected to develop different colour lines and an Indian Karakul strain was evolved. In Indian Karakul, the percentage of Jacket type pelt was 47.71 (10.72% less than Karakul) and black colour was 95.06 (3.71% less than Karakul) however, the Indian Karakul lambs had more colours such as steel grey, sur and brown than Karakul lambs (Singh, 1990). It was observed that the Indian Karakul lambs had significantly lower values for pelt length by 4.95% and were near to Karakul in pelt width and weight. The pelt quality index was also quite close to Karakul. It is unfortunate that the project was closed down because of pressure from the Society for Beauty without Cruelty to Animals, in spite being explained to the Select Committee of the Parliament of India at the time of their visit to Bikaner regarding no breach of Indians laws of prevention of cruelty to animals as lambs were removed from their mothers immediately after birth and slaughtered in a separate chamber and the pelts removed. The meat was used for human consumption and was similar in taste as chicken meat with little fat. All the Karakul sheep were removed from Bikaner and transferred to the Society for Beauty without Cruelty on the orders of the Union Minister of Agriculture and were allowed to die. Even the crossbreds that were retained were not used for pelt production and eventually were decimated and the project was closed. Sheep rearing for pelt production was thus closed without making any impact on pelt production in the country. It is brought to notice that large numbers of lamb pelts are being imported for making caps and other products especially in Jammu and Kashmir and there is growing demand of pelt for fashionable products in the country. The project on pelt production may be again initiated at Jammu and Kashmir for meat and pelt production with strengthening of small industries for pelt processing and marketing in the country.

Future trends in pelt production

The interest for sheep breeding for high quality pelt production will increase in future with growing demand by the consumers in different parts of the world. The labour cost and the pelt prices may fluctuate between years and periods, which will makes profitable pelt production unstable. The infrastructure for processing and marketing may be strengthened for avoiding price fluctuation. The increased demand for meat in many parts of the world will strengthens the focus for sheep breeding for twin objective of meat and pelt production. This can be seen in the prolific breed, for which the current breeding goal does not include pelt traits. Better pelt price and demand may create interest among farmers for raising sheep for pelt breeding. In India, meat production is as important as pelt production and when the lambs are slaughtered at an age of 4-6 months both the pelts and the carcasses will provide more remunerative income to farmer.

Conclusion

Pelts from sheep in future are expected to retain its status as a by-product from meat and wool production in the country. Karakul is choice of breed for pelt production in desert areas with scanty feed resources. Hair quality, size of curl, and weight of pelt are traits of importance in Karakul breeding. Breeding goal should include increased growth rate, pelt quality and feed efficiency. The hardiness of the breed and its adaptation to marginal grassland resources are also important to retain Karakul sheep in hot arid climate. Indian coarse wool producing sheep like Malpura, Sonadi and Marwari may be crossed to develop Indian Karakul with desirable pelt production. Efforts are required to develop different colour lines by interbreeding the half breds and ¾^{ths}. Moreover *Fec B* gene from Garole / Kendrapada breeds may be introgressed in the Karakul sheep to produce twin and triplets where one lambs can be used for pelt production and other lambs can be raised for meat production.

References

Adalsteinsson, S., 1983. Inheritance of colours, pelt characteristics and skin quality traits in North European sheep breeds: a review. Livestock Production Science 10: 555-567.

Adalsteinsson, S., Sigurðsson, I.G., Steingrímsson Tr, J. and Hjaltadóttir, K.R. 1982. Erfðir feldgæða og skinngæða. Journal of Agricultural Research Iceland 14: 69-83.

Albertyn, J.R. and Schoeman, S.J. 1993. Factors influencing the quality of Karakul pelts, with emphasis on discrete characteristics. South African Journal of Animal Science 23: 183-186.

Bray, A.R. and Gonzalez-Macuer, E. 2010. New Zealand sheep and wool industries. In: International Sheep and Wool Handbook (D.J. Cottle, Ed.), Nottingham University Press, pp. 73-83.

Cottle, D.J. 2010. Australian sheep and wool industries. In: International Sheep and Wool Handbook (D.J. Cottle, Ed.), Nottingham University Press, pp. 49-71.

Eythorsdottir, E. 1999. Genetic variation in woolskin quality of Icelandic lambs. Livestock Production Science 57: 113-126.

FAOSTAT, 2011. http://faostat.fao.org/site/569/default.aspx#ancor

Flamant, J.C., Boutonnet, J.P., Dyrmundssom, O., Jankowski, S., Morand-Fehr, P., Robinson, J.J., Treacher, T. and Valls Ortiz, M.V. 1982. Sheep and goats. Livestock Production Science 9: 163-196.

Gordon, P.G. 1995. Australian woolskins-their value and processing. Wool Technology, Sheep Breed 43: 141-165.

Greeff, J.C., Faure, A.S., Minnaar, G.J. and Schoeman, S.J. 1993a. Genetic trends for pelt traits in Karakul sheep I. Direct responses. South African Journal of Animal Science 23: 164-169.

Greeff, J.C., Faure, A.S., Minnaar, G.J. and Schoeman, S.J. 1993b. Genetic trends for pelt traits in Karakul sheep II. Correlated responses. South African Journal of Animal Science 23: 170-175.

Ibragimov, Y., Svitojus, A., Yusupov, S. and Baltrenaite, L. 2007. Management, use and conservation of Karakul sheep in traditional livestock farming systems in Uzbekistan. In: People and Animals. Traditional Livestock Keepers: Guardians of Domestic Animal Diversity. Food and Agricultural Organization of the United Nations, Rome.

Jolley, D.J., Wright, R., McGowan, S., Hickey, M.B., Campbell, D.A., Sinclair, R.D. and Montgomery, K.C. 2004. Preventing pressure ulcers with the Australian Medical Sheepskin: an open-label randomized controlled trial. Medical Journal of Australia 180: 324-327.

Martins, C. and Peters, K.J. 1992a. Alternative use of Karakul sheep for pelt and lamb production in Botswana. I. Reproduction and growth performance. Small Ruminant Research 9: 1-10.

Martins, C. and Peters, K.J. 1992b. Alternative use of Karakul sheep for pelt and lamb production in Botswana. II. Pelt produciton. Small Ruminant Research 9: 11-19.

Martins, C. and Peters, K.J. 1992c. Alternative use of Karakul sheep for pelt and lamb production in Botswana. III. Economic evaluation. Small Ruminant Research 9: 21-26.

Nanekarani, S., Amirinia, C., Amirmozafari, N., Torshizi, R.V. and Gharahdaghi, A.A. 2010. Genetic variation among pelt sheep population using microsatellite markers. African Journal of Biotechnology 9: 7437-7445.

Näsholm, A. 2005. Genetic study on pelt quality in the Gotland sheep breed. Acta Agriculturæ Scandinavica, Section A 55: 57-65.

Näsholm, A. 2008. Genetic relationships between pelt quality, maternal ability and lamb production in the Gotland sheep breed. Livestock Science 117: 93-100.

Nel, J.A. 1991. Pelt breeds of sheep. In: Genetic Resources of Pig, Sheep, and Goat. World Animal Science (A. Karakul, and K. Maijala, Eds.), B8, Elsevier Science Publishers B.V., Amsterdam, The Netherlands, pp. 291-299.

Passman, A. and Sumner, R.M.W. 1987. Effects of breed and level of feeding on leather produced from export lambs reared on hilly country. New Zealand Journal of Experimental Agriculture 15: 309-316.

Schoeman, S.J. 1998. Genetic and environmental factors influencing the quality of pelt traits in Karakul sheep. South African Journal of Animal Science 28: 125-137.

Scobie, D. 2010. Skins. In: International Sheep and Wool Handbook, (D.J. Cottle Ed.), Nottingham University Press, pp. 661-675.

Scobie, D.R., Young, S.R., O'Connell, D. and Eythorsdottir, E., 2005. Skin wrinkles of the sire adversely affect Merino and half bred pelt characteristics and other production traits. Australian Journal of Experimental Agriculture 45: 1551-1557.

Singh, V.K. 1990. Genetic evaluation of performance of Karakul and its crosses with indigenous coarse wool breeds in north western arid region. Ph.D. Thesis, Rajasthan Agricultural University, Bikaner (Rajasthan).

□□□

Chapter 25

Recent Advances in Wool and Woollen Processing

V.S. Goud and J.S. Udakhe*
Wool Research Association, P O. Sandoz Baug, Kolshet Road
Thane (W)- 400 607 (Maharashtra)

Wool is a keratin fibre that has a very complex physical structure which makes it a difficult fibre for processing. Wool being natural in origin has some inherent limitations like outer hydrophobic cuticle structure, harsh feel in case of coarser wools and lower spinnability in fibres like Angora and few other animal fibres. These limitations act as impediments to enhance features such as anti-wrinkle, anti-shrinkage finishing and dyeing. Wool's water repellency on the surface also hinders its ability to absorb moisture and in humid condition makes wool garments feel sweaty. Current treatments to make wool hydrophilic, shrink proof, antibacterial, moth proof etc. may not last long, may damage fabric and are not eco-friendly. Conventional wool processes such as scouring, dyeing, finishing, etc. can be improved with the help of novel technologies such as plasma, ultrasonic, nano-technology, bio-processing, supercritical fluids, combined processes etc. This paper describes the developments that occur in other branches of engineering and technology are being utilized to improve the conventional chemical based wool processing to meet such requirements.

Ultrasound assisted processing

Ultrasound is the sound with frequencies above 18 KHz which is above the limits of human audibility. Ultrasonic energy offers many potential advantages such as energy savings, and reduced processing times, environmental improvements, process enhancement and lower overall processing costs (Awad, 1993). Ultrasound appears to be a very promising alternative technique to provide a far more efficient stirring or mixing mechanism for the immediate border layer of liquid at fibre surface (Sivakumar *et al.*, 2009). Generally, sonication of liquids causes two primary effects: cavitation and heating. As the ultrasound passes through a liquid, it produces compression and rarefaction regions in it. During the rarefaction phase, the liquid is literally torn apart, creating millions of microscopic cavity bubbles in it. When these bubbles collapse at the surface of the solid substrate (e.g. textile fibre), they generate powerful shock waves which remove the contaminants adhered to the substrate (Beckham *et al.*, 1996; Moholkar, *et al.*, 2003). Cavitations are generated in the order of microseconds. It is estimated that the pressure is about 35-70 K Pascal and the transient localized temperatures are about 5000°C with the velocity of micro streaming around 400 Km/hr. These conditions tremendously improve the cleaning process (Awad, 1997). In textiles, ultrasound has successfully demonstrated its usefulness in processes such as bleaching, dyeing, washing, etc for saving in time and temperature. Heat induced by the ultrasonic process is adequate for dyeing process and thus eliminates the need for external heating in many cases. It has been reported that ultrasound can promote the dyeing process of textile materials made of wool, polyamide or cotton with acceleration of process, deeper colouration and higher levelness. Advantages of ultrasonics include energy saving by reduced processing temperature, time and lower consumptions of auxiliary chemicals and further processing enhancement by overall cost control. Ultrasound is also said to boost the enzymatic activity. Ultrasonic has also been used for washing the fabrics and garments. Attempts have been made to analyze the effect of ultrasonic in dyeing processes on almost all types of fibre using direct, reactive, acid and disperse dyes (Thakore, *et al.*, 1990; Moses and Jagannathan, 1996). Ultrasonic waves accelerate the rate of diffusion of the dye inside the fibre with enhanced wetting of fibre. Acoustic irradiation of the liquor results in a higher and more uniform concentration of dyestuff on the fibre surface, making it available for ready diffusion into the fibre interior. The influence of ultrasonic on the dyeing system has three fold effects namely, dispersion effect, i.e., breaking up of micelles and high molecular weight aggregates into uniform dispersion in the dye bath, degassing by the removal of dissolved or entrapped gas molecules or air from fibre capillaries and interstices at the cross over points of the fabric into liquid thereby facilitating a dye-fibre contact and accelerating the rate of diffusion of the dye inside the fibre by breaking the boundary layers covering the fibre and accelerating the interaction between dye and fibre (Saligram *et al.*, 1993; Moses and Jagannathan, 1996; Yachmenev *et al.*, 2001; Canoglu, *et al.*, 2004; Ramachandran *et al.*, 2008).

Ultrasound assisted scouring

Wool is a natural fibre which in raw form comprises nearly 30% of its weight by contaminants. These contaminants consist of 5-25% grease, 2-15% suint and 5-20% dirt and vegetable matter. These impurities need to be removed before any further processing. This is done by scouring the wool. The conventional methods of wool scouring utilize high amount of chemicals, detergent, alkali etc which create some serious problems; both, for the environment and the industry while effluent treatment and disposal. A study carried out by Wool Research Association on application of ultrasonic technology for scouring of raw wool found that ultrasonic scouring can be done at lower temperature and chemical concentration. The scouring efficiency in terms of grease and suint removal was doubled in presence of ultrasonic irradiation. This was attributed to the cavitation effect of ultrasonic energy. As the microscopic cavity bubbles implode, they liberate shock waves which help in removal of contaminants from the surface of wool fibres (Goud *et al.*, 2011). The method of scouring greasy wool by ultrasonic technique recently developed by Wool Research Association is under consideration for patenting (Application No.1795/MUM/2011).

Plasma technology

Plasma is the forth state of matter apart from solid, liquid and gaseous state. The coupling of electromagnetic power into a process gas volume generates the plasma medium comprising a dynamic mix of ions, electrons, neutrons, photons, free radicals, meta-stable excited species and molecular and polymeric fragments, the system overall being at room temperature. This allows the surface functionalisation of fibres and textiles without affecting their bulk properties. These species move under electromagnetic fields, diffusion gradients, etc. on the textile substrates placed in or passed through the plasma. This enables a variety of generic surface processes including surface activation by bond breaking to create reactive sites, grafting of chemical moieties and functional groups, material volatilisation and removal (etching), dissociation of surface contaminants/layers (cleaning/scouring) and deposition of conformal coatings. In all these processes a highly surface specific region of the material (<1000 Å) is given new, desirable properties without negatively affecting the bulk properties of the constituent fibres. It is a dry process and is an effective and versatile technique for modifying homogeneously the uppermost atomic layers of a material surface leaving the bulk characteristics unaffected, due to its very low penetration (Simpson, 2002).

Plasma technology in dyeing and printing: The partial removal of surface lipids, the increase in carbonyl and single bonded CO groups, the conversion of cystine to cysteic acid in the fibre surface and the increase in surface roughness results in an increase in the wettability of wool. The improved dye-uptake of plasma-treated wool described by different authors (Binias *et al.*, 2004; Chi-wai, 2007) can be therefore related to the plasma-induced degradation of the natural diffusion barrier of the fibre. This obviously facilitates an accelerated, more even and more complete dye-uptake, resulting in significant enhanced final bath exhaustion and thus in significantly reduced effluent discharges during dyeing.

Plasma technology in shrink proofing: Felting is a special property of wool that occurs when wool is subjected to mechanical agitation in water. Though this behaviour is required for creating felts or fabrics with special optical appearance, the well-known irreversible shrinkage during washing is one of the principal drawbacks of textiles made of wool. Felting and shrinkage are the result of movements of individual fibres within the textile, always taking place towards the fibre root. The phenomenon of unidirectional fibre movement primarily is related to the unique scale structure (from the root to the tip) of the wool fibre surface, which is responsible for a different coefficient of friction in the with-scale and against-scale direction. As a consequence of the reduction in the difference in the coefficient of friction, plasma-treated wool shows a significantly diminished felting behaviour. Complete shrink proofing of woollen garments cannot be achieved using plasma treatment alone and hence this requires an additional coverage of the fibre surface to further decrease the difference in coefficient of friction by masking the scale edges. Since commercially available resins do not show the expected positive influence on the felt free performance of plasma-treated wool, new resins have been tailored for the plasma-treated fibre surface. Two different wool-compatible resin types have been developed by BAYER, allowing the generation of machine-washable wool after GD or BD treatment. One type consists of a water-dispersible isocyanate-bearing resin which is able to permanently coat each individual fibre. The differences in the degree of felting after different plasma-only treatments can be equalized by the resin application, to an extent which meets the value for Chlorine/ Hercosett treated samples. The second resin is a polyurethane type which does not coat the fibre completely, but is deposited at the scale edges instead. This also results in significantly decreased shrinkage behaviour. DBD treatment of tops followed by application of one or both resins guarantees the specifications set by the Woolmark Company in their Technical Method 31 (Thomas, 2007).

Plasma and enzyme technology for itch-proofing of woollen garments: Wool Research Association has recently completed a project 'To develop itch free woollens to be worn next to the skin by improvement of surface topography of wool fibres with the help of plasma technology' sponsored by the Ministry of Textiles, Government of India. The objective of the project was to make woollen garments wearable as next to skin inner garments. Itching due to woollen garments worn next to skin can be attributed to prickling due to protruding coarse fibres and friction with skin due to sharp scales on wool fibre. To study the effect of yarn hairiness on the itching propensity of woollen knitwear, 2/24 Nm double yarn (23 µm wool) having hairiness index of 6.73, 6.98, 7.62, 7.95 and 8.37 were used for making knitwear and these knitwear were tested by wearer trials for assessing their itching propensity. It was found that, irrespective of yarn hairiness itching propensity of these knitwear were very high and these knitwear were found to be unbearable as next to skin innerwear. Itching propensity was found to increase with increase in the yarn hairiness index. Knitwear made from 2/24 Nm double yarn having yarn hairiness index 8.37 were further treated with 1, 2, 3, 4 and 5% (owf) sebalkaline protease enzyme. In another set of experiment, the knitwear were pre-treated with air plasma and then further treatment was carried out with 1, 2, 3, 4 and 5% (owf) sebalkaline protease enzyme. OFDA-100, SEM and tensile tests were carried out on the fibre samples from the knitwear to study change in average fibre diameter, surface morphology and mechanical properties along with critical buckling load respectively. These enzyme and plasma + enzyme treated knitwear were tested for itching propensity using wearer trials. It was found that enzyme treatment reduces the average fibre diameter, damages the scales, and reduces the mechanical properties along with critical buckling load. Plasma and enzyme treatment are found to work synergistically. It was found that 4 and 5% enzyme treated and 3, 4 and 5% plasma + enzyme treated knitwear becomes completely itch-free and could be worn next to skin, without wearing the intermediate cotton garment. This has been correlated with critical buckling load for these fibres which was found to be below 70 mg. The method developed by WRA to reduce the itching propensity of woollen garments with the help of plasma and enzyme treatment is under consideration for Indian patent (Application No. 1794/MUM/2011).

Bio-processing of wool

Enzymes are natural biocatalysts that have great potential in catalysis of chemical compounds decomposition and synthesis. Enzymes speed up the rates of reactions without themselves undergoing any permanent change. The utilization of enzymes in the textile industry has been known and applied commercially for many years, principally in cellulosic fibres, like the use of amylases for desizing of cotton and cellulases for indigo abrasion on denim (Cavaco-Paulo and Almeida, 1994; Cavaco-Paulo *et al.*, 1996; Eriksson and Cavaco-Paulo, 1998). However, for protein fibres, there are other possibilities for enzyme application, including the use of proteases for wool and silk processing and for the surface modification of cashmere fibres (Cavaco-Paulo *et al.*, 1998, 1999). Mixtures of cellulase, pectinase and xylanase enzymes have been successfully used for bio-carbonizing of wool without affecting the inherent properties of wool fibres (El-Sayed, 2010). Proteolytic enzymes can be use to replace the oxidative processes like pre treatment using chlorination and will be an eco friendly alternative. Rybicki *et al.* (2000) suggested enzymatic pretreatment and chitosan deposition on wool fabric as a new ecological method for shrink-proofing of wool fabrics. Based on the results, it was concluded that enzymatic pre treatment itself greatly improved the shrink proofing property by partial destruction of the fibre scales, and the post application of chitosan enhanced the shrinkproofing and ensured an increased dyeability of wool fabrics by reactive dyes (Rybicki *et al.*, 2000; Onar and Sariisik, 2004; Xie *et al.*, 2009).

As enzyme treatment causes weight and strength loss of wool fibres, other possible solution for this problem is that either the enzyme has to be controlled (for example, diffusion control by enzyme immobilization) or the enzyme has to be specially "designed" (for example, by genetic engineering) in such a way that only a distinct part of the substrate is altered like scales on wool fibre surface (Xie *et al.,* 2009). Silva *et al.* (2005) and Paulo and Silva (2006) studied the diffusion of native subtilisin and bigger molecular weight polyethylene glycol (PEG)-subtilisin into the wool fibres. It was found that, the alkaline peroxide pre-treatment improves the enzyme diffusion on wool. Subtilisin-PEG, the big protease, hydrolyzed just the cuticle layer of wool thus resulting in the higher tensile strength and lower felting of the fibre; on the other hand native subtilisin penetrates deep into the fibre core and causes more strength loss. Another way of recovering the strength loss of wool is to cross link glutamine and lysine protein residues in the wool fibre using transglutaminases (TG) enzymes to form covalent bonds. Transglutaminases (TG) belong to a class of enzymes known as aminoacyltransferases that catalyze calcium-dependent acyl transfer reactions between peptide-bound glutamine residues as acyl donors and peptide-bound lysine residues as acyl acceptors, resulting in the formation of intermolecular e-(g-glutamyl) lysine crosslinks (Griffin *et al.,* 2002; van der Vlist and Loos, 2010). Wool fibres contains, 450(μmol/g) of glutamine - $(CH_2)_2$-$CONH_2$ and 250(μmol/g) of lysine - $(CH_2)_4$-NH_2, so there is a fare chance of cross linking between glutamine and lysine initiated by TG (Hocker, 2002) This covalent isopeptide crosslink is stable and resistant to proteolysis, thereby increasing the resistance to chemical, enzymatic and mechanical disruption (Greenberg *et al.,* 1991).

Application of biopolymers

Polymer deposition on wool fibers to coat the scales is one method to prevent laundering-shrinkage of wool fabrics by felting. Lim and Hudson (2003) in their polymer review described different methods of applying chitosan biopolymer on the wool fabrics to achieve the shrink proofing properties. In a two-step application, chitosan solutions in dilute acids were padded on wool fabrics and dried. The chitosan-deposited fabrics were further treated with cross-linkers, such as glyoxal or glutaraldehyde, which react with chitosan as well as with functional groups on the wool, e.g., lysine, arginine, histidine, or serine residues. In a single-step application, mixtures of chitosan solution and cross-linkers, such as glyoxal, glutaraldehyde, or DMDHEU, were padded on the fabrics, dried, and then cured. Both application methods improved resistance to laundering-shrinkage of the fabrics. In another study wool fabrics were pretreated with hydrogen peroxide (H_2O_2) either under alkaline or acidic conditions. The purpose of the pretreatment was to increase the number of cysteic acid groups (-SO_3H) by the oxidation of the disulfide bonds on wool fibers and, consequently, increase the anionic charges on the fiber surface, which could enhance the sorption of chitosan with cationic charge. It was found that both acidic and alkaline H_2O_2 treatments generated similar amounts of cysteic acid groups on the fibers. The pretreated fabrics were padded with chitosan (MW 70,000) solution in dilute acetic acid and dried at room temperature. The laundering shrinkage measurements revealed that the best shrink resistance was obtained from the wool fabric pretreated with H_2O_2 under alkaline condition. It was concluded that the shrink resistance and chitosan sorption were related to the hydrophilicity rather than the cysteic acid content of the wool. Alkaline H_2O_2 pretreatment generates more hydrophilic fibre surface than acidic H_2O_2 pretreatment and hence shows better shrink resistance properties. Effect of chitosan MW on the shrink resistance of H_2O_2 pretreated (at pH 9.0) wool fabrics was studied. It was found that, the higher molecular weight chitosan gives better shrink resistance. To promote the sorption of chitosan on wool fabric, fabric was first pretreated with an anionic surfactant sodium lauryl sulfate (SLS) at different pH conditions. In an acidic condition (pH 2.2), the highest adsorption of SLS on wool was observed. This was explained by the formation of a double layer of SLS on the wool surface. The protonated amino groups of wool at acidic pH are ionically linked by SLS, and the second layer is formed by hydrophobic interaction between the hydrocarbon chains of SLS. Finally, the fiber surface acquires a substantial amount of negative charge. All SLS pretreated fabrics were treated with chitosan (MW 70,000) solution. The lowest laundering-shrinkage was obtained from the fabric pretreated with SLS at pH 2.2. In another study (Hsieh *et al.*, 2004), citric acid was used as a cross linking agent for biopolymer chitosan on potassium permanganate pretreated wool fabric. It was found that the surface cross links of the oxidized woolen fibre were relatively coarse, which was undesirable for shrink-proofing and yet beneficial for the antimicrobial and antiseptic effects of the woolen fabrics. A new process for felt proofing of wool fibers based on the biopolymer sericin was reported by Allam *et al.* (2009). The susceptibility of wool to sericin has been enhanced by creation of new active sites along the wool keratin molecules, such as cysteic acid and S-cystine sulphonate residues, by pretreatment with hydrogen peroxide and sodium sulphite. The sericin-combining capacity of wool has been even enhanced by carrying out the reaction in the presence of different cross linkers namely dimethylol dihydroxy ethylene urea, dimethyl dihyroxy ethylene urea, and epichlorohydrin, which are able to link sericin with the available sites of wool. The felting resistance of wool tops treated with the system H_2O_2 /Na_2SO_3/sericin/ECH (felt ball density 0.045 g /cm^3) was close to that of the machine washable wool obtained commercially (felt ball density 0.039 g /cm^3).

Supercritical processing

Dyeing in medium other than water has always been looked as a good alternative to conventional dyeing due to saving of energy and lesser pollution. A new dyeing procedure was developed where carbon dioxide in supercritical conditions was used instead of water (Lewis, 1999; Bach *et al.*, 2002; Fernandez Cid *et al.*, 2004; Hou and Dai, 2005). Though several gases can be used as supercritical fluids but carbon dioxide has been the most preferred one due to easily accessible critical conditions (31 °C, 7.4 MPa), the viscosity (10.5-10.4 Pa s) and diffusion coefficient (10.8-10.7 m^2 s) values are similar to those of water, making it suitable for use as a dyeing medium, ease of availability from industrial combustion and fermentation processes, ammonia synthesis and mineral springs, inexpensive and other properties such as non-toxicity, non-flammability and recyclability. Further carbon dioxide above critical point has excellent penetration properties as it retains free mobility of the gaseous state and density is more towards that of liquid with increasing pressure and thus is important in dyeing. Further in this process, drying of substrate is not required making the process economically more feasible. Thus supercritical dyeing process can be looked as a cleaner technology which is economically attractive to dyers (Aiqin Hou *et al.*, 2010). A schematic representation of the textile dyeing equipment in SC-CO_2 can be seen in Figure1.

Supercritical dyeing of wool: The biggest limitation of SC-CO_2 is its poor solvent properties for a wide range of hydrophiles because of its low permittivity (Schmidt *et al.*, 2003). Water soluble dyes are insufficiently soluble in SC-CO_2. Dyeing of textile fibers in SC-CO_2, therefore, has been limited to synthetic fibers using SC-CO_2 soluble disperse dyes. Thus dyeing of wool fibres with these dyes directly in SC-CO_2 medium is not feasible. However, Different methods are being worked out to overcome this problem. The most current and promising technique has been the addition of an entrainer like water or ethanol to SC-CO_2 which can increase the polarity and solvent power to dissolve polar solvents and thus make the dyeing of natural fibres feasible (Sawadaa and Uedab, 2004). Earlier, Giehl *et al.* (1999) dyed wool in the presence of water and methanol using non-polar natural, disperse and vat dyes and obtained a higher colour depth than in the absence of co-solvent. Guzel and Akgerman (2000) impregnated wool with metal cations [Cr (III) or Fe (II)] from water and used CO_2 soluble mordant dyes which formed complexes with the metal ions, producing dyeing of excellent wash fastness. Another possibility is to use reactive disperse dyes e.g. C.I. Disperse Yellow 23 modified with 2-bromoacrylic acid and 1, 3, 5-trichloro-2, 4, 6-triazine as reactive groups. Experiments shown that, a high colour depth was obtained along with good wash, rub and light fastness properties. The highest colour yield obtained when dyed at 160 °C for 240 mins but fibre damage was observed. Dyeing at 120 °C for 240 mins also yield good colour depth and lesser fibre damage (Schmidt *et al.*, 2003).

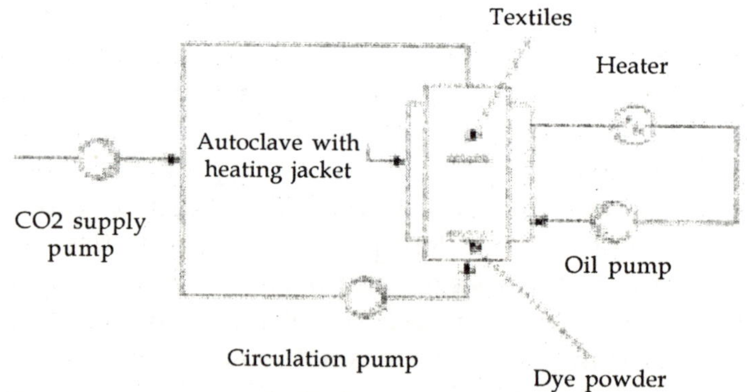

Fig. 1 : SC-CO_2 dyeing equipment (Fernandez Cid *et al.*, 2007)

Foam finishing

The wet processing of textile materials includes highly energy consuming operations, amounts approximately to 80% of total energy requirement of all the operations. Out of this, about 66% of the energy is consumed in heating and evaporation of water from the fibres. Invariably, the liquor retained in the fabric is distributed (Srivastava, 1993; Morton and Hearle, 2000; Pleva, 2002) within and between the fibres in the form of capillary liquid in the available spaces between the yarns and also on the surface of the textile material, ie, surface bound water. Squeezing the fabric between the nips eliminate the excess liquor available on the surface of the fabric and the interstices of the yarns, which depends on the nip pressure, hardness of rubber, roller diameter and machine speed or fabric speed. The concept of low add-on is based on the controlled transfer of a reduced quantity of liquor from a dipping roller to the fabrics. Moreover foam application is different from the low add-on technique since air is used to dilute the liquor, which is not the case in the earlier ones. In the foam process the liquor is diluted using the air instead of water that is normally used to apply the chemicals over the textile materials. In foam finishing, most of the water is replaced by air that leads to a reduction of energy requirements in the drying processes resulting in substantial savings in energy cost. Foam is a colloidal system comprising of mass of gas bubbles dispersed in the liquid continuum (Pleva, 2002). Foam can be generated by mechanical air blowing, through excess agitation or chemically by introduction of foaming agents or combination of these methods. The relative proportions of air and liquid phases in the foam are designated by blow ratio. Foam stability, density and diameters are the important parameters that need constant attention (Harrison, 1986). A varying bubble size represents an unbalanced bath density. Foam density in general, varies between 0.14 - 0.07 g/cc for the foam finishing and 0.33 - 0.20 g/cc in the foam printing. The selection of the density of the foam depends on the fabric weight and needs to be increased with increasing fabric weight. Foam viscosity depends on the foam density and viscosity of the un-foamed liquor. Increase in foam viscosity results increased foam stability. Bubbles with smaller size are more stable than bigger bubble size and the bubble diameter ranges, generally, from 0.001 - 2.0 mm depending on the generation systems. Bubbles or foams, inherently, do not thrive in higher energy environment since higher energy levels results in the destability of the foam Destabilization of the foam is also caused by creation of the faults in the foam structure at the air/liquid/air interface. The destruction of foam after application on to the fabrics can be achieved by conventional padding or vacuum application or combination of both. Foam application technique can be used (Sohl, 1999) in the fabric preparation, dyeing and printing, DP finish, softening, soil-release finish, water, oil repellant finish, FR finish, anti-static finish, mercerisation, etc. The foam can be applied either on one or both sides of the fabrics. Horizontal padder, kiss roller coating, knife over the roller coating, knife on air system and slot applicator system are commonly employed in foam applications. Conservation of water and energy has been the centre of research during the past and today also (Srivastava, 1993), foam finishing process can be used to achieve 80% of water consumption the energy consumption by 60-65% in the form of gas, electricity depending upon the type of finishing treatment used, obnoxious gases and their related pollution can be minimized (Levy, 2004).

Conclusion

The developments that occur in other branches of engineering and technology are being utilized to improve the conventional methods of wool processing. Processing of wool with the help of eco-friendly technologies such as plasma, ultrasonic, bio-processing, supercritical fluids, etc, can be used to save huge amount of energy, reduce effluent load as well as endow the wool based textiles with value added properties to survive in a highly competitive market. However, more research and developmental work is still required in order to utilize the benefits of such technologies on an industrial scale.

References

Aiqin Hou, Bo Chen, Jinjin Dai and Kai Zhang. 2010. Using supercritical carbon dioxide as solvent to replace water in polyethylene terephthalate (PET) fabric dyeing procedures. Journal of Cleaner Production 18: 1009-1014.

Allam, O.G., El-Sayed, H., Kantouch, A. and Haggag, K. 2009. Use of sericin in felt proofing of wool. Journal of Natural Fibers 6: 14-26

Awad, S.B. 1993. An ultrasonic semi-aqueous alternative to vapor degreasing. Precision Cleaning I: 75.

Awad, S.B. 1997. Method for Cleaning and Drying of Metalic and Nonmetallic Surfaces. U.S. Patent, 5397397, 1997.

Bach, E., Cleve, E. and Schollmeyer, E. 2002. Review Progress Coloration 32: 88-102.

Beckham, H. W., Carr, W.W., Michielsen S., Good, J., Merriman, T. and Zhan, J. 1996. Fundamental investigation of ultrasonic effects in textile wet processing. National Textile Center Annual Report: G95-13: 143-151.

Binias, D., W³ochowicz, A. and Binias, W. 2004. Fibres and Textiles in Eastern Europe, 12: 46.

Canoglu, S., Gultekin, B.C. and Yukseloglu, S.M. 2004. Effect of ultrasonic energy in washing of medical surgery gowns. Ultrasonic 42: 113-119.

Cavaco-Paulo, A, and Almeida, L. 1994. Applications of enzymatic technologies in cotton finishing. Nova têxtil 32: 34-37.

Cavaco-Paulo, A., Almeida, L. and Bishop, D. 1996. Indigo backstaining during cellulase washing. Textile Chemist and Colorist 28: 28-32.

Cavaco-Paulo, A., Morgado, J., Almeida, L. and Kilburn, D. 1998. Backstaining during cellulase washing. Textile Research Journal 68: 398-401.

Cavaco-Paulo, A., Morgado, J., Andreaus, J, and Kilburn, D. 1999. Interaction of cotton with CBD peptides. Enzyme and Microbial technology 25: 639-643.

Chi-wai, KAN. 2007. Effect of low temperature plasma on different wool dyeing systems AUTEX Research Journal 8: 255-263.

El-Sayed, H., El-Gabry, L. and Kantouch, F. 2010. Effect of bio-carbonization of coarse wool on its dyeability. Indian Journal of Fibre and Textile Research 35: 330-336

Eriksson, K. and Cavaco-Paulo, A. 1998. Enzyme application in fibre processing. ACS Symposium Series Book, Washington DC, 687:180-189.

Fernandez Cid, M.V., Gerstner, K.N., Spronsen, J., van Kraan, M. van der, Veugelers, W.J.T., Woerlee, G.F. and Witkamp, G.J. 2007. Novel process to enhance the dyeability of cotton in supercritical carbon dioxide. Textile Research Journal 77: 38-46.

Fernandez Cid, M.V., Veugelers, W.J.T., Woerlee, G.F. and Witkamp, G.J. 2004. Kinetics study of a dichlorotriazine reactive dye in supercritical carbon dioxide. Journal of Supercritical Fluids 32: 147-152.

Giehl, A., Giebmann, M., Schafer, K. and Hocker, H. 1999. In: Proc. 4th International Symposium Extraction for Sample Preparation, University GH of Siegen, Siegen, pp 29-30.

Goud V.S., Honade, S.P., Bardhan, M.K. and Rao, T.R. 2011. Ultrsound assisted scouring of raw wool. In: National Seminar Cum Workshop on Recent R & D Initiatives and Development Schemes of Wool and Woollens, May 2011, p.25

Greenberg, C.S., Birckbichler, P.J. and Rice, R.H. 1991. Transglutaminases: multifunctional cross-linking enzymes that stabilize tissues. *The FASEB Journal*, 5: 3071-3077.

Griffin, M., Casadio, R. and Bergamini, C.M. 2002. Nature's biological glues. Biochem Journal 368: 377-396.

Guzel, B. and Akgerman, A. 2000. Mordant dyeing of wool by supercritical processing, Journal of Supercritical Fluids 18: 247-252.

Harrison, P.W. 1986. Textile Progress 14: 2: 17.

Hocker, H. 2002. Fibre Morphology In: Wool: Science and Technology (W.S. Simpson and G.H. Crawshaw, Eds), Woodhead Publishing Limited, Cambridge, p. 60-79.

Hou, A. and Dai, J. 2005. Coloration Technology 121: 18-20.

Hsieh, S.H., Huang, Z.K., Huang, Z.Z. and Tseng, Z.S. 2004. Journal of Applied Polymer Science 94: 1999.

Levy, B. 2004. International Dyer 10: 18.

Lewis, D.M. 1999. Review Progress Coloration, 29: 23-28.

Lim, S.H. and Hudson, S.M. 2003. Review of chitosan and its derivatives as antimicrobial agents and their uses as textile chemicals, Journal of Macromolecular Science. Part C - Polymer Reviews C43: 223-269.

Moholkar, V.S., Nierstrasz, V.A. and Warmoeskerken, M.M.C.G. 2003. Intensification of mass transfer in wet textile processes by power ultrasound. AUTEX Research Journal 3: 129-138.

Morton, H.E. and Hearle, J.W.S. 2000. The Textile Institute 61.

Moses, J.J. and Jagannathan, K. 1996. Bleaching of cotton using hydrogen peroxide in ultrasonic energy and dyeing, Colourage 11: 19-24.

Onar, N. and Sariisik, M. 2004. Application of enzymes and chitosan biopolymer to the antifelting finishing process. Journal of Applied Polymer Science: 93: 2903-2908.

Paulo, A.C. and Silva, C.J.S.M. 2006. U S Patent 2006/0121595A1, (8 June 2006)

Pleva, R. 2002. International Textile Bulletin 2: 62.

Ramachandran, T., Karthik, T. and Saravanan, D. 2008. Novel trends in textile wet processing. Journal of Institution of Engineers 89: 3.

Rybicki, E., Filipowska, B. and Walawska, A. 2000. Application of natural biopolymers in shrink-proofing of Wool. Fibres and Textiles in Eastern Europe 8: 62-65.

Saligram A.N., Shukla S.R., and Mathur Manisha. 1993. Dyeing of polyester fibres using ultrasound.Journal of Society of Dyers and Colourist, 109: 263-266.

Sawada, K. and Uedab, M. 2004. Evaluation of the dyeing mechanism of an acid dye on protein fibers in supercritical CO_2. Dyes and Pigments 63: 77-81.

Schmidt, A., Bach, E. and Schollmeyer, E. 2003. The dying of natural fibres with reactive disperse dyes in supercritical carbon dioxide. Dyes and Pigments 56: 27-35.

Silva, C.J.S.M., Prabaharan, M., Gubitz, G. and Cavaco-Paulo, A. 2005. Treatment of wool fibres with subtilisin and subtilisin-PEG. Enzyme and Microbial Technology 36: 917-922.

Simpson, W.S. 2002. Wool production and fibre marketing. In: Wool: Science and Technology (W.S. Simpson and G.H. Crawshaw, Eds.), Woodhead Publishing Limited, Cambridge p 215.

Sivakumar, V., Chandrasekaran, F., Swaminathan, G. and Rao P.G. 2009. Towards cleaner degreasing method in industries: ultrasound-assisted aqueous degreasing in leather making. Journal of Cleaner Production 17: 101-104.

Sohl, K. 1999. AATCC 11: 31.

Srivastava, C.P. 1993. Man Made Textile in India 12: 513.

Thakore, K.A., Smith, C.B. and Clapp, T.G. 1990. Application of ultrasound to textile wet processing. American Dyestuff Reporter 10: p 30-44.

Thomas, H. 2007. In: Plasma Technologies for Textiles (R. Shishoo ed.), Woodhead publishing Limited Cambridge, pp 228.

van der Vlist, J. and Loos, K. 2010. Transferases in polymer chemistry. Advances in Polymer Science 237: 21-54.

Xie, T., Wang, A., Huang, L., Li, H., Chen, Z., Wang, Q. and Yin, X. 2009. Review: Recent advance in the support and technology used in enzyme immobilization. African Journal of Biotechnology 8: 4724-4733.

Yachmenev, V.G., Bertoniere, N.R. and Blanchard, E.J. 2001. Effect of sonication on cotton preparation with alkaline pectinase. Textile Research Journal 71: 527–533.

□□□

Chapter 26

Advances in Wool Based Non Woven Technical Textiles

G.Thilagavathi[1], V.R. Giridev[2] T. Senthilram[2] and A.S.M.Raja[3]
[1]Department of Textile Technology, PSG College of Technology, Coimbatore- 641 004 (Tamil Nadu), [2]Department of Textile Technology, Anna University, Chennai- 600 025 (Tamil Nadu), [3]Central Sheep and Wool Research Institute, Avikanagar- 304 501 (Rajasthan)

Wool fiber occupies an important part in the annals of textile fibre process. The uniqueness of wool has led to various technical applications apart from being used as clothing. The present paper provides an insight about the wool and its properties along with the potential applications in the technical textiles. The unique fiber arrangement and the presence of the amino acids have led to its usage as insulation, UV protective, flame retardant and in antimicrobial technical textiles.

Wool is a natural protein fibre that grows from the follicles of the sheep's skin. Throughout history, wool fibre has enjoyed widespread popularity as an apparel fibre and in interior textiles. Today wool remains a premium, sought after apparel fibre with an impressive set of technical attributes. Similarly, for carpets, rugs and home textiles, wool remains the benchmark of quality and performance with which other fibres are compared. Efforts are also being made to utilize wool for technical applications (Johnson *et al.*, 2003). The unique physical and chemical characteristics of this fibre provide a range of unique properties like warmth and coolness, breathability, moisture absorption and buffering, resilience, low odour and odour absorption, softness, flame resistance, biodegradability and recyclability to the apparel fabrics which can be advantageously utilized for making technical textiles (Radetic *et al.*, 2003). The potential application for the animal fibre based technical textiles are filtration of toxic gases, oil spills, thermal and sound insulation, shock absorbent and wound protective textiles, fire resistant products, high altitude weather protective materials, interiors in automobiles, aircrafts, buildings.

Macro and micro structure of wool

Wool has complex morphological structure (Fig. 1). The fibre contains two major components in its structure namely cuticle, the hydrophobic outer layer of the fibre with scales and cortex, the inner layer of the fibre which contains micro fibrils. Medium fine and coarse wools contains a third component in their fibre structure called medulla, which is the central canal filled with air running along the fibre axis. The cuticle and cortex differ in confirmations in their polymer

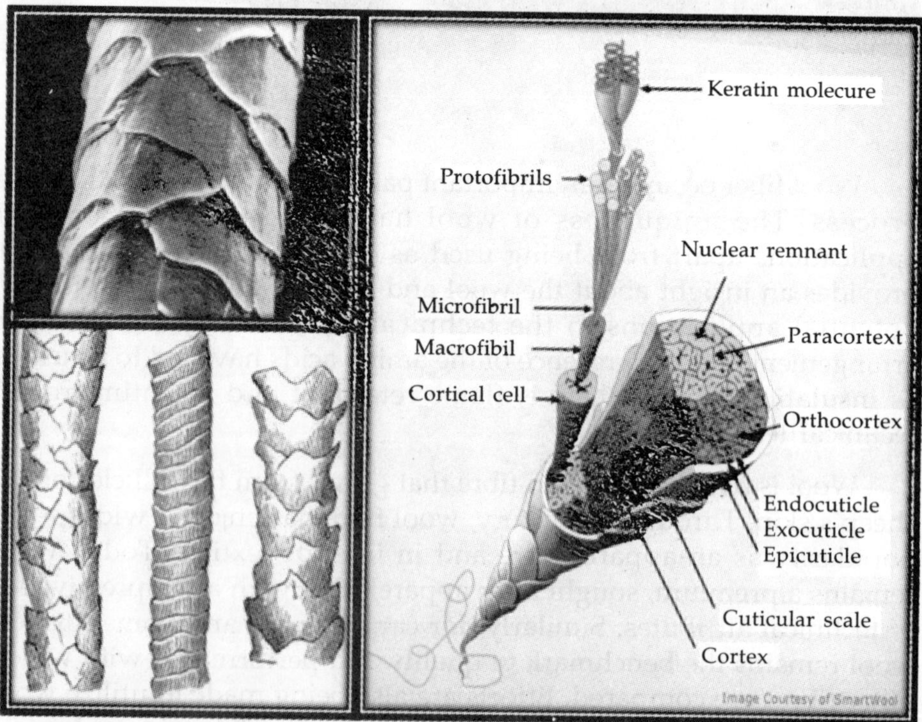

Fig. 1 : Macro and Micro structure of wool

chains as well as amino acid compositions. The cortex, comprising 90% of the fibre, consists of different kinds of cortex cells, ortho (60-90%) and paracortex cells (40-10%). Paracortex contain larger amount of sulphur than orthocortex cells (Kulkarni *et al.*, 1971; Jones *et al.*, 1990). The cortical cells (macrofibrils) are found to be higher in á-helical content as compared to the cuticle cells, which has increased disorder content. Each cortial cell is composed of 100-300nm embedded into the intermcrofibrillar matrix material comprising cytoplasmatic and nuclear remnants of the keratinocytes. The macrofibrils are composed of bundles of 500-800 microfibrils.

Wool polymer system

Wool is chemically a polypeptide polymer made up of 18 amino acids with á- keratin arranged in helical structure. The repeating unit of the wool polymer is the amino acid which has the general formula (Fig. 2). The side groups of amino acids vary in size and can be grouped, according to their chemical properties: hydrocarbons, which are hydrophobic (water-hating); hydrophilic (water-loving); acidic; basic; and amino acids that contain sulphur. Amino acids are linked to each other by peptide bond (that is -CO-NH-) to form the wool polymer.

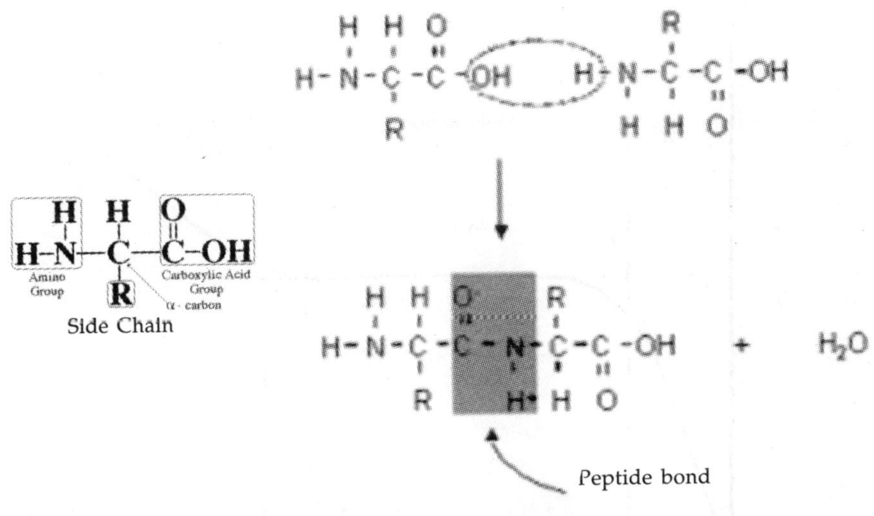

Fig. 2 : Wool Polymer System

Wool polymers have carboxylate (-COO-) as side groups, while others have amino ($-NH_3^+$) as side groups. Between these two groups, that is acidic and basic groups, salt linkages or ionic bond will form.

The sulphur containing amino acids present in wool, makes the wool polymer system the only one with cystine linkages, also known as disulphide bonds. Finally, the polymer system of wool is extremely amorphous: it is about 25-30% crystalline, correspondingly, 70-75% amorphous (Hocker, 2002).

Mechanical property of wool

Wool has a unique form of stress-strain curve (Fig. 3). One of the key features is the long flat yield region, where the fibre extends at constant stress. It has been shown that this mechanical feature is associated with the conversion of á helical rods to extended structures known as â-pleated sheets (which are also strongly hydrogen bonded). The á-â conversion is an important feature of wool behaviour. At the same time as the helices are extended, the matrix is also stretched. The retractive force of the strained disulphide-bond network, much like rubber, assists recovery of the fibre when the stress is released. This ability of wool to change configurations reversibly (i.e. its high degree of elasticity and resilience) compensates for the relatively low tensile strength of the fibre. The Young's modulus of wool in the Hookean region is about 1.4 GPa (Feughelman and Haly, 1960).

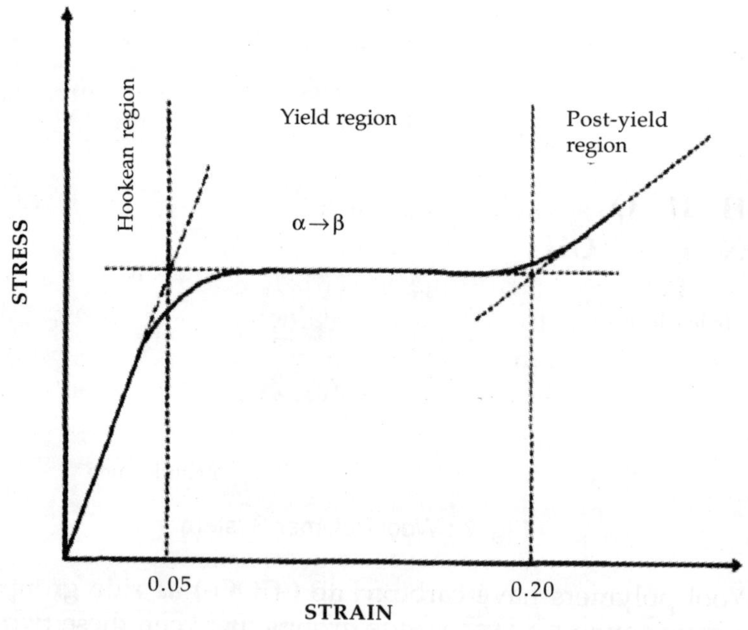

Fig. 3 : Stress-strain curve of fine wool

Chemical properties of wool

Wool is more resistant to acids than alkalis. This is because acids hydrolyse the peptide groups but do not damage the disulphide bonds. The disulphide bonds are very important to keep the wool polymer intact. Although the polymer system of wool is weakened under acid conditions, the fibre does not dissolve, but it is vulnerable to further degradation. It is therefore important that wool be neutralised after any acid treatment. Wool dissolves readily in alkaline solutions, which hydrolyse the disulphide bonds, hydrogen bonds, and salt linkages and cause the polymer chains to separate from each other. Prolonged exposure causes hydrolysis of the peptide bonds of the polymer chains, leading to polymer fragmentation and complete destruction of the fibre (Maclaren and Milligan, 1981).

Functional properties of wool

Thermal Insulation: Wool as such is exothermic in nature because of the various reactive groups in its structure and in wet condition it is able to release heat. In case of high humid conditions such as in winter, it absorbs the moisture and provides us the warmth. Warmth property of the woolen product is also due to entrapped air in the fabric structure, which insulates/prevents our body temperature to move out along with the exothermic nature of the wool (Baxter, 1946).

Flame retardant: Among the different natural fibres, wool has natural flame retardant property due to 14% nitrogen content in its chemical constituent. Wool fibre also contains sulphur. Due to the presence of nitrogen and sulphur, wool materials require large amount of oxygen for combustion. The limiting oxygen index (LOI) of wool is 25.2. The LOI of cotton is about 18.4. Similary due to complex morphological structure already explained the wool after ignition, the flame spread very slowly and the char produced has self extinguishing property. The higher levels of moisture content also contribute to the flame retardant properties of wool. The flame retardant property of wool is advantageous for development of technical products like airline furnishings, interior technical textiles etc (www.csiro.au/files/files/pa29.pdf).

Anti- static nature: Wool can absorb as much as 15% moisture without feeling wet. Due to this property, the static energy generation in the woolen products is very less (Gohl and Vilensky, 2005).

UV-protection: When ultraviolet radiation hits the textile materials, different types of interactions occur depending upon the substrate and its conditions. It is established that wool fibre can give very good protection against the UV light. The physical and chemical interactions of the fiber also decide the UV absorption property. The UPF of pure wool is calculated to be more than 30 units. Wool absorbs strongly in the region of 280 nm-400 nm and even beyond 400 nm. This is due to the presence of the aromatic amino acids and cysteine.

Feltability: The wool fibre has the unique properties called felting due to differential frictional effect of surface cuticle cells. This property is used to produce different felted products for technical applications (Albrecht, 2003).

Toxic gases, odour and sound absorbing: Wool has the capacity to absorb toxic cases like sulphur dioxide, ammonia, nitrogen oxides, formaldehyde etc from the environment and woollen materials have best sound absorption capability (Wang *et al.*, 2003).

Biodegradability: The wool fibre is completely biodegradable and sustainable making it environmentally safe.

Wool in technical textiles

The technical textiles form wool can be produced from different methods as follows

- Pressed felt using the natural felting behavior of wool
- Non woven manufacturing using needle punch technique, spun lace techniques
- Composite materials using molding technology.

The technical textile produced from the pressed felt of wool and non-wovens is discussed in the following section.

Pressed felt and its application

Pressed felt is produced by using the natural felting properties of wool. Briefly, this process consists of carding, web formation, laying of web into bat form and hardening with the application of moisture, heat etc., and finally fulling using hammers. Technical pressed felt using wool has a wide range of applications in industrial and domestic surroundings which include:

- Sound absorption
- Vibration absorption
- Oil reservoirs and applicators
- Removal of unwanted liquids (wiping) and solids (filtration)
- Removal of mists from gases.
- Polishing
- Padding and packing
- Gaskets and Spacers
- Air Seals (for example, in tumble driers, vacuum cleaners and sliding windows)
- Garment stiffeners
- Medical uses such as corn plasters.

Wool nonwoven formation techniques

Needle punching technology: Needle punching is a process of bonding nonwoven web structure by mechanically interlocking the fibres through the web. The principle of needle felting is based on the reorientation of a portion of horizontally located fibres or filaments into the vertical plane in form of fibre tufts through the use of barbed needles. The barbed needle carries tuft fibres into a vertical direction and tuft ends remain outside the fibre batt during return of the needles. This results in a condensation of the reoriented fibres into bundles, which increases the friction between fibres so that the fibre consolidation is achieved through shape and friction (Fig. 4). During fibre reorientation to the vertical plane, a fibre movement takes place within the felt as the fibres caught by the needles slide by each other and change their position. The majority of fibres or fibre sections which are not consolidated into fibre tufts remain in their horizontal position. The fibre movement within the fibre batt, caused by the needling action, results in length and width changes of the area mass influenced by the process conditions (Gohl and Vilensky, 2005).

Spunlace technology: The mechanical process of entangling fibre webs by means of water jets. Spunlacing uses high-speed jets of water to strike a web so that the fibers knot about one another. As a result, nonwoven fabrics made by this method have specific properties, as soft handle and drapability. Japan is the major producer of hydrogen tangled nonwovens in the world. In this process, entangling a web of loose fibers on a porous belt or moving perforated or patterned screen to form a sheet structure by subjecting the fibers to multiple rows of fine high-pressure jets of water (Fig. 5).

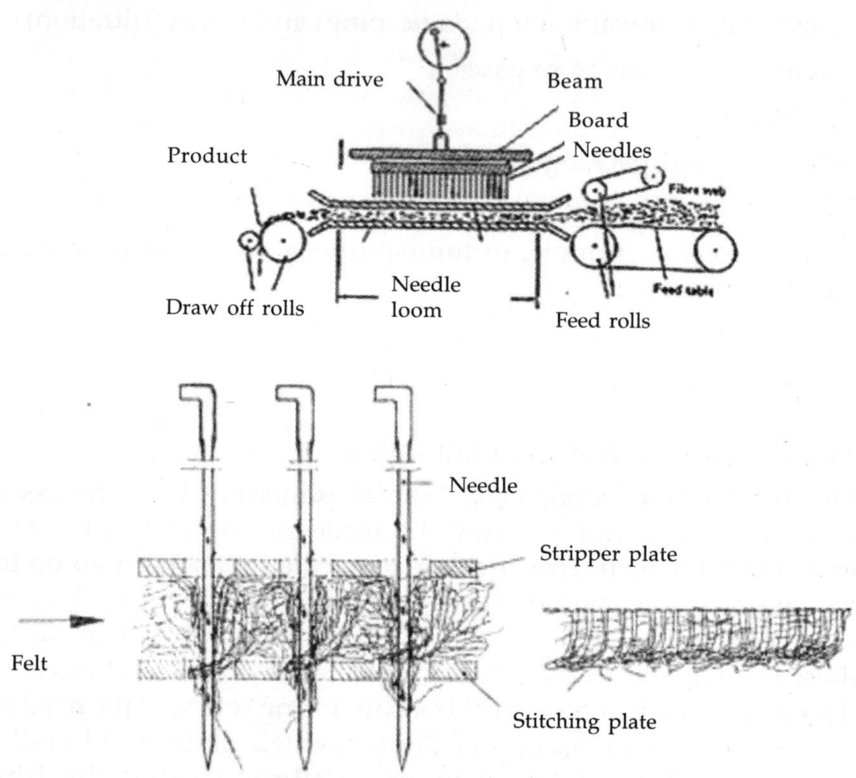

Fig. 4 : Needle punching process

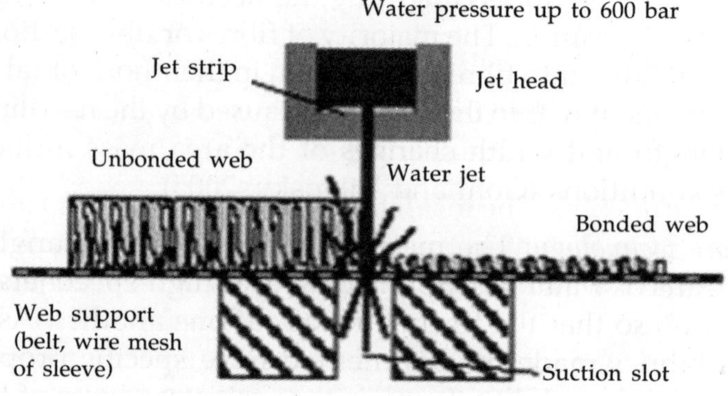

Fig. 5 : Spunlace bonding process

The formed web (usually air-laid or wet-laid, but sometimes spun bond or melt-blown, etc.) is first compacted and pre-wetted to eliminate air pockets and then water-needled. The water pressure generally increases from the first to the last injectors. Pressure as high as 2200 psi are used to direct the water jets onto the web to form the nonwoven (http://www.engr.utk.edu/mse/Textiles/Spunlace.htm). Crimp promotes cohesion in carded webs prior to bonding, it also influences the strength of fabrics produced by low to medium pressure hydrogen tanglement systems. As a consequence of the high resistance to compression, helically crimped fibres require higher energy inputs to obtain fabrics with acceptable strength. The effect of crimp is particularly noticeable in the hydrogen tanglement of fine wool, which has a high crimp frequency and requires high pressure to produce a coherent, abrasion-resistant structure (Russell, 2007; Moschler, 1995).

Dry laid nonwovens

The first dry laid systems owe much to the felting process known since medieval times. In the pressed felt industry, cards and web lappers were used to make a batt containing wool or a wool blend that is subsequently felted (hardened) using moisture, agitation and heat (Albrecht, 2003).

Applications

The major areas of application of wool technical textiles are

- Aircraft/ Automobile interior materials eg. Carpets, liners etc
- Fire proof jackets/uniforms
- Thermal insulation jackets and roofs, sound absorption panels
- Electro static filters, filtration material for toxic gas, oil spill
- Medical bandages, Skin injury prevention materials
- Shock absorbing material
- Scaffolds for tissue engineering

Automobile interiors: The insulation, flame retardant and absorption of toxic gases from the environment properties of wool makes it more suitable material for automobile liners, carpets etc. Tufted and needle punch carpets are the two major product choices of floor coverings for automobiles. Commercially, the needle-punched non woven material out of wool – ramie blend is used in automobile industries as liners. This process consists of opening and blending, followed by carding, cross-lapping, needle punching and finishing. The range of fibre weight is between 225 gsm to 350 gsm.

Insulation bat as roof liners: Wool bat has been used as thermal insulation liners for roof since ancient times. Wool is converted into bat form mechanically and laminated with rubber latex. This form wool bat is used as roof liners for insulation. When nonwovens are composed of wool fibres, Baxter expanded Schuhmeister's equation and found that the thermal conductivity of the wool fabric is as follows:

$$k_m = x(k_1v_1 + k_2v_2) + y\left(\frac{k_1k_2}{k_1v_2 + k_2v_1}\right)$$

Where $x = 0.21$, $y = 0.79$, $k1$ is the thermal conductivity of air ($k_1 = 0.0264$), k_2 is the thermal conductivity of wool fibre at a certain regain ($k_2 = 0.2226$ at a regain of 0.7%, $k_2 = 0.1933$ at a regain of 10.7%) and v_1 and v_2 are the fractional volumes of air and the wool fibre, respectively (Baxter, 1946).

Geo textiles: It is reported that needle punched non woven wool mat can be used as grass-strike germination mat. The non woven mat is used as a cover fabric after seed has been shown. By this way the germination of seed is increased. It is also reported that the non woven mats has been used for mulching purpose (Johnson, *et al.*, 2003).

Absorbent materials: Wool has good absorbing properties for hydro carbons. Based on this property, the recycle wool has been converted into non woven materials. The material can be used for absorbing oil spill in the sea and removing/cleaning oils from the machines (Radetic, 2003) and removal of heavy metal like copper, zinc, chromium etc (Wang *et al.*, 2003).

Sport wear: Hydrogen tangled fabrics composed of merino wool has been developed and such fabrics have been incorporated in performance outerwear products such as outdoor clothing. Sports shirts and vests have also been produced from hydrogen tangled fabrics (Russell, 2007).

Shock absorbing material: The pressed felt products of wool are being used as shock absorbent, mounting pads and vibrant damper materials in different fields.

Sound absorption pads: Wool felt absorbs more sound per thickness than other materials making it the leading choice in applications where space is limited.

Electro static filters: Fine particles of pollutants from the air can affect the human lungs. Wool is considered for making electrostatic filter materials due to its absorbing properties. Electrostatic filter is a device attached with air cleaners to remove the dust particles from the flowing air. Wool and polypropylene blend of 50:50 ratio was used to produce electrostatic filter. The filter made out of wool showed optimum performance with high particulate loading capacity (Schutz and Humphries, 2010).

Wool composite materials: Wool based composite materials using wool as filling material and resins are mainly used for thermal insulation and fire retardant composites. Wool fibre was mixed with bast fibres for making flame retardant composites.

Wool based medical textiles: Pressure relieving devices can protect the skin from the effects of pressure, friction and moisture. They provide excellent protection when placed under the back, calves and heels.

(i) Bedsore and pressure sore prevention: The dense 30mm wool pile medical sheepskins provides an interface between the patient and the bed that reduces pressure, friction and skin moisture- the primary causes of pressure or bed sores (http://www.medicalsheepskins.com/medical.htm).

(ii) Wool-pile (Nursing fleece): It is a cheaper alternative to sheepskin. It does have a number of advantages. It is made from sheared very-fine wool and provides the benefits of wool; without size restrictions. Machine Washable nursing fleece is easy to wash and can be dried quickly (http://www.medicalsheepskins.com/medical.htm).

(iii) Foot care: It is very-fine combed wool that can be used around toes for pressure reduction and improved comfort. To cushion toes for relief from corns and shoe pressure and also used in the toes of ballet shoes. It is very ideal for diabetic foot care ((http://www.medicalsheepskins.com/medical.htm).

Antimicrobial and scaffolds for tissue engineering: Wool due to the presence of amino acids presents excellent wound healing and antimicrobial properties at mild acidic pH. The authours have attempted coating of wool with chitosan followed by dyeing with natural dyes such as henna and turmeric. Excellent antimicrobial resistance was observed and the presences of chitosan provide two layers of defense at the infected site. Wool fiber due to the presence of the amino acids provides excellent cell adhesion for the fibroblast cells.

The cells rapidly proliferate and multiply compared to the TCP. The images of cells cultured on the wool scaffolds are given in Fig. 6.

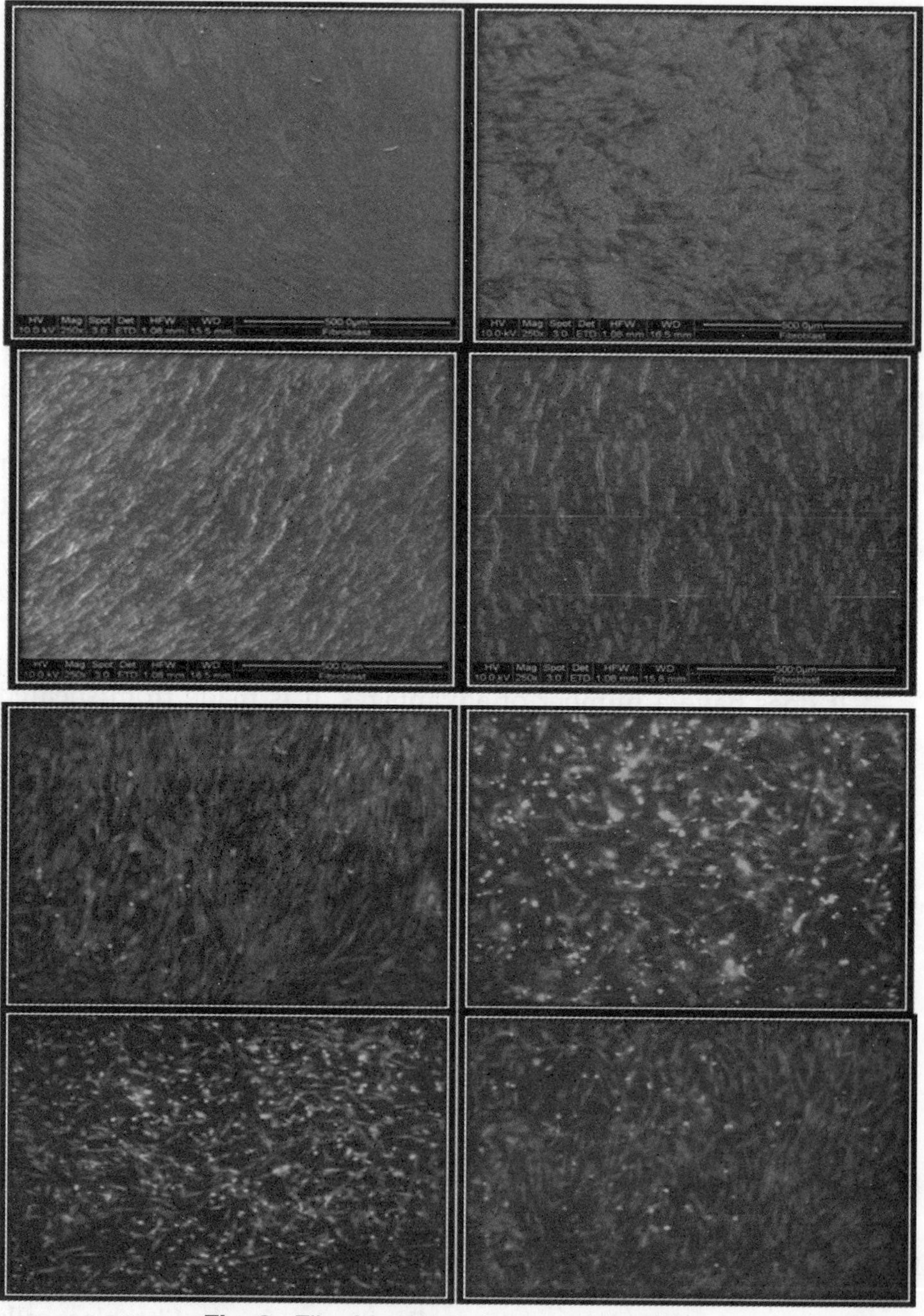

Fig. 6 : Fibroblast growth on wool scaffolds

Conclusion

The overall high extensibility of wool, its natural waviness and ability to trap air has a coordinated effect of comfort and warmth, which also make it an ideal insulating material. The sophisticated dual morphology of wool produces the characteristic crimp which has also been an inspiration for the development of some highly technical synthetic fibres. Wool is inherently fire retardant, but further improvements can be achieved by a number of fire-retardant treatments. Wool inherent chemical and physical properties, it has large scope in future technical textiles (Simpson and Crawshaw, 2002; http://uk.sheepwoolinsulation.com/why_wool; http://www.technical-textiles.net/archive/html).

References

Albrecht, W., Fuchs, H. and Kittelmann, W. 2003. Nonwoven Fabrics. Wiley Publications, ISBN 3-527-30406-1, pp 270-271.

Baxter, S. The thermal conductivity of textiles. In: Proc. Physical Society, 58: 105-118.

Feughelman and Haly, H.R. 1960. The mechanical properties of wool keratin and its molecular configuration. Colloid and Polymer Science 168: 107-115

Gohl, E.P.G. and Vilensky, L.D. 2005. Textile Science. CBS Publishers and Distributors, New Delhi.

Hocker, H. In: Wool: Science and Technology. (W.S. Simpson and G.H. Crawshaw, Eds.), Woodhead Publishing, Cambridge.

Johnson, N.A.G., Wood, E.J., Ingham, P.E., McNeil, S.J. and McFarlane, I.D. 2003. Wool as a technical fibre. Journal of the Textile Institute 94: 26-40.

Jones, L.N., Cholewa, M., Kaplin, I.J., Legge, G.J.F. and Ollerhead, R.W. 1990. In: Proc. Eighth International Wool and Textile Research Conference, Christchurch, 1: 246.

Kulkarni, V.G., Robson, R.M. and Robson, J. A. 1971. Polymer Science Application. 18: 127.

Maclaren, J.A. and Milligan, B. 1981. Wool science, the chemical reactivity of the wool fibre. Science Press, Marrackville, N.S.W., Australia.

Moschler, W. 1995. Some results in the fields of hydrogen tanglement of fibrous webs and their thermal after-treatment. In: International Nonwovens Symposium, EDANA.

Radetic, M.M., Jocic, J.M., Jovanc, P.M., Zoran, I.C., Petrovic, L.J. and Thomas, H.F. 2003. Recycled wool-based nonwoven material as oil sorbent. Environmental Science and Technology 37: 1008-1012.

Russell, S. J. 2007. Hand Book of Nonwovens. Woodhead Publishing Limited.

Schutz, J.A. and Humphries, W. 2010, A study of wool/polypropylene nonwovens as an alternative to the hansen filter. Textile Research Journal 80: 1265-1277.

Simpson, W.S. and Crawshaw, G.H. 2002. Wool: Science and Technology", Woodhead Publishing Limited, pp 67-68.

Wang Yuen-Hua, Lin Su-Hsia, Juang Ruey-Shin. 2003. Removal of heavy metal ions from aqueous solutions using various low-cost adsorbents. Journal of Hazardous Materials B102: 291-302.

□□□

Chapter 27

Non-Conventional Utilisation of Wool and Other Animal Hairs

D.B. Shakyawar and A.S.M. Raja
Division of Textile Manufacturing and Textile Chemistry,
Central Sheep and Wool Research Institute, Avikanagar-304 501
Rajasthan

Wool and other animal hairs/fibres are playing an important role in Indian economy despite of small share as compared to cotton and synthetic fibres due to their special virtues. Hairy wool produced in southern region and hair obtained from goat, camel, equine and pashmina guard hairs are coarse and hairy type. These fibres/hairs could not be utilized commercially due to lack of desirable characteristics required for yarn formation. As a result, they are not fetching any value to farmers. Therefore, there is a need to explore the possibilities of utilization of these fibers for suitable products i.e. packing, technical textile in pure or blend forms. Development of non-woven products using needle punched felting machine will be potential application in civil construction and other industrial uses. Bio-composites from animal fibres are also have good potential application for producing eco-friendly high functional composites such as films, bio materials for wound dressing, drug delivery bio plastics, heavy metal absorbents, keratin scaffolds and hygiene fabrics. Extraction of protein from coarse wool and application as bio-fertilizer will also a new area of application. Protein powder is now also produced commercially as an additive in cosmetic products and functional foods. Other potential applications of protein powder such as surface coating, fibre treatment, fillers in films, ink wound care, enzyme immobilisation, composite scaffold for cell growth and drug delivery have also been reported.

Wool based non-woven technical textiles

Needle punching is one of the important eco-friendly processes of nonwoven production systems. It is by far the most versatile and commonly used method of fibre. Nonwovens with higher porosity and absorbency are most suitable for agricultural and industrial application such as oil reservoirs, washers, filters. Thus for desired functional end use, mixture of fine and coarse fibre is required to produce nonwoven felts with higher compressibility, recovery characteristics and low energy loss. The Indian wool found most suitable for such end use having medium to coarse fineness (diameter- 25-45 μm) and fibre length (40-70 mm). The high areal density felts can able to engineered by optimizing blend of fine and coarse wool or other fibre mix for needle punched nonwoven felts. The excellent biophysical properties i.e. hygroscopicity, thermal insulation, flame retardency and sound absorption of wool provides active breathing, regulating humidity and permeable structures in form of needle punched woolen felts which will be the solution of barrier materials in construction and building industry for centuries. These wool based needle punched nonwoven structures, besides transmitting water vapour, let pass also other gases, e.g. carbon dioxide. This way, gaseous contaminants in the air are removed from interiors not only by air exchange but also through natural breathing of walls when used as environmental friendly filling insulation materials and as facing insulation material for housing, interior and furnishing and giving users a real feeling of building comfort. The inherent thermal insulation characteristics wool specially the coarse wool having medullation i.e. air filled fibres provides extra bulk and thermal insulation to the needle punched nonwoven felts can be use as bio materials for wound dressing, drug delivery bio plastics heavy metal absorbents, keratin scaffolds and hygiene wipes. Wool and specialty hair fibres such as Angora and yak are quite suitable for apparel application. These fibres in the form of nonwoven using needle punching system with low areal density will be more appropriate for manufacturing of multi layered garments suitable for cold region of country.

Non-woven insulation made from natural fibrous raw materials can be classified in the group of environmentally friendly materials for thermal and acoustic insulation. Needle punching is by far the most versatile and commonly used method of bonding accounting for 20-25% of the nonwovens. Needle punched fabric forms the base in making many composites. The nonwovens made ups of synthetic materials are not eco-friendly in processing and liberate high volatile organic chemicals (VOCs), more over they are not breathable and biodegradable. The wool fibre is characterized by good biophysical properties such as hygroscopicity, thermal insulation, fire retardency etc. At present very few products are made of wool nonwovens. Though, there are good potential to develop suitable wool based non woven to use in compartment/ multi-stake/ vertical cropping system, the hygroscopicity (high moisture holding capacity 200-300%) and thermal insulation to restrict heat transfer from bottom give better germination condition to plants.

The high bulk properties thermal insulation and fire resistant properties of wool can also be not yet fully exploited in as environmental friendly filling insulation materials and as facing insulation material for housing, interior furnishing and transport. Flexible needle punched wool based nonwoven has good potential to act as insulating nonwovens in construction and building materials as barrier for thermal conduction, fire protection and acoustic insulation. The commercial produced woolen nonwoven i.e. woolen felt is used by different medium and small industries for their various processing raw material such as, oil reservoirs, washers, brushing and polishing of ornaments etc. There is limitation of areal density to these felt prepared by chemical and mechanical process which may possible to improve with needle punched nonwoven felts to make suitable for more industrial applications. Nonwoven products provide high thermal insulation as compared to woven. Light weight multi layered wool based needle punched fabrics will be developed for cold regions of Leh/Ladhakh.

Wool based bio-composites

Composites are cohesive structures made by physically combining two or more compatible materials provide multifunctional characteristics not obtainable from any discrete material such as electrical and thermal insulations etc. Most of the present fiber reinforced composites are composed of ceramics and glasses such as small mineral particles, metal particles such as aluminum and amorphous materials, including polymers and carbon black and if from natural fibrous source than based of cellulosic materials. The composites made up of synthetic materials are not eco-friendly and liberate high VOCs. Moreover, they are not breathable and fire retardant like that of wool. The highest fire and thermal resistant properties of wool did not exploit in reinforced composites, though wool is quit flexible as compared to present non biodegradable fibrous sources used in composites. There is vast potential for using wool for the end uses like, fire retardancy, thermal insulation, antimicrobial, biomaterials, drug delivery, bio plastics, heavy metal absorbents properties and bio-composites in construction and building materials. At present very few products are made of wool composites. Therefore, there is good potential to develop suitable wool composite having unique properties.

The higher amorphous structure of the wool make it highly hygroscopic in nature and high ammonia content make it highest fire resistance capability (limiting oxygen index, LOI value- 26.3) among all the natural and synthetic fibres. It has capability of self extinguishing the fire at low level but higher level of fire flame will propagate. The application of flame retardant finishes such as borax or boric acid improved the fire resistance characteristics but in apparel end use it reduces the moisture properties of fabric. The application of these finishes as micro/nano composites with wool will improve fire resistant properties without affecting its natural behavior. The scale structure wool provide poly functional properties exploit immobilize the micro and nano particles and provides desired functional properties in wool based micro, nano and bio-composites. Due to keratinous fibre wool inherentially resistance against micro-organisms except wool moth but like other natural fibres most commonly prone to accumulation, multiplication and proliferation of micro-organisms into their surrounding environment. In fact, several factors such as suitable temperature and humidity, entrapping of dust, soil, spilled food and drink stains etc. on the textile surfaces can make textile optimal enrichment cultures for a rapid multiplication of micro-organisms. Application of inorganic nano-particles and their nanocomposites would be a more hygiene alternative of present apparel. The regeneration of wool based keratin for bio-fibre through electro or wet spinning may used to reinforced with carbon nano tubes, clays has vast applications. The wool keratin is annually renewable, abundant available as used carpet, rugs, apparels, from woolen industries etc. may found suitable for producing eco-friendly high functional composites such as films, bio materials for wound dressing, drug delivery bio plastics heavy metal absorbents, keratin scaffolds and hygiene fabrics.

Wool beyond textiles

When considering the application of wool beyond textiles and fibres it is important first to consider the materials from which wool is made up. Both biological characteristics and practical considerations are of importance to evaluate future application of wool. The simple non conventional application of wool is for stuffing the dolls. As per the EU guidelines, the dolls need to be stuffed with biodegradable and flame retardant fibres. Most of the doll manufacturers are using wool for this purpose. Wool is also used for making the mob yarn. The mob yarn is made up of other fibres with 5-10% wool to enhance the water absorbing properties. The other major applications and their potential in future are summarized below.

Extraction of amino acid from wool and hairy fibres

Advanced applications of wool beyond the fibre utilize the keratin protein from which the fibre is constructed. The first step in the development of these materials is isolation of that protein in a versatile form that can be further manipulated into desired application. The primary component of hairy wool fibre (HWF) is keratin proteins constituting 65 to 95% of total hair protein. The sulphur in cysteine molecules in adjacent keratin proteins are link together in disulfide chemical bonds which are strong and very difficult to break apart. These are largely resistant to the action of proteolytic enzymes and acids but the disulfide bonds can be broken apart by hot alkali solutions and the hydrolyzed peptide bonds eventually broken down into its constituent amino acids. There are two possible methods of hydrolysis i.e. hot sodium hydroxide treatment and hydrolysis with HCl having strength greater than 20% for 6 hrs at 100°C. Both the methods followed by sequential activated carbon filtration, crystallisation and drying.

Although these are seldom used exclusively as fertilizer, they can be used in combination with other compost material. The major difference of such fertilizers compared to inorganic fertilizers comes from their slow degradation. Hence, their use as sole fertilizer, specifically for fast growing plants is discouraged. Their use as slow N releasing mats is a newly introduced idea that can be used with orchid plants, ornamental plants, nursery pots and roof top gardens. Such mat contains about 15% nitrogen that slowly releases over a period to provide nutrients to plants at a steady rate and highly biodegradable. Hydrolysates of HWF are safe as long as they do not carry contaminants (Papilloma viruses, Picorna viruses etc). It is necessary to reduce the risk before its use. Before hydrolysis, HWF are washed, dried at 62°C for >5 min and sterilized by dry steam at 150°C. Extractions of only few amino acids (cystein, serine and glutamic acid) are more economical from HWF. However, proline has use in cosmetic products that makes its extraction economically feasible. Keratin peptides have formed a core part of many familiar products including fire fighting foams, as protein foam concentrates, as moisture retardants in building plaster and most significantly as hair and skin care products. Beyond cosmetic enhancement of skin and hair is biological enhancement of skin and other tissues. The use of keratin materials for medical applications, to enhance the repair of tissues both within and on the surface of the body, has been subject of both research and commercial endeavor.

Powder technology

Protein fibres i.e. wool and silk macromolecules have been extensively studied in recent years as biomaterial for a number of different non-textile applications (Rajkhowa *et al.*, 2008, 2009; Xu *et al.*, 2004). This has been done through re-fabrication of protein fibres as nano fibres, films, hydrogels, foams, coating materials and powders. Among these forms, powder is now produced commercially as an additive in cosmetic products and functional foods. Other potential applications of protein powder such as surface coating, fibre treatment, fillers in films, ink wound care, enzyme immobilisation, composite scaffold for cell growth and drug delivery have also been reported. Powder can be prepared either by a solution route or by a mechanical method. In a typical solution route, fibres are dissolved by concentrated chaotropic salts and then the solution is dialyzed to remove salts. Particles are regenerated from the aqueous solution by self assembly and freeze drying or spray drying. Alternatively, aqueous silk /wool solutions can be dehydrated and pulverised. Chemical and enzymatic hydrolysis during powder preparation to get low molecular weight water soluble edible silk/wool powder and silk peptide powder is also reported. Though useful for certain uses, e.g. food additive and encapsulation, particles prepared through the solution route do not fulfil many desired requirements for applications in cosmetics, filler, coating and fibre treatment. This is due to partial solubility of powder and the formation of lumps of particles on wetting. Moreover, in the solution route, â crystalline structure of silk fibroin is changed to random coil and á form. Hence, a further treatment with methanol is usually required to induce crystallinity and impart stability in silk particles. Solution routes have inherent bottlenecks in the preparation process, such as long time of dialysis, high production costs, safety and environmental constraints. The mechanical method, on the other hand, avoids lengthy, costly and environmentally sensitive production procedures associated with the solution route. In contrast, mechanical attrition method can avoid these problems and fabricate insoluble silk particles directly. It also retains the crystallinity and water insolubility of particles. Unlike inorganic materials such as metals and ceramics, organic polymer materials are very difficult to mill into fine particles. A recommended mechanical method involved chopping fibres with a suitable machine, followed by crushing the chopped fibres in a media mill, for example, a ball mill. Jet mill is recommended at the final stage to get fine powder. However, protein fibres are viscoelastic and not easy to crush. Long milling time (up to 20–40 hr) and restricted fineness (d (0.5)=10-20 ìm) remain the major issues in mechanical silk/wool milling processes. To overcome these, various pre-treatments were used to reduce fibre strength. To reduce the particle size further down to 2-3 ìm, severe pre-treatments were employed prior to mechanical attrition, such as alkali degradation, exposure to high temperature, radiation or steam explosion. Similarly, pre-treatment before mechanical attrition to prepare wool powder was also reported. These treatments weakened the fibres and thus helped their milling. Even with harsh pre-treatments, the average particle size of silk powder prepared by ball and jet milling remained greater than 1 ìm. Preparation of nanoscale silk/wool particles through a special device using a working pressure of 1000 kgf/cm was revealed. However, fabrication of submicron silk particles by standard mechanical attrition has not been reported. Availability of such ultrafine powder may also open out new application avenues of powdered wool.

Advance applications in medical textiles

If wool is considered as a source of durable biopolymer material for which application development to parallel synthetic polymer is possible, then the possibilities for advanced applications of wool are boundless. Future advanced uses of wool keratin lie in two distinct areas. The first is medical technology. Developments will be driven by science and improved healing outcomes. Keratin in the body plays more than a physical role for the growth and differentiation of cells. Coupled with developing technology for creation of medical devices from wool keratin will be advance area of medical research (Kelly, 2009). The major applications of wool keratin in medical are wound care and orthopaedics. The second area of advanced use of keratin is in industrial technology. Keratin is one of the nature's most successful materials; it was evolved to be versatile, tough and protective and as a natural protein, there are wide opportunities in a range of industrial areas.

References

Kelly, R. 2009. Application of wool keratins ranging from Industrial materials to medical devices. Advances in Wool technology 323-331.

Rajkhowa, R., Wang, L. and Wang, X. 2008. Ultra-fine silk powder preparation through rotary and ball milling, Powder Technology 185: 87-95.

Rajkhowa, R., Wang L., Kanwar, J. and Wang, X. 2009. Fabrication of ultrafine powder from eri silk through attritor and jet milling. Powder Technology 191: 155-163.

Xu,W., Cui,W., Li, W. and Guo, W. 2004. Development and characterizations of super-fine wool powder. Powder Technology 140: 136-140.

□□□

Chapter 28

Developments in Processing and Product Development of Speciality Hair Fibres (Pashmina)

Sarfaraz A Wani[1], DB Shakyawar[2] and Asif H Sofi[1]

[1]Division of Livestock Products Technology, Faculty of Veterinary Sciences and Animal Husbandry, Sher-e-Kashmir University of Agricultural Sciences and Technology of Kashmir, [2]Division of Textile Manufacture and Textile Chemistry, Central Sheep and Wool Research Institute, Avikanagar (Rajasthan) 304501

The world's annual production of all luxury fibres is only 30 m kgs which is very negligible in comparison to total textile fibre production of 50,000 m kgs. If natural silk is included in luxury and rare fibres the total annual production reaches upto 100 m kg which is only 0.2% of total fibre production. The production and harvesting of luxury fibres are difficult and labour intensive as these often come from remote area of the world where access and transport are difficult, and their prices are high to very high. Nevertheless their fineness, softness, warmth and pleasurable handle have secured them a firm places in the niche areas of luxury apparel and furnishing fabrics. If these fibres are allowed to disappear, thousands of people in developing countries will suffer a loss of an income, which contributes significantly towards their financial security even if it is less as per developed countries standard.

Speciality Fibres

Goat family

Angora goat	Mohair
Cashmere goat	Cashmere wool
Common goat	Goat hair

Camel family

Camel	Dromedary Bactrian
Llama	Guanaco Llama Alpaca Vicuna
Rabbit	Rabbit hair

Pashmina goats, Yak and Mithun prevalent in north Himalayan region have been producing fibres and are used locally. Improvement of goat for mohair producing was started as early as 1867 by importation of Angora goats and crossing with the local animals in Himachal Pradesh and Maharashtra and met little success. In the year 1980, the CSWRI was the pioneering Institute to start Angora rabbit breeding at its Northern Temperate Regional Station, Garsa (Kulu) using imported stock. The rabbit breeding for hairs has now been well-accepted in Himachal Pradesh, Jammu & Kashmir and hilly parts of Uttar Pradesh. Similarly, research on improvement of Pashmina production was started at Indian Veterinary Research Institute's centre, Mukteshwar (Uttaranchal) using Chegu and Changthangi goat breeds.

In view of the economics of speciality hairs and their capacity to generate employment in cottage and small sectors as well as the handsome prices fetched by the finished products, the speciality hair have drawn active attention in the recent past. The present status with respect to the research, achievements, production levels and utilization programmes of these hairs as well as the expected scope is given below:

Pashmina Production and Processing and Value addition

Pashmina, the "King of Fibres" is known all over the world for its fineness, warmth, softness, desirable aesthetic value, elegance and timelessness in fashion. It has occupied a unique position among the fibres of animal origin due to its fineness, warmth, softness, handle and its ability to absorb dyes and moisture (Ryder, 1987). It is a down fibre/undercoat derived from domestic goat known as *Capra hircus* which is native to India. It has derived its name from the Persian word *"pashm"* which means *"soft gold"*, the King of fiber (Anon, 2005).

Pashmina goats are distributed throughout the mountainous regions of Central Asia ranging from China proper through Xinjing into Tibet, Mongolia, Kirghizia, Russia, Afghanistan and Iran (Ryder, 1987). China is the leading Pashmina producing country in the world followed by Mongolia. In India, Pashmina is produced in Jammu and Kashmir state (Ladakh region), Himachal Pradesh (Lahul and Spiti valley) and Uttaranchal (Uttar Kashi, Chamoli and Pithoragarh).

The total world Pashmina production is 15000-20000 T (Anon, 2009). Out of this, China alone is producing 70% followed by Mongolia (20%) where as India contributes only less than 1%. Out of 50 tons of Pashmina produced in India, Jammu & Kashmir alone produced 40 tons of Pashmina (Wani and Wani, 2007) which is considered as best of the lot. In India, Pashmina is produced by two breed viz; Changthangi in Jammu and Kashmir and Chegu in Himachal Pradesh. The average Productivity of Pashmina varies from 100 gm/ animal/ year in Chegu goat to 250 gm/animal/year in Changthangi as against world average of 700-1000 gm/year (Singh, 2004).

Fibre Quality

Pashmina is a fine fibre possessing scales of cylindrical nature. The quality of fibres in terms of fineness varies as reported by various workers e.g. 11.30μ (Sahni, 1981) 13.20±0.20μ (Deb, 1998), 12.16-12.55μ (Ganai *et al.* 2004), 13.51μ (Wani *et al.* 2004). Like fibre diameter, fibre length also shows considerable variation. The fibre length has been reported as 4.0-6.20 cm (Sahni, 1981), 5.80 cm (Deb, 1998), 4.86 cm (Ganai *et al.*, 2004), 4.95± 0.11 cm (Darokhan and Tomar, 1983).

Pashmina fibres are non medullated and are lacking crimps. It is having scale width to length ratio of 2:3. The internal cortical structure comprises of ortho and meso cortical cells, which is quite distinct from mohair and wool as they possess ortho surrounded by para and bilateral ortho structure respectively. In contrast to wool, Pashmina fibres are having little felting property. The fibre is slightly weaker than wool and is more susceptible to wetting (Ryder, 1984). The strength of

Cashmere fibres is about 10% below the finest sheep wool and 40% below Mohair. Breaking length has been reported as 6.92 g wt/km for Kazaki goats (Dauletbaev and Aryngaziev, 1980), 3.776±0.012 gwt/ km for *Changthangi* Pashmina (Ahmad and Gupta, 1989). On equal weigh basis, it is having 3 times more insulating capacity as that of wool. On wetting, Pashmina is having 80% retention of breaking strength (Ahmad and Gupta, 1989) compared to wool having 50-60%. The commonest natural colours of Pashmina are gray, brown, black while white being rarer. Among all shades, white one is fetching highest price because of rarity (Balleli, 1982).

The quality of *Changthangi* Pashmina as reported by Ahmad and Gupta (1989) & (Nazir *et al.*, 2011a) are presented in following table 1.

Table 1 : Quality of Changthangi Pashmina

Quality Parameter	Mean ± S.E	Mean ± S.E
Under coat percentage (w/w)	71.07± 1.917	76.01±0.32
Fibre Diametre (μ)	13.37± 0.049	12.25±0.11
Fibre length (mm)	55.86± 0.377	49.04±0.19
Tex (g wt)	0.319± 0.007	0.33 ± 0.17
Breaking Strength (gwt/tex)	11.81 ± 0.148	3.0 ± 0.01
Breaking Extension (%)	34.58± 0.377	30.33 ±1.23
Grease content (%)	5.61±0.278	-
Suint content (%)	6.94±0.794	-
Vegetable matter (%)	0.54±0.072	-
Tenacity (g/tex)	-	7.60 ± 0.98
Compressibility (%)	-	50.3±2.57
Compressional Resiliency (%)	-	45.10±1.32

Source : Ahmad and Gupta, 1989, Nazir *et al.*, 2011a

Under National Agricultural Innovation Project entitled "A Value Chain on Enhanced Productivity and Profitability of Pashmina", the quality characteristics of pashmina produced in different areas of Changthang viz; karjung, tsaga, samdoo, anlay, chomar, kharnak, korzok, koyal and samad has been assessed. It is reported that the undercoat, guard hair and dusting loss percentages (evaluated manually) were reported highest in pashmina of tsaga (67.55±2.27), samdoo (28.76±5.83) and samad (54.37±2.48) respectively. Fibre diameter (μ) and fibre length (mm) ranged from 12.94±0.21 (koyal) to 14.49±0.29 (karjung) and 56.28± 3.05 (koyal) to 75.76±2.05 (kharnak) respectively. The grease content (%) showed non-significant difference with a range from 5.75±1.38 to 8.64±0.35. The study revealed that the pashmina showed variation in quality from different areas of rearing due to the difference in their environmental conditions viz; temperature, wind velocity, altitude, vegetation cover etc (Sofi *et al.*, 2011).

Pashmina is utilized for the development of aesthetic products like knitwear and woven fabrics. In India, majority of Pashmina is utilized for preparation of shawls in Kashmir valley which is mostly hand spun and hand woven. Processing of Pashmina is an age old practice. Pashmina products prepared in Kashmir are known for its quality throughout the world. Not only the quality of the fibres but the process of manufacturing involving sorting, dusting, spinning and especially weaving has given these Pashmina products a special importance in the world.

Developments in Processing and Product Development

Under the ICAR funded National Agricultural Innovation Project (NAIP) subproject entitled "A Value Chain on Enhanced Productivity and Profitability of Pashmina Fibre" with SKUAST-K as lead centre and CSWRI-Avikanagar, CSK HP KVV Palampur and Sheep Husbandry Department as Partners, various developments have been achieved in processing and product development from pashmina fibre.

1. Sorting/ Dehairing

Sorting/dehairing means separation of guard hair from undercoat/pashmina from which is done with great care, so as to minimize the loss of valuable fiber. This sorting of pashmina was traditionally being done manually, mostly by women folk. Now with the introduction of machines, this sorting/ removal of guard hairs is carried out by the dehairing machines. The comparative quality of pashmina dehaired manually and with machine are presented in Table 2 and 3.

Table 2: Effect of Dehairing Methods on the Physico-chemical Quality of Pashmina.

Type	Fibre diameter (μ)	Medullation (%)	Fibre length (cms)	Scouring yield (%)	Guard Hair (%)	Fine fibre (%)
Machine Dehaired	12.66 ± 0.16	Nil	6.27±0.23	75.80±1.12	58.51	41.49
Manually Dehaired	13.19 ± 0.62	Nil	8.07±1.33	72.92±0.00	26.09	73.91

Source: Wani *et al.*, 2004

Table 3 : Effect of Machine Dehairing on the Quality of Pashmina Fibre

Parameter	Manually dehaired	Machine Dehaired
Fiber diameter (μ)	12.57 ± 0.64[a]	12.25 ±0.11[a]
Fiber Length (mm)	60.33 ± 0.21[b]	49.04 ± 0.19[a]
Bundle strength (g/tex)	10.1 ± 0.11[a]	9.03 ± 0.28[a]
Coefficient of friction (μ)	0.61 ± 0.005[b]	0.58 ± 0.007[a]

Source: Nazir *et al.*, 2011b

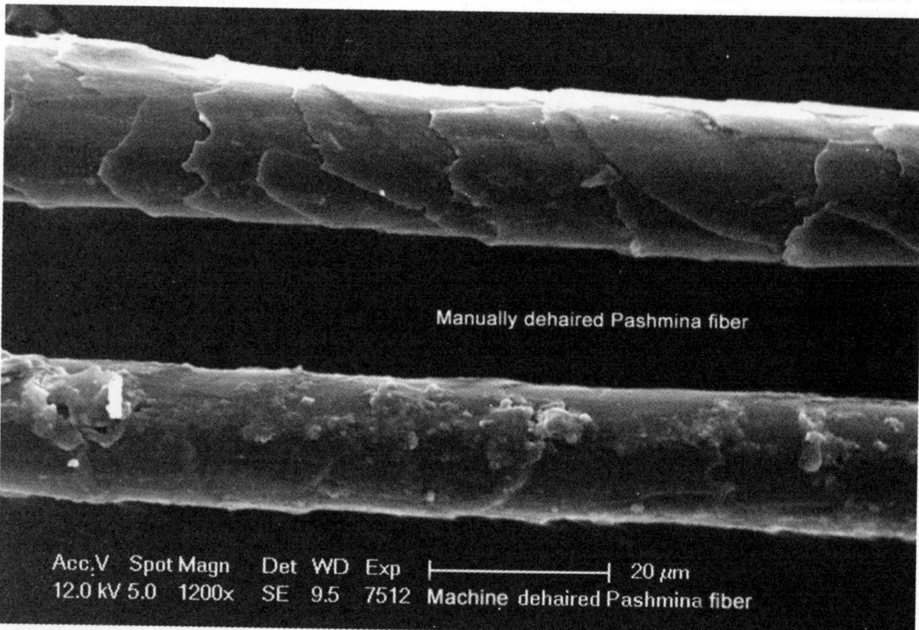

Fig 1 : Surface property of Pashmina Fibre Dehaired Manually and with a Machine
Source: Nazir *et al.*, 2011b

Although with the introduction of machine dehairing, there is reduction in processing time i.e. dehairing but at the same time it leads to the reduction in strength of fibres and also damages the surface structure due to the repeated passage of fibres through dehairing machine as is evident from SEM images. Due to the damage of delicate fibres, the final product may have a short life as compared to the product developed from manually dehaired fibres. Thus, there was a need to develop a dehairing system where in maximum recovery is possible with minimum passage through dehairing machine/rollers or any recovery system. Keeping in mind, the improvisation in the dehairing machine has been carried out where the number of passages of pashmina fibre between the rollers of dehairing machine has been reduced from 5 to only 3 with maximum recovery of undercoat. Initial trails have shown promising results and are under further study.

2. Spinning

Spinning is a processing step where fibre is being converted into a yarn which is usually done by women folk on a traditional spinning wheel known as *Yander*. It is a difficult task as it leads to a lot of physical stress in the form of backache, numbness in the legs etc besides being less remunerative to the artisans. Keeping in view the importance of Pashmina shawls, made from hand spun Pashmina and physical stress to the artisans, attempts were made to reduce the stress and increase remuneration by fabrication of an innovative Charka without compromising with the quality of yarn. Four types of charkhas (small size model, ball bearing model, paddle operated model and Table top model) were fabricated. Out of these, Table Top Model proved efficient. The charka comprises of two parts. One being Table Top and another is small spinning wheel. The spinner sits on a stool and operates the charka with her foot. The fabrication of innovative charkha resulted in a reduction of physical drudgery to the artisans, increased remuneration as against traditional one without deterioting the quality of yarn. Tables 4 shows the Percentage increase in spinning Efficiency of Improved Charkha over traditional one.

Table 4 : Spinning Efficiency of Improved Charkha over Traditional One.

S. No.	Parameter	Traditional Charkha	Innovative Charkha
1.	Time taken to spun 10 gm of Pashmina **(hours)**	27.8±0.49	15.95±0.43
2.	Increased efficiency of innovative charkha over traditional one (%)	-	**74.29**
3.	Spinning Charges /10 gms **(Rs)**	160	160
4.	Amount earned by a spinner/hr **(Rs)**	5.57	10.03
5.	Working hrs/day	7	7
6..	Working hrs/month	210	210
7.	Income/month **(Rs)**.	1169	2106
8.	Increase in income over traditional one **(Rs)**.	-	**937**
8.	Increase in net return/ month for improved Charkha over traditional one (%)	-	**80.15**

Table 5 presents the comparative quality of pashmina yarn spun on the both traditional and innovative charkha is as follows:

Table 5 : Comparative Quality of Pashmina Yarn Spun on Traditional and Innovative Charkha

Parameter	Yarn spun on Traditional Charkha	Yarn spun on Innovative Charkha
Actual Count (Nm)	61.18 ±1.53	68.80±0.76
Actual Tex (gm/Km)	17.35±0.95	14.57±0.35
Conditioned Count(Nm)	63.58±1.55	70.28±0.81
Tex (gm/Km)	16.65±0.91	14.27±0.37
No. of fibres/cross section	68.13± 0.89[b]	58.42± 0.69[a]
No. of Twists /inch	10.42± 0.24[b]	8.76± 0.21[a]
Breaking Load (gm. wt.)	42.107±0.36	42.25±0.37
Percent Elongation (%)	4.123±0.14	4.174±0.13
Tensile Strength (N/mm^2)	3824±4.51	2350±2.77
Tenacity (gm wt./ tex)	2.53	2.35

Source: Wani *et al.*, 2011

3. Dyeing of Pashmina

The pashmina fabrics are being dyed with a synthetic colouring agent besides some natural materials. These synthetic dye materials are very harmful as far as environmental safeguard is concerned. Furthermore, there are some naturally available plant materials which otherwise goes waste has a great potential to be used as a dyeing material for pashmina fabrics. Keeping in view these facts, the waste material like pomegranate rind, walnut husk, saffron flower waste, onion peel etc have been used for dying of Pashmina fabrics/yarn. The results are very promising with good colour fastness to washing and light (4-5) and are in line with BIS standards (Raja *et al.* 2010). Table 6 indicates the colour fastness results of pashmina shawls dyed with natural colouring materials from plant sources.

Table 6 : Colour Fastness of Dyed Pashmina Shawls using Natural dyes

S. No.	Detail of dye and mordant	Colour fastness to Dry cleaning		Colour fastness to washing		Colour fastness to light
		Staining on solvent	Change in colour	Staining on cotton/wool	Change in colour	
1.	Walnut mordanting with Ferrous sulphate	4	4	4/4-5	3-4	3.5
2.	Onion mordanting with stanus chloride	3-4	4	4/4-5	3-4	3
3.	Onion mordanting with Ferrous sulphate	3-4	4	4/4-5	3	4
4.	Saffron mordanting with stanus chloride	4	4	4/4-5	3	3
5.	Pomegranate with mordanting Ferrous sulphate	3-4	4	3-4/4	3-4	4
6.	BIS Standards for dyed worsted shawl	3-4 or better	3-4 or better	3-4 or better	3-4 or better	4 or better
7.	Wool marks (TWC)	3	3-4	4	3-4	3 or better

4. Developments in Machine Spinning of Pashmina

Pashmina fibres are very delicate and fragile, hence cannot be spun on a machine as there is a breakage of fibres, hence the fibres are blended with a carrier fibre viz; Nylon which increase its strength for machine spinning. Table 7 presents the comparative quality of hand spun and machine spun yarn after blended with nylon:

Table 7 : Comparative Quality of Hand Spun and Machine Spun Yarn.

Parameter	Hand spun yarn	Machine spun yarn
No. of fiber in cross-section (*Double ply yarn*)	39.10 ± 2.23^a	56.6 ± 2.61^b
Twist per inch	4.23 ± 0.31^a	4.70 ± 0.20^a
Actual count (Nm) (*Double ply yarn*)	56.65 ± 1.19^b	49.02 ± 2.22^a
Actual count (Nm) (*Single ply yarn*)	112.69 ± 0.47^a	98.04 ± 0.01^b
Tex (g/km)	17.75 ± 0.33^a	20.0 ± 1.04^a
Breaking strength (g.wt)	60.9 ± 0.003^a	56.2 ± 0.002^a
Elongation (%)	33.13 ± 2.37^a	50.21 ± 4.31^b
Tenacity (gwt/tex)	3.41 ± 0.20^b	2.80 ± 0.14^a
Bending length (gwt/cm^3)	21.83 ± 1.95^a	29.20 ± 3.10^a
Coefficient of friction (μ)	0.93 ± 0.006^b	0.76 ± 0.004^a

Source: Nazir *et al.* (c)

The biggest disadvantage with the nylon is that it can be removed from pashmina yarn by dipping in HCl solution which indirectly damaging the fibre resulting in reduction in life of a product. Efforts are being made to replace the nylon with PVA as carrier fibre with the objective that the life of the product made from machine spun yarn will improve as the PVA can be removed from the final product by dipping the shawl in boiling water instead of HCl as was the case with Nylon. Initial trails have shown very promising results.

5. Weaving

Traditionally the pashmina shawls are being developed from the king of fibres on traditional handlooms. Although the shawls prepared in this way are known all over the world for their aesthetic feel, handle and touch, but is painstaking and time consuming. Attempts have been made to develop these shawls on woolen handlooms from both hand spun and machine spun pashmina yarn which should increase the efficiency without detiorting the quality of a fabric. The Total hand value of pashmina shawls developed from hand spun and machine spun yarn on both traditional and woolen handlooms is presented in Table 8 revealing that the THV of Pashmina shawls prepared from hand spun pashmina yarn is significantly superior to machine spun yarn. It further has revealed that the THV of shawls woven on traditional loom are non-significantly different that shawls woven on woolen looms.

Table 8 : Total Hand Value of Pashmina Shawls (Source: Nazir *et al.* 2010)

Parameter / Fabric Type	Total Hand Value (score out of 5)*		
	Female	*Male*	*Overall Average*
HSTL	4.7±0.30[c]	3.8±0.58[a]	**4.25±0.34[b]**
HSWL	3.6±0.25[a]	3.6±0.60[a]	**3.60±0.30[b]**
MSTL	3.2±0.20[a]	1.4±0.40[b]	**2.30±0.36[a]**
MSWL	2.1±0.01[b]	3.0±0.36[ab]	**2.55±0.34[a]**

6. Value addition

Value addition means the aesthetic exquisite and attractive appearance of the products which one intends to buy and in reciprocal it will begets more sales, better customer's satisfaction, resulting in repeat customers and spin-off of good reputation. Value addition can be done by number of ways including. Cost of production can be reduced by blending of Pashmina with fine merino tops, angora, silk etc. which can be achieved immediately after dehairing. Studies on this aspect carried out at Sher-e-Kashmir University of Agricultural Sciences and Technology of Kashmir, wherein it was reported that Pashmina wool blend ratio of 80:20, 70:30, and 50:50 reduced cost up to 30-40%. It was concluded that up to 30% blending, products are of comparative quality at both yarn and fabric level. The effect of blending on properties of Pashmina yarn/fabric is presented in Tables 9, 10 and 10.

Table 9 : Effect of Blending on Properties of Pashmina Yarn

Sample	Fibre Diameter (μ)	Theoretical Count (Nm)	Metric count (Actual Nm)	No. of fibres / cross section
Pure	13.51 ± 0.01	132.18	56.72	31.88
70:30 wool	14.42 ± 0.04	116.02	81.54	41.66
80:20 wool	15.66 ± 0.86	98.37	74.49	32.33
80:20Angora	14.86 ± 1.12	109.25	30.62	35.66
50:50 wool	16.33 ± 0.38	90.47	38.7	42.33

Source: Wani, 2003

Table 10 : Effect of Blending on Physical Quality of Pashmina Shawls

Type	No. of samples	Fibre Diameter (μ)	Wrap (No of ends per inch)	Weft (No of ends per inch)	Weight (gm)
Pure	11	13.51± 0.01	18.4±0.29	13.6 0.24	210
70:30 wool	14	15.66+0.86	27.82 9.82	13.7 9.17	209.58
80:20 wool	11	14.42± 0.14	28.86 0.92	18.43 0.89	182.23
80:20 Angora	11	14.86±1.12	33 0.12	18.35 0.20	173.33
50:50 wool	10	16.33±0.38	34 0.14	18.40 0.22	178.75

Source: Wani *et al.* 2004

Angora Rabit Hairs Production, Processing and Value Addition

Many types of Angora rabbits viz., Russian, British and German have been introduced in the country in order to enhance the hair productivity. The present level of production ranges between 200 to 600 g per animal per year depending upon the type of animals and sells at an average price of about Rs.500/- to 600/- per kg. Of the three types introduced in the country, the German Angora has been found to give highest production as well as better and longer fibre with less coarse (guard) hair content both in selective as well as crossbreeding with other Angora types. As in case with other speciality fibres the processing/utilization techniques need special attention. Angora rabbit hair blends with compatible fibres for textile use were introduced in India about few years back. The CSWRI also developed processing technology for utilization rabbit hair fibres. Research results achieved so far indicate that rabbit hair can be utilized in blends with wool, silk and polyester in order to improve product performance as well as reduce the production cost. The results on processing trials indicate that rabbit hair polyester blends can be processed on cotton spinning systems. Appropriate rabbit hair blended yarns can be used for producing suitable knitwears, shawls etc. Utilization of rabbit hair blends can be efficiently and profitably used in the decentralized sectors with the help of Charkha and other Khadi Spinning Units for enhancing rural employment potential. The research and development efforts need to be strengthened for enhancing the production as well as evolving product utilization technologies particularly for eliminating the problems of static electric charge and abrasion losses during processing the fibres.

Table 11 : Effect of Blending on Mechanical Quality of Pashmina Shawls

Type	Shrinkage %		Air permeability $m^3/m^2/min$	Thermal conductivity Wm^0K	Water permeability (Cone test)
	Wrap way	Weft way			
Pure	0.13	(-)0.66	65.7	0.0142	Leakage
70:30 wool	0.67	(-)0.93	74.6	0.0150	....″....
80:20 wool	0.61	(-)1.07	92.8	0.0119	....″....
80:20Angora	(-)0.13	(-)0.67	80.8	0.0114	....″....
50:50 wool	0.93	(-)0.94	81.8	0.0172	....″....

Source: Wani *et al.*, 2004

The Khadi system hand spinning and handloom weaving is favoured for rabbit processing because it requires less quantity of fibre for processing with negligible waste and is a high labour intensive system. Moreover the processing machinery can be made available in rural parts. Rabbit hair with limited production cannot meet the requirement of large mills. Its use is more appropriate in the decentralized Khadi sector. As rabbit hair rearing has been started by CSWRI and considering all aspects, some experimental processing trails were undertaken to study the processing performance of rabbit hair fibre in blends with cotton, wool and polyester in Khadi machinery.

Blending with Cotton

Angora rabbit hair and Hybrid-4 cotton were taken for experiments. Rabbit hair and cotton in proportions of 25/75, 50/50 and 75/25 were thoroughly opened and blended manually. Rabbit hair is very strongly charged in comparison to wool. Antistat finishes reduce the electrostatic charge to almost half. So to avoid the development of electrostatic charges 2% cirrsol, an antistatic agent was sprayed on all over the blends. These blends were processed in different Khadi preparatory machines for opening, carding, drawing, roving and then spun on Amber Charkha. While processing these blends on cotton Khadi system, no difficulty was encountered except some problem in the case of cent per cent rabbit hair at drumming stage. It was due lack of interfibre cohesion and light weight of rabbit hair which hindered the formation of proper web and its winding on the drum. Absence of crimp in rabbit hair is also one of the main factors responsible for its poor cohesion. There was no difficulty in spinning yarn up to 21 tex from 25/75 rabbit hair cotton blend. It is observed that rabbit (10.4 m) are quite similar in fineness. The yarn results in table show that with the increase in the proportion of cotton in the blend, the yarn tenacity increases and the percentage extension decreases. This is mainly due to higher breaking stress and lower breaking strain of cotton fibre.

Blending with Wool

Rabbit hair and finer wool were opened thoroughly and the vegetable matter present in wool was removed manually. They were further opened and blended in Khadi opener. Rabbit/hair/wool were blended in the proportion of 25/75, 50/50 and 75/25. These blends were also processed on a Torigoe, Japan make worsted card having two cylinders two doffer arrangements. The sliver and the carded web of these lots were taken for spinning on Bhageshwari, Ghantaria and Amber Charkhas. These blends were tried on cotton Khadi system also. Yarns could be prepared out of two rabbit hair-wool blends viz.

25/75 and 50/50 on Ghantaria and Bhageshwari Charkhas. The blend having 75% rabbit hair could not be converted into yarn because the preparatory process employed failed to give a thorough blend and subsequently the yarn prepared was highly uneven having distinct dominating lumps of rabbit hair and wool at places. The yarn spun on Bhageshwari Charkha out of worsted card web or sliver was better than the yarn prepared out of the blend made on Khadi preparatory openers. In general, wool tops prepared on worsted set of machinery are used for spinning on Amber Charkhas. The sliver prepared on worsted card was drawn twice on Khadi preparatory machine and taken for spinning. Since this process omits combing the sliver prepared had short fibres and hence its spinning on Amber Charkha resulted in an irregular yarn. But a combination of worsted sliver and decentralized charka spinning found to provide spinnability of around 50 tex yarn. Finer (29 tex) and stronger yarn could be spun from polyester/rabbit hair blends. The polyester blended yarn has exhibited a superior tenacity of 19.0 as compared to 7.8 of Merino yarn (Table 13). Muffler cloth and shawls were woven on handloom out of two plied yarns. Also knitted sweater was prepared on hand flat 6 gauge knitting machine out of pure wool and rabbit hair blends with polyester and wool. On overall judgment of fabrics it is observed that 25-50% inclusion of rabbit hair in blended fabrics makes a superior fabric in comparison to all wool fabrics in respect of softness, whiteness, fullness, warmth, stretch and recovery properties.

Table 12 : Rabbit hair Cotton Blended Yarn properties

Blend Proportion %	Linear density, tex	Tenacity g/tex	Extension %
Rabbit hair: Cotton			
100: 0	43.3	2.27	7.4
75: 25	44.7	5.25	7.6
50:50	39.6	5.50	6.6
25:75	21.3	6.34	4.8
0:100	24.2	7.52	2.8

Spinning of Wool-Angora rabbit hair on modified cotton card

Bharat Merino wool from Southern Regional Research Centre of Central Sheep and Wool Research Institute (CSWRI), Mannavanur having 22μ diameter, 40-50 mm staple length and Angora rabbit hair

Table 13 : Rabbit hair Wool Blended Yarn properties

Yarn sample/ Proportion	Tex	Tenacity g/tex	Extension %	Charkha used
Rabbit hair: Wool (100 : 0)	43.3	2.29	7.4	Amber
Rabbit hair : Crossbred Wool (25 : 75)	80.5	1.57	7.3	Bhageshwari (Spun from open fibres)
	52.5	2.00	7.2	Bhageshwari (Spun from sliver)
	52.5	5.33	16.1	Worsted sliver and Charkha combination
Rabbit hair : Crossbred Wool (50 : 50)	64.7	2.20	7.6	Bhageshwari Charkha (Spun from open fibres)
Rabbit hair : Nilgiri Wool (50 : 50)	55.4	4.48	14.9	Worsted sliver and Charkha combination
Rabbit hair : Nilgiri Cross (50 : 50)	45.6	6.02	17.6	-do-
Rabbit hair : Merino (0 : 100)	44.6	7.81	17.0	-do-
Rabbit hair : Polyester (50 : 50)	28.6	18.99	12.5	-do-

from North Temperate Research Station of CSWRI, Garsa having 12ì diameter and 60 mm staple length were used for this study. Rabbit hair (RH) was blended with Bharat Merino (BM) wool in three different proportions i.e. 28:72, 40:60 and 60:40 at carding stage using modified cotton card at slow speed to avoid breakage of fibres and produce homogeneous blend. Antistatic agents were not used during carding stage. The blends were then spun into yarn on semi worsted system using gill box, roving frame and worsted ring frame. All the three blended yarns were then used to prepare the shawls using wool-polyester (60:40) blended yarn (2/70 Nm, 8.54 g/tex tenacity, 10% extension and 177 tpm) as warp in 3/1 twill weave pattern on powerloom. During spinning, it was observed that rabbit hair could be blended up to 60% without any difficulties. The developed yarns were used to produce shawl fabric using powerloom, followed by dyeing with reactive dye and finishing with cationic softener. The performance of the shawls showed that softness and thermal insulation of the shawls was increased with the increase in the proportion of Angora rabbit hair from 28 to 60%. The abrasion loss was also less when the rabbit hair proportion was increased in the shawls (Raja et. al, 2011). Another study, the Bharat merino wool was blended with rabbit hair in the proportion of 50:50, 40:60 and 30:70. This study further confirms earlier results.

Knitwear Garments

Knitted garments were developed out of Rabbit hair acrylic blended yarns which posses unique properties like smoothness, bulkiness and brightness. Blends of Rabbit hair, Acrylic non shrinkable and Acrylic shrinkable fibres in the proportion of 20:60:20 is having better knitted fabric properties with 7.07 cm/bulk, 174.2 g/cm hardness, 4.42 cal/C Mt. Hr. then conductivity as compared to other blends. It also reveals that elongation at break is 10_15% higher in the blend of rabbit hair ANS: AS (20:60:20) than others. It may be summarized that excellent knitted garments could be developed out of Rabbit has acrylic blended yarns, which may encourage rabbit hair utilization in organized worsted sector. It helps Rabbit woolgrower for getting high price for Rabbit wool with increasing demand in knitting sector.

References

Ahmad Sarfaraz and Gupta. N.P. 1989. Studies on Changthangi Pashmina I. *The Indian Textile Journal*. Pp 80-89.

Anonymous, 2005. Princess Draperies. *Darpan*. Sep-Oct, 2005: pp 70-72.

Anonymous, 2009. Cited from *www. Natural Fibres.org*.

Beileli, T 1982. High quality wool and hair fibres. Some special animal fibres. Industrial Textiles No. 1122. pp 423-426.

Deb, S.M. 1998. Performance of Pashmina (Cashmere) Goat on Kumaon Himalayas. *Indian Journal of Animal Science*. 68: 954-956.

Darokhan, M.D.; Tomar, N.S. 1983. Studies on Pashmina Yield of Changthangi Goats. *Indian Veterinary Journal*. 60 (8): pp 650-653.

Dauletbaev, B.S.; Aryngaziev, S. 1980. Yield and quality of undercoat in cross bred goats. *In Rezultaty soveshenstvouniya porod ovets Kazakhstana*, pp 139-141

Ganai, T.A.S, Kiramani, M.A., Ganai, N.A. and Tundup, T. 2004. Pashmina (Changthangi) Goats beyond period of the longest and shortest day. *Proceeding of the Conference of India Society of Animal Genetics and Breeding and Nutritional Symposium on Conservation of Livestock and Poultry:* pp: 16-17.

Miller, P, 1986. The Performance of Pashmina Goats. *Animal Breeding Abstracts.* 54: 181-199.

Nazir, A; Shakyawar DB; Wani Sarfaraz A and Sofi Asif H, 2010. Comparative study on Total hand Value of pashmina shawl developed by using hand and machine spun yarn. *Proceedings of 39th Textile Research Symposium.* IIT Delhi. 16th -18th Dec. pp: 526-528.

Nazir, A; Wani Sarfaraz A; Shakyawar DB and Sofi Asif H; Ishrat Yaqoob and Sheikh FD. 2011a. Physico-mechanical Quality of Changthangi pashmina. *VetScan- Online journal. (In Press)*

Nazir, A; Wani Sarfaraz A; Shakyawar DB and Sofi Asif H; Ishrat Yaqoob and Sheikh FD. 2011b. Effect of machine Dehairing on Quality of pashmina. *Indian Journal of small ruminants. (In Press)*

Nazir, A; Wani Sarfaraz A; Shakyawar DB and Sofi Asif H; Ishrat yaqoob and Sheikh FD. 2011c. Comparative study on quality of shawls made from hand and machine-spun pashmina yarns. *Indian Journal of Fibre and Textile Research. (In Press)*

Raja, ASM; Shakyawar DB; Pareek PK and Wani, Sarfaraz A, 2010. Comparative study on Total hand Value of pashmina shawl developed by using hand and machine spun yarn. *Proceedings of 39th Textile Research Symposium.* IIT Delhi. 16th -18th Dec. pp: 298-301.

Raja A.S.M., Ammayappan L., Shakyawar D.B. and Gupta N.P. 2011. Production and performance of angora rabbit hair- bharat merino Wool blended shawls. Indian Journal of Small Ruminants 2011, 17(1): 79-82

Ryder, M.L. 1984. Prospects for cashmere production in Scotland. *Wool record.* Nov. 1984. pp 37, 43.

Ryder, M.L. 1987. Cashmere, Mohair and other luxury animal fiber for breeders and spinner. *Ospreyclose.* Southampton. So18Ex.

Sahni, K.L. 1981. Project Coordinators report 1980. Central Institute of Research on goat Makhdoom.

Sofi Asif H; Wani Sarfaraz; Sheikh, F.D; Matoo F A; Ishrat Yaqoob, Kirmani, M. A. and Khan A A, 2011. Comparative Study on Quality of Pashmina from Different Areas of Changthang Region of Ladakh. *National Seminar on Prospects and retrospect of small ruminants and rabbit production: Contribution to Socio-economic security.* ISSGPU. 7th to 10th Dec 2011.

Singh, V.K. 2004. Polices for research/development of Angora rabbit/Pashmina production in the changing scenario of the country. *Souvenir of National Seminar on Angora Rabbit Wool and Cashmere Production and Utilization:* pp, 8-24.

Wani, S.A. 2003. National Agricultural Technology Project Report on "Processing of wool/ Hair for Value Added Products".

Wani, S.A., Ishrat, Y., Salahuddin, M. and Malik, A.H. 2004. Processing and Product development from Cashmere fiber. *Souvenir of National Seminar on Angora Rabbit Wool Cashmere Production and Utilization:* 25-26.

Wani, S.A. and Wani, M.H. 2007. Economics of Pashmina Production under pastoralist nomadic system of management in cold arid region of Jammu and Kashmir. *World Journal of Agricultural Sciences.* 3 (6): 788-795.

Wani Sarfaraz A, Sofi Asif H, Ishrat Yaqoob and Shayawar D.B. 2011. Comparative Quality of pashmina yarn spun on traditional and innovative charkha (Unpublished).

❑❑❑

Chapter 29

Advances in Eco-Friendly Processing of Woollen Textiles

A.S.M. Raja and Ajay Kumar
Division of Textile Manufacture and Textile Chemistry
Central Sheep and Wool Research Institute, Avikanagar-304 501 (Rajasthan)

Textile wet processing industry consumes large quantity of water and it is based on chemical application for scouring, bleaching, dyeing and finishing of textile materials. The industry is considered as one of the major environment polluting industries. The textile wet processing industries use harmful chemicals and release of large quantities of acids, alkalis and organic dyes into water channels. Another concern with this industry is the emission of green house gases (GHG) on earth, owing to its huge size and scope. Many processes and products that go into the making of fibers, textiles and apparel products consume significant quantities of fossil fuel. Apparel and textiles account for approximately 10% of the total carbon impact. The estimated consumption of electricity and water for an annual global production of 60 billion kg of fabrics was estimated at 1 trillion kilowatt hrs and 9 trillion liters of water (Valerio, 2010). Hence, textile based industries are the prime targets of the environmentalists for their crusade against pollution.

Woollen sector constitutes about 4% of the total textile industries. Even though small in size, the sector requires huge amount of water especially for scouring, carbonization, bleaching and dyeing. Therefore, lot of efforts has been taken to develop eco-friendly methods for processing of wool fibres. Most of the eco-friendly process aims at developing a method which will

- Reduce the water consumption,
- Require lesser energy,
- Use of eco friendly chemicals, dyes and reagents for processing in place of harmful chemicals and dyes,
- Use of green processes like microwave, plasma, supercritical carbon dioxide etc and
- Produce minimum damage to wool during processing.

In order to attain above goal, several research programmes have been taken up. Briefly, the eco- friendly processing methods of wool can be classified into

- Enzyme based wool pretreatments, dyeing and finishing
- Solvent scouring
- Low temperature dyeing
- Natural dyes/additives for dyeing and finishing
- Plasma assisted processing
- Supercritical Carbon dioxide based chemical wet processing

Wool preparatory treatments

The shorn wool from sheep contains grease, a waxy substance and lot of acquired impurities like skin flakes, suint, sand, dirt and vegetable matter. These impurities are removed before the fibre is subjected to spinning operations. The following processes are employed for the above such purposes.

Scouring of wool: It is first process for removing the dirt, grease and other impurities from raw wool. The scouring of wool is normally carried out with hot solution of sodium carbonate and non-ionic surfactants (Dominguez *et al.*, 2003). The scouring loss depends on the grease content of wool. Generally, fine wool fibres exhibit 50% weight loss compared to 5-10% in the case of carpet and coarse wools. The grease that is removed (lanolin) from wool is considered as a valuable byproduct and can be used in the manufacture of many cosmetics and pharmaceuticals. Lanolin consists of a highly complex mixture of esters, alcohols, and fatty acids. The scouring wool needs large quantities of water and leads to environmental problem. Another problem related to wool scouring is fibre entanglement. These problems have renewed interest in solvent scouring using trichloroethylene. Though the solvent scouring process is slightly costly, the process use lower water and energy. The solvent can be recovered and can be reused.

The other important development in the eco-friendly scouring process is the use of enzymes. Different enzymes like xylanase, protease and pectinase either alone or in combination were found to scour the fibers as efficiently as soap, but without causing any physical damage to the fibers (Das and Ramaswamy, 2006). The grease, wax obtained from the enzyme based scouring process is requiring minimum refinement compared to the soap/detergent based scouring process. After removing the grease, the water can be reused. For Indian wools which contain only 5-10% grease, it is proposed to use suint scouring process. In this process, the suint present in the wool can be acidified to produce soap which will clean the fibres. Though this process is time consuming, it is most suitable process for Indian wools. Some of the industries in India use this process for scouring.

Carbonizing of wool: Scouring does not always eliminate vegetable matter such as burrs and seeds. Heavily contaminated wool must go through a process known as carbonizing. If burrs are not removed at this stage, they can cling to the wool fibres and not be noticed until the process is complete. The process of carbonizing is the treatment of the vegetable matter with sulphuric acid followed by baking. The wool is steeped in the sulphuric acid solution, which causes the burrs to break up. The wool is then subjected to heat, which converts the disintegrated material into carbon. The burrs are then finally removed, firstly by crushing and then shaken out of the wool by a machine rotating at high speed. Any remaining impurities are thus blown out of the fibre. Following carbonizing, the wool should be rinsed and neutralized with mild alkali by a wet process. Such neutralization should be carried out immediately after baking; otherwise fibre damage will occur during storage of the wool in such an acidic state (Lewis, 1992). Like scouring, this process also requires large amount of water and chemicals for carbonization as well as neutralization of sulphuric acid. In addition, the disposal of sulphuric acid also poses very big problem for the industries. In order to solve this problem, it is attempted to use the combination of acid cellulose, pectinase and xylanase enzymes for carbonization application (El-Syed *et al.,* 2010). The enzyme based process is eco-friendly, require less energy and minimum damage to wool. There is no need for sulphuric acid. However, the cost of enzymes and complex processing are the limiting factors.

Bleaching of wool: Wool is generally bleached with an alkaline peroxide solution. Hydrogen peroxide and peroxy compounds damage wool fibres, due to progressive oxidation of disulfide bonds ultimately forming cysteic acid. This chemical change can lead to adverse effects on the fibre mechanical properties. The process also required to be carried out at higher temperatures for activation of hydrogen peroxide. There are some studies in literature, which shows that wool can be bleached using hydrogen peroxide in acidic condition with Prestogen W, a peroxide stabilizer from BASF containing organic acid salts (Gacen and Cayuela, 2000), as well as a mixture of citric acid and sodium acetate (Karunditu *et al.,* 1994). The bleaching of wool at acidic condition leads to lesser damage compared to alkaline condition.

Alternatively, the use of reducing agents for bleaching also proposed. However, the use of traditional textile reducing agents such as hydrosulphite, thiourea, tiourea dioxide, formamidine sulphinic acid, zinc formaldehyde sulphoxylate and sodium formaldehyde sulphoxylate for bleaching are problematic, since, even during minimal storage times, they lose strength through oxidation and generates environmentally hazardous by-products, using certain of those procedures. Furthermore, they also have dosage, storage, and odour and dust problems. As an alternative, sodium borohydride based bleaching process is developed. Sodium borohydride is a mild reducing agent with excellent stability in alkaline solution. Sodium borohydride based bleaching process was developed and patented by CSIRO and the process named as Colourclear™. The borohydride based bleaching process can be carried out in low temperature without much damage to wool compared hydrogen peroxide based bleaching process.

Dyeing of wool: Dyes used for dyeing the wool are either acid, metal complex, metal containing acid or reactive in nature. Wool fibre has large number reactive groups due to its heterogeneous side chain. Wool is needed to be dyed at boiling condition because of its higher glass transition temperature. Several research studies are reported in which wool is subjected to enzyme (Cardamone and Damert, 2006), UV light (Xin *et al.,* 2002) and plasma treatments (Kan and Yuen,

2006; Wakida *et al.*, 1993) in order to dye it in lower temperatures. Similarly, dyeing auxiliaries like leveling agents and dye penetration facilitating agents were developed to carry out the dyeing at low temperature with lesser time so that fibre entanglement and damage are at minimum.

Chromium either used in metal complex dyes or used as a mordant, is present in the majority of dyed wools. The threat to chrome dyeing systems from environmental legislation appears to have been reduced by the widespread adoption of optimized dyeing methods (Clarke and Steinle, 1995) and, in many cases, the installation of improved dye-house effluent treatment plants. The major dyestuff manufacturers have responded to the concerns over chromium by promoting alternative metal-free dyes. New reactive dyes (e.g. Lanasol CE – Ciba) and optimized ranges of metal-free acid dyes (Sandolan MF – Clariant) have been developed to achieve a balance of economy and performance comparable to chrome dyes in targeted applications such as piece and hank dyeing, especially bright fashion shades. Another important development in the dyeing of wool at low temperatures is liposome assisted dyeing. Liposome is a vesicle made up of lipid. Liposomes can be used to encapsulate the dye molecules and engineered for slow releasing process. It is reported that liposome assisted dyeing of wool with dyes produced higher exhaustion of dye at lower temperature (Montazer *et al.*, 2009).

Natural dyes: Wool is the most suitable fibre to be dyed with natural dyes due to its heterogeneous chemical structure. Wool materials have been traditionally dyed with henna extract since ancient time. The wool materials dyed with natural dyes exhibits good shade and fastness properties. Recently, the natural dyes extracted from different plants were converted into ready to use powders just like synthetic dyes using different drying techniques such as spray drying and freeze drying. Such developed natural dyes are available for all shades of colours. The wool materials can be comprehensively dyed with natural dyes. Another important aspect of the readymade natural dyes is that the dyes are certified under Global Organic Textile Standards (GOTS). The important dyes in this category are indigo, henna, lac, ratanjot, anotta etc. Several new sources were also identified for dyeing of wool like onion skin, saffron, silver oak, dhol kanali etc. The problem associated with the natural dyes is limited availability resources for extraction of dyes. In order to address this problem, it was attempted to use tannin containing deciduous plant leaves for extraction of dye and application on wool. The leaves of silver oak, wattle, tanners' senna and flame of forest were identified for extraction of dyes (Raja and Thilagavathi, 2008).

Wool finishing

Finishing to wool materials is done to enhance inherent unique properties and to impart several new functional characteristics like shrink resistance, handle, microbial resistance, and water repellency etc.

Shrink resistant finish for wool: This is the most commonly used finish for wool, which draw the attention of most of researchers on wool finishing. The major cause of wool shrinkage is overlapping of surface cuticle scales and this process is called as "differential frictional effect". This differential friction effect arises from the ratchet-like nature of the wool scales, with the pointed scale edges all pointing towards the tip. Movement of the fibres against any surface in the root to tip direction results in contact with the "smooth" surface of the scale and a low resistance to sliding. The basic mechanism of this type of finish is to remove the surface scales present in the wool fibre (approximately 10% of the total weight of the fibre) partly/completely, which are the major cause of shrinkage. The most widely used method is the use of chlorine/ chlorine salts, which disintegrates keratin molecules in the cuticle and removes the surface scales by oxidation. The action of this oxidative chemical is not restricted to the surface scale but also disintegrates keratins in the cortex of the wool leading to loss in tensile strength and weight and also leads to AOX (Absorbable Oxy Halides) formation in the effluents (Brady, 1997). Efforts have been made to use only polymer based shrink resistant finishes without the use of any oxidative chemicals like chlorine. The polymers like Synthappret BAP and Impranil DLV (Bayer), Protolan 367 and Terolin 352 (Rotta) can be applied by pad-dry cure process to wool. However, the hydrophobicity of the fibre surface has created difficulties in obtaining satisfactory adhesion of polymer during shrink resist treatments (Byrne, 1996). Over all, this finish introduced an important advantage of machine washability and tumble dryability (total easy care wool) to the wool materials like knitted goods and worsted fabrics.

Enzyme based shrink resistance and handle improvement processes for wool: With the advent of biotechnology, several enzyme based shrink resistance and handle improvement processes have been developed for wool materials. Most of them utilize the proteolytic properties of enzymes like protease (especially serine proteases) capacity to degrade the cuticle cells of the wool fibre. This protease enzyme treatment partially or completely removes the wool cuticle to impart shrink resistance. This process is considered as environmentally safe process compared to the chlorine-based process commonly used in wool industry. The protease enzyme treatment with lower concentration can be used to enhance the handle related properties of wool like softness, reduced prickliness, reduced pilling etc (Bishop *et al.*, 1998; Heine and Hocker, 1995).

It is well documented that papain, a proteolytic enzyme form plant origin was used for shrink proofing of wool in earlier years. However, the wool had to be pretreated with reducing agent like sodium sulphite to achieve effective shrink resistant property before enzyme treatment. The efficiency of the proteolytic enzyme papain in conferring shrink-resistance to wool tops and woven fabrics has been enhanced by pretreatment of the wool with lipase/sodium monoperoxyphthalate/ sodium sulphite (El-Syed *et al.*, 2001). The wool fabric is subjected to an alkaline protease (Perizym-AFW) treatment, which improved shrink resistance, whiteness, pilling behaviour, dyeability and washability. This process is called as Lanazym process, which is based on purely enzymatic anti felting finishing of wool (Brier, 2000). Levene (1997) found that sodium bisulphite pretreatment enhanced the activity of alkaline bacterial protease enzyme and had conferred better shrink resistance to wool tops and fabric. Among enzymes, Esperase was found to be most active while causing the least damage.

One of the major problems associated with the use of this enzyme is the excessive weight and strength losses in the treated wool materials. The enzyme due to its high reactivity and relatively small size (MW approximately 14–20 kDa for most proteases) penetrates into the cortex of the wool and hydrolyze the proteins and cell membrane complexes, which leads to higher weight loss and strength loss in the treated wool materials (Jovancic *et al.*, 2001). The surface of the enzyme treated wool is not smooth and uniform due to the uneven damage to the wool cuticle. Hence, it is necessary to give softening treatment with silicone or cationic-based finishing agent. At CSWRI, Aviaknagar it was attempted to use medium fine Chokla wool for making tweed fabrics. The developed fabric was treated with alkaline protease enzyme followed by silicone finishing treatment. By this treatment, the handle of the fabric was improved and could be used as a quality serge fabric. Similarly, it was attempted to reduce the pilling behaviour of Angora-Wool blended shawls using enzyme treatment.

Immobilized protease enzymes treatment: The activity of the enzyme can be restricted to the outer surface of cuticle in order to minimize the loss of weight and strength. For this purpose, the native enzymes were immobilized with polymers. A commercial protease, Esperase, was covalently linked to Eudragit S-100, a reversible soluble–insoluble polymer by carbo-diimide coupling. When compared to the native enzyme, the immobilized form presented a lower specific activity towards wool but a higher thermal stability at all temperatures tested. The optimum pH of the immobilized protease was shifted towards the alkaline side by about one pH unit while there was no change in optimum temperature between the free and immobilized protease. The immobilized protease exhibited a good storage stability and re-usability (Silva *et al.*, 2006). Similarly, proteases were modified with the soluble polymer polyethylene glycol (PEG) in the bio-finishing process of wool fibres, to target enzyme action to the outer parts of wool fibres. Different proteolytic enzymes from *Bacillus lentus* and *Bacillus subtilis* in native and PEG-modified forms were investigated and their influence on the modification of wool fibres morphology surface, chemical structure, as well as the hydrolysis of wool proteins, the physico-mechanical properties, and the sorption properties of 1:2 metal complex dye during dyeing were studied. SEM images of wool fibres confirmed smoother and cleaner fibre surfaces without fibre damages using PEG-modified proteases. Modified enzyme products have exhibited beneficial effect without severe fibre damage measured in terms of tensile strength and weight loss of the fibre (Jus *et al.*, 2007; Silva *et al.*, 2005).

In order to limit the action of protease within wool cuticle, the wool was pretreated with alkaline peroxide in the presence of high concentration of common salt. The presence of salt in the outer surface of wool improved the susceptibility of the outer surface scale protein for enzyme degradation (Lenting *et al.*, 2006).

Application of acid protease: The activity of alkaline protease enzymes on wool is depending on the pH of the treatment. The enzyme action is taking place between pH of 8.0-9.5 and a slight variation in the above pH range leads to deactivation of the enzyme. This problem is further aggravated by the fact that weak acids are rapidly released from wool during alkaline protease treatment due to the protein hydrolysis action of enzyme. Hence, during alkaline protease treatment on wool, the drop in pH towards acid side is evident and an optimum alkaline pH is maintained by intermediate addition of mild alkali to retain the enzyme activity. In order to avoid this problem, wool was treated with *Aspergillus usamii* L86 enzymes including acid protease and CMCase in acidic pH (Yu *et al.*, 2001) to improve the shrink resistance and handle. An acid protease enzyme from fungai source was applied on wool serge fabrics to improve the handle and shrink resistance and compared with the conventional alkaline protease. The results indicated that acid protease enzyme improved the handle as much as the alkaline protease but not shrink resistance (Raja and Thilagavathi, 2010).

Enzyme treatment and dye uptake: Enzyme pretreatment on wool fabric decreased the resistance of the fibre to dye diffusion and so it increased the adsorption rate constant and decreased in the apparent activation energy for the dyestuff when compared to untreated fabric (Riva *et al.*, 2002). Enzyme pretreatment of wool fabric with trypsin increased exhaustion of natural dye like crocin, beta-carotene, curcumin, chlorophyll and carmine without change in fastness property (Liakopoulou *et al.*, 1998; Tsatsaroni and Liakopoulou 1995).

Plasma processing of wool

The low temperature plasma (LTP) technique is used to modify wool surface to provide hydrophilicity, shrink resistance, etc. This is regarded as an environmental friendly process as no chemicals are used. Plasma is an ionized gas composed of charged and neutral particles. When this plasma is applied to the wool, the free electrons or other meta stable particles, upon collision with the substrate, break the chemical bonds, create free radicals like C=O,C–O, O–C=O, SO_3- on the polymer surface. These free radicals can undergo additional reactions depending on the gases in the atmosphere. Thus, the substrate can be coated with different kinds of gases without changing the fabric's bulk characteristics. Plasmas containing CF_4, C_3F_6, argon, or other hydrocarbon gases can provide hydrophobicity to the fabric. Similarly plasmas containing oxygen and nitrogen can provide hydrophilicity to the fabric. Several attempts were also made to give shrink resist finish using plasma as a pre treatment. The wool fabric was first treated with oxygen or nitrogen or mixture of nitrogen and hydrogen plasmas which resulted in the enhanced wettability of the surface due to the formation of more ionisable / free radical groups in the fibre surface. Then the shrink resistant finish was given using different kind of silicone polymers. The wool treated by this process showed increased shrink resistant property compared to the untreated one (Rajpreet *et al.*, 2004; Kan and Yeun, 2006).

Super critical carbon dioxide based processing wool

Chemical processing of textile materials in supercritical carbon dioxide has been identified as one of the alternatives to water-based conventional process. A supercritical fluid actually has physical properties somewhere between those of a liquid and a gas. Supercritical fluids are able to spread out along a surface more easily than a true liquid because they have lower surface tensions than liquids. At the same time, a supercritical fluid maintains a liquid's ability to dissolve substances that are soluble in the compound, which a gas cannot do. Supercritical fluids are by definition at a temperature and pressure greater than or equal to the critical temperature and pressure of the fluid. The critical pressure of carbon dioxide is about 1,070 pounds per square inch (psi) and critical temperature is about 31°C, so supercritical applications using carbon dioxide typically operate at temperatures between 32°C and 49°C and pressures between 1,070 and 3,500 psi. A pressure-temperature (P-T) phase diagram (Fig. 1) illustrates the nature of a supercritical fluid (Anon, 2011). Based on the above facts, the wool can be scoured and dyed using supercritical carbon dioxide medium instead of water. Separating residual dye from the CO_2 and recycling of CO_2 are easy. Energy is saved because processed materials do not need to be dried after the dyeing process. An additional advantage of supercritical CO_2 is the high diffusivity and low viscosity that allow the dye to diffuse faster towards and into the textile fibres. This results in a faster dyeing process.

Conclusion

The use of eco friendly methods for processing of wool is very much essential and need of the hour. There are several methods are available for greener processing route. The enzyme based processes, low temperature dyeing additives, natural dyes are well taken up by the industries. However, the adoption of the process like, plasma and supercritical carbon dioxide etc by the industries is very low due to the requirement of completely different set of costly machineries.

References

Anon. 2011. Basics of super fluid carbon dioxide cleaning. www.pprc.org/pubs/techreviews/co2/co2intro.html

Bishop, D.P., Shen, J., Heine, E. and Hollfelder, B. 1998. The use of proteolytic enzymes to reduce wool fibre stiffness and prickle, Journal of the Textile Institute 89: 546-553.

Brady, P.R. 1997. A Guide to the Theory and Practice of Finishing Woven Wool Fabrics. Brady P.R. (Ed.), CSIRO Wool Technology, Australia.

Brier, R. 2000. Lanazym process: Purely Enzymatic Antifelt Finishing of Wool. Melliand Textilberichte, 81: 298-302.

Byrne, K. 1996. Easy care wool woven products, Coloration Technology, 112: 350-353.

Cardamone, J.M. and Damert, W.C. 2006. Low-temperature dyeing of wool processed for shrinkage control. Textile Research Journal 76: 78-85.

Clarke, E.A. and Steinle, D. 1995. Health and environmental safety aspects of organic colorants, Review of Progress in Coloration 25: 1-5.

Dominguez, C., Jover, E., Bayona, J.M. and Erra, P. 2003. Effect of the carbon dioxide modifier on the lipid composition of wool wax extracted from raw wool. Analytica Chimica Acta 477: 233-242.

El-Sayed, H., Kantouch, A., Heine, E. and Hocker, H. 2001. Developing a zero-AOX shrink-resist process for wool: Part-1: Preliminary results. Coloration Technology 117: 234-238.

El-Sayed, H., Gabry, L. EI. and Kantouch, F. 2010. Effect of biocarbonisation of coarse wool on its dyeability. Indian Journal of Fibre and Textile Research 35: 330-336.

Gacen, J. and Cayuela, D. 2000. Comparison of wool bleaching with hydrogen peroxide in alkaline and acidic media. Coloration Technology 116: 13-15.

Heine, E. and Hocker, H. 1995. Enzyme treatments for wool and cotton. Review of Progress in Coloration 25: 57-63.

Jovancic, P., Jocic, D., Molina, R., Rosa Julia, R. and Erra, P. 2001. Shrinkage properties of peroxide-enzyme–biopolymer treated wool. Textile Research Journal 71: 948-953.

Jus, S., Schroeder, M., Guebitz, G.M., Heine, E. and Kokol, V. 2007. The influence of enzymatic treatment on wool fibre properties using PEG-modified proteases. Enzyme and Microbial Technology 40: 1705-1711.

Kan, C.W. and Yeun, C.W.M. 2006. Surface Characterization of low temperature plasma treated wool Fibre. Journal of Materials Processing Technology 178: 52-60.

Karunditu, A.W., Carr, C.M., Dodd, K., Mallinson, P., Fleet, I.A. and Tetler, L.W. 1994. Activated hydrogen peroxide bleaching of wool. Textile Research Journal 64: 570-572.

Lenting, H.B.M., Schroeder, M., Guebitz, G.M., Cavaco-Paulo, A. and Shen, J. 2006. New enzyme-based process-direction to prevent wool shrinking without substantial tensile strength loss. Biotechnology Letters 28: 711-716.

Levene, R. 1997. Enzyme enhanced bleaching of wool. Coloration Technology 113: 206-210.

Lewis, D.M. 1992. Wool dyeing. Society of Dyers and Colorists, Bradford, UK, ISBN 0901956538, 4.

Liakopoulou, K.M., Tsatsaroni, E., Laderos, P. and Geogiadou, K. 1998. Dyeing of cotton and wool fibers with pigments from *Crours sativs* - effect of enzymatic pretreatment. Dyes and Pigments 36: 215-221.

Montazer, M., Zolfaghari, A., Toliat, T. and Moghadam, M.B. 2009. Modification of wool surface by liposomes for dyeing with weld. Journal of Liposome Research 19: 173-179.

Raja, A.S.M. and Thilagavathi, G. 2008. Dyes from the leaves of deciduous plants with a high tannin content for wool. Coloration Technology 124: 285-289.

Raja, A.S.M. and Thilagavathi, G. 2010. Comparative study on the effect of acid and alkaline protease enzyme treatments on wool for improving handle and shrink resistance. Journal of the Textile Institute 101: 823-834.

Rajpreet, K.V., Gita, N.R., Bourham, M. and Bures, B.L. 2004. Plasma and antimicrobial treatment of nonwoven fabrics for surgical gowns. Textile Research Journal 74: 1073-1079.

Riva, A., Algeba, I. and Prieto, R. 2002. Dyeing kinetics of wool fabric pretreated with a protease. Coloration Technology 118: 59-63.

Silva, C.J.S.M., Prabaharan, M., Gübitz, G. and Cavaco-Paulo, A. 2005. Treatment of wool fibres with subtilisin and subtilisin-PEG. Enzyme and Microbial Technology 36: 917-922.

Silva, C.J.S.M., Zhang, Q., Shen, J. and Cavaco-Paula, A. 2006. Immobilization of proteases with a water soluble-insoluble reversible polymer for treatment of wool. Enzyme and Microbial Technology 39: 634-640.

Das, T. and Ramaswamy Gita N. 2006. Enzyme treatment of wool and specialty hair fibers. Textile Research Journal 76: 126-133.

Tsatsaroni, E. and Liakopoulou, K.M. 1995. Effect of enzyme treatment on the dyeing of cotton and wool fibres with natural dyes. Dyes and Pigments 29: 203-209.

Valerio, Z. 2010. www.textileworld.com/Articles/2010/July/July_August_issue/Features/Climate_Change_Carbon_ Mitigation_In_Textiles.html

Wakida, T., Tokino, S. and Niu, S. 1993. Dyeing properties of wool treated with low-temperature plasma under atmospheric pressure. Textile Research Journal 63: 438-442.

Xin, J.H., Zhu, R., Hua, J. and Shen, J. 2002. Surface modification and low temperature dyeing properties of wool treated by UV radiation. Coloration Technology 118: 169-173.

Yu, X.W., Guan, W.J., Li, Y.Q., Guo, T.J. and Zhou, J.D. 2005. A biological treatment technique for wool textile. Brazilian Archives of Biology and Technology 48: 675-680.

□□□

Chapter 30

Development of Woolen Khadi Spinning System

R. Chattopadhyay, D. B. Shakyawar[1] and Nishant Kumar
[1]Principal Scientist, Textile Manufacturing and Textile Chemistry, CSWRI, Avikanagar
Department of Textile Technology
Indian Institute of Technology, Huas Khas, New Delhi-11016

Woollen Khadi plays an important role in Indian economy by providing large scale employment in rural areas. During pre-independent era, Khadi products were symbol of national pride. Earlier, woollen Khadi products were made from indigenous wool available in Rajasthan, J&K, Himachal Pradesh and other parts of country. The present infrastructure set up of the Khadi sector in India speaks volumes about its importance in the Country's Economy (Anon, 2009).

Woollen Yarn Manufacturing

Yarn from fibre is an important intermediate stage of fabric manufacturing. There are four basic yarn-manufacturing systems that have become fairly well standardized. These stems are ring-carded cotton, ring combed cotton, woollen and worsted. Among four spinning systems, woollen spinning system is extensively used for spinning of coarse yarn of 2-12 Nm count. However, semi-worsted and worsted spinning systems are used for fine yarn production of

14-100 Nm. Later 60's, some new spinning systems have been developed with high production speed and some special features. Among them Siro and Solo-spinning systems have shown some potential for development of yarn from wool fibre (Ishtiaque, 1988).

Yarn manufacturing in Khadi Sector

Khadi sector employed charkha for yarn manufacturing from wool and wool blends. Spinning wheel is used to spin yarn from very coarse to fine count. The productivity of this system is very low due to single spindle. However, the quality of yarn is very good and finest yarn of 120 Nm could be spun from pashmina wool. Recently some modification has been made and paddle operated charkha has been developed.

New Model Charkha

In order to enhance the productivity, 4-8 spindle charkha has been developed. Roving sliver is used as a feed material and fibre passes through 3/3 drafting system and further twisting and winding is done. The only major difference between New Model Charkha (NMC) and other spinning system is that it is driven by human muscle and in other case it is driven by mechanical source. The overall processing sequences divide into two sections viz. worsted roving making and NMC spinning. The basic function of roving making is to remove the various natural or acquired impurities in the raw wool and to mechanical manipulate and mix the fibres to produce a roving sliver, a uniform, coherent sliver of parallel fibres free from entanglement and short fibres. The roving sliver provides the raw material for drafting and spinning where the mass per unit length is progressively reduced to produce a NMC yarn. The detail flow-chart of conversion from fibre to NMC yarn is shown in Figure 1. The amount of twist put into a yarn varies considerably and depends on the grade of the wool and type of yarn; long fibres generally require less twist than short ones. Wool grades based on the American blood count, English metric count, and the micron system; maximum possible finest yarn can be spun on worsted system.

The roving was further utilized for making yarn on New Model Charkha (NMC) varying different draft and twist level to achieve desire yarn count. New model charkha is a modified version of Amber charkha used in Khadi system for woollen spinning. The input material to the charkha is roving which contains 1000-2000 fibres in their cross section. In order to get optimal spinnability on spinning system, the numbers of fibres in the yarn cross section must be reduced to about 100. The reduction of fibres in the cross section is effected through drafting. In new model charkha, three rollers single-apron drafting system is used (Figure 2). During drafting the fibres are firmly nipped between the bottoms steel fluted roller and the weighted top pressure roller. The pressure is applied by spring weighting system. The roller pairs rotate at an incremental speed resulting stretch (i.e. draft) in the material nipped between the rollers. The controlled two stage stretching operations (i.e. drafting) elongate the feed roving and bring it to the required yarn dimension from the point of view of mass per unit length (Chattopadhyay *et al.,* 2003).

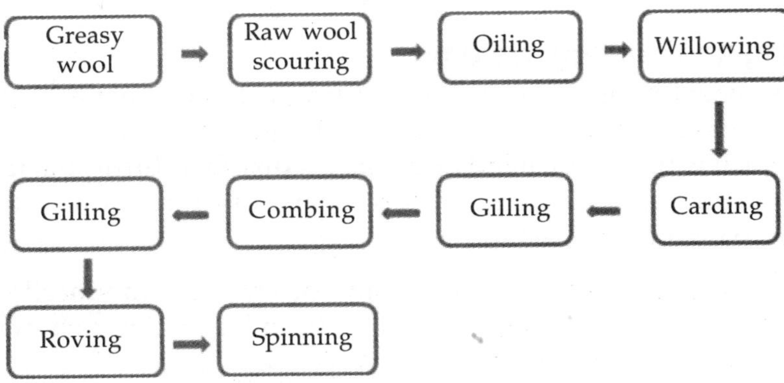

Fig. 1 : Flowchart of worsted system of processing

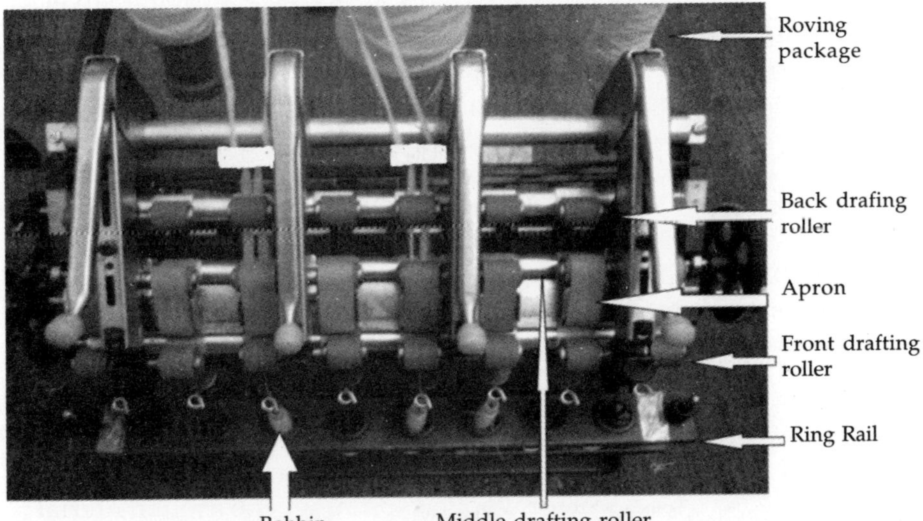

Fig. 2 : Systematic diagram of New Model Charkha (NMC)

Once the drafted product emerges from the nip of the front rollers, it is to be twisted to impart strength to the fibre matrix. Twist is imparted by the combination of ring and traveller. The spindle which holds the package (bobbin) causes the traveller to rotate on a ring. The yarn loop between the front rollers to the bobbin via the traveller causes required force to be imparted on the traveller by the spindle. Every revolution of traveller causes the yarn to be twisted around its own axis. The twisted yarn is simultaneously wound on the package. The ring rests on a platform which is made to oscillate from bottom to top of the package at a certain frequency. As the ring moves up and down, the traveller also follows the same and hence the yarn is guided from bottom to top of the bobbin for laying.

Gearing and drafting system

The charkha is operated by turning a handle usually. Pedal operated charkhas are also available. The prime mover is the main shaft which is turned by hand or pedal. As this shaft turns, the motion gets transmitted through a series of gears and pulleys to different rotating parts of the machine.

The bottom drafting rollers made of steel are mounted on an inclined roller stand having fixed brackets. In Figure 3 it is shown that

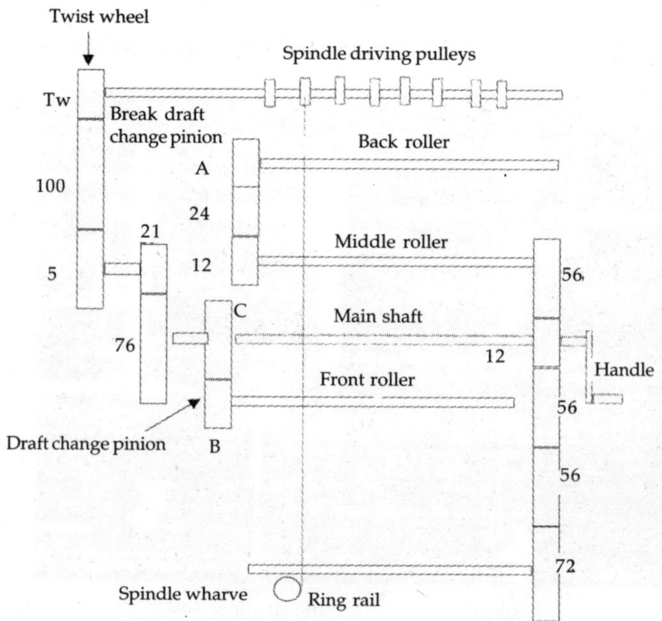

Fig. 3 : Gearing arrangement of NMC

the top rubber covered rollers are mounted in a pendulum lever arm which is pivoted in the machine frame. The lever can be swung to lift all the rollers together. The top rollers are pressed against the bottom steel rollers by spring pressure. The bottom rollers are positively driven and top rollers are surface driven. Certain flexibility in fixing the values of draft is required to be able to spin yarns of different fineness from the same feed material and hence while designing drive to the rollers change gears needs to be incorporated. Nip to nip distance between rollers shown in Figure 4.

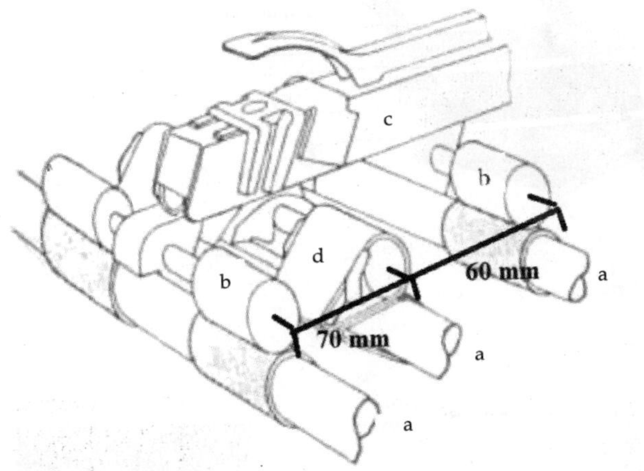

a. Bottom fluted roller, b. Top roller, c. Pendulum lever arm, d. Apron

Fig. 4 : Drafting System of NM Charkha

Siro Spinning system attachment for NM charkha

A SIRO spun yarn is produced on ring spinning frame by twisting together two strands, which have been separated in drafting zone. It produces a yarn with two strands and resultant yarn is essentially a single yarn. It is found to have greater abrasion resistance than equivalent single worsted yarn. It can thus be used directly as a warp for weaving without the usual two plying operation, resulted reduction in production cost of warp yarn as compared to conventional two plied yarn. Apart from low production cost, SIRO spun yarn also provides better handle and thermal insulation as compared to conventional worsted yarn (Ishtiaque, 1988).

NM Charkha has been used for spinning single yarns of 24-36 Nm in Khadi system using Australian merino top. The single yarn is essentially to be doubled for making waevable on handloom. In order to reduce cost of yarn production, SIRO technology is introduced in New model charkha. In SIRO spinning, two roving are fed simultaneously using Siro attachment (Roving Guide) having 10 mm spacing to achieve better the yarn uniformity.

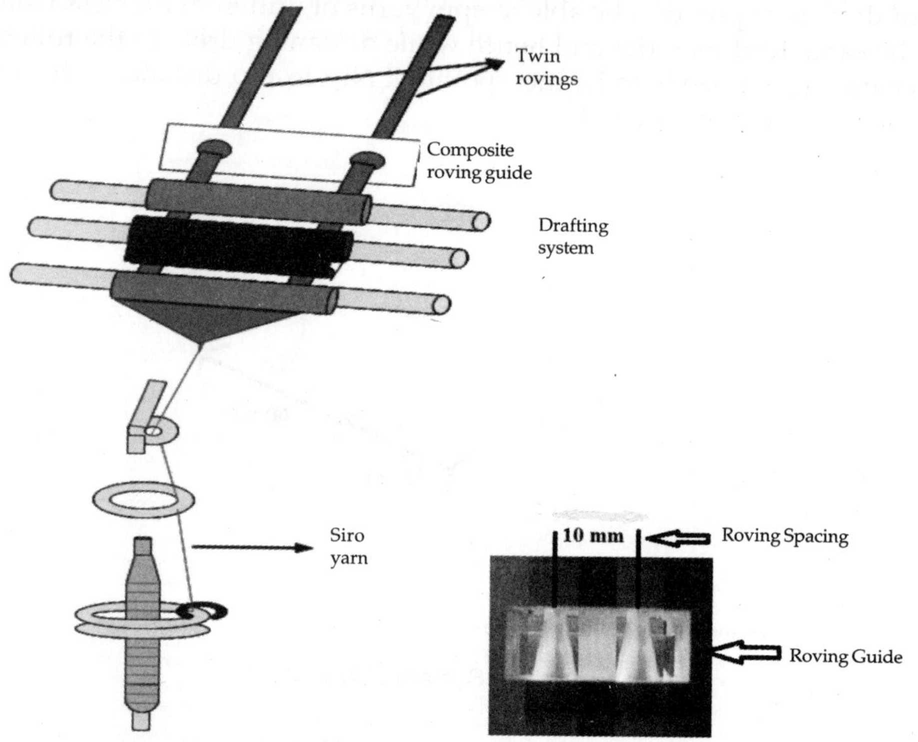

Fig. 5 : Diagram of Siro Spinning **Fig. 6 :** Roving Guide for NM Charkha.

Solo-Spinning

The Solospun™ process is a joint development by the Woolmark, CSIRO and WRONZ (Prins, 2009). It is a versatile, cost effective and highly efficient alternative to the two-fold, Sirospun™ process offering significant benefits in terms of efficiency, productivity and return on investment. As compared to two-fold yarn production, spinning costs and processing times are dramatically reduced, efficiency is improved; there are no plying (two-folding) costs and coarser micron wool can be used (within comfort constraints). The Solospun™ technology is concerned with the attachments, which consist of a pair of rollers mounted on a bracket, illustrated below in Fig. 7. The bracket clips onto the top front roller shafts of the drafting arms. Each consists of a wire spring frame with a friction pad on one side and the roller shaft bearing on the other. The clip is fitted by squeezing the pad towards the bearing and pushing the clip over the top draft roller shaft (Fig. 8). When the drafting arm is locked down the spring squeezes the rollers against the bottom (metal) draft roller through the pressure pad (Fig. 8). This pad runs on the back of the bottom roller between the fluted areas. It is made from a low friction, hard wearing plastic.

Besides reducing the cost of manufacturing, Solospun™ technology also allows the use of finer yarns for lighter fabrics, opening up new possibilities in product design. Simplicity is central to the success of Solospun™. Simple plastic rollers are clipped in pairs to the drafting arms of the spinning frame. The rollers split the roving and prevent twist reaching the nip. The sub-strands are recombined in such a way as to increase dramatically the fibre security, resulting in a yarn that is visibly indistinguishable from a normal singles yarn, but is sufficiently resistant to abrasion to be weavable in the warp. Solo-spinning attachment can easily mounted on front roller of NMC Charkha. This system can produce single weaveable yarn from crossbred wool produced in India. It is having good potential to employ in NMC Charkha in khadi system.

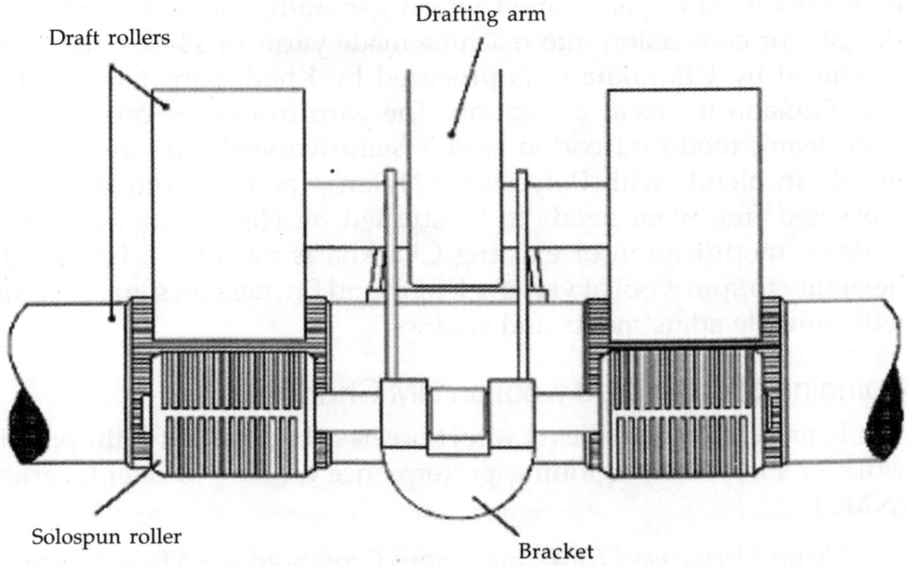

Fig. 7 : Schematic of solospun roller

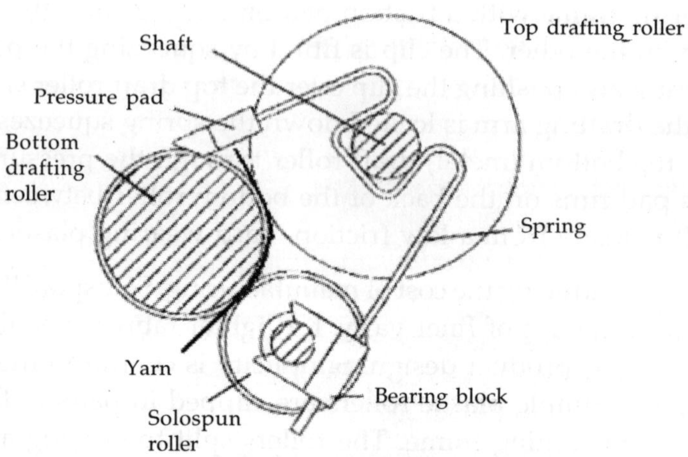

Fig. 8 : Drive to solospun roller

Research and development on Khadi system

Crossbred wool produced in this region is very much suitable for apparels in terms of fineness but is shorter in length and not suitable for worsted spinning system. Presently such wool is used for making shawl in handloom sector of HP. HP Wool federation procures wool from farmers. Similarly J&K sheep and Sheep product Development Board, Srinagar, procures wool directly from farmers, grades it and then sells it into open market which generally comes to Ludhiana, Punjab, for conversion into machine made yarns of 24-42 Nm. Wool produced by Uttarakhand is procured by Khadi Sansthan, Garwal and Kumaon for local utilization. The yarn from crossbred wool is spun using modified cotton card / semi-worsted spinning system mostly in blends with Polyester / Nylon / acrylic. Spinnabality of crossbred fine wool needs to be studied on New Model Charkha. Suitable modification of existing Charkha is needed to further the flexibility to spin wool of varying length and fineness on same Charkha with suitable adjustments and settings.

Spinning of crossbred wool on NM Charkha

Four different varieties of wool fibre have been taken for the present work to study their spinning performance on New Model Charkha (NMC).

Bharat Merino wool (BM): Ingenuous Crossbred wool from Southern peninsular having fibre diameter 24.6 μm.

Indian Farm wool (IFW): Ingenuous Crossbreed from North temperate having diameter 23.43 μm.

Australian Merino wool (AM): Imported wool from Australia having 22.46 μm.

Chokla wool (CH): Ingenuous wool from north western region having diameter 31.94 μm.

From four different wool, all 14 different yarn prepared on New Model Charkha having different fineness level 11, 22 and 44 Nm including three Siro yarn using Siro attachment on NM Charkha.

Yarn quality

The tensile properties such as tenacity determined on Instron tensile tester for all woollen yarn are shown in Table 2. Yarn made of Bharat Merino wool shows higher yarn tenacity than Australian Merino followed crossbred Indian farm wool followed Chokla woollen yarn in all three different yarn counts. Yarn made of Bharat merino wool having highest tenacity value for all three different yarn count, Chokla wools possess lowest tenacity value for 11 and 22 Nm yarn counts and 44Nm yarn of Indian wool having lowest tenacity value. As yarn count increases yarn tenacity decreases due decrease in number of fibres in yarn X-section. Even though Chokla wool is having highest fibre tenacity (1.80 g/d) but impact of number of fibres in yarn cross section has greater in case of Chokla. Indian farm wool possesses lowest fibre tenacity (1.17 g/d) value among four different wools and having shorter mean fibre length (69.63mm) as compared to others, leads lower yarn tenacity. The decrease in tenacity with increase in yarn count is due to increase in mass variation in yarn and decrease in no of fibre in yarn X- section. The breaking extension of Australian Merino (AM), Chokla (CH) and Bharat Merino (BM) is found to be almost same but Indian farm wool (IFW) shows lowest breaking extension among all four wool varieties and yarn count. The decrease in elongation is due to non-uniformity in the yarn which affects both tenacity and breaking elongation of yarn.

Yarn evenness: Yarns made of Chokla wool with 11 and 22 Nm show highest Uster CV% followed Bharat Merino and then Indian Farm wool and Australian Merino wool. Among 44Nm count yarns, IFW possesses highest yarn CV% (37.25 %) followed Bharat Merino (37.19%) and AM yarn shows lowest yarn CV% (33.03%). Higher yarn CV% of Chokla yarn is mainly due to higher fibre diameter variation (36.99%) which causes more numbers of thick-thin places and end breakage in the yarn. Lower mean fibre length (69.63mm) of Indian farm wool yarn also causes higher yarn CV%.

Table 2 : Yarn tenacity and elongation of different wool yarn.

Yarn count	Yarn tenacity (g/tex)				Elongation (%)			
	Bharat Merino (BM)	Indian Farm wool (IFW)	Australian Merino (AM)	Chokla (CH)	Bharat Merino (BM)	Indian Farm wool (IFW)	Australian Merino (AM)	Chokla (CH)
11 Nm	8.73	7.47	8.51	6.09	16.89	8.38	15.75	15.08
22Nm	6.94	6.31	6.78	5.64	9.50	7.31	10.52	10.92
44Nm	3.57	2.91	3.51		7.06	6.49	6.60	

Table 3 : Yarn evenness

Yarn count	Wool variety Yarn properties	Bharat Merino wool (BM)	Indian Farm wool (IFW)	Australian Merino wool (AM)	Chokla wool (CH)
11Nm	Thin place (-50%)	461	2115	196	1408
	Thick place (+50%)	219	149	3	96
	Neps(+200%)	22	5	2	72
	CV%	21.38	15.18	13.66	24.09
22Nm	Thin place (-50%)	1547	304	827	2347
	Thick place (+50%)	769	310	416	767
	Neps(+200%)	439	189	10	610
	CV%	27.43	26.49	24.44	36.5
44Nm	Thin place (-50%)	1950	1085	1090	
	Thick place (+50%)	1070	1114	769	
	Neps(+200%)	250	115	107	
	CV%	37.19	37.25	33.03	

Yarn hairiness: Yarn hairiness test were perform on Zweigle G566. Coarser count (11 Nm) has higher S3 value than finer count in all three variety of wool. From all four different variety of wool, yarn made of Chokla wool shows highest S3 value for 11 and 22 Nm yarn count followed Indian farm wool and then Bharat merino and

Australian merino woollen yarn shows almost same S3 value (Figure 9). For 44Nm yarn, Indian Farm wool (2181) shows higher S3 value followed Bharat Merino (2018) and Australian Merino woollen yarn having lowest S3 value (1873). Chokla woollen yarn having higher S3 value is higher fibre diameter causes high fibre bending rigidity. Due to presence of shorter length fibre in case of Indian farm wool causing more number of protruding fibre on yarn surface. As yarn count increases hairiness value decreases due to positive impact of yarn twist and decrease in number of fibres in the yarn cross-section.

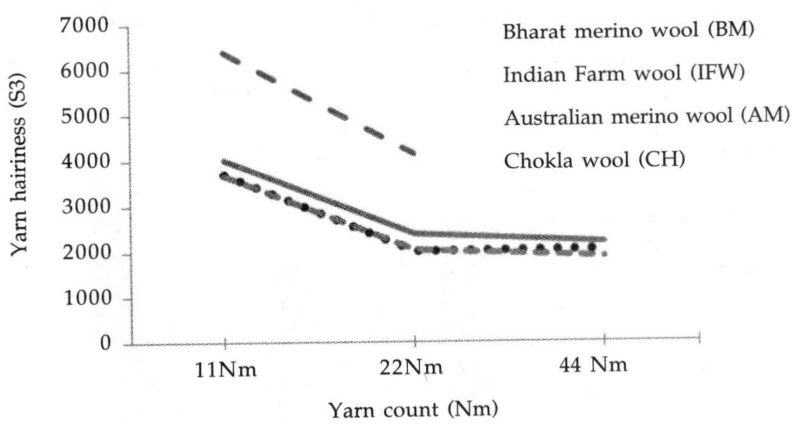

Fig. 9 : Yarn hairiness vs. yarn count.

Performance of NM Charkha: Sirospun yarn

NMC Sirospun yarn gives higher tenacity value followed NMC Single yarn for all different variety of wool fibre. Sirospun yarn made of Bharat merino (7.29 g/tex) gives higher tenacity value followed Australian merino (7.14 g/tex) and then Indian farm wool (6.29 g/tex). Significant improvement found in tenacity value at 95% confidence limit in sirospun yarn from single NMC yarn. It is mainly due to doubling effect. The yarn uniformity increases which results in higher yarn tenacity value of sirospun yarn compare to single yarn.

NMC Sirospun yarn also gives higher yarn elongation value followed NMC Single yarn for all different variety of wool fibre. Sirospun yarn made of Australian merino (17.43 %) gives higher extension value followed Bharat merino (14.48%) and then Indian farm wool (12.09%).Significant improvement found in tenacity value at 95% confidence limit in sirospun yarn from single NMC yarn.

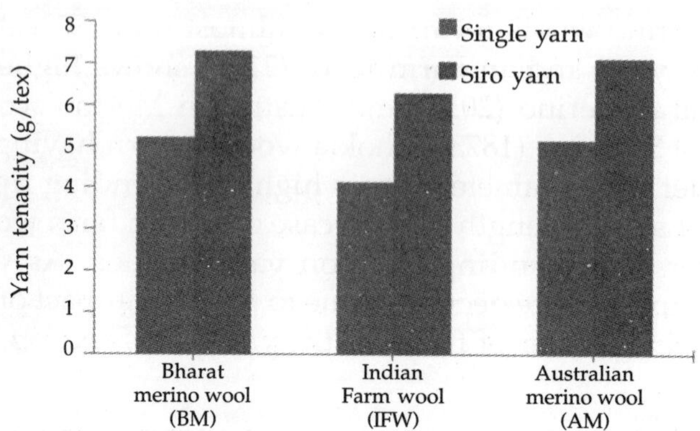

Fig. 10 : Yarn tenacity: Siro yarn vs Single yarn

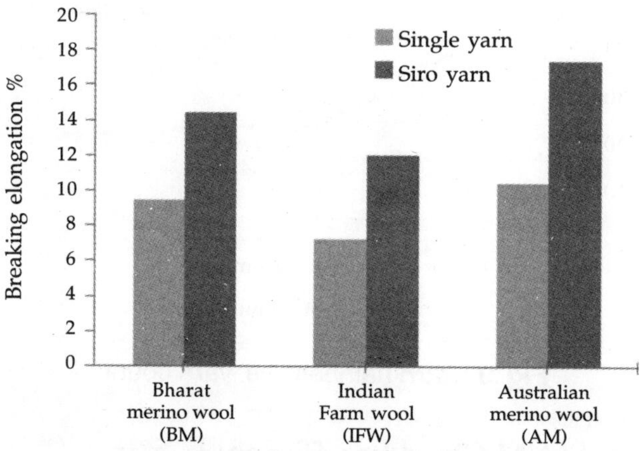

Fig. 11 : Yarn Elongation: Siro yarn vs Single yarn

Yarn evenness and hairiness

NMC Sirospun yarn gives lower yarn mass CV% value than NMC Single yarn for all different variety of wool fibre. Sirospun yarn made of Indian farm wool (25.69 %) gives highest yarn mass CV% value followed Bharat Merino (22.65%) and then Australian Merino (22.21%) Significant improvement found in tenacity value at 95% confidence limit in sirospun yarn from single NMC yarn. There is marginal change in S3 value of Siro yarn compare to single yarn. Indian Farm wool (2398) shows higher S3 value followed Bharat Merino (1953) and Australian Merino woollen yarn having lowest S3 value (1880). Siro yarn made of Indian Farm wool shows more hairy yarn than other due to presence of shorter fibre length which has tendency to migrate towards surface of yarn.

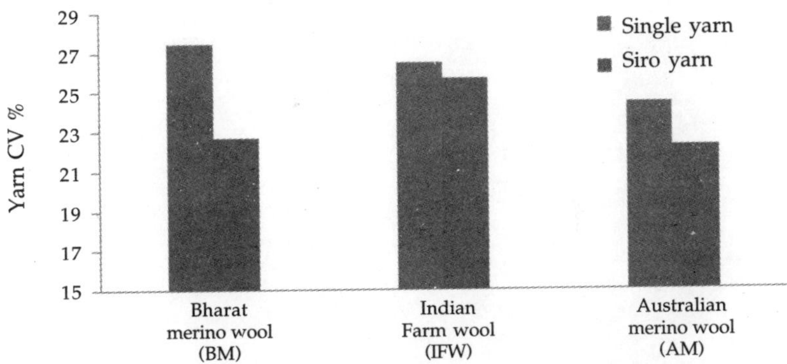

Fig. 12 : Yarn evenness: Siro yarn vs Single yarn

Table 4 : Yarn Hairiness (S3): Siro yarn vs Single yarn (22 Nm)

Yarn count	Bharat merino wool (BM)	Indian Farm wool (IFW)	Australian merino wool (AM)
Normal yarn	1989	2359	2045
Siro yarn	1953	2398	1880

Conclusion

The new techniques of yarn manufacture in Khadi sector can produce yarn with modified structure and add different characteristics to the yarns, which are translated into affordable lightweight fabrics with a fresh new look. It also helps in enhancement of productivity of yarn in Khadi system. It is hoped that they will continue to produce distinct yarn structures unique products from time to come.

References

Anon, Annual Report, KVIC, (Govt. of India), 2009-10

Chattopadhyay. R., Chavan. R. B. and Nayak. R. K. 2003. NMC Charkha: A Design Analysis from Technological Considerations, Indian Institute of Technology, Delhi, India.

Ishtiaque, S. M., Dhawan, K., Saxena, A., and Jai Prakash. 1988. Siro Yarn Mechanism, Text Asia, 118.

Prins, M. W. 2009. Advances in wool spinning technology In: Advances in wool technology, (Editors Johnson, A. G. and Russell, I. M., Woodhead publishing Ltd, Cambridge, England.

□□□

Chapter 31

Scope, Performance and Current Status of Broiler Rabbit Production in India

Rajeev Gulyani
Division of Transfer of Technology and Social Sciences
Central Sheep and Wool Research Institute, Avikanagar-304 501 (Rajasthan)

Animal protein intake is dismally low in lesser developed countries and not adequate in developing countries as compared to developed countries. The FAO recommends a minimum of 70g of protein daily per capita, out of which at least 35g (50%) should come from animal protein. The average Indian consumption of protein is low and that of animal protein is still lower. As such all reasonable options for increasing animal protein in the diet of people deserves through consideration. Micro-livestock such as rabbit has been suggested as a rapid means of obtaining animal protein for the expanding population of lesser developed countries and which appears to be the most sustainable means of producing high quality protein. Rabbit production has the potential to provide the improvised urban population and the resource poor rural dwellers the opportunity to meet part of their total protein intake and earn additional income. The rabbit can be a potential money spinner if properly managed. Prospect for increased livestock production in developing countries would have to involve short cycle animals like rabbit kept by small scale farmers. Rabbit production thus appears as an attractive proposition for the supply of high quality meat especially in developing countries with no cereal surplus. In recent times rabbit farming is becoming more and more attractive due to its high production potentials like high mothering ability, adaptability to a wide range of conditions, high genetic variability, high roughage utilization, high rate of reproduction, early maturation, rapid growth rate, limited competition with man for similar foods and high quality nutritious meat. In addition, its skin is soft and luxurious and can be used in the production of garments and toys in cottage industries. It is estimated that a family raising 5-6 does on locally available grain, forage and household waste can obtain 2 rabbits or 2.5 kg meat every week for domestic consumption or sale. Hence small scale backyard rabbit rearing can be a useful enterprise to improve the health and socio-economic condition of the tribals, rural and urban poor in our country. Commercial rabbit production also has a great scope in and around metropolitan cities. Moreover, there are no religious inhibitions for the consumption of rabbit meat among non-vegetarian population. Studies at temperate, sub-temperate and semi-arid regions have demonstrated that broiler rabbits can be raised successfully almost all over the country with some variation in managemental practices to suit the local climatic condition.

National status

Taking in to consideration, the scope and potential of rabbit rearing in our country, the Central Sheep and Wool Research Institute (CSWRI), Avikanagar (Rajasthan) imported 60 New Zealand White rabbits (10 males+50 females) from U.K. in March 1978. Again during November 1979 another lot of 25 males and 100 females each of Soviet Chinchilla, Grey Giant and White Giant were received under Indo-USSR protocol for agricultural development as *gratis*. These rabbits were initially reared at North Temperate Regional Station (NTRS), Garsa (Himachal Pradesh) and later shifted to Avikanagar and Southern Regional Research Station (SRRC), Mannavanur (Tamil Nadu) to study their adaptability and performance in different agro climatic condition of India. As per the livestock census (2003), the total rabbit population of the country is estimated to be 406000. Most of the states and union territories are having rabbit population. Kerala has the highest number (148233) of rabbits followed by Nagaland (38408), Bihar (29380), Rajasthan (22929) and Uttar Pradesh (22191). The broiler rabbits are also concentrated in the states of Andhra Pradesh, Orissa, West Bengal, Maharashtra, Madhya Pradesh and other North

Eastern States. Thus in states which have a sizable tribal population and also have a sizable meat eating population, which is desirous of eating healthy meat, rabbit meat production has a great scope as a small backyard enterprise as well as a medium to large scale enterprise. In backyard and small scale system one can expect higher outputs at lower inputs involving no off-farm purchase that would supply inexpensive meat for the family, improve farm productivity, and supplement income through the sale of surplus stock.

An important by product obtained from broiler rabbits is the skin which is covered with soft luxurious fur. At present most of the demand for fur pelts for making fur garments is met out of illegal trade in pelts from wild animals and through import. Therefore, there is a good scope for obtaining good quality pelts at cheaper rates from broiler rabbits reared under farm conditions. Our country also has a large and thriving domestic fur industry mainly centered in Jammu and Kashmir. About 5 million fur skins are estimated to be imported every year, mainly from France, of which more than half are rabbit skins as they are cheaper alternatives to high priced furs and are affordable to the majority. Farm reared rabbits, particularly in high altitudes, can thus fulfill this domestic demand for rabbit skins and also relieve pressure on illegal hunting of animals and save valuable foreign exchange. Moreover, the fur produced in temperate regions is of superior quality as it is thick and has higher hair density and insulation capability.

At present the major constraints is the shortage of germplasm. The available germplasm of broiler type rabbits with the CSWRI Avikanagar and its stations at Garsa and Mannavanur falls much short of the demand. Moreover, the breeders from farfetched areas have to bear high transportation cost who in turn charges a heavy price on the sale of these rabbits to new breeders. Thus it is desirable that State Animal Husbandry Departments start rabbitries locally so that the new entrepreneurs may readily get the stock. The other major constraint is non-availability of a well-organized market for rabbit meat. The rabbit breeder either utilizes the product himself or sells it in the neighborhood. Marketing of rabbit meat and fur skins deserves due attention from the development agencies in order to popularize broiler rabbit breeding in the country. There is also need to educate the law enforcement agencies like Forest Department and Police not to confuse domestic rabbit with wild rabbit and allow free trade in rabbits and its products. Another problem is that people think of rabbit as a pet and fancy animal. They have to be educated about the rabbit as a producer of quality meat.

Scope of rabbit production

The domestic rabbit by virtue of its special features, possessed by none other domestic livestock species, merits due consideration to be exploited as an important livestock spęcies. The body size of the rabbit is small and requires comparatively lesser amount of feed which has little direct competition with human food. Further, it can be housed in small, inexpensive and easily constructed sheds/ houses. There are no religious inhibitions for the consumption of rabbit meat among non-vegetarian population. The gestation period of rabbit is short (one month) and it can be rebred within 24 hours of kindling. This super-imposed with its high prolificacy (average litter size 6-8) provides an opportunity for fast multiplication. Four to six kindlings /doe/year can be taken under routine managemental conditions. The animal is fast- growing and slaughter weight of approximately 2 kg live weight can be achieved within 12 to 15 weeks of age if managed properly.

Rabbits can be reared on grain free diets comprising of forages, by-products etc. Reasonable performance of rabbits can be achieved on feeding grain-free diets including forages, tree leaves, leguminous plants, waste vegetables, fruits etc., with supplementation of by-products like cakes, wheat bran, etc. The rabbit meat is low in fat, cholesterol and sodium as compared to other meats like mutton, chevon, beef and pork and as such a boon for patients with heart condition and hypertension. The skin of rabbit is a valuable by-product used to manufacture fur garments, toys, decoration pieces etc. It is soft and luxurious and commands a good price. With above features, broiler rabbits have a great scope to be exploited for profitable meat and fur skin production in addition to its other utilities. Rabbit rearing is a fast return proposition.

Broiler rabbit breeds in India

Exotic breeds of broiler rabbits like Soviet Chinchilla (SC), White Giant (WG) and Grey Giant (GG) were imported from former USSR While New Zealand White (NZW) from UK in the year 1978. Later two new colour segregates viz., Black Brown (BB) and Dutch were evolved from GG and SC breeds (Table 1). These segregates were selected strictly over the years for their colour and type and are now breeding true to their characteristics. In 1983, a rabbit research unit was established at Avikanagar to study the performance of broiler rabbits as the semi-arid region constitutes about 50% of the geographical area of the country.

Table 1 : Broiler rabbit breeds and their characteristics

Breed	Fur color	Adult weight (kg)	Country of origin	Availability at
Soviet Chinchilla	Chinchilla, steel grey	3.5-4.0	Former USSR	CSWRI, NTRS, SRRS
Grey Giant	Greyish brown	3.5-4.0	-do-	CSWRI, NTRS
White Giant	White	4.0 kg	-do-	CSWRI, NTRS, SRRS
New Zealand White	White	3.0-3.5	U.K.	NTRS
Black Brown	Blackish Brown	3.5-4.0	India	CSWRI, NTRS
Dutch	Dutch pattern	3.0	India	CSWRI, NTRS

International scenario

As per FAO estimates, India has 36700 females producing 7.50 tons of rabbit meat with a per capita consumption of 0.009 kg and that at least 82% of world's production of rabbit meat occurs in the developed countries. There are an estimated 64 million rabbit does in the world and 709 million total rabbits. Rabbit meat is consumed mainly in the European Latin countries (1.9 to 5.6 kg/head/year) and secondarily in East European countries (1.04 kg/head/year). The average world rabbit meat consumption is 0.3 kg/head/year. Rabbit meat constitutes 5.6% of the world meat production and is dominated by Italy, China, Hungary, France, Germany, Belgium, USA, Egypt and Indonesia. The European Union is best organized in the terms of rabbit meat production and marketing in the world. Rabbit meat is included in the Common Market Organizations (CMO) related to agricultural products in the European Treaty. The CMO are based on common prices regime to protect community producers. Formation of producer groups are encouraged for smooth supply and marketing of rabbit products. Sanitary measures are strictly followed and it is a compulsory requirement that rabbit should come from holdings free of rabies, myxomatosis, viral haemorrhagic disease and tularaemia. The EU is the main consumer, producer and importer of rabbit meat and meat products in the world. In the EU, Italy, Germany, France and Netherlands are the major producers, consumers and importers of rabbit meat. The imports are mainly from China (47.05%) and Hungary (23.65%).

The six countries producing more than 100,000 tons/year are Italy, France, Ukraine, China, Spain and Russia (representing 58% of world rabbit meat production) and eleven countries producing more that 20,000 tons/year are Indonesia, Nigeria, Egypt, USA, Germany, Belarus, Belgium, Poland, Morocco, Portugal and Czech Republic (representing 32% of world rabbit meat production). It was observed that 43% of the rabbit producers are in West Europe, 24% in East Europe, 14% in Far East Asia and 19% in the African continent. The productivity of rabbit does is also the highest in West Europe (36 kg rabbit meat/doe/year), followed by East Europe (27.5 kg), Far East Asia (17.5 kg) and African continent (14.0 kg). For every thousand inhabitants in the world there are 12 rabbit does.

Broiler rabbit production under climate change scenario

Climate change and stress, in all likelihood, are going to impact seriously on animal productivity over the next decade and beyond. Production losses due to impaired physiology is quiet distinct. Thus there is an urgent need to understand these complex issues so that we can device suitable managemental practices to reduce the adverse effects of climate change. Proper shelter management has been known to mitigate climate related stress to a great extent. This assumes particular significance in rabbits as these animals are generally housed indoors where the micro-climate can be controlled. When productivity of other livestock becomes impaired, rabbits can play a crucial role in filling this gap. Day length plays a crucial role in rabbits and is responsible for the seasonality in reproduction observed in rabbits. This seasonality in reproduction can be overcome by providing artificial light to breeding does during short day length periods. At the same time, more emphasis can be given on selecting rabbit genotype which is more adapted to high ambient temperature and has better feed efficiency under stress. High ambient temperatures can cause infertility in breeding rabbits, bucks being more sensitive than does. Therefore, it is always advisable to provide a cooling system in the rabbitry during the hot periods to prevent male rabbits (bucks) from becoming sterile resulting in lower conception rates in females (does). The does also exhibit poor receptivity, lower litter size, early embryonic deaths and decreased fetal growth if exposed to heat stress. Kits and weaners are particularly sensitive to hot and humid conditions, which causes rapid spread of coccidiosis and thereby heavy mortality due to enteritis. To overcome this problem, prophylaxis is employed against coccidiosis or breeding schedule planned in a manner so as to avoid kindling and weaning during the hot-humid months and instead intensive rabbit breeding and production is practiced during the remaining good part of the year to maintain the overall production. However, if the exposure is over long periods, the rabbits get acclimatized to constant stress situations, also termed as adaptation, to withstand the onslaught of adverse climate. Such adaptive changes are of advantage in terms of disease resistance and ability to withstand climatic stress but disadvantageous in terms of production performance. In general, growth rates of rabbits range from 10-20 g/day in the tropical regions compared to temperate countries where growth performance typically is between 35-40 g/day.

The universal distribution of rabbits throughout the world, from cold temperate to hot tropical regions, speaks favorably about the adaptability of rabbits to different climatic conditions. The broiler rabbit breeds available in the country were imported from cold temperate former USSR and the UK. These were initially introduced into our country in the Kullu Valley of Himachal Pradesh at NTRS, Garsa. Later in 1982, these were introduced in the hot semi-arid region at CSWRI Avikanagar to study their adaptability and performance. The performance over the years at Avikanagar has shown that broiler rabbits can be reared successfully in the hot semi-arid regions of our country which constitute roughly 65% of the total geographical area of our country and where temperatures reach 45-47°C during peak summer. Since Broiler rabbits are mostly reared indoors, these become most suitable for livestock production under prevailing and future global warming conditions. With a few modifications in their shelter management, they can tide over the difficult summer phase, which may extend beyond the two to three months period at present, but at an increased cost of production.

The severity of heat stress experienced by rabbit depends on a number of factors. The key ones include the actual temperature and humidity inside the shed, housing type, the length of heat stress period, water availability, the degree of night cooling, ventilation and air flow, the size and age of animal, breed (native, exotic or crossbred), and density of fur and the level of production. In tropical areas, environmental temperature along with relative humidity is the environmental factor that has the most profound impact on the efficiency of rabbit production and welfare conditions. The ranges of temperature and relative humidity recommended for laboratory rabbits (16 to 22°C and 30 to 70%) are often exceeded under natural conditions. Housing systems for rabbit should minimize the negative effects of natural environment on the animals.

Rabbits are highly susceptible to heat stress as they have few functional sweat glands and have a difficult heat output situation when the environmental temperature is high. In a study undertaken at Avikanagar on the effect of season and breed on the thermoregulatory responses of broiler rabbits in hot semi-arid environment, we observed that winter and spring seasons are relatively comfortable than summer for broiler rabbits on the basis of their respiration rate (RR), which could go up to 450-500 breaths/min. during hot summer temperatures of 35-45°C. It was also observed that SC rabbits could maintain relatively lower rectal temperature as compared to WG during peak of thermal stress by increasing the respiratory evaporative cooling through increase in RR, and that this breed characteristic in SC could be of help to tolerate high environmental temperature, which was manifested in lower mortality (15%) as compared to WG (40%).

Role of nutrition in augmenting reproduction in rabbits

Reproduction being the most important characteristic of the rabbit deserves special attention and sustaining such a high rate of reproduction requires a high plane of nutrition and a high level of management skill. Among the methods available for maintaining good fertility, improved nutrition is the most important in rabbits, though regular breeding and photoperiod are also important. The correct nutrition of a rabbit is one of the most important aspects of rabbit keeping. A good rabbit can be ruined by poor nutrition and a poor one improved by good feeding. Since the greatest cost of rearing rabbits lies in their feeding, the importance of correct feeding cannot be over emphasized. On the other hand rabbits also have the ability to convert forage into meat efficiently. This is of special significance in developing countries where population pressures and food shortages are greatest. A few does can be kept by villagers on a backyard scale to produce enough meat to satisfy the needs of a family using weeds, tropical forages, vegetable tops and table scraps as feed for rabbits. In such a scenario, a larger gap is required between subsequent kindlings to recoup the female from previous kindling and lactation stress. Intensive breeding cannot be practiced under such a feeding regimen, as a balanced nutrition is essential for exploiting their reproductive potential for commercial purposes.

Fertility and good body condition are closely related. One of the first bodily functions to suffer from poor feeding is the reproductive system. The ration should be properly balanced and proper amount of feed given to keep the rabbits in desired breeding condition. Rabbits that are abnormally fat or thin have impaired fertility, or they may become sterile. The ration, therefore, should be adjusted and breeding delayed until they are in proper physical condition. For those that are too fat, restrict pelleted diet and increase good quality greens/hay. For those that are too thin pellet ration and greens should be fed in increased amounts. The does should, therefore, be checked regularly for their body condition by weighing them at regular intervals and through physical check-up. By passing the hand over the back of a rabbit one can determine the level of fatness. If the vertebras on the back are not felt easily on the palm, the doe is termed fatty and if the vertebras are felt easily and prick the palm, the doe is in poor body condition. In the commercial rabbit breeds available at our Institute (SC, WG, GG and NZW), the ideal body weight of a good reproductive doe is between 3.0 to 3.5 kg in the semi-arid region and between 3.25 to 3.75 kg in the sub-temperate region. Overly fat does are more likely to abort their fetuses. Molting or the development of new coat may tax the animal's vitality, which may lead to delayed conception in rabbits.

Higher percentages of fertile mating occur during autumn and spring in the semi-arid region. This is probably due to the adequate availability of good quality green fodder at these times. In contrast, a decrease in conception in the winter is usually observed in rabbits. This may be caused by inadequate feeding. In unheated rabbitries, the rabbits use more of their daily ration to produce heat to keep warm. Therefore, less energy is available for the reproduction processes. To meet this increased body heat demand, it is recommended that the daily feed allotment to does should be increased by about 25% during winter. Studies on reproductive efficiency of broiler rabbits in the semi-arid region revealed that the overall conception rate was 50.25% and number of services/conception was 1.98.

Some does show vices such as cannibalism i.e., eating its own young ones just after birth. In most of the cases a doe may bite her kit accidentally while cleaning it but then proceeds to devour it completely as it may eventually die and contaminate the nest. This vice is generally associated with first litter does but may also be due to bad nutrition, particularly the lack of B group vitamins and water. It is always essential that plenty of feed and water are available to a kindling doe as she is very hungry and thirsty just after kindling. Level of nutrition is also very essential for bucks and does to reach sexual maturity in time. After weaning, the food supply has a considerable influence on the rate of growth. Rabbits may be permanently stunted if their nutrition is poor, which may affect their overall productivity as adults. In such rabbits usually their sexual organs are stunted. In the breeds available at the Institute, the age of sexual maturity is 6 to 7 months in does and 7 to 8 months in bucks, but a minimum body weight of $\geq$ 2.5 kg is essential for the initiation of reproduction activity in these breeds. A breeding male should be fed approximately 10 to 15% above maintenance ration to keep it vigorous and in good health. A doe usually consumes less than normal for 2 to 3 days before kindling (parturition), and this is normal as the developing fetuses exert pressure on the stomach to decrease appetite. She should be given small amounts of greens each day to tempt her appetite and to have a beneficial effect on the digestive system as when lactation begins, their feed intake will increase markedly. It is desirable to gradually increase the amount of feed offered to the doe for the first week following kindling until full feed intake is reached. Over feeding of the doe in lactation is not good as excessive milk production by an overfed doe may cause 5 to 6 day old kits to die of milk enterotoxaemia.

Diseases account for only a small percentage of the mortality that occurs in the first week following kindling. Most of the losses during this time are due to improper feeding and management methods. Some losses may also be due to the doe failing to produce milk, which may be because the ration she received during gestation period was inadequate in quantity and quality.

The diets and feeding techniques of reproducing does have changed considerably over the years. A diet suited to both growing rabbits and does, though more commonly used can be substituted by reproduction diets that feature higher protein and energy levels for breeding females throughout the reproductive cycle. The reproduction diet can be further diversified for various phases of reproduction viz., for young, pregnant, lactating and simultaneously pregnant and lactating does. Despite the rapid development of reproduction activity in the rabbit and the overlapping of certain phases, the energy and protein metabolism and utilization of body reserves for milk synthesis and fetal growth vary and depend on the physiological state and breeding rhythm adopted, and requires highly diversified strategies.

Performance of broiler rabbits in the semi-arid region of India

Rabbits are highly susceptible to heat stress as they have few functional sweat glands and have a difficult heat output situation when environmental temperatures are high. In the semi-arid region, the rabbits show lower body weights from April to August and improvement in body weights as environment becomes favorable (Table 2). The rabbits maintain a lower body weight in the semi-arid region as compared to the temperate and sub-temperature regions of the country, indicating that during the course of adaptation to harsh environment there is a reduction in their adult body weights. The survivability of rabbits varies among different age groups (Table 3). The mortality in kits (0-6 weeks) was highest in all the breeds, particularly in the first week of life as the kits are naked and depend totally on the mothering ability of the doe as well as the climatic conditions prevailing at that time. During winter kits generally die of hypothermia and in summer due to hyperthermia. The overall survivability was high in GG and SC breeds and low in WG breed.

Table 2 : Average adult body weight (kg) of broiler rabbits

Breed	Jan	Feb	Mar	Apr	May	Jun	Jul	Aug	Sep	Oct	Nov	Dec
WG	3.36	3.33	3.40	3.36	3.19	3.05	3.07	3.21	3.24	3.34	3.34	3.51
GG	3.04	3.05	3.09	3.02	2.90	2.69	2.70	2.74	2.78	2.81	2.98	3.01
SC	3.20	3.25	3.22	3.25	3.07	2.79	2.84	2.80	2.90	3.12	3.17	3.27

Table 3 : Survivability (%) in rabbits among different age groups

Age group	WG	NZW	GG	SC
0-6 Weeks	79.82	70.83	78.15	83.17
7-12 weeks	89.32	95.85	92.24	82.89
13-24 Weeks	92.56	95.48	93.70	97.38
Adults	82.44	85.73	88.25	88.13

Growth is an important aspect of broiler rabbit production. The growth performance of different broiler rabbit breeds is presented in table 4. The growth of the young during the suckling period, especially during the first three weeks, greatly affects their later performance. Apart from milk yield, the liter size and doe's nursing ability also influence the pre-weaning growth. The 12-week weight ranged from 1711.11 g to 1853.00 g showing marginal breed difference. The body weight at 12 weeks is of crucial significance as the broiler rabbit is usually marketed and slaughtered at this age. The growth is fastest during 7-12 weeks period. The higher the body weight at 12 weeks, the more the carcass yield and profitability. Under experimental *ad libitum* complete diet feeding system, average weight of 2.0 to 2.3 kg at 12 weeks has been achieved at this Institute.

Table 4 : Growth performance of broiler rabbits

Breed	Body Weights (g)			
	At birth	6 weeks	12 weeks	24 weeks
WG	54.05	806.41	1853.00	2645.30
SC	54.57	876.98	1788.46	2502.80
BB	46.08	769.76	1711.11	2448.60

The reproductive performance of broiler rabbits is presented in table 5. The litter size at birth (LSB) ranged from 6.46 to 7.26 while the litter size at weaning (LSW) ranged from 4.92 to 6.17 in different breeds. High LSB and LSW were recorded in GG and WG breeds. Similarly, high litter weights at birth (LWB) and weaning (LWW) were recorded in GG and WG breeds. The average LWB and LWW ranged from 325.34 to 390.82 g and 3023.80 to 3488.22 g, respectively. Rabbits are induced ovulators and can be bred within 24 hrs of parturition. The average number of kindling/doe/year and average number of offspring/doe/year achieved in the semi-arid region under the semi-intensive production system was 3.5 and 23.9, respectively, while under intensive system it was marginally higher (4.0 litter/doe/year). However, in the temperate region it was possible to achieve an average of 5.16 litters/doe/year (range- 4 to 9) or 35-40 offspring/doe/year under the intensive production system.

Table 5 : Reproductive performance of broiler rabbits

Breed	Litter size at		Litter weight (g) at	
	Birth	Weaning (6 weeks)	Birth	Weaning (6 Weeks)
GG	7.26	6.17	374.19	3488.22
WG	7.23	5.70	390.80	3681.09
NZW	6.46	5.18	345.99	3300.50
SC	6.65	5.26	258.00	3023.80
BB	7.06	4.92	325.34	3304.34

Studies on milking ability of broiler rabbit does revealed that milk yield and nursing ability of doe increased with parity order. The total milk yield of SC does was higher (4370.90 g) as compared to WG (4326.43 g) and BB (4179.00 g) in a 35 days lactation period (Table 6). There was, however, a sudden decline in milk production in all the three breeds from 31 to 32 days onwards if lactation is continued beyond 28 days. Therefore, in order to take more number of kindlings per doe per year, it is recommended to go for early weaning at 28 days as by this time the young start consuming some solid feed as well as roughage and the role of milk in their diet declines. Milk production by a rabbit doe is an important indicator of growth and health of young rabbits in their first month of life and is intimately related to the body weight achieved at the slaughter age of 12 weeks of age. The pre-weaning growth of kits is entirely dependent upon the does milk yield, particularly during the first 21 days of life.

Table 6 : Milk production in broiler rabbit does

Lactation period (Days)	Milk yield/doe (g)		
	SC	WG	BB
0-7	531.38	561.25	527.14
8-14	903.33	797.50	808.57
15-21	1055.83	923.75	892.50
22-28	941.11	975.45	915.83
28-35	700.00	680.00	725.00
0-28	3481.66	3278.18	3205.00
0-35	4370.90	4326.43	4179.00

Slaughter studies conducted at CSWRI showed that the Killing out percentages of 55-60% saleable meat yield is achievable in rabbit

(Table 7).The first step in slaughtering rabbit is stunning before bleeding. In small scale operations, dislocation of neck is generally the method of choice, while on a commercial scale electrical stunning is mostly used. Feed is withheld at least 12 hrs before slaughter to ensure an almost empty gut. After separation of head, the whole body is suspended by inserting the hook in the hock joint of the hind leg and skinning is carried out carefully to avoid any cut on the skin as it reduces the value of the skin, which is an important by-product of rabbit. This is followed by evisceration of all the visceral organs and separation from the carcass.

Some 70% of rabbit carcass is composed of edible meat as compared to 50% in chicken. Rabbit meat is also comparable to chicken in terms of low fat content (3.8%) and high protein (20.7%) and these values are favorable than most other meats. Moreover the digestibility of rabbit meat is as high as 98.9%. Rabbit meat is in fact appreciated for its low content of total fat and cholesterol and high proportion of polyunsaturated fatty acids (PUFA) and phospholipids, as presently nutritional value and safety have gained great importance among factors that determine meat quality. Rabbit meat is a lean meat, rich in proteins of a high biological value, low in sodium, contains no uric acid, has low content of purines and is characterized by high levels of essential amino-acids. The amount of cholesterol in rabbit meat is about 59mg/100g of muscle which is lower than meats from other species.

Table 7 : Carcass traits of broiler rabbits

Traits	Soviet Chinchilla	Grey Giant	Pooled
Pre-slaughter weight (g)	2131.90	2206.60	2169.20
Blood weight (g)	80.40	80.60	80.50
Head weight (g)	186.40	191.90	189.20
Skin Weight (g)	224.00	238.40	231.20
Inedible offal weight (g)	477.10	516.20	496.60
Edible offal (g)	81.40	80.10	80.70
Head meat weight (g)	61.70	58.40	60.10
Leg cut weight (g)	423.40	422.50	422.90
Loin cut weight (g)	249.40	237.90	243.60
Rack, neck and BF cut weight (g)	409.80	433.00	421.40
Total cut weight (g)	1082.60	1099.30	1090.90
Saleable meat yield (g)	1225.70	1237.80	1231.80
% PSW	57.45	55.68	56.57

Conclusion

Studies at the Central Sheep and Wool Research Institute and its sub-stations in different parts of the country have shown that broiler rabbits have wide adaptability and have the potential to become an alternate source of meat in the country.

□□□

Conclusion

Studies at the Central Sheep and Wool Research Institute and its sub-stations in different parts of the country have shown that broiler rabbits have wide adaptability and have the potential to become an alternate source of meat in the country.

Chapter 32

Existing Technology Transfer System - Where We Stand ?

Hema Tripathi[1] and Shabeer Ahmad Hamdani[2]
[1]Principal Scientist and Program Coordinator KVK [2]Doctoral Student, Division of Extension Education, Indian Veterinary Research Institute, Izatnagar 243 122 (UP)

Agriculture in India is characterized by a symbiosis of crop and livestock husbandry. Despite only 15.7% contribution to gross domestic product (GDP) by agriculture, its role remains critical as it provides employment to around 52% of the workforce. Livestock constitutes an important sub-sector of Indian agriculture and contributed over 4.07% of the total GDP along with fisheries sector during the year 2008-09. India possesses great potential in animal husbandry sector being the largest milk producing country in the world with the current production of about 112.5 million tonnes (Economic Survey, 2009-10). India also has the largest buffalo population, while it stands second in cattle population of the world. The per capita availability of milk has increased from 112 g in 1968-69 to 258 g in 2008-09 (DAHD, 2010). On the other hand, sustained economic growth, increasing urbanization and a shift in diets are fuelling the growth in demand for livestock products. In view of the increasing demand for milk and milk products by the growing population and also the scope for exports, an assessment has been made by the Planning Commission and National Dairy Development Board (NDDB) that the milk production need to be enhanced from 100.9 million tonnes for 2006-07 to 180.0 million tonnes by 2021-22 (National Dairy Plan, 2010).This increased demand will have to be largely met by increasing the productivity of the milch animals as the option of increasing their number is undesirable.

However, the current levels of productivity of milch cattle remain an area of concern in the given circumstances. The productive potential of animals depends crucially on the genetic material, quality of nutrition provided and animal health system where unfortunately India has a poor record (Ahuja *et al.*, 2008). In order to utilize the vast opportunities prevalent with the livestock resources of the country, there is a strong need for efficient livestock technology delivery system which includes mainly animal health, breeding and other veterinary and extension services. Transfer of technology (TOT) can be understand by referring the entire process of technology development, processing, dissemination and integration through research, extension and farming systems, keeping in view the resources, organizational limitations and capabilities of the three systems to solve the problem of society. Thus, transfer of technology (TOT) is not a linear process with push button shifting of technologies as people are rational and adopt new technology if they are convinced about its utility along with compatibility to social and cultural system. It is thus a collaborative effort of all the three partners viz. farming, extension and research system. There are three major trends in the way transfer of technology is carried out. The oldest and most common approach is known by many names like as *top down* or *conventional model,* next followed by *feedback model* with due consideration to farmer's reaction and the third recent approach as *participatory model*. There are other supporting models and tenets used in the classification of transfer of agricultural technology. Besides these models, the transfer of technology can be studied under general agricultural extension approach, commodity specialized approach, training and visit approach, agricultural extension participatory approach, project approach, farming systems development approach, cost sharing approach and educational institution approach.

Conventional Model is the most prevalent model so far, ever since the beginning of agricultural research and extension. Technology generation is the sole responsibility of the researchers, and the interaction with farmers or extension person is not seen as relevant. Here the farmers are seen as passive recipients of technology. There is little or no contact between farmers and scientists. The role of extension is to persuade the farmers to adopt new technologies. Thus, this model suffered from the feeling of superiority about scientists and technologies, without any due consideration to solve of problems of users and look into their views. This type of approach was seen especially during Green Revolution. The feedback model received much impetus after Green Revolution due to the failure of conventional model to reap much benefit without farmer's involvement. Farming systems research / extension (FSR/E) was evolved in 1970s as an alternative to conventional research and extension which had propagated technologies requiring high external inputs. FSR/E is farmer-based, problem solving, comprehensive, interdisciplinary, complementary, iterative, dynamic and responsible to society. FSR involves a set of activities beginning from target and research area selection to problem diagnosis and development of relevant agenda, planning and design of on-farm research and extension of research results. As a basic element of the scheme, constant collaborations and rapport among researchers, extension personnel and farmers' extension personnel have important role to play at each of the steps of FSR/E. Thus, farming system conceptually is an integrated set of elements or components and activities that farmer perform in their farms under their resources and circumstances to maximize the productivity and net farm income on a sustainable basis. It takes into account the various components of farm family with the family at the centre of managing the agriculture and related activities. The farming system approach is a problem solving, holistic approach, complex in nature i.e interrelated matrix of soil, plant, animal, power, implement, labour, capital and other inputs, influenced by political, economic, institutional and social forces.

Existing livestock technology transfer system

The agricultural and livestock technology development process involves three major systems viz. research system, linking/extension system and client/farmer system. It is necessary that these three systems must participate, interact and collaborate with each other. The National Agriculture Research System (NARS) is at the forefront to guide the technological breakthrough in agriculture through ICAR Institutes, State and Central Agricultural Universities, while the National Agriculture Extension System (NAES) has established the largest extension service at national, state, district, block and village level. Besides, the technology generation and human resource development, NARS is also involved in technology assessment, refinement and dissemination. The Ministry of Agriculture, Government of India, through its Department of Agricultural Research and Education (DARE) and Department of Agriculture and Cooperation (DAC) coordinate the agricultural development work. The DARE looks after agriculture research and education, while DAC looks after extension works through its well established network from national to grass root levels.

Since the independence in India, the public sector continues to be the main livestock service provider for free of cost or with heavy subsidies. However, increasing fiscal constraints on government, concerns raised about the efficiency and efficacy of the public sector veterinary services and the diverse demand of farmers have together led to a search for alternative ways of providing these services. Privatization of veterinary services, as one alternative strategy for providing efficient service is finding acceptance in developing countries including India. Thus, the privatization of various livestock services has started in many parts of the country in recent past as a part of new economic policy with a view to enhance greater role for rationalization of government fiscal deficits and disinvestments of public sector.

State level animal husbandry departments

Livestock extension service is a mandate of the state level animal husbandry departments. State animal husbandry departments throughout the country have 7415 veterinary hospitals/polyclinics, 14573 veterinary dispensaries, 23682 veterinary aid and 43782 Artificial insemination (AI) centres spread out widely throughout the country to carry out various activities of the departments (Sasidhar and Chandel, 2003). In general, this department at its apex has the directorate of animal husbandry at state level, while it has a veterinary dispensary at panchayat union level (headquarter for cluster of villages / hamlets) and further down has animal breeding centres / sub centres which covers few villages. At the district level, the Deputy Director / Joint Director are responsible for animal husbandry activities and at grass root level veterinarians and para veterinarian represent the animal husbandry departments. Currently more than 10000 cattle unit heads are taken care by one veterinarian (Sudeepkumar, 1999) against the recommendation of per 5000 cattle unit per head (NAC, 1976). Similar conditions exist in case of supporting staffs. As per the job chart, veterinarians need to carry out regular services such as treatment, breeding, record keeping, administrative works and extension activities with the support of para staff. But with this work load the probability of carrying out extension activities become limited (Sudeepkumar, 1999). On the other hand, under the guidelines of donor agencies (World Bank, International Monitory Fund, Asian Development Bank etc) structural policy changes in government makes state governments reluctant to recruit new human resources in place of existing vacancies and for the last few years there was almost no new recruitments of human resources. State governments are in tempo of privatization of various services including extension services. For example as per Orissa state livestock policy, the extension will be restructured to promote convergent approach involving various technical training, the financial service organization and delivery of quality services at the doorstep moving from free services to payment for quality and timely services. This can be said as initiation of privatization on extension from complete free service to cost recovery. Secondly the budget allotted to extension services very limited (Morton *et al.*, 1997). This fact holds good now also. Pondicherry animal husbandry department spends around 2.6% of its total expenditure in 2002-03 while the adjoining state Tamil Nadu has spent 0.04% in 2003-04 of total departmental budget. Central and State government in the past allocated inadequate funds for agricultural research programmes and public sector extension services of crop and animal husbandry.

Besides, the other factors like low budgeting along with lack of human resources, infrastructure and adequate financial support gets reflected in the whole extension system (Bhat and Das, 2002; Ravikumar and Chander, 2006). It is further reported that the current extension system provides inferior services and meagre attention on small ruminant. Thus, the state governments are in tempo of privatization of various services including extension services to overcome the poor performance at the field level.

Agricultural technology management agency (ATMA)

Now, Agricultural Technology Management Agency (ATMA) is being implemented in almost all states of India as one of the new extension innovations after Training and Visiting System. This initiative at state level has working groups coordinating various departments of agriculture including animal husbandry departments and state agricultural and / or veterinary universities while at district level similar working groups are set with their representatives of the above institutes. At a lower level, it has farm information and advisory centres, which has established links and formed various sub committees with representation from farmers and community-based organization. The farmer information centre has an agricultural extension officer, livestock extension officer and horticultural extension officer. This whole new initiative in extension attempts to cover all activities under an umbrella to give a single window for extension system and also works out model for complete cost recovery mechanisms. One of the aims of ATMA programme is to recover partial or complete cost of extension services through a phased manner. In addition under ATMA, public private partnership for extension services is being established. Under this, the farmers are mobilized into small groups based on the commodity they produce (Commodity Interest Groups) and linked to contact farming firms, procurement agencies, input suppliers, food processors and corporate retail outlets. This all together force the farming community to rely more on corporate for extension services. Corporate engaged in this process will recover the cost through indirect/direct mechanisms.

Agri-clinics

The Government of India, under the Ministry of Agriculture, MANAGE (Hyderabad) and NABARD initiated new concept called agri-clinics to privatize livestock services including livestock extension along with agriculture. The main objective of the programme was to provide input services including extension services to farming community through private individuals / groups. Under this initiative, private veterinary clinic are being established throughout the country. Since agri-clinic is owned by the individuals (private) they are charging for whatever service they provide to the livestock farming community. Besides, the start-up training of graduates in agriculture and allied subjects will support in establishing self-employment activities by the agri-tech graduates and develop linkages for sustainable growth in agriculture.

Krishi Vigyan Kendras (KVKs)

These are farm science based centres playing an important role in application of innovative agricultural technologies in different agro-ecological situations. The KVKs pursue participatory mode of planning and implementation of its programmes which may be realized by streamlining active involvement of farmers, line departments, research institutes, NGOs and others at different levels. KVKs emphasize on technology integration and process development for large scale adoption.

Over time, change in mandate of KVK has taken place. The revised mandate of KVK (XI plan) aims at 'assessment, refinement and demonstration of technology/products and its dissemination through training of farmers and extension personnel, besides the responsibility to work as knowledge and resource centre of agricultural technology. Over the years, the KVKs have grown in number and intensity of programmes, along with the conceptual changes in its approach from (i) sporadic to cluster approach, (ii) individual to group approach, (iii) institution to change agent approach, (iv) training to technology application, (v) technology to knowledge and resource management and (vi) independent to convergence mode of action. In addition to the above mentioned activities, there are other numerous growing areas where the KVKs have their role like the distance mode of technology dissemination and capacity building of KVK trainers with the help of basic IT facilities required in distance mode. Presently more than 585 KVKs are working in the country at district level (Singh and Singh, 2009).

Agricultural Technology Information Centre (ATIC)

ATIC is a "single window" support system linking the various units of a research institution with intermediary users and end users (farmers) in decision making and problem solving exercise. The rationale for establishment of ATIC includes, providing diagnostic services for soil and water testing, plant and livestock health, to supply research products such as seeds and other planting materials, poultry strains, livestock breeds, fish seed, processed products, etc, emerging from the institution for testing and adaptation by various clientele, to provide information through published literature and communication materials as well as audio-visual aids and providing an opportunity to the institutes/ SAU's to generate some resource through the sale of their technologies. Thus these centres provides a 'balanced scorecard' in terms of (i) financial- resource generation and financial sustainability, (ii) customers- measures on performance of the technology from the customer's point of view, (iii) process- the performance of key internal processes in terms of providing quality services, seed and other inputs materials, (iv) linkage with district extension system and spread of improved technology and productivity in the area and (v) learning- the ability of the research organization to improve continuously and innovate in its products, services and processes.

Information and Communication Technology (ICT) based tools/ approaches/centres for technology transfer

ICT is an umbrella term which includes different sets of tools / equipments that excel technologically and contain resources for creation, proper dissemination and management of knowledge to the end users. In general, the ICT tools encompass computers, internet, broadcasting technologies (radio and television), telephony and other applications associated with them, such as video-conferencing and distance learning. The ICTs are being increased used by governments to deliver services at the locations convenient to the citizens at their village door steps. Besides, it can be used by wide number of organizations in technology transfer e.g women self help groups (WSHGs) in Kerala using (i) COMBACC (Cell phone Operated Mobile Audio Communication system), (ii) ASLICS (Automated and Self Learning and Interactive Communication System) and (iii) VAKTHRAM (Visual Assistant and Knowledge Transferring Automated Mechanism).

Extension organizations are working as medium between communication technologies and the target groups. In this role they must be able to examine the appropriateness of various ICTs, the accessibility of ICT in rural and remote areas, how to best to reconcile costs and benefits and how to ensure ICT access. However, ICT projects come with a range of weakness, which can be overcome by agriculture extension (Rajeev *et al.*, 2009).

Cell phone an ICT tool has great potential especially under Indian conditions as no other technology has spread as faster as is the case with it. The tiny handsets in the developing countries like India act as hubs for mobile banking, entrepreneurship, fact checking and public health announcements. In many parts of the country farmers are already using mobile phones to find the latest market price on the products like buffalo milk and information on agricultural practices from various service providers, without much cost of calling.

Community radio is one more ICT tool which can play a vital role in providing local information needed for social and economic development and empowerment of women. Studies show that farmers prefer interpersonal and local source or mass media in many places. Ordinary people have used community radio to revitalize local communities. There are numerous studies on its efficacy in transfer of technology reported over worldwide.

Web based technology, expert systems and information kiosks are the other important areas whereby we are harvesting the immense potential of the ICTs in the field of agricultural technology utilization. The web based expert system is used in dissemination of agricultural information to the farmers and helps in decision making like the expert system developed by Birsa Agricultural University, Ranchi. It comprises of fifteen modules and is presented in seven languages with architecture of 3 tier MySQL system working behind it. Similarly, the information kiosks spread in many parts of the country play vital role in development of agriculture as a whole and livestock in particular. The Dairy Information Service Kiosk (DISK) under the National Dairy Development Board falls in this category. This case describes the automation of the milk buying process at 2500 rural milk collection societies. The application user personal computers at the milk collection centre of the Dairy Cooperative Societies (DCS) have connectivity to an Internet Service Provider (ISP), with the two components as – a Dairy Portal (DP) and DISK. There other related systems and kiosks working under non-governmental organizations like the aAQUA, e-chaupals and ikisan or the public sector common service centres working under broad programme of e-governance system in the country.

Information technology based village information centres are emerging as a important media centres in rural areas. Development of VSAT and corDECT technology made the internet connectivity easier and cheaper to the rural India and facilitates easy access to the markets, in addition to organizing contract farming / procurement of primary goods (Prahalad and Hart, 2002). Corporate houses such as ITC (Indian Tobacco Company), HUL (Hindustan Unilever Limited) and Mahindra and Mahindra are tapping the rural market opportunity through IT innovations in India. ITC alone has reached out to more than 2.4 million farmers in 21000 villages and six states through 4100 e-Choupals, which are IT based rural village information and service centres of ITC (Anonymous, 2004). While HUL has started to experiment in its iSakthi project by selling its veterinary drugs with support of Andhra Pradesh e-Seva (IT based rural village Information and service centres) centres. Many new initiatives by governments, private and NGOs are in pipeline. In this background the government of India started to pool the efforts of above stakeholders to bring out IT based village knowledge information centres for more than half a million villages within few years. Emerging of IT in the rural backdrop as a new media is likely to play predominant role in agriculture and livestock extension.

Traditional folk media

'Traditional folk media' is term used to denote the 'people's performances'. The traditional media means the mediums through which the cultural traits passed from generation to generation. Folk media is the creative dissemination of information through culture and performance art. In traditional societies, folk media: drama, skits, poems, stories, riddles, songs and dance have been popularly and successfully used to disseminate messages and even to pass wisdom of older generation to youth. Folk media can overcome the difficulty of languages, speech, words and other barriers of communication especially in Indian context with the prevalence of almost forty types of languages and dialects. Therefore, the rural people are logically, psychologically and mentally attached to these traditional media like Ram leelas, Bhajan, Jhanki, Allaha, Nukad, Natak etc.

Market led extension system

It is the strategy in which a farming system seeks to determine what products a consumer might want and then moves the farm to develop those products. It relies heavily on market research along with activities like value addition supported by proper knowledge and facilities for pre and post harvest practices. Thus the extension strategy for this system can have emphasis on items like client-oriented and demand led participatory research for development of appropriate technology, promoting pluralistic extension system in public-private partnership mode, area approach for integrated development, reorienting functioning of KVKs, reorienting the extension role of SAUs/ICAR institutes, involving farmers and their groups/association in marketing and trading and village based integrated models for market led agriculture.

Producer's cooperative societies

Dairy cooperatives carry out dairy extension services as part of their mandate. The federation apex body at the state level has a centralized publications unit, which produces extension materials based on the problems encountered in the fields of union. At the district level the union organizes exposure visits, audio visual shows and distribution of extension materials through Milk Producer's Cooperative Societies (MPCS) and establishes demonstration units on dairy and fodder. The MPCS are the grass root level organization of the dairy cooperatives and receive backend support from the dairy unions and state level federations. In turn the state federations and unions get support from NDDB. On comparison with crop producer cooperatives and other stakeholders in extension (agriculture departments, animal husbandry departments, state agricultural universities, NGOs) has better contact intensity and manpower for extension activities (Sulaiman and Sadamate, 2000). But still they are able to cover only 20% of the total milk produced in the country. But recent developments in dairy cooperative sector especially the conversion of dairy cooperatives to more autonomous institutions forces them to run the business with a limited support from government. Under Andhra Pradesh Mutually Aided Cooperative Societies Act-1995, the diary cooperatives in Andhra Pradesh province became autonomous and the support of central and state becomes scanty. Currently six milk unions in the above state start operate on their own without any support from state federation. They are operating on complete cost recovery mechanisms. Bihar, Jammu and Kashmir and Madhya Pradesh are few states following Andhra Pradesh model. Thus cooperatives are forced up to pass on the cost of dairy extension services to farming community. In this background dairy unions started to charge the dairy farming community for the extension services (Chapman and Tripp, 2003). In coming days, cooperative sectors are expected to fall in similar lines and the cost of dairy extension services would eventually fall on shoulders of dairy farmers.

Veterinary / agricultural educational institutes and their substations

The prime agenda of the veterinary and agricultural universities are three folds namely; education, producing skilled human resources, research and extension services. These universities addresses livestock and fodder related extension activities through associated bodies. These bodies are principally extension and communication departments, regional stations, KVK, ATIC and farmers training centres. The Extension and Communication Department along with Directorate of Extension of the university provides training, conducts postal courses, and produces mass media programmes on livestock husbandry. But activities of these institutes were restricted to a limited number of local areas (Sulaiman and Van den Ban, 2003). Generally KVK operates through central government funding under the supervision of the local agricultural / veterinary sciences universities and NGOs. One of the mandates of KVKs is to update extension personnel on emerging advances in research.

Private industries

Private industries carry out the information dissemination through direct contacts and mass media. e.g. in poultry sector the private industries / corporate houses play a predominant role. As corporate work with poultry farming community under various levels of production and their relation also varies. In broiler farming, a high degree of contract farming starting from supply of day old chick to procurement of marketable broiler and selling to final consumer exists (i.e from hatchery to dining table). But in case of egg production private companies participate at different levels. The companies engaged in contact farming or supplying of inputs or procurement of outputs play major role in dissemination of poultry information. Contract companies, hatcheries, feed manufactures; drug producers through their representatives or marketing agents push up the information for increased business turn out in favour of the firm.

Implementation of Milk and Milk Products order 1992 and later amendments resulted in opening of dairy sector for organized private sector participation. This resulted in entry of organized private dairies on a large scale under contract system. Well known examples are Nestle, Smithkline, Hindustan Unilever, Heritage and Hatsun Agro Limited. These corporate houses operate with farming community through a contract agreement. They provide a variety of input services to dairy members, including dairy extension (Thirunavukkarasu and Sudeepkumar, 2005). These private dairies organize mass contact programmes such as animal health camps, dairy educational tours and also publish a number of printed materials on dairy husbandry. Similar to poultry sector the dairy feed companies are also started to push the information through direct contacts and mass media. Drug and vaccine companies organize similar type of activities with the support of their marketing people and local sales agents and also participate in agricultural exhibitions in order to create awareness on their products. In recent years reluctance of the government to invest in livestock sector and on the other hand intensive promotion of private investment has resulted in entry of corporate. Entry of Charoen Pokphand, Hindustan Lever and diversification of Venky, Suguna, Shanthi fortunes etc to various sub sectors of livestock field (Example- Venky an Indian monopoly in poultry sector expanding from hatchery business to vaccines and broiler contract farming). This all indicates in coming days, more intensive participation from business houses likely to take place in this sector. Private / corporate participation pushes (corporate pro information to the farming community rather than rational information on new livestock technologies and innovations) its own commercial interest information resulting in hardship to farming community and risk to the environment in the long run. The character of information has already started to take "U" turn from pro poor to corporate pro i.e. from information to advertisement.

Non-governmental organizations (NGOs) and others

In general, the role of NGOs in livestock extension and other livestock services were limited to few geographical areas in the past. But in the context of new structural policies the NGOs participation in livestock sector has increased. Various state governments stated to sub contract various livestock services to NGOs. It can be recollected from the initiation of DANIDA (Danish International Development Agency) and Tamil Nadu Animal Husbandry Department collaborated programme, which involved in enwrapping NGOs to create a pool of private extension workers. The popular NGOs engaged in these activities were BAIF (Bharathiya Agro Industrial Federation), Anthra, JK Gram Vikas Yogana Trust and Pradan etc. These NGOs work on development of community based animal health workers and inseminators. This Para staffs also takes care of disseminating information on various livestock issues. Some of the NGOs provide their service on cost basis, while others provide it as a social service.

According to Ahuja (2004) the NGOs activity in this field organizes and mobilizes the latent market demand for animal health services. This means in future, the NGOs will facilitate consolidation and organization of livestock services for private participation or NGOs on its own will mature as a private party and capitalize the emerging markets. This all together will end up in adding cost burdens for farming community and when private players come into the scene with the support of NGOs corporate pro messages will be in the forefront. Some freelance publications include study materials for livestock farmers in the local language. The local newspaper "Eenadu" in Andhra Pradesh and "Dinamalar" in Tamil Nadu provinces has a regular agricultural section in it. Currently in many of the local languages farmer's magazine are also available. While the central ministry and National Institutes' namely National Dairy Research Institute, Indian Veterinary Research Institute and other ICAR institutes on livestock and fodder and their sub stations organize various training programmes on livestock issues for farmers and supporting staffs of cooperatives and animal husbandry departments.

Challenges of transfer of technology system

The existing extension system of India is at crossroads. As we are in 21st century, the extension faces not only the challenge of meeting the increased demand for food but also the issues related to sustainable development, environmental protection, conservation of natural resources as well as improving the socio-economic status of weaker sections of society. Vijayaragvan (2001) emphasized the need for shift in extension paradigm to meet the challenge for efficient transfer of efficient transfer of technology (Table 1).

Table 1 : Needed shift in extension paradigm at a glance (source: Vijayaragvan, 2001)

S. No.	Components	Traditional Extension	Extension for 21th century
1.	Goal	Transfer of technology	Enhancing the overall capacity of farmers
2.	Need assessment and programme planning	Top down approach and rigid	Bottom up approach and flexible
3.	Source of technology	Mainly government research institutions	Multiple sources – governments, private and farmers knowledge
4.	Nature of technology	i. Input intensive, crop based and general recommendations	i. Knowledge intensive, broad based, farming system perspective and location specific
		ii. Fixed package information	ii. Provision of choices

5.	Dissemination of technology	i. Individual approach with lack of participation of farmers ii. NGOs not involved	i. Group approach with increased participation of farmers and their organization ii. Greater involvement of NGOs
6.	Clients	Mostly male farmers	Efforts to reach both male and female farmers, rural youth and farm labourers.
7.	Farmers activity	Routine application of technology/ inputs	Encouraging farmers experimentation and learning
8.	Role of extension agents	Information transfer	Facilitation of learning
9.	Rewards and incentives for extension personnel	Rewards not linked to performance	Rewards linked to performance
10.	Financial sustainability	Very low	High
11.	Role of extension agents	Knowledge transfer	To help to build overall capacity of farmers.

Thus there is need and stress on farmers' participatory model of technology transfer under present scenario. The farmers are seen as active partners in research and extension with due consideration to the valued indigenous wisdom possessed by them. The research is seen as a joint endeavor involving farmers and researchers to solve the problems being faced by the farmers, with the emphasis on need for scientists to become more sensitive to understand, communicate and collaborate with farmers. Further the establishment of physical infrastructure and educational facilities for strengthening local experimentation is an essential aspect of participatory model.

Henceforth, we see the case of Participatory Technology Development (PTD) as a process of bringing together the local communities with their own knowledge and capacity for research, on one platform with the researchers and other professionals. Thus PTD as a process is aimed at strengthening existing experimental capacity of farmers in search of sustainable innovation generation system. It requires the development of social skills in professionals along with exposure to anthropological and social tools with due respect to Indigenous Technological Knowledge (ITK).

Revitalizing transfer of technology system

There is an urgent need to revitalize the present extension system for better utilization of the resources to meet our demands on sustainable basis as continuous focus on organizing technology oriented programmes addressing local priorities. Thus, there is a need for strong technological support between KVKs, SAUs, ICAR Institutes and other such organizations like NGOs. There is need for initiative on process development by various organizations along with work on developing mechanisms, processes, models and cases which could be replicated for other locations. There has to be a considerable thought on shouldering off the unwanted responsibility from various technology transferring bodies for their effective working by concentration on the actual role expected from them. Enhancement of technical manpower and creation of some specialist positions needed for looking into the requirement of various areas especially in case of KVK and other field level organizations and improved monitoring of technical programmes with the strengthening of links among various concerned organizations for development of quality programmes. There are other issues as well into which all the stakeholders should reflect upon to have the results on ground level in due course of time, with a holistic view of the prevalent situations.

References

Ahuja, V. 2004. The economic rationale of public and private sector roles in the provision of animal health services. Revue scientifique et technique / Office international des epizooties, 23: 33-45.

Ahuja, V., Kurup, M.P.G., Bhasin, N.R. and Joseph, A.K. 2008. Assessment and reflections on livestock service delivery systems in Andhra Pradesh. In: Proc. Wworkshops and Consultations, Mehboobnagar, Chittoor, Annavaram, Nalconda and Rampachodavaram.

Anonymous. 2001. Issues in perspective. In: NDRI Vision 2020. All India business directory (Dairy year book), 2001 (Special millennium issue).

Bhat, P.N. and Das, N. 2002. Report of working group on animal husbandry and dairying for the tenth five year plan (2002-2007), Government of India, Planning commission.

Chapman, R. and Tripp, R. 2003. Changing incentives for agricultural extension-A review of privatized extension in practice. Agricultural Research and Extension Network Paper No. 132.

DAHD. 2010. Annual Report, Department of Animal Husbandry and Dairying, Ministry of Agriculture, New Delhi, Government of India.

Economic Survey. 2009-10. Economic Division, Ministry of Finance, New Delhi, Government of India.

Morton, J., Matthewman, R. and Barton, D. 1997. Livestock production extension: Issues, case studies and policy options. NRI Socio-economic Series 12. Chatham, UK, Natural Resources Institute.

National Dairy Plan. 2010 Department of Animal Husbandry and Dairying, Ministry of Agriculture, New Delhi, Government of India, 2008-09.

Prahalad C.K and Hart Stuart, L. 2002. The fortune at the bottom of the Pyramid. Strategy + business, First quarter.

Rajeev, T.S., Ramkumar, S., Marshal, C.R. and Rajesh, K.R. 2009. ICT based tools for dissemination of technology among women self help groups engaged in livestock rearing for effective modification of behavioural attributes. In: Proc. ISEE National Seminar, IVRI, Izatnagar, U.P., 29-30 December.

Ravikumar, R.K. and Chander, M. 2006. Extension educational efforts by state department of animal husbandry (SDAH), Tamil Nadu: SWOT analysis. Livestock Research for Rural Development. Volume 18.

Sasidhar, P.V.K. and Chandel, B.S. 2003. Rational delivery of private livestock extension services - Interventions. MANAGE Extension Research Review 3: 121-131.

Singh, A.K. and Singh, L. 2009. Emerging role of KVKs in development of technology and process modules. In Proceedings: ISEE National Seminar, IVRI, Izatnagar, U.P., 29-30 December.

Sudeepkumar, N.K. 1999. Manpower planning of veterinary personal in Tamil Nadu. Ph D thesis, TANUVAS, Chennai, Tamil Nadu, India.

Sulaiman, V.R. and Sadamate, V.V. 2000. Privatizing agricultural extension in India, Policy paper 10, National Centre for Agricultural Economics and Policy Research, New Delhi.

Sulaiman, V.R. and Van den Ban, A.W. 2003. Funding and delivering agricultural extension in India. Journal of International Agricultural and Extension Education 10: 21-29.

Thirunavukkarasu and Sudeepkumar, N.K. 2005. Milk procurement systems and services to the dairy farmers in the open economy of India: A case study. Afro Asian Journal of Rural Development 38: 87-95.

Vijayaragvan, K. 2001. Agricultural Extension - A vision 2020. Division of Agricultural Extension, IARI, New Delhi.

□□□

Chapter 33

Linking Goat Farmers and Markets for Improving Productivity and Livelihoods

Shalander Kumar, Khem Chand and M.M. Roy
Central Arid Zone Research Institute, Jodhpur-500 059 (Rajasthan)
* The work was carried out at CIRG, Makhdoom, Mathura, UP

Goat rearing plays an important role in the food and nutritional security of millions of rural landless, marginal and small farmers especially in the rain fed areas of the country having low agricultural productivity. Under the prevailing production system goats are mostly raised under extensive system on common property resources (CPRs). They have distinct economic and managerial advantages over other livestock species particularly for the resource poor rural people. The requirement of less initial investment, less management problems due to small body size and docile nature, low input, higher prolificacy, early sexual maturity at 8-12 months of age, almost equal market value of male and female goats, easy marketing and unprejudiced social acceptance of their products are few of many advantages of this activity that provides assured higher income. Goats can efficiently survive on available shrubs and trees in adverse environment in less fertile lands. In a state like Rajasthan where agriculture production is severely affected by frequent droughts, the livestock rearing is the most stable economic activity for the rural people. Further the goats with their inherent ability to perform under adverse conditions, constitute the largest share (34%) of the total livestock in the state making them more important in the rural economy. The rural poor who can not afford to maintain a cow or a buffalo find goat as the best alternative source of supplementary income and milk. This is one reason why poor rural households maintain a few number of goats. Unlike a cow or buffalo, a few goats can be maintained easily and can be easily sold in the years of drought. In recent experience, goat enterprise has also shown promise of its successful intensification and commercialization (Kumar, 2007). But, the existing goat production system is under pressure because of continuous decline in the quantity and quality of CPRs on which goats mainly depend for their feeding. In spite of having potential in goat rearing to generate good economic returns the paradox however is that, the goat keepers are poorest among the rural poor people. Feed scarcity, poor access to market and non-adoption of improved technologies including preventive health schedule are the major reasons of low income from goat rearing. At the same time due to increased domestic demand and resultant spiralling price of goat meat, which at present is Rs. 200 to Rs. 300 per kg, there appears to be good prospects for goat production.

This paper has documented two cases of innovative arrangements for linking goat farmers and market. The innovation-I is about 'Linking the goat farmers of feed scarce region in Rajasthan to resource poor goat keepers mainly women in Uttar Pradesh, Bihar, Jharkhand and West Bengal which are relatively fodder rich regions'. In the process, the goat kids are transferred from feed scarce region to the area with relatively better feed availability for goats. The innovation-II is 'Creation of an informal network of goat farmers belonging to different states for improving access to market, technology and critical inputs'

Case- I: Linking the goat keepers of feed scarce Rajasthan and feed and fodder rich regions

Issues, communities and location

Faced with low productivity and high uncertainty in crop production, majority of rural people in Rajasthan are dependent on common property resources (CPRs) based livestock especially small ruminant rearing. Among the small ruminants, the goats are economically more important in eastern semi arid zone of Rajasthan consisting Ajmer, Tonk and Jaipur districts, where one of the two good practices has emerged. This zone along with Nagaur, Sirohi, Bansbara districts is also the home tract of one of the most economically important and widely adapted goat breed of India 'Sirohi'. The animals of this breed are hardier, have medium to large body size, milk yield of 1.5 to 2.5 liters per day and have good demand for meat and ceremonial sacrifices. Goat rearing which is one of the major sources of livelihood for majority of the rural people in this rainfed region has been facing a major constraint in terms of feed and fodder scarcity. The productivity of goats under the prevailing traditional extensive production system has been very low, where they are maintained on natural vegetation in degraded common grazing lands and tree lopping. Even these degraded grazing resources are also shrinking continuously.

Under the feed scarcity situation in Rajasthan, the goats had access to only limited feed resources available in CPRs and some supplementary feed and fodder occasionally. As a consequence there is a trade off that either the farmers use the limited feed and fodder only for rearing the adult female goats producing milk and kids or thinly spread the limited feed and fodder for raising all the goats that is adult females, male as well as the kids up to the economic age of slaughter 6 to 8 months resulting in poor productivity of all the animals in terms of less growth of body weight, lower milk yield, poor conception rate in female goats, etc. Among the two options, the farmers have opted to feed their adult female goats and sell the kids at the earliest age of 2-3 months (at weaning: age at which generally a goat kid stops suckling mothers milk and starts taking feed and fodder). Another major reason to sell the kids at an early age was that in the absence of proper housing structures for goats, the young goat kids continue to suck mother's milk even up the age of 5-6 months. This results in direct loss of milk and finally income of the farmer. In this process the farmers have been selling goat kids at the age of 2-3 months to the trader/butchers, which were mostly slaughtered for meat. However in this arrangement where farmer want to get rid of the goat kids at an early age, on the one hand the kids are sold at very low price resulting in loss to the goat farmers and on the other hand, it is a loss to the national economy by losing the potential production due to slaughtering of under age kids instead of raising them up to economic age of slaughter, which should be 6-8 months.

Development of linkages

With CPRs continuously declining in terms of area and productivity, it has been felt for quite some time by the experts that an institutional arrangement should be developed so as to transfer the young kids of goats and sheep after weaning (at about 2.5 to 3 months age) from feed scarce regions to the relatively feed and fodder rich regions for raising them under intensive or semi-intensive system of production. Such a good practice has emerged out of its necessity due to market forces.

Origin and institutional arrangement in innovation: As a result of increasing market demand and price of goat meat during the past one and half decade and consequent increased potential of higher profitability from goat rearing, increasingly large number of resource poor rural people especially women in Uttar Pradesh, Bihar and West Bengal have taken up goat rearing as a mean of supplementary source of income. These households are interested to rear 1-2 or 3 goats especially males under intensive or semi-intensive systems wherein male kids are fed on leftover food of the family and also some supplementary feed and fodder. They are largely sold for ceremonial scarifies like Eid and Durga Puja. These goat keepers wanted to rear such male kids which have good look and relatively large body size in order to get premium price of male goats during Eid festival.

As a part of the existing marketing channel, traditionally *'Sirohi'* goats are collected by the traders from Ajmer, Tonk, Jaipur and Bharatpur districts of Rajasthan and transported and sold in Uttar Pradesh, Bihar and West Bengal. The Sirohi goats are preferred because of their hardiness, better milk yield, large body size and good colour (brown). The traders who were collecting Sirohi goats from Rajasthan and selling in other states, occasionally also purchased small kids (2-3 months age) of Sirohi goats and sold them to the women goat keepers in Uttar Pradesh, Bihar and West Bengal. These small kids of Sirohi goats were very well received by the farmers and performed well under the new agro-climatic conditions. The goat kids which were transferred from feed scarce Rajasthan got better access to feed and fodder and individual care by the goat keepers and consequently showed better body weight growth rate and finally attracted very good market price. As a result, a good demand was created for young males of Sirohi goats of 2-3 months in Uttar Pradesh, Bihar and West Bengal. That further encouraged the middlemen / traders to take up the trade in small goat kids. With the ready demand in these states and supply from Rajasthan, the marketing channel for trading of young goat kids got strengthened. However, this inter-state trade of small goat kids was completely in the hands of private middlemen/traders, who are interested only in their profit margins. The traders from Uttar Pradesh purchase the goat kids either directly from the farmers in the villages of Rajasthan or often they make purchases from local traders of Rajasthan. Consequently, the kids are transported and sold in Uttar Pradesh, Bihar and West Bengal. The market forces thus have helped in creating an arrangement for transferring the goat kids from feed scarce Rajasthan to the areas with relatively better feed availability, where they could be better reared.

Impact of linking goat farmers of Rajasthan and Uttar Pradesh, Bihar and West Bengal

The impact of linking the goat keepers of feed and fodder scarce region and feed and fodder rich region has been multi-dimensional and has benefited different stakeholders. This arrangement for marketing production benefited both the goat farmers in Rajasthan as well as in Uttar Pradesh, west Bengal and parts of Bihar and the goat economy as such by providing an opportunity to rear the male kids up to the economic age of their slaughter.

Benefits to farmers of feed scarce region (Rajasthan): On account of severe scarcity of feed and fodder, the farmers in Ajmer, Nagaur, Tonk, Jaipur districts of Rajasthan wanted to get rid of the goat kid at an early age and use the available feed to feed the milking goats. Consequently they were selling the goat kids at the age of 2-3 months to the trader / butchers, which were mostly slaughtered to produce meat. Before this arrangement came into effect, taking the benefit of compulsion of the farmers, the traders used to purchase the goat kids at very low price resulting in the loss of the poor farmers. As this good practice evolved, a lot of demand was created for the goat kids of 2-3 months age of Sirohi breed; as a result the price of these young kids suddenly rose from about Rs. 400-500 to about Rs. 700-900 per kid during the year 2006. Now the present price of each goat kid of 2-3 month age is Rs. 1000-1200. That has resulted in direct increment in the returns from goat rearing to the farmers. This arrangement of linking the goat keepers of feed and fodder scarce Rajasthan and feed and fodder rich region of Uttar Pradesh, Bihar and West Bengal not only resulted in increase in returns from goat rearing for the farmers of Rajasthan but also enhanced the sustainability of the goat production system in Rajasthan which has been under pressure due to continuous shrinkage of common feed resources. It is well documented that major part of income from goat rearing activity is accrued from the sale of surplus live animals. Before this arrangement came into effect, very low price for surplus male kids and higher grazing incidence in Rajasthan was threatening the viability and sustainability of the goat production system.

Benefits to the goat economy: Besides benefits to the goat farmers and enhancing the sustainability of the goat production system, this arrangement of linkages has benefited the national goat economy. Before the linkage among the goat farmers of Rajasthan and goat breeders of UP, Bihar and West Bengal, the male kids of Sirohi goats produced in Rajasthan were slaughtered at an uneconomic age of 2-3 months and it was a direct loss to the national economy by loosing the potential production due to slaughtering of under age kids instead of raising them up to economic age of slaughter, which 6-8 months. However with this arrangement in place the sold out small male goat kids from Rajasthan are reared up to their economic age of slaughter in other states resulting in more than 3 fold increase in meat production per male kid. That is benefiting the national economy as such.

Benefits to the goat keepers in Uttar Pradesh, Bihar and West Bengal: To take the benefit of lucrative market for festive sale of male goat, the small and marginal farmers and landless households especially the women in western Uttar Pradesh, west Bengal and parts of Bihar are interested in rearing 2-3 male kids of larger breed particularly 'Sirohi' from Rajasthan under intensive and semi intensive system. Through development of linkages, these goat keepers have got an opportunity to buy male kids of Sirohi goat and raise them up to one year of age for their sale during the festival of Eid. In response to the market demand, the traders from Uttar Pradesh were buying small Sirohi male kids of 2-3 months age at about Rs. 700-900 per kid and sold it to the rearers in UP, Bihar and West Bengal. These goat rearers in Uttar Pradesh, west Bengal and Bihar were able get a male goat kid of Sirohi of 2-3 months age at the rate of Rs. 900-1200 per kid from the traders. A well fed male of Sirohi breed is large in size and bear good look and colour, it fetched good price of Rs.3500 to Rs.5500 during the Eid festival during 2006-07. Although the transfer of young kid from Rajasthan to UP , Bihar and West Bengal for raising them has been an unorganized effort, but it has surely benefited the goat farmers and goat economy as such.

In this system, the small kids are being shifted from feed scarce region to the area with relatively better availability of feed resources and were raised properly on relatively low cost feeds resulting in higher efficiency of resource use (feed and fodders), and prevented the slaughter of under-age animals. Therefore, it would be appropriate to make some organized efforts to encourage the farmers and entrepreneurs to adopt kid rearing for commercial chevon (goat meat) production by purchasing the weaner kids (when kid stops taking mother's milk at 2.5 to 3 months age) from the traditional breeders of feed scarce regions and rear them under intensive or semi intensive system for achieving a target finishing weight of 25-30 kg at 6-7 months of age.

Case - II: Linking goat farmers across states (rearing goats under intensive and semi-intensive system)

Issues, communities and location

Due to increased human population, rising income levels and changing consumer preferences, the demand for goat meat and its market price has swiftly increased in the recent past and that increased from Rs. 80 to Rs. 200-300 per kg over a period of past one decade. That has created a greater attraction towards goat production. The goat rearing under traditional extensive system may not be able to produce enough to meet the rising demand because of continuous shrinkage in the common grazing/feeding resources. Hence the traditional system of goat production under extensive grazing programme based on CPRs has to undergo a substantial transformation towards intensification. With these prospects on the horizon, many farmers during the past one decade started intensification of goat production after acquiring some training on improved methods of production. Most of these goat farmers tried to select and rear pure animals under semi intensive system of management and used improved packages of practice to a considerable extent.

Since the marketing of live goats is completely in the hands of middlemen, traders and butchers, they did not offer reasonable price even for good quality pure breed animals produced by these farmers and continued to earn handsome margins. The farmers also did not have any other regulated market or opportunity to sell their surplus animals at reasonable price. Most of these goat farmers belonging to Uttar Pradesh, Madhya Pradesh, Maharashtra, Rajasthan, Chhattisgarh and other states were forced to sell the surplus goats during the year 2004-05 at a low price of about Rs. 50 to 65 per kg of live body weight to the middlemen traders (Kumar, 2007). Consequently many of these farmers started incurring loss mainly due to realization of lower price for the produce and also because of mortality in goats due to non-availability of required veterinary support and critical inputs like vaccines, and non-availability of good quality breeding stock was also a major constraint.

Creation of informal network of goat farmers

In order to address some of the constraints of the goat farmers scattered over different states, the initiative for creation of a network of goat farmers was undertaken by under ICAR Ad-hoc Research Project on 'Commercialization of goat farming and marketing of goats in India' with the technical support provided by Central Institute for Research on Goat, Makhdoom, Mathura, Uttar Pradesh. The goat farmers from different states actively participated and cooperated in this process. The objective was to create an informal network of these goat farmers without having any structure, and create an opportunity for the farmers to know about that what the other farmers were doing, their access to market and technology.

Bringing the goat farmers on a common platform and setting the stage for creation of the Network

Initially the efforts were made to identify the goat farms operating under semi-intensive or intensive system of management mostly producing pure bred animals in different states and rapport was developed with these farms. Information on extent and process of intensification, marketing and constraints thereof were solicited from all the identified farms through questionnaire. The questionnaire responses were collected from 61 goat farmers. Based on the preliminary analysis of data of these 61 farms an initial view on intensification of goat farming in the country was formed. The status of constraints mentioned by the farmers like realization of lower prices, losses due to diseases, scarcity of feed & fodder, lack of knowledge and lack of availability of breeding stock, critical inputs and credit are summarized in Figure 1. In order to comprehend the whole system, thereafter an in-depth study covering 18 goat farms from different states was carried out. This study analyzed information on the following aspects: socio-economic information of goat farmers, source of information, incentives in intensive system of goat farming, level of technology adoption, type of business - production, supports, constraints and opportunities, marketing behavior and pattern and marketing strategy, source of market information and type of competition, price structure of live goats, products and by products in different seasons, marketing costs and value addition, type of market demand for goats & its products, type of support needed for intensification of goat farming and constraints and opportunities in marketing of goats and their products.

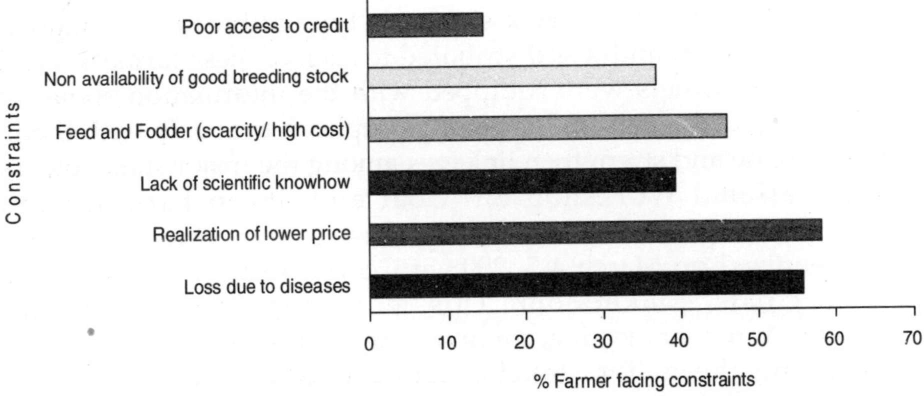

Fig. 1 : Constraints faced by farmers during initial stage of intensification of goat production

Finally employing different methods of collecting information such as personal contact, published and internet sources, Animal Husbandry Departments, farmers, NGOs, key informants and other agencies, a total of 157 goat farms spread over 16 states operating under semi-intensive or intensive system of management mostly producing pure bred animals were identified. These farms were rearing goats of different breeds as per the production objectives and suitability of agro-climatic conditions. They consisted of 38 farms with Barbari goats, 24 with Osmanabadi goats, 26 with Sirohi goats, 18 with Bengal goats, 16 with Jamunapari goats and rest with other breeds and non-descript animals.

- The goat farmers' perception and views on strengthening linkages among them were ascertained. It was revealed that the sixty seven percent of the farmers understand the benefit and wanted to strengthen the linkages among the farmers. The farmers were particularly interested in exchanging technical and market information and breeding bucks among the different farms. Some farmers in Maharashtra and Madhya Pradesh were sharing technical knowledge on improved goat farming with the local traditional goat farmers.

- The experiences of success and failure of intensification of goat farming undertaken in different parts of the country were documented for sharing this experience with the farmers.
- At the outset a directory containing addresses with phone number and email (if existed) of identified 157 goat farms spread over 16 states, their flock size and type of breeds maintained was prepared and was distributed to each of these farmers. With this the farmers were equipped with the information about all other goat farmers and type of germplasm available with them. To create and strengthen linkages among the major stakeholders a National Workshop on 'Goat and Sheep Farming and Marketing: Farmer–Industry–Researcher Interface' was organized on March 4-5, 2006 at Central Institute for Research on Goats, Makhdoom. This workshop provided a rare opportunity of meeting, communication and information sharing among the major stakeholders including traditional and commercial goat farmers, researchers, NGOs working with goats, state animal husbandry officers, entrepreneurs and industry. The most important outcome of this workshop was that all the participants including goat farmers from different states could know the magnitude and number of operating and up-coming goat farming projects under intensive and semi-intensive system of management through out the country. With the help of the directory of addresses of goat farms and meat processors and exporters provided by us (Kumar and Sharma, 2009), they got instant basis to start developing linkages among them. These farmers started making communication among them.
- During the Workshop, we shared the results of our study covering experiences of success and failure of intensification of goat farming in different parts of the country, investment pattern, factors influencing the economic viability of goat farming, innovative marketing methods and strategies for enhancing profitability of the goat rearing activity. During the workshop, a number of goat farmers also shared their good and bad experiences related to goat farming intensification.
- Such Multi-stakeholder Workshops consisting goat farmers from different states, researchers, NGOs, goat traders, industry and extension agencies were organized continuously for four years i.e. 2006, 2007, 2008 and 2009. That really strengthened the

linkages among the goat farmers. Moreover the Directory of addresses of goat farmers was further updated and distributed to the existing farmers and put up as a priced publication for sale for interested stakeholders.

This process has really helped in creation of an *Informal Network* among these goat farmers and that is still continuing. There are no fixed members, no structure, no executive but interaction, communication and exchange of information and breeding animals still continuing because of the tremendous benefits it has provided to these farmers and goat farming as such. Now many of these farmers have also hosted their website (www.goatwala.com; http://www.goatpeople.com; Gaganvfn2001@yahoo.com; pankajbpl1q@yahoo.com; www.ajaputra.com; http://www.nadurgoatfarm.com.).

With the opportunity available for interacting and communicating the goat farmers started interacting more frequently with the farmers of their region/ state or with farmers who were rearing the same breed of goat. Besides interacting across states, the interactions among farmers within the state, for example in Maharashtra, Madhya Pradesh were more frequent. Majority of the farmers in a state were rearing goats of the same breed, e.g. all the farmers in Maharashtra mainly rear goats of Osmanabadi breed and had similar constraints and requirement related to got rearing that resulted in higher interaction among the goat farmers of a state.

Impact of linking goat farmers across states

Creation of an informal network of goat farmers has tremendously contributed towards the process of intensification of goat production in the country. As part of stakeholder workshops, goat farmers' interface with various relevant NGOs, meat processing industry and animal husbandry departments was also initiated. Strengthened linkages among the goat farmers provided them better access to improved technologies, breeding stock, critical inputs and market. As a result of interaction among the goat farmers and information available through the 'directory of addresses of goat farmers' a large number of existing as well as aspirant goat farmers, NGOs working with goats and state animal husbandry departments started requisitioning breeding goats of different breeds from the goat farmers who were part of the informal network. That resulted in creation of a large demand of breeding goats for the existing goat farmers rearing good quality Sirohi, Osmanabadi, Barbari, Jamunapari, Black Bengal and Boer cross goats. As a result the farmers who were producing pure breed goats of different breeds started getting premium price for their animals. Before the creation of linkages among the farmers, they were forced to sell even their pure breed animals at very low price to the traders/ butchers. But now the goat farmers who were earlier getting market rate of Rs. 60 to 70 per kg of live body weight for their goats started getting a price of Rs. 100 to 150 per kg of live body weight in the year 2006-07 and started earning good profit. Many farmers rearing goats under semi-intensive/ intensive system and who were in loss also started earning reasonable profit from the activity because of realization of better price of the produce.

The increased prices of breeding goats due to strengthened linkages have not only created large opportunities and interest for private investment in goat farming projects under intensive/ semi-intensive system but have also encouraged the such existing goat farmers to produce pure-breed good quality animals (germ plasm) of different goat breeds, which would be critically important for the development of goat enterprise in the country. Before this project there were number of farms rearing goats under intensive/ semi-intensive system were operating in the country. It was natural that the cost of goat rearing under intensive and semi intensive system on these farms was higher than the traditional flocks, but the prices of their live goats received from the butcher/traders were low and hence many of them were becoming unsustainable. Through this innovation these goat farmers were not only exposed to the improved technologies of goat production but also of success stories of similar goat rearing units operating in different parts of the country. The farmers could learn that what makes the goat farming as a viable and profitable enterprise and what factors are responsible for losses in this enterprise. Level of adoption of improved technology in goat production in the country has been very low. That mainly attributes to non-existence of relevant extension agency, lack of resources, awareness and knowledge of farmers and poor access to critical inputs and output market. With the creation of this network the goat farmers could have access to improved technologies and knowledge on goat production. They could know what improved practices and inputs other farmers were using and what was the source of those inputs. For example certain vaccines against diseases like PPR (peste des petits ruminants) and goat pox and appropriate mineral mixture were not easily available in the market, but the farmers could help themselves through exchanging information. Some innovative low cost methods of production like different combination of feeds, low cost feeders etc. used by many farmers also benefited the other farmers. Exchanging information among the farmers also helped them in timely diagnosis of certain diseases in their goats. Because of the awareness created through this project and network, about 200 new entrepreneurs have started goat farming under intensive/ semi-intensive system of management during the next one and half year. Since most of these farmers were producing pure breed goats, nearby traditional goat farmers' access to good breeding stock have also increased. Moreover all these goat farmers have started selling their live goats on body weight basis and using most of the recommended package of practices for goat production.

Conclusion

The phenomenon of linking the goat keepers of feed and fodder scarce region in Rajasthan and relatively feed and fodder rich regions tremendously improved the economic viability and sustainability of goat production in Rajasthan and provided good economic opportunity to the resource poor rural people especially women in Uttar Pradesh, Bihar and West Bengal to rear goats quite profitably. It has also contributed towards intensification of goat production which is desirable to some extent on account of continuous shrinkage of common grazing resources. This arrangement which has been evolved due to market forces needs to be institutionalized not only in Rajasthan but in all other regions of the country linking feed scarce and relatively feed and fodder rich areas. In that order the self help groups (SHGs) especially women SHGs in different states may be encouraged to undertake goat kid fattening/ rearing by adopting similar arrangement.

Creation of an informal network of goat farmers has tremendously contributed towards the process of intensification of goat production in the country. Because of continuous interaction among them, the goat farmers have been immensely benefitted in terms of better access to improved technology and critical inputs and increased demand for their breeding goats especially good quality Sirohi, Osmanabadi, Barbari, Jamunapari, Black Bengal and Boer cross goats from the existing as well as aspirant goat farmers, NGOs and animal husbandry departments and as a result higher price for their animals. The increased market price for breeding goats have also encouraged the existing goat farmers to produce such good quality pure breed animals (germplasm) of different goat breeds, which would be critically important for the development of goat enterprise in the country. The goat farmers were also exposed to the success stories of goat rearing units operating in different parts of the country. In order to promote multiplication of superior germplasm, the farms managed on scientific lines should be encouraged to become the centres of production of superior quality breeding animals and need to be supported. The research and extension institutions should make efforts and facilitate in creating such networks of producers and providing them technical support. That would go a long way in realizing the potential of this sector.

References

Kumar, Shalander. 2007. Commercialization of Goat of Goat Farming and Marketing of Goats in India. Final Report of ICAR Ad-hoc research scheme 2004-07, CIRG, Makhdoom, Mathura.

Kumar, Shalander and Sharma, M.C. 2009. Directory commercial goat farms in India. CIRG, Makhdoom, Mathura, Uttar Pradesh.

□□□

Chapter 34

Current Status and Role of Extension in Promotion and Development of Sheep in India

Rajeev Gulyani and L.R.Meena
Division of Transfer of Technology and Social Sciences
Central Sheep and Wool Research Institute, Avikanagar-304 501 (Rajasthan)

The role of sheep is very important in the animal husbandry sector, especially in rural agrarian economy of semi-arid and arid regions. Millions of small and marginal farmers and landless labourers are solely dependent on sheep production for earning their livelihood. Sheep rearing is most suitable to drought prone areas of the country. This enterprise is a boon for the farmers who are not dependent upon agriculture land and other livestock. Moreover, sheep farming can be run by the farmers who do not have grazing land of their own, but can raise their sheep on community grazing lands and uncultivable wastelands. The sheep farming is considered as a multifaceted utility because it produces wool, meat, skin, milk and manure. The sheep population in India was estimated to be 65 million in 2007, ranking 6th in the world and accounting for about 5-6% of the world sheep population. It is estimated that about 0.14 million metric tones of mutton is produced annually from sheep along with 45 million kg of wool and 15% hides and skins. The consumption of wool in India is about 135 million kg/annum. In India approximately 12 lakh persons are associated with the sheep farming activities. The improved practices of sheep rearing, if adopted by farmers, can increase the production of mutton and wool quantitatively and qualitatively and thereby increase the income of sheep farmers. The research results if passed on to the farmers and adopted by them can accelerate this process. But adoption is not a simple process. The major factors contributing to the low productivity of sheep includes poor exploitation of genetic potential of indigenous animals, inadequate resources of feed and fodder, insufficient health cover and inadequate marketing facilities and credit support and due to lack of focused developmental efforts for improvement of sheep. There are many social, economic and organizational constraints, which kgay a vital role in the adoption of improved practices developed by the research organizations. Hence, the study of constraints and their removal through adoption of developed techniques is the need of the hour.

Sheep and wool scenario in the seventh plan period

According to 1972 census India possessed 40.39 million sheep and ranked 6th among the countries of the world in sheep population. The contribution of sheep production to the gross national product exceeded Rs. 160.00 crores/year. In 1970, India exported raw wool and manufactured goods, specially carpet and hosiery worth Rs. 237.97 million and imported fine wool worth Rs. 171.62 million/year. The total installed capacity in the worsted sector required on two shift basis around 34 million kg and about 18 million kg fine wool was imported on scoured basis. Assuming that the imports would continue on this level, the estimated gap between the requirement and availability would be to the extent of 12 million kg of fine wool on clean basis in the worsted sector alone. However, the position in the woolen sector was not so unsatisfactory and the internal production of wool was sufficient to meet the requirement of the industry. There was great demand for superior quality carpet wool in the international market. There was also serious gap between the availability and requirement of mutton considering the contribution of mutton to the total meat produced in the country and the requirement of animal protein in human diet. The estimated annual number of sheep slaughtered was around 12.38 million and contributed 17% to the total meat production in the country (1967-68).

Operational research project on sheep and wool development scheme (1975-81)

Sheep substantiates the rural income to a great extent in arid and semi-arid areas of the country. It has multifaceted utility as it produces wool, mutton, skin, milk and manure. The improved methods of sheep farming, if adopted by farmers, can increase the production of wool and meat quantitatively and qualitatively and thereby can raise income of the farmers. The research results, if passed on to the sheep owners and adopted by them, can accelerate this process. But adoption is not a simple process. There are many social, economic and organizational constraints, which play a vital role in adoption of new technologies. These need to be studied and removed to enhance the adoption process. Keeping this in view the Operational Research Project (ORP) on Sheep and Wool Development Programme was initiated at this Institute in 1975. There were twenty villages under the coverage of the project. The objectives of the project were (i) to study the sheep production practices, their economics vis-à-vis other livestock and crop farming, (ii) to demonstrate the usefulness of improved sheep production technology and (iii) to study the socio-economic constraints in transfer of technologies.

The major findings of this project were:

Flock size and structure: The flock size varied from 10 to 150 sheep. On an average the flock comprised of 48 ewes, 21 lambs and one ram at the time of survey (1975). Bigger flocks had 1-3 rams but smaller flocks normally did not have rams. The body weight of ewes varied from 20 to 25 kg and rams weighed up to 45 kg. The lambs continued to suckle for 5 to 6 months.

Migratory practices: There are very few migrating flocks in the area. Only 22% flocks do migrate to smaller distance say up to 20 Km during the lean periods (April to June).

Watering of flocks: The flocks were usually taken to ponds for watering. However, they were totally dependent on wells in summers. The flocks were watered 2-3 times in a day in summers and once in rest of the seasons.

Grazing management and supplementary feeding: The sheep were grazed around watering points for about 11-12 hrs in lean periods and for about 8 hrs during rainy season. The lambs were grazed with sheep. About 18% sheep farmers fed pala and 19.5% fed methi to their sheep during summer season. The quantity of green fodder did not exceed 350 g/ewe/day. During very lean periods, when sufficient grasses were not available, some breeders fed cluster bean stover, barley and wheat straw etc. and about 50% sheep breeders offer supplementary feeding to rams during breeding season and lean periods. They are always kept with the flock. No concentrate mixture or green fodder was given to flush ewes.

Housing and provision of shelter: Usually no good shelter was provided to sheep. Only 22.5% breeders had small kaccha houses and 37.5% had small thatched roofs to save their sheep from rainy and cold weathers. The covered area was hardly 9 square feet per sheep.

Breeding season: Though the sheep came into heat round the year but the major breeding season was after rains when about 42% sheep came into heat. About 35% sheep came into heat during February to April. The sheep were covered with natural service with native rams only. Artificial insemination was not practiced in the area.

Care and management of pregnant ewes and lambs: The ewes in advance pregnancy were kept in the flock. They delivered the lambs either in pasture or sheep enclosures. No treatment was given to naval cords of the lambs' after birth. The average birth weight of the lambs was 1.93 kg. The average marketing age of the lambs was around 10 month. No concentrate mixture was given to male lambs raised for marketing. Most of the breeders sold the lambs to khatiks on each head basis instead of their weight basis.

Shearing and marketing of wool: Most of the breederskgashed their sheep before shearing but they did not use sheep dip after shearing. Shearing was done by khatik only, no shearing machine was practiced. Shearing was done twice a year except in few cases a third shearing was also done in June before rains. An average flock of 48 sheep yielded 38.25 kg wool with an average of about 800 g/head/yr. Skirting of wool was unknown to the farmers. Most of the breeders sold the wool to khatik, while the wool was still on sheep, on the basis of per animal.

Docking and castration: The breeders did not practice docking and castration in sheep and they did not know about vasectomy in rams. Teaser rams were not kept in the flocks.

Disease incidence and measures adopted: Most common diseases were enterotoxaemia, worm infection, ecthyama, naval ill, piroplasmosis and FMD etc. The mortality in sheep flocks was 18.78% before initiation of ORP. Enterotoxaemia was reported after grazing of sheep in rabi harvested fields and its occurrence continued up to September. Nearly 90-100% sheep, which showed symptoms of the disease died. Bottle jaw was seen round the year; however, it was more prevalent in February-March and July to September. Foot infection and piroplasmosis were prevalent in rainy season. FMD occurred mostly in winter months. Thiabandazole was known to farmers and they were using it against most of the diseases. Some breeders also knew Terramycin (not by name but by colour of the carton).Vaccination against enterotoxaemia and sheep pox was not much known amongst the breeders. These findings formed the basis for application of improved technologies in the field.

Institute village linkages programme (IVLP) for sheep improvement

In the prockgs of technology generation sheep farmers' participation along with their resources, social and economic aspects and perception are often ignored, particularly in case ofkgarginal, sub-marginal and landless farmers. This has resulted in inappropriate technology generation. Realizing this, a participatory research was implemented on farmers' flocks in semi-arid agro-ecosystem to identify the problems (using matrix analysis) and their prioritization based on their need and available rekgurces. Interventions were designed to test the technology for solving the constraints in sheep rearing. Under this programme two sets of treatments (i) sheep owners' practices and (ii) institute evolved practices were used. In case of verification trials, simikgr set of treatments were tested under shepherd management andkgesources situation and replicated according to convenience. Inkguch a way shepherd and institute participatory approach enabled us to solve the constraints being faced by the sheep owners with generation of considerable additional revenue (Mann and Dhaka, 2003). Non-adoption of improved technologies is one of the major reasons for low productivity of sheep. Inappropriateness of technologies resulting from non-consideration of farmers' real life situations is recognized as main reason for non-adoption. After going through the results, it was felt that such model of sheep production should be replicated in every village to increase the prosperity in rural areas (Mann and Meena, 2004).

Benefits derived from application of transferable technologies in sheep

The farmers supplement their wages by keeping small ruminants to meet the day to day and emergent type of expenditures. The main advantage of sheep and goats in livestock-crop production system is their distinguished ability to utilize natural grasses, bushes, shrubs, crop stubbles and tree leaves and to produce saleable products. Sheep is an important species mainly on account of their short generation interval and multifaceted utility as producer of wool, meat, skin manure and milk to some extent. The mutton is the first priority of sheep rearing and wool, hide and skins are the next priority (Gupta, 2004).

Use of superior germplasm for improving productivity in sheep

The improved germplasm of sheep are regularly distributed to interested farmers for breeding purposes. The survey of crossbred produced in the villages in and around CSWRI, Aviaknagar indicated that there are mainly three typeskgf sheep, native (Malpura), crossbreds and mixed type akgilable with the farmerskgThe crossbreds weighed more atkg and 6 month of age than the other two types. The wool yield was 25% higher in crossbreds than natives. The wool quality in terms of diameter and medullation was better in the crossbreds. However, due to lack of grading and organized marketing, the crossbred wool does not fetch better price. The farmers find it difficult to adopt crossbreeding because of poor availability of feed resources and they have to migrate with the flock in search of feed resources. Only well to do farmers come forward to rear crossbred sheep. Attempts have been made to establish field units of the improved germplasm of sheep. Bharat merino, Avikalin and selected Malpura sheep are used as improver breeds for the indigenous sheep. It was also observed that farmers prefer Marwari and Kheri type of sheep as they are sturdy and well adapted for migration. Marwari rams are being supplied to interested farmers and government agencies in order to bring improvement. Gaddi synthetic sheep is preferred by the farmers to improve their Gaddi flocks in order to attain more and better quality wool. In breed improvement programme the carpet wool strain-Avikalin has been developed. Bharat Merino, a superior fine wool sheep has been developed through crossing Rambouillet/Russian Merino with native Chokla, Malpura, Nali and Jaisalmeri ewes and stabilizing exotic inheritance at 75 % level. Gaddi synthetic, another fine wool sheep has been developed by crossing Gaddi sheep with Russian Merino and Rambouillet Ram at regional station of the Institute at North

Temperate Regional Station, Garsa (Himachal Pradesh). Avikalin ram which need special care during lean period (April-June) in dry areas has shown considerable improvement over its native contemporary Malpura breed with regard to greasy fleece yield and wool quality. Avikalin can be used as an improver breed for cross breeding the coarse wool breeds of sheep to increase carpet wool production. The breed is quite suitable as a dual purpose sheep for carpet wool and mutton production. The results obtained from Bharat merino revealed that the genotype is promising to substitute the import of fine wool sheep as an improver breed. Its performance has been found satisfactory in sub-temperate climate at Kodai hills (Tamil Nadu) where this breed achieved 25 and 35 kg body weight at the age of 6 and 12 months, respectively. Some new high producing strains have also been evolved under All India Coordinated Research Project on Sheep Breeding. At TANVASU, Sanynallah a fine wool sheep, Nilgiri synthetic has been evolved which meets the requirement of worsted spinning. At GAU, Dantiwada, Patanwari crosses have shown their performance better than native. At APAU, Palamner, new mutton sheep, Nellore Synthetic lambs were found superior to Nellore lambs on intensive feeding. Results of AICRP on sheep breeding have indicated that fine wool production and quality can be improved through introduction of exotic inheritance from Rambouillet and Russian Merino and stabilizing exotic inheritance up to 50% in North Western region and around 75% in Temperate region of the country. The comparison of growth performance of genetically improved rams distributed to the farmers' under the project and their base line appraisal was made at farmers' level (Table 1). From these results it is evident that the performance of progeny of genetically improved rams was better than base line under local feeding system. These results clearly establish the superiority of genetically improved rams over local bred under local conditions.

Table 1 : Growth performance of progeny from distributed improved rams as compared to base line information

Birth weight (kg)	3 month weight (kg)			
	Base line	Progeny of distributed sires	Base line	Progeny of distributed sires
Male	3.50 (204)	3.78 (112)	13.63 (76)	14.69 (46)
Female	3.24 (216)	3.34 (106)	13.41(120)	13.53 (56)

Physiological manipulation for enhancing reproduction efficiency in sheep

CSWRI, Avikanagar has developed protocol for freezing semen and utilization of the same in artificial insemination with sheep. This technology can provide speedier multiplication of exotic germ plasm of sheep as well as produce more useful animals from indigenous surrogate ewes. With more facilities in terms of infrastructure the semen of better quality animals can be preserved and supplied to the field flocks. The technology has been tested in field conditions and a large number of ewes can be inseminated using chilled semen from superior ram to produce more productive animals. On average semen from one ram (1ml) can be used for 25-30 ewes. The field studies on artificial insemination have showed about 55% successes in farmers flocks (Table 2).

Table 2 : Performance of artificial insemination in farmer flocks

	1995	1996	1997	2009	2010	Overall
No. of ewes inseminated	112	84	37	45	44	322
Lambing (%)	58.03	69.04	37.83	46.66	65.90	55.49

Indigenous practices for sheep health care

Indigenous knowledge and technologies are considered to be the outcome of survival strategies of the disadvantaged people in the risk prone and vulnerable regions. Over a period of time, a vast repository of knowledge has been developed by the farmers. These traditional practices play vital role in sheep husbandry (Mann *et al.*, 2002). The indigenous sheep health care practices assume considerable significance in sheep rearing because of non-availability of doctors and medicines when the flocks are migratory and there is lack of resources with the poor shepherds. These practices are being used extensively and effectively to keep animal healthy and productive since long from generation to generation. They use some common materials like alum, guar, groundnut oil, acacia bark, hool jhari etc. for various diseases. However, their use did not appear to be of much profit, though turmeric power in groundnut oil was useful in control of impaction in lambs caused by licking of soil.

Morbidity and mortality reduction in field through adoption of health calendar

Due to continuous efforts of the Institute in educating the farmers as well as by applying different prophylactic measures, the mortality of sheep in the field condition has been reduced from 18% in 1987 to 5% (2010). The farmers have been motivated and thereby regularly contact the Animal Health technologists for solving the flock health problems. Prophylactic and curative health services to sheep flocks in transfer of technology areas are being adopted over the years.

Nutritional interventions for sheep improvement

The Institute has developed various technologies for utilization of various feed resources, agricultural waste and industrial by-products in sheep feeds. This has resulted in increasing the growth rate as well as the yield of meat and wool. The CSWRI, Avikanagar has evolved various feeding technologies to improve the growth rate in mutton type lambs after weaning at appropriate stage and feeding intensively under feedlot. These developed technologies related to animal feeding with concentrate ration and other types of feeds during different phases such as gestation, early and late lactation caused significant increase in body weight as well as lambing percentage. The body weight gain by lambs during 4 to 6 months age was very fast, so the market value of these animals can be increased with supplementary feeding to ewes. Commonly available roughages and crops residues with farmers are generally deficient in protein and energy and animals cannot be maintained on them. So supplementary feeding of ewes during critical stages of production is essential to enhance the general condition of ewes and birth weight and growth performance of lambs. Ewes in advanced pregnancy should be supplemented @ 1% of their body weight to achieve better performance. In field condition the surplus lambs should be marketed at 20 to 25 kg body weight achieved at 9 to 12 months of age. Under intensive feeding 25 kg finishing weight could be achieved at the age of 125 days with protocol of 60 days weaning and 65 days of intensive feeding on 50:50 concentrate and roughages based ration. Any progressive farmer raising 100 lambs for mutton production will invest Rs. 9200 in non recurring (housing, feeding trough and buckets) and Rs. 66000 in recurring (purchase value of lambs, kgst of roughages and concentrate, health coverage, kgbour charge and POL for lamb purchase) expenditure with total receipt of Rs. 71250 form live animal sale to contractor and Rs. 82500 if slaughtered with net profit of Rs 5250 and 16500, respectively in 90 to 100 days of feeding. In addition to routine grazing, the concentrate supplementation @ 1 % of the body weight improved the body weight of lambs which was successfully demonstrated at different production stages. Supplementation to sheep during later part of pregnancy resulted in 31.54% increase in birth weight of lambs over the control which gave Rs 493.00 as net return with 3.95 B: C ratio (Table 3). It is clear that economic returns of this simple and easy to adopt technology are very high. Similar observations were also observed by Chaturvedi *et al.* (2000) in a participatory research under field condition. The IVLP paved a new path for economic up-liftment of resource poor farmers through participatory approach. The farmers generated additional revenue from their available resources.

Table 3 : Effect of improved feeding practices on the body weight of lambs

Treatment	Birth weight (kg)	% increase in birth weight over the control	Net return (Rs/animal)	B:C ratio
Control	2.98	-	315	-
Supplementation during later part of pregnancy	3.92	31.54	493	3.95
Supplementation during early part of lactation	3.50	17.45	425	2.85
Supplementation throughout later part of pregnancy to early part of lactation	4.07	36.58	4872.42	

Feed resource development and feeding practices

Efforts have been made to demonstrate and educate the farmers regarding the various agronomical practices to establish grass pasture and grow different fodder crops. Fodder tree saplings were distributed. The farmers have been demonstrated how to enrich low quality fodders such as wheat straw, bajra kadbi by urea-ammonia treatment. Utilization of different feed resources, salt and mineral licks were demonstrated. The improvement in nutritional status of livestock especially sheep is possible through improvement of common rangeland, establishment of pasture and silvi-pasture systems and introduction of fodder trees on farmers fields through agroforestry and horti-pasture systems. Moreover, in fodder production, inclusion of high yielding varieties of fodder crops in existing crop rotations and judicious conservation of grasses, legumes, shrubs, bushes and tree leaves in the form of hay, silage and loom or pala is needed for commercial sheep farming because maximum expenditure (70%) is incurkgd on their feeding. Therefore, studies were conducted with major emphasis on development of fodder production technologies to reduce the cost of sheep rearing. Results showed that a good Anjan (*C. ciliaris*) or Dhaman grass (*C. setigerus*) pasture may provide sufficient grazing material for 6 sheep/ha, while protected grazing land may stock 2-3 sheep/ha and uncared pasture may hardly be sufficient for one sheep/ha. The seeds of grasses should be sown at 1-2 cm below the surface with 50 cm apart in rows. Application of sheep manure @ 10 t/ha once in three years has been found sufficient. Sheep manure @ 10 t/ha with 20 kg N and 40 kgP_2O_5/ha is sufficient to maintain biomass productivity for four years. The biomass productivity of common grazing lands is hardly 1-2 t/ha against 5-6 t/ha. The productivity of common rangelands can be increased through single, two and three-tier systems of fodder production than open system. Meena *et al.* (2001) reported that forage yield of rangeland could be doubled within two years by protecting them from the biotic factors. Under silvi-pasture system 100 ardu (*Ailanthus excelsa* Roxb) trees with the combination of *Cenchrus*: cowpea in 1:2 ratio have been suggested for semi-arid regions of the country. In the horti pasture system, legumes such as cowpea (*Vigna unguiculata*), guar (*Cymopsis tetragonoloba*), and moth bean (*Vigna aconitifolia*) have been tested for their production potential on the farmers' fields. Its results exhibited that productivity of grass can be increased by inclusion of legumes as one of the component in intercropping /stripping or mixed cropping with other species. Subsequently additional economic gain can be obtained from fruit trees like aonla (*Emblica officinalish* L.) and ber (*Zizyphus mauritiana* Lank) under this system. Since last few years berseem (*Trifolium alexzanrium*) has been acclimatized in TOT area. It showed very encouraging results pertaining to black soil. Improved seeds of fodder crops *viz.* jowar (*Sorghum bicolor*), maize (*Zea mays*), bajra (*Pennisetum typhoideum*), cowpea, popat (*Dolichos lab lab*), titli matar (*Clitoria ternatea*), oats (*Avena sativa*), lucerne (*Medicago sativa*) and grasses seeds were also verified. The production potential of improved fodder crops varieties was superior over traditional ones. The response of balance doses of chemical fertilizers in fodder crops was significant. To increase the popularity among the farmers for plantation of multipurpose tree species as farm boundary or as an intercrop with field crops in agroforestry system has been emphasized. The overall survival of provided fodder and fruit trees saplings was about 30% during severe drought condition while it was more in good rainfall years but it varied over the years due to change in climate.

Composition of community pasture and their carrying capacity

The available land with sheep owners was comprised of uncultivated (11%), under forest (4%), grazing land (11.5%) and fallow land (9%). The irrigation sources were available for 12.8% land and rest fall under unirrigated or rainfed (dry lands). The grazing lands in the area are very poor. They are never reseeded. All types of animals graze on them. The stocking rate is very kggh (1.87 cattle, 0.69 buffalo, 2.06 sheep and 1.10 goats per acre). The community grazing lands species were *Eragrostis, Crotolaria, indigofera, Dicanthium, Aristida, Apluda, Themdeda, Cyprus, Digitaria, Vernonia, Cenchrus, Cynodon, Euphorbia, Digera, Chloris, Sporobolus, Urochloa, Launea, Tribulus, Commelina, Eclipta, Plycarpia etc. Amongst the bushes Zizyphus* species were common. The animals got stubble grazing after the harvest of crops. The animals were mostly dependent on top feeding from January to March. The trees available in the area were Neem, Babool, Orangia, Kakera, Khejri, Peepal, Siris, Bar, Sanzana, Ardu, Bergad, Imli etc. The number of trees in community land was small. The trees were severely lopped by the sheep farmers every year. Production potential of natural grasslands open to grazing is quite low (5.0-9.5 q/ha). Several management and biological techniques viz. closure sowing, introduction of improved grasses and legumes, fertilization and cutting techniques have been standardized for enhancing biomass production and quality of these grasslands. Ahuja (1977) felt that natural succession of superior species of grasses in arid and semi-arid regions is a slow process. Hence, reseeding with suitable high forage producing species suiting to different agro climatic tract is thkgonly solution. Dhir (1987) concluded that 2/3 of the open pasture are severely degraded. Ahuja (1977) has shown that with 2 years of protection and controlled grazing, forage yield increased by 148.3, 91.9 and 116.3%, respectively from poor, fair and good rangelands.

Wool quality evaluation and utilization

The wool quality of different types of sheep in the operational research project villages were evaluated to educate the farmers regarding the important changes brought about in the wool due to crossbreeding programmes in their flocks. Village artisans were trained regularly on the utilization of wool for better utilization in the cottage sector. In recent years, women in particular were trained to spin Bharat Merino wool on hand charkhas and knit them into sweaters and pullovers. Efforts were made to dye Bharat Merino wool by using vegetable colours. Our past experience has indicated that through some technologies were developed for utilizing wool as such and in blends with other fibres, the technologies could not be much utilized by the weavers, artisans and even by the industrialist because these do not match according to their requirement (Table 4).

Table 4 : Technologies developed for wool processing and utilization by CSWRI and industry requirements

Institute developed technologies	Industry requirements
The institute has developed technologies to use wide range fibre, which is having 25- 45-µ diameter and 20-70 mm staple length. The textile technology and wool science division of the institute developed processing technology for effective utilization of the wool produced in the country. The technology on various blend of natural and synthetic fibres *viz.* wool, polyester, wool acrylic and wool plant fibre has been developed. In such a way coarse Indian wool can be used through blending. Technologies also on handloom woven blankets, wool camel hair blended products, development of handmade felts and manufacturing low cost handloom woven carpets were also developed.	The wool should have 35±5 µ diameter and 50-70 mm staple length which is most suitable for carpet industry to get premise prices of Rs. 70-80 /kg from wool. The industry requires good quality of wool, which is having white colour, free from burr/ vegetable contaminants and any other matter. The industry requires wool which has 30% medullation.

The CSWRI has been trying to solve the problems of the people through supply of low cost input and technologies, which are more feasible and economically viable. In the traditional system of wool shearing the sheep breeders are shearing sheep by using scissors which is time consuming and are not able to cut the fleece in most economical manner i.e. in a single long cut. Adoption of new technology by introducing shearing machine will help sheep owners to get more wool in each clip with better staple length which fetches better price. The industry will be able to get long staple wool, which is not available in sufficient quantity at present. Shearing machine will avoid double cutting of staples hence approximately 50 g of extra wool will be obtained from each animal. This will lead to increase of 5% in wool production. Regarding value addition at the raw wool stage, awareness on sheep preparation for shearing, practical skill in selection of shearing tools, equipments, shearing site and preparation of clip and marketing of wool has been developed among the sheep farmers. In general 20-25% farmers sold their wool on weight basis against the sheep head basis (80-75%). Sale of wool on weight basis thereby enhanced the income by Rs 5-6/kg wool as compared to sheep head basis. The wool on sheep head basis has been sold for Rs. 12-13/sheep head for three clips and Rs.18-20 for two clips. The wool on weight basis has been sold for Rs. 55-60 /kg wool. The major constraints were the low price of wool. The price of wool is declining mainly due to the import of carpet grade wool at a lower price from countries like New Zealand and China. Carpet industries are not well developed in many wool producing countries from where cheaper wool is imported to India. The imported wool is better priced compared to the domestically produced one even after accounting for the high percentage of impurities present in the domestic wool (Ray, 1999). Indian wool producers are at a disadvantage in comparison to them. Lack of proper grading of wool before marketing coupled with the highly unorganized nature of the farmers expose them to the exploitation by the buyers who are few in number and organized. In case of live -sheep marketing, markets are traditional and the price spread is high (Rathore, 1993).

Survey of sheep breeders

The socio-economic survey conducted on 144 sheep breeders in TOT areas indicated that out of the total adopted sheep breeders 28.4 and 7.0% belonged to schedule caste and schedule tribe communities. Sheep farming and agriculture were the main occupations of 45.8 and 53.5% farmers, respectively, while 55.6 and 24.8% have sheep husbandry and agriculture as subsidiary occupations respectively. Further 52.1 and 47.9% were joint and nuclear sheep breeders families, respectively. The average land holding of the sheep breeders was 4.02 hectares out of which 22.83% was irrigated land. Survey conducted in 1991-92 revealed that 5.67% sheep were crossbred. The average flock size was 64. The birth weight of crossbreds was higher than the native breed like Malpura. Similarly body weights at different growth stages as 6, 9 and 12 month was higher in crossbreds than local breeds. The greasy fleece production of cross breeds was also higher than native breeds and ranged from 340 and 648 g/clip. The visual appraisal of the wool indicated that the fibre diameter and medullation were lower in crossbreds. The fibre diameter of native and quarter bred sheep wool was 41 and 26 micron with medullation of 70 and 30% in two groups, respectively indicating the improvement due to crossbreeding. Crossbred in the adopted area had wool of 32 micron and mixed flocks wool had of 36 micron. Overall morbidity in adopted villages ranged from 43.8-64.9% while mortality in adopted villages varied from 2.44 to 8.65%. At present the emphasis is on rearing of native breed of sheep. Magra sheep was reared mostly with flock size ranging from 20-600. The wool yield ranged from 615-640 g/sheep with staple length 44.02-83.50 mm. The sheep breeders were aware of the modern health technology practices like vaccination. The wool yield of these animals in 3 clips ranged from 2-3 kg/sheep.

Cost and returns from sheep, goat and bovine farming

The cost of rearing animals mainly consists of fixed and variable cost. The fixed cost is the value of animal purchased, investment made on house/shed to keep the animals, equipments *viz.* feedings troughs, bucket, spade etc for day to day work. The variable cost consists of feed, fodder, labour and veterinary charges, investment on fixed and working capital etc. and miscellaneous charges like electricity and water. The small ruminants are generally penned under the open sky which is fenced with thorny hedge and are grazed in the outskirts of the villages and on stubbles in the fields of harvested kharif and rabi crops. Whereas, the large animals (buffalo, cow, camel etc.) are provided with Kachha / Pakka shed, stall feeding management with or without grazing in the fields with proper veterinary treatment. In order to compare the viable economics of small ruminants with other livestock (cow, buffalo and both) only variable cost components and returns thereof have been taken into account. The fixed cost components like depreciation on assets, interest on capital were not taken into account, as the assets are heritable in nature. The CSWRI has conducted socio-economic surveys of households in the villages from time to time, who possess small ruminants. The sheep and goats are generally reared in the extensive system of management in our country. However, the large ruminant (cow and buffalo) are usually reared in the semi-intensive or intensive system of management. The survey study conducted in Tonk district of Rajasthan in 1990 indicated that Malpura and Kheri breeds of sheep are prominent breeds in the surveyed area. Sirohi goats are predominant breed and bovines are non- descript breeds. The animals were kept sole on grazing. Mostly, sheep are non-migratory in this area, however, a few flocks go for short duration of migration for a short distance during the summer months. Rawat *et al.* (1993) reported that the annual gross cost of sheep, goat and bovine rearing is Rs 71, 57 and 422 per animal, respectively and the net returns are 44 from sheep, 67 from goat and 298 from bovine (Table 5). This resulted in the benefit: cost ratio of 1.62, 2.18 and 1.71 for sheep, goat and bovine, respectively. It showed that goat is more economically viable than sheep and bovine. Devendra (1992) also reported that marginal farmers also recorded a high net income from goats than other large animals. Another study conducted by Rawat *et al.* (1998) reported that the component wise average cost per animal of sheep and goat rearing in the extensive system of management (Table 6) is Rs. 3.59 and 21.13, respectively. The cost component consisted of green and dry fodder, veterinary charges and other (salt, gur and oil). The cost component does not include the labour cost on account of own family labour employed in raising the livestock. The component wise income from small ruminants (Table 7) shows the maximum return through sale of live animals followed by milk, wool and manure respectively. The gross average return per animal has been Rs. 228 from sheep and 281 from goat respectively. The net returns from sheep, goat, buffalo and cow (Table 8) have been reported Rs. 204, 260, 970 and 377, respectively. Therefore, the benefit: cost has been found highest in goat (12.28), followed by sheep (9.66), buffalo (2.05) and cattle (1.50). However, a net return was highest in buffalo (970) followed by cattle (377), goat (260) and lowest in sheep (204).

Table 5 : Annual cost and return from livestock rearing in Tonk district of Rajasthan in 1990

Particulars	Sheep	Goat	Bovine
Number of animals	6319	1513	445
Gross cost	71	57	422
Gross return	115	124	720
Net Return	44	67	298
B:C ratio	1.62	2.18	1.71

Source: Wool and woolens of India, October-December 1993

Table 6 : Component wise average cost (Rs/head) of sheep and goat rearing in Tonk district of Rajasthan in 1997

Cost components	Sheep	Goat
Dry fodder	5.76	13.41
Green fodder	0.50	-
Feed	5.28	3.51
Veterinary charges	10.94	3.3
Others	1.12	1.06
Total	23.59	21.13

Source: A report on socio-economic status of sheep and goat breeders and agriculture farmers covered under IVLP/TOT programme, Statistics and Economics and Marketing Section CSWRI, Avikanagar (1998)

Table 7 : Component wise average income (Rs/head) from sheep and goat in Tonk district of Rajasthan in 1997

Income components	Sheep	Goat
Sale of animals	99.71	137.73
Sale of wool	40.66	-
Sale of milk	47.70	102.98
Sale of manure	39.74	40.00
Total	227.81	280.71

Source: A report on socio-economic status of sheep and goat breeders and agriculture farmers covered under IVLP/TOT programme, Statistics and Economics and Marketing Section CSWRI, Avikanagar (1998)

Table 8 : Average cost and returns from, goat and other livestock in Tonk district of Rajasthan 1997

Particulars	Sheep	Goat	Buffalo	Cattle
Number of animals	1215	798	96	103
Number of household	27	57	26	35
Average cost/ animal (Rs)	23.59	21.13	922.02	756.33
Average income/ animal (Rs)	227.81	280.71	1891.72	1133.80
Net return(Rs)	204.22	259.58	969.70	377.47
Benefit: cost ratio	9.66	12.28	2.05	1.50

Source: A report on Socio-Economic status of sheep and goat and agriculture farming covered under IVLP/TOT programme, Statistics, economics and marketing Section CSWRI, Avikanagar (1998)

Technical literacy and extension education

The efforts were made to motivate the farmers by making extension approaches and using different media. Some of the salient ones were publication of pamphlets, prassar patra, organizing and participating in exhibitions, fairs, kisan gosthies, talks and news coverage on radio and television are being taken up regularly. Besides Institute activities, news was regularly published in newspapers particularly in Hindi. Farmers and women trainings are also being organized regularly to develop the skill among the farmers in adopting newer technologies. Providing flock health facilities, training in sheep production, investigation of sheep diseases and field trips of subject matter specialist were found most important in TOT programme being carried out by CSWRI Avikanagar. The impact of Institute in terms of gain in knowledge, attitude and socio-economic status of adopted farmers was found significant as compared to non-adopted farmers. Socio personal traits *viz.* education and socio-economic status (SES) has a positive and significant relationship with knowledge level of respondents about improved sheep production technology. Majority of adopted respondents (98%) had medium to high knowledge level while in case of non-adopted respondents majority of respondents (86%) had low and medium knowledge level. This showed that CSWRI Avikanagar had a significant influence on the knowledge level of sheep breeders. The survey conducted to study the benefits derived out of the technology passed on to sheep farmers revealed that the estimated average annual gross income of sheep breeders was Rs 7650/ from a flock of 72 in 1975. The gross income increased by an annual rate of 8% from Rs 8800 in 1981 to Rs 26100 in 1989. Highest benefit: cost ratio was observed to be 2.38 in case of small farmer category with a livestock configuration of 66 sheep, 24 goats and 4 bovine and with land holding size of 1-2 hectares. This combination of livestock configuration and land holding size along with free grazing area has generated maximum net returns of Rs.13400/ per sheep breeder in 1990 in the semi-arid areas. Different queries received from the farmers on problems faced by them regarding sheep production were regularly answered and whenever required scientific and technical personnel visited such farmers flocks to alleviate their problems. Several trainings were held at periodical intervals on different production aspects for farmers, extension workers, development officers and other government agencies engaged in sheep production. State level discussions were also held to identify the different aspects of sheep production that can be undertaken in the different states.

Attitude of sheep farmers towards transferred technologies

It was evident that majority of the sheep farmers (80%) had a favourable attitude towards transferred technologies. Further, it was noted that about 20% of the sheep farmers showed neutral attitude towards supplied technologies but none of the sheep farmer had showed unfavourable attitude towards supplied technologies (Dhaka and Mann, 2003). The data of surveyed flocks showed that improved rams for flock improvement obtained higher score (117.45) followed by the supplied seed of T-9 variety of lucerne (113.57). Farmers showed less interest regarding infertility management (69.10) and artificial insemination practices in sheep. Practices like infertility management and artificial insemination in sheep received comparatively low score indicating thereby greater need for improvement in these two practices. Overall it can be concluded that respondents (sheep farmers) were satisfied with the philosophy, principles, objectives, services, linkages, field workers and technologies suggested under TOT programme of the CSWRI. However, technologies like infertility management and use of artificial insemination in sheep need to be refined as per need and requirement of the farmers (Table 9).

Table 9 : Semantic differential scores of innovation on various attributes

Innovation	Relative advantage	Compa-tibility	Comp-lexity	Practic-ability	Total
Panacure (Endoparasite)	25.89	31.59	29.33	26.76	113.57
Nilverm (Endoparasite)	24.92	28.59	29.18	27.58	110.27
Sheep pox vaccine	23.85	22.22	28.15	19.52	93.74
Enterotoxaemia vaccine	23.72	22.89	29.13	18.08	93.82
Improved rams in flock	26.12	36.56	33.12	21.65	117.45
Infertility management	16.10	19.23	21.22	12.55	69.10
Artificial insemination	18.96	15.49	14.59	26.89	75.88
Supplementary feeding	23.66	27.59	28.44	24.22	103.91
Urea treatment of straw	25.47	28.19	26.17	23.15	102.98
T-9(Lucerne) variety	23.7	25.85	32.43	31.33	113.31

Conclusion

Operational Research Project on sheep and wool development was under taken in 1975 in 20 villages around CSWRI, Avikanagar. Survey conducted in 1975, 1980 and 1985 indicated that the crossbred population increased upto 26.65%. There was no significant difference in body weight of cross bred and native sheep at different ages in similar sex. However, cross bred ewes and hoggets produced 33 and 20% more wool than the native breed and cross bred produced fine wool than native. The regular preventive and curative sheep health programme at farmers door the mortality rate was considerably reduced from 18.78% in 1975 to 5% in 2010. The mortality rate in crossbred lamb was higher in comparison to contemporary native lambs. The feed and fodder production programme has readily been accepted by the farmers. The survivability of multi purpose fodder trees was around 25%. Pasture plots were maintained successfully under proper protection but Gram Panchayat could not maintain when these plots were handover to them. Field demonstrations on fodder crops were adopted successfully. The dissemination of information and technology to farmers' field depends on how the technology is taken at the farm level. The farm level approach should be holistic and interdisciplinary and it should include farmers' participation in its (technology) generation, assessment, refinement and transfer. If technology is taken properly at the farm level it can have tremendous impact on sheep productivity. Marketing of sheep and its by products have been a major constraints for the breeders. Lack of organized market yards is keeping the sheep breeders away from obtaining justified profits. Formation of sheep breeders' cooperatives and their organization may be helpful in getting the maximum benefits of increased production through adoption of improved viable technologies in different region of various states. Developed technologies paved a new way for economic up-liftment to resource poor farmers through participatory research approaches. The famers generated additional revenue from their available resources. The crop and sheep based interventions enabled the farmers to produce considerable amount of additional tonnage as well as the revenue. The farmers were satisfied with the recommended packages regarding development of sheep husbandry in arid and semi-arid parts of the country.

The CSWRI extension system functions like as action research and plays a catalytic role in accelerating the process of transfer of technology among sheep farmers. This complementary role to the main extension system of the Ministry of Agriculture/State departments of Agriculture and Animal Husbandry needs to be fully appreciated and utilized by State extension machinery and NGO's. Looking into the favorable response of the sheep farmers towards adoption of new technologies developed by CSWRI Avikanagar and the proven effectiveness of these technologies in the field, a KVK solely devoted to sheep needs to be established at Avikanagar to widen its area of influence and strengthen the existing extension system for the overall benefit of the sheep farmers of Rajasthan and the country as a whole.

References

Ahuja, L.D. 1977. Improving rangeland productivity. In: Desertification and its control. ICAR, New Delhi, pp. 203-214.

Chaturvedi, O.H., Mishra, A.S., Karim, S.A. and Jakhmola, R.C. 2000. Effect of supplementary feeding on the growth performance of lambs under field condition. Indian Journal of Small Ruminants 6: 110-112.

Devendra, C. 1992. Goat production: An international prospective. In: 5th International Conference on Goats, IASRI, Pusa, New Delhi, 2-8 March, pp 64-81.

Dhaka, B.L. and Mann, J.S. 2002. Participatory way to increase production: Extend summaries. In: proc. 2nd International Agronomy Congress on Balancing Food and Environmental Security-Continuing Challenge, New DelhiVol.2: p.1490.

Dhir, R.P. 1987. Land Degradation in Arid Zone. Unpublished.

Dhaka, B.L. and Mann, J.S. 2003. Attitude of farmers towards technologies suggested under IVLP . Indian Journal of Extension Education 49: 94-96.

Gupta, D.C. 2004. Economics of sheep and goat farming in comparison to other livestock. In: Training manual on advances in sheep, goat and rabbit production and their production utilization. Pp.176-183.

Mann, J.S. and Dhaka, B.L. 2003. Institute village linkage programme- a participatory approach for farmers' upliftment. SAARC Journal of Agriculture 1: 105-110.

Mann, J.S., Dhaka, B.L. and Solanki, V.K. 2002. Indigenous practices for sheep heath care. In: 5th National Seminar on Strength, Challenges and Opportunities in Small Ruminant Diseases in New Millennium, Jaipur 30-31, December, p 154.

Mann, J.S. and Meena, L.R. 2004.Transfertable technology for sheep improvement. In: Proc. National Seminar on opportunities and Challenges in Nutrition and Feeding Management of Sheep, Goat and Rabbit for Sustainable production, CSWRI, Avikanagar, 10-12 February. Pp 298-304.

Meena, L.R., Mann, J.S .and Mehta, R.S. 2001. Grassland improvement in semi-arid tropics of Northern India. Indian Farming 58: 15-18.

Rawat, P.S., Riyazuddin and Sharma, S.C. 1993. Economic status of sheep farmers in semi-arid region of Rajasthan. Wool and woolen in India . pp 7-13.

Rawat, P.S., Riyazuddin, Kumar, A. and Singh, R.N.1998. A report on socio Economic Status of Sheep and Goat Breeders and agriculture farmers covered under IVLP/TOT programme. CSWRI, Avikanagar (Rajasthan).

Rathore, M.S. 1993. Marketing of Goats in Rajasthan. Study Report. Institute of Development Studies, Jaipur, Rajasthan.

Ray, S.1999. Declining production conditions of raw wool: Analysis of emerging conflicts in sheep husbandry in Rajasthan. Economic and Political Weekly. May15, 1209-1214.

□□□

About the Editors

Dr A. Sahoo, Principal Scientist and Head, Animal Nutrition Division, Central Sheep and Wool Research Institute, Avikanagar, completed his B.V.Sc. & A.H. (1987-88) from Orissa University of Agriculture and Technology, Bhubaneswar and M.V.Sc. (1990) & Ph.D. (Animal Nutrition) (1994) from Indian Veterinary Research Institute, Izatnagar, UP. He joined Agriculture Research Service (ARS) in 1993. He has more than 22 year of research experience in the field of 'Animal Nutrition' with specialization in rumen metabolism and manipulation, feed resource evaluation, assessment of nutritional adequacy, and clinical and therapeutic nutrition. He has published 80 research papers, 16 books/ compendium/manuals, five book chapters, 61 general articles, 14 popular articles and 170 contributory papers. He has guided several post-graduate students. He is a member of several important Professional and Academic Bodies and Research Advisory committee.

Dr. S.K. Sankhyan did his B.Sc. (Ag.)From University of Rajasthan in 1986, M.Sc. and Ph.D in Animal Nutrition from Himachal Pradesh Krishi Vishva Vidhyalaya, Palampur in1988 and 1991 respectively. He was awarded University merit fellowship during M.Sc. and Ph.D. programme. He joined Agricultural Research Services as Scientist in 1991 at Central Sheep and Wool Research Institute, Avikanagar and presently working as Principal Scientist (AN) and I/C ARIS Cell. He has 18 year of research experience and pursued the research in the area of nutrition of sheep and goats on pasture and mineral nutrition of field animals for the last fifteen years. He is presently conducting research in AICRP on "Improvement of feed resources and its utilization in raising animal, production". He has published 4 Books, 58 research papers in National and International Journals, 12 leads / invited papers and presented 54 abstract papers in National Seminar. He is life member of five National Societies of Animal Science

Dr. C.P. Swarnkar, Scientist (Selection Grade) CSWRI, Avikanagar has extensively worked on epidemiology, anthelmintic resistance and management of gastrointestinal nematodes in sheep. He has published 90 research papers in journals of national and international repute, 72 abstracts, 7 book chapters, 28 popular articles, 21 lead papers, 3 training manuals and two books. He developed technologies like regional worm management programme, targeted selective treatment, forecasting system (FROGIN) for GI nematodes. He has conferred with ICAR Award for Outstanding Team Research for the Biennium 2003-04 and 8 professional societies' awards. He is also assistant editor of Indian Journal of small Ruminants.

Dr A.K. Shinde did his M.V.Sc and A.H. and Ph.D. in Livestock Production and Management from College of Veterinary Science and Animal Husbandry, Madhya Pradesh Pashu Chikitsha Vigyan Viswavidyalaya Jabalpur in 1983 and 1996.

He started his career in 1983 as Veterinary Officer in Ujjain Dugdh Mahasangh, Ujjain. Later he jointed Agricultural Research Services as Scientist in 1989 at Central Sheep and Wool Research Institute, Avikanagar and now holding position of Principal Scientist. He pursued research on nutrition of sheep and goats on pasture and mineral nutrition since last 20 years. He has published 55 research papers in national and international journals, three books, four bulletins and presented 70 papers in conferences / seminars. He has written a book on Applied Animal Husbandry in Hindi and contributed chapters in several book. He is member of four scientific societies of animal science and Editor of Indian Journal of Sheep and Goat Production and Utilization. He has received Dr Rajendra Prasad Award from ICAR, New Delhi and Rajiv Gandhi Rashtriya Award Gyan Vigyan Molik Pushtak Lekhan Puruskar from Ministry of Home Affair, New Delhi for Technical Book.

Dr. S.A. Karim, Director, Central Sheep and Wool Research Institute, Avikanagar, completed his B.V.Sc. & A.H. and M.V.Se. (Animal Nutrition) from Orissa Veterinary College Bhubaneswar in the year of 1974 and 1976, respectively. He was awarded University Gold Medal for securing first position in M.V.Sc. (AN). He completed his Ph.D. degree in Animal Nutrition from National Dairy Research Institute, Karnal in the year of 1991. He joined Agriculture Research Service (ARS) in 1978. He has more than 26 year of research experience in the filed of ruminant nutrition with specialization in nutrition environment interaction, growth maximization of lambs, range managed small ruminants' nutrition and carcass evaluation. He has published 140 research papers, 45 invited papers, 15 popular articles and 200 contributory papers. He has guided several Ph.D. students. He is a member of several important academic bodies and as Board of Studies, Academic council, Research Advisory committee.